The Founders of Operative Surgery

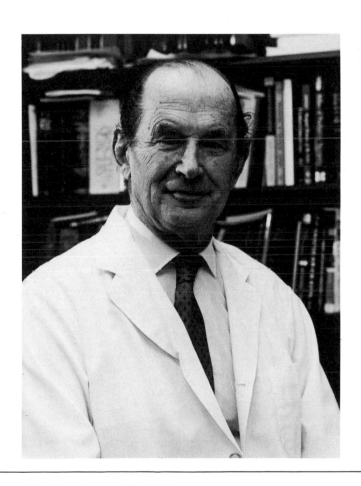

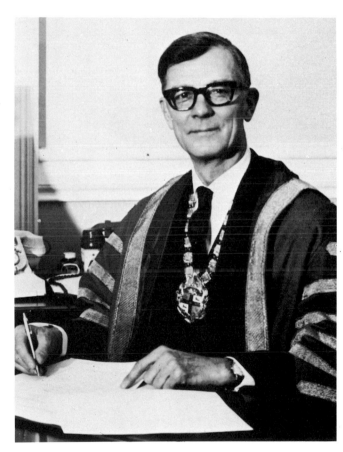

Charles Granville Rob MC, MChir, MD, FRCS, FACS
Professor of Surgery, Department of Surgery, Uniformed
Services University of the Health Sciences, F. Edward Hébert
School of Medicine, Bethesda, Maryland
Quondam: Professor of Surgery, St Mary's Hospital Medical
School, London 1950–1960;
Professor and Chairman, Department of Surgery, University of
Rochester, New York, 1960–1978;
Professor of Surgery, East Carolina University, 1978–1983

Lord Smith of Marlow KBE, MS, FRCS, Hon DSc
(Exeter and Leeds), Hon MD (Zurich), Hon FRACS,
Hon FRCS(Ed.), Hon FACS, Hon FRCS(Can.), Hon FRCSI,
Hon FCS(SA), Hon FDS
Honorary Consulting Surgeon, St George's Hospital, London
Quondam: Surgeon, St George's Hospital, London,
1946–1978;
President of the Royal College of Surgeons of England,
1973–1977

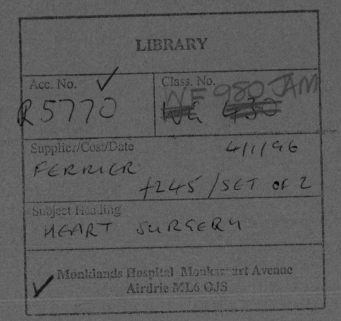

Rob & Smith's
Operative Surgery

Cardiac Surgery

Fourth Edition

Rob & Smith's

Operative Surgery

General Editors

Hugh Dudley ChM, FRCS(Ed.), FRACS, FRCS
Professor of Surgery, St Mary's Hospital, London, UK

David C. Carter MD, FRCS(Ed.), FRCS(Glas.)
St Mungo Professor of Surgery, University of Glasgow;
Honorary Consultant Surgeon, Royal Infirmary, Glasgow, UK

Rob & Smith's
Operative Surgery

Cardiac Surgery

Fourth Edition

Edited by

Stuart W. Jamieson MB, FRCS, FACS
Professor and Head, Cardiothoracic Surgery,
University of Minnesota, Minneapolis, Minnesota, USA

and

Norman E. Shumway MD, PhD, FACS, FRCS(Hon)
Professor and Chairman, Department of Cardiovascular Surgery,
Stanford University Hospital, Stanford, California, USA

Illustrations by Barbara Hyams

Butterworths
London Boston Durban Singapore Sydney Toronto Wellington

© Butterworths 1986

First edition published in eight volumes 1956–1958
Second edition published in fourteen volumes 1968–1971
Third edition published in nineteen volumes 1976–1981
Fourth edition published 1983–

British Library Cataloguing in Publication Data

Rob, Charles
    Rob & Smith's operative surgery. – 4th ed.
    Cardiac
    1. Surgery, Operative
    I. Title   II. Smith, Rodney Smith, *Baron*
    III. Jamieson, Stuart W.   IV. Shumway,
    Norman E.   V. Rob, Charles. Operative surgery
    617'.91   RD32

    ISBN 0-407-00660-5

Library of Congress Cataloging in Publication Data
(Revised for volume 5)

Rob & Smith's operative surgery.

    Rev. ed. of: Operative Surgery. 3rd ed. 1976–
    Includes bibliographies and indexes.
    Contents; [1] Alimentary tract and abdominal wall.
    1. General principles, oesophagus, stomach, duodenum,
    small intestine, abdominal wall, hernia/edited by
    Hugh Dudley – [5] Cardiac/edited by Stuart J. Jamieson
    and N. E. Shumway.
    1. Surgery, Operative. I. Rob, Charles.
    II. Smith of Marlow, Rodney Smith, Baron, 1914–
    III. Dudley, Hugh A. F. (Hugh Arnold Freeman). IV. Pories,
    Walter J. V. Carter, David C. (David Craig)
    VI. Jamieson, Stuart W. VII. Shumway, N. E.

Library of Congress Cataloging-in-Publication Data

(Norman Edwards), 1923–. VIII. Operative surgery.
[DNLM: 1. Surgery, Operative. WO 500 061 1982]
RD32.06   1983   617'.91   83-14465
ISBN 0-407-00651-6 (v. 1)

Photoset by Butterworths Litho Preparation Department
Printed by Blantyre Printing Ltd, London & Glasgow
Bound by Robert Hartnoll Ltd, Bodmin, Cornwall

Volumes and Editors

Alimentary Tract and Abdominal Wall

1 **General Principles · Oesophagus · Stomach · Duodenum · Small Intestine · Abdominal Wall · Hernia**

Hugh Dudley ChM, FRCS(Ed.), FRACS, FRCS
Professor of Surgery, St Mary's Hospital, London, UK

2 **Liver · Portal Hypertension · Spleen · Biliary Tract · Pancreas**

Hugh Dudley ChM, FRCS(Ed.), FRACS, FRCS
Professor of Surgery, St Mary's Hospital, London, UK

3 **Colon, Rectum and Anus**

Ian P. Todd MS, MD(Tor), FRCS, DCH
Consulting Surgeon, St Bartholomew's Hospital, London;
Consultant Surgeon, St Mark's Hospital and
King Edward VII Hospital for Officers, London, UK

L. P. Fielding MB, FRCS
Chief of Surgery, St Mary's Hospital, Waterbury, Connecticut, USA;
Associate Professor of Surgery, Yale University, Connecticut, USA

Cardiac Surgery

Stuart W. Jamieson MB, FRCS, FACS
Professor and Head, Cardiothoracic Surgery,
University of Minnesota, Minneapolis, Minnesota, USA

Norman E. Shumway MD, PhD, FACS, FRCS(Hon)
Professor and Chairman, Department of Cardiovascular Surgery,
Stanford University School of Medicine, Stanford, California, USA

The Ear

John C. Bailantyne CBE, FRCS, HonFRCSI, DLO
Consultant Ear, Nose and Throat Surgeon,
Royal Free and King Edward VII Hospital for Officers, London, UK

Andrew Morrison FRCS, DLO
Senior Consultant Otolaryngologist, The London Hospital, UK

General Principles, Breast and Extracranial Endocrines

Hugh Dudley ChM, FRCS(Ed.), FRACS, FRCS
Professor of Surgery, St Mary's Hospital, London, UK

Walter J. Pories MD, FACS
Professor and Chairman, Department of Surgery, School of Medicine,
East Carolina University, Greenville, North Carolina, USA

Gynaecology and Obstetrics

J. M. Monaghan MB, FRCS(Ed.), MRCOG
Consultant Surgeon, Regional Department of Gynaecological Oncology,
Queen Elizabeth Hospital, Gateshead, UK

The Hand

Rolfe Birch FRCS
Consultant Orthopaedic Surgeon, PNI Unit and Hand Clinic,
Royal National Orthopaedic Hospital, London and
St Mary's Hospital, London, UK

Donal Brooks MA, MB, FRCS, FRSCI
Consulting Orthopaedic Surgeon, University College Hospital
and Royal National Orthopaedic Hospital, London, UK;
Civilian Consultant in Hand Surgery to the Royal Navy and
Royal Air Force

Neurosurgery

Lindsay Symon TD, FRCS, FRCS(Ed.)
Professor of Neurological Surgery, Institute of Neurology,
The National Hospital, Queen Square, London, UK

David G. T. Thomas MRCP, FRCSE
Senior Lecturer and Consultant Neurosurgeon,
Institute of Neurology, The National Hospital,
Queen Square, London, UK

Kemp Clarke MD
Professor and Chairman, Division of Neurological Surgery,
Southwestern Medical School, Dallas, Texas, USA

Nose and Throat

John C. Ballantyne CBE, FRCS, HonFRCSI, DLO
Consultant Ear, Nose and Throat Surgeon,
Royal Free and King Edward VII Hospital for Officers, London, UK

D. F. N. Harrison MD, MS, PhD, FRCS, FRACS
Professor of Laryngology and Otology,
Royal National Throat, Nose and Ear Hospital, London, UK

Ophthalmic Surgery

Thomas A. Rice MD
Assistant Clinical Professor of Ophthalmology,
Case Western Reserve University School of Medicine,
Cleveland, Ohio, USA;
formerly of the Wilmer Ophthalmological Institute

Ronald G. Michels MD
Professor of Ophthalmology, The Wilmer Ophthalmological Institute,
The Johns Hopkins University School of Medicine,
Maryland, USA

Walter W. J. Stark MD
Professor of Ophthalmology, The Wilmer Ophthalmological Institute,
The Johns Hopkins University School of Medicine,
Maryland, USA

Orthopaedics (in 2 volumes)

George Bentley ChM, FRCS
Professor of Orthopaedic Surgery, Institute of Orthopaedics,
Royal National Orthopaedic Hospital, London, UK

Paediatric Surgery

L. Spitz PhD, FRCS
Nuffield Professor of Paediatric Surgery and Honorary
Consultant Paediatric Surgeon, The Hospital for Sick Children,
Great Ormond Street, London, UK

H. Homewood Nixon MA, MB, BChir, FRCS, HonFAAP
Consultant Paediatric Surgeon, The Hospital for Sick Children,
Great Ormond Street, London and Paddington Green Children's
Hospital, St Mary's Hospital Group, London, UK

Plastic Surgery

T. L. Barclay ChM, FRCS
Consultant Plastic Surgeon, St Luke's Hospital,
Bradford, West Yorkshire, UK

Desmond A. Kernahan, MD
Chief, Division of Plastic Surgery,
The Children's Memorial Hospital, Chicago, Illinois, USA

Thoracic Surgery

J. W. Jackson MCh, FRCS
Formerly Consultant Thoracic Surgeon, Harefield Hospital, Middlesex, UK

D. K. C. Cooper MD, PhD, FRCS
Department of Cardiac Surgery, University of Cape Town
Medical School, Cape Town, South Africa

Trauma

John V. Robbs FRCS
Associate Professor of Surgery,
Department of Surgery, University of Natal, South Africa

Howard R. Champion FRCS
Chief, Trauma Service;
Director, Surgery Critical Care Services,
The Washington Hospital Center, Washington DC, USA

Donald Trunkey MD
San Francisco General Hospital, San Francisco, California, USA

Urology

W. Scott McDougal MD
Professor and Chairman, Department of Urology, Vanderbilt
University, Nashville, Tennessee, USA

Vascular Surgery

James A. DeWeese MD
Professor and Chairman, Division of Cardiothoracic Surgery,
University of Rochester Medical Center, Rochester, New York, USA

Contributors

Pietro A. Abbruzzese MD
Chief Resident, Division of Cardiopulmonary Surgery, Oregon Health Sciences University, Oregon, USA

Robert H. Anderson BSc, MD, MRCPath
Joseph Levy Professor of Paediatric Cardiac Morphology, Cardiothoracic Institute, Brompton Hospital, London, UK

Avenilo P. Aventura MD
Director, Philippine Heart Center for Asia, Quezon City, The Philippines

John C. Baldwin MD
Department of Cardiovascular Surgery, Stanford University School of Medicine, Stanford, California, USA

William A. Baumgartner MD
Associate Professor of Surgery, The Johns Hopkins Hospital, Baltimore, Maryland, USA

Wayne H. Bellows MD
Staff Anesthesiologist, Cardiovascular Anesthesia, Permanente Medical Center, San Francisco, California, USA

A. Gerald Brom MD
Head of Cardiac Surgery, Mafraq Hospital, Abu Dhabi, United Arab Emirates

David B. Campbell MD
Assistant Professor of Surgery, Division of Cardiothoracic Surgery, The Pennsylvania State University College of Medicine, The Miltons Hershey Medical Center, Hershey, Pennsylvania, USA

Alain Carpentier MD
Professor of Cardiac Surgery, University of Paris; Chief, Department of Cardiovascular Surgery, Hôpital Broussais, Paris, France

Denton A. Cooley MD
Surgeon-in-Chief, Texas Heart Institute, Houston, Texas, USA

Richard Cory-Pearce MB, BS, FRCS, FACC
Senior Research Fellow, British Heart Foundation; Consultant Cardiothoracic surgeon, University of Cambridge and Papworth Hospital, Cambridge, UK

Gordon K. Danielson MD
Professor of Surgery, Mayo Medical School and Consultant in Thoracic and Cardiothoracic Surgery, Mayo Clinic, Rochester, Minnesota, USA

William M. Daggett MD
Professor of Surgery, Harvard Medical School; Visiting Surgeon, Massachusetts General Hospital, Boston, Massachusetts, USA

Wayne Derkac MD
Instructor in Surgery, Harvard Medical School; Assistant in Surgery, Massachusetts General Hospital, Boston, Massachusetts, USA

Marc de Leval MD
Consultant Cardiothoracic Surgeon, The Hospital for Sick Children, Great Ormond Street, London, UK

J. P. Dhasmana FRCS
Senior Registrar in Cardiac and Thoracic Surgery, United Bristol Hospitals and Frenchay Hospital, Bristol, UK

Terence A. H. English MB, BSc, MA, FRCS
Consultant Cardiothoracic Surgeon to Papworth and Addenbrooke's Hospitals, Cambridge, Cambridgeshire, UK

Francis Fontan MD
Hôpital Cardiologique du Haut-Leveque, Universite de Bordeaux, Bordeaux (Pessac), France

Robert Fowles MD, FACC
Adjunct Associate Professor of Medicine, Cardiology Division, University of Utah Medical Center and Salt Lake Clinic, Salt Lake City, Utah, USA

J. Kent Garman MD
Staff Anesthesiologist, Sequoia Hospital, Redwood City, California; Clinical Associate Professor, Stanford University School of Medicine, Stanford, California, USA

Vincent A. Gaudiani MD
Sequoia Hospital, Redwood City, California, USA

David I. Hamilton FRCS
Cardiac Surgeon, Royal Liverpool Children's Hospital, Liverpool, UK

Stuart W. Jamieson MB, FRCS, FACS
Professor and Head, Cardiothoracic Surgery, University of Minnesota, Minneapolis, Minnesota, USA

W. R. Eric Jamieson MD, FACC, FACS, FRCS(C)
Clinical Associate Professor, Division of Cardiovascular and Thoracic Surgery, Department of Surgery, University of British Colombia, Vancouver, Canada

John R. W. Keates MB, BChir, FRCS
Consultant Cardiothoracic Surgeon, King's College Hospital, London,
UK

Hillel Laks MD
Professor and Chief, Division of Cardiothoracic Surgery, UCLA School
of Medicine, Los Angeles, California, USA

Christopher Lincoln FRCS
Consultant Cardiothoracic Surgeon, Brompton Hospital, London;
Senior Lecturer in Paediatric Surgery, London University, London, UK

Floyd D. Loop MD
Chairman, Department of Thoracic and Cardiovascular Surgery, The
Cleveland Clinic Foundation, Cleveland, Ohio, USA

Bruce W. Lytle MD
Staff Surgeon, Department of Thoracic and Cardiovascular Surgery,
The Cleveland Clinic Foundation, Cleveland, Ohio, USA

John A. Macoviak MD
Chief Resident in Cardiac Surgery, Stanford University Medical
Center, Stanford, California, USA

Bonnie G. Massing MD, FRCP(C)
Clinical Assistant Professor, Department of Pathology, University of
British Columbia, Vancouver, and Associate Pathologist, British
Columbia Children's Hospital, Vancouver, Canada

D. Craig Miller MD
Associate Professor of Cardiovascular Surgery, Stanford University
School of Medicine, Stanford, California, USA

Charles H. Moore MD
Humana Hospital, San Antonio, Texas, USA

Andrew G. Morrow MD
Formerly Chief, Clinic of Surgery, National Heart Institute, Bethesda,
Maryland, USA

Jan M. Quaegebeur MD
Assistant Professor, Department of Thoracic Surgery, University
Hospital, Leiden, The Netherlands

Noel F. Quenville MD, FRCP(C)
Head, Division of Anatomical Pathology, Vancouver General
Hospital; Clinical Professor, Department of Pathology, University of
British Columbia, Vancouver, Canada

William J. Rashkind MD
Director, Cardiovascular Laboratories, The Children's Hospital of
Philadelphia, One Children Center, Philadelphia, Pennsylvania, USA

Allen K. Ream MS, MS, MD, FACA
Associate Professor of Anesthesia; Director, Institute of Engineering
Design in Medicine, Stanford University School of Medicine, Palo
Alto, California, USA

Bruce A. Reitz MD
Professor of Surgery, Cardiac Surgeon-in-Chief, The Johns Hopkins
University School of Medicine, Baltimore, Maryland, USA

John Rohmer MD
Head, Department of Pediatric Cardiology, University Hospital,
Leiden, The Netherlands

Sir Keith Ross MS, FRCS
Consultant Cardiac Surgeon, Wessex Regional Cardiothoracic Centre,
Southampton, Hampshire, UK

Albert Starr MD
Professor of Surgery and Chief, Division of Cardiopulmonary Surgery,
Oregon Health Sciences University, Oregon, USA

J. Stark MD, FRCS, FACS
Consultant Cardiothoracic Surgeon, Thoracic Unit, The Hospital for
Sick Children, Great Ormond Street, London, UK

Panagiotis N. Symbas MD
Professor of Surgery, Emory University of Medicine, Atlanta, Georgia,
USA

John A. Waldhausen MD
John W. Oswald Professor of Surgery, Chairman, Department of
Surgery, The Pennsylvania State University College of Medicine,
Pennsylvania, USA

David J. Wheatley MD, ChM, FRCS (Ed and Glas)
Professor of Cardiac Surgery, University of Glasgow; Honorary
Consultant Cardiac Surgeon to the Greater Glasgow Health Board,
Glasgow, UK

James D. Wisheart MCh, FRCS
Cardiothoracic Surgeon, Bristol Royal Infirmary, Bristol, Avon, UK

Benson R. Wilcox MD
Professor and Chief of Cardiothoracic Surgery, University of North
Carolina, Chapel Hill, North Carolina, USA

Magdi H. Yacoub FRCS, DSc (Hon)
Consultant Cardiac Surgeon, Harefield Hospital, Harefield,
Middlesex; National Heart Hospital, London, UK

Contributing Medical Artists

Daniel S Beisel MA
Medical Illustrator, Department of Educational Resources, The Milton
S. Hershey Medical Center, Hershey, Pennsylvania 17033, USA

Barbara Hyams MA, AMI
Medical Illustrator, 'Poynings', Northchurch Common, Northchurch,
Berkhamsted, Herts, UK

Siew Yen Ho BSc, PhD
Senior Lecturer in Paediatric Cardiac Morphology, Cardiothoracic
Institute, Brompton Hospital, London SW3 6HP, UK

Contents

Introductory

The assessment of cardiac disease   1
Robert E. Fowles

Surgical access to the heart and great vessels   17
Terence A. H. English

Anaesthesia for cardiac surgery   32
J. Kent Garman
Wayne H. Bellows

Cardiopulmonary bypass and circulatory support   51
Allen K. Ream

Myocardial protection for cardiac surgery   65
Stuart W. Jamieson

Postoperative care   71
John A. Macoviak

Cardiac pacemaker implantation   77
Vincent A. Gaudiani

Paediatric cardiac surgery

The anatomy of congenital heart disease   88
Robert H. Anderson
Benson R. Wilcox

Shunt procedures   107
Hillel Laks

Pulmonary artery banding   117
Charles H. Moore

Total anomalous pulmonary venous connection: surgical anatomy   122
Robert H. Anderson

Total anomalous pulmonary venous drainage: surgical repair   129
J. Stark

Atrial septal defect: surgical anatomy 138
Robert H. Anderson

Atrial septal defect 143
John R. W. Keates

Atrioventricular septal defect: surgical anatomy 151
Robert H. Anderson

Atrioventricular septal defect 160
Alain Carpentier

Double inlet ventricle 173
Robert H. Anderson

Tricuspid atresia: surgical anatomy 184
Robert H. Anderson

The Fontan operation 191
John C. Baldwin
Francis Fontan

Ebstein's anomaly: surgical anatomy 204
Robert H. Anderson

Ebstein's anomaly: surgical treatment 208
Gordon K. Danielson

Ventricular septal defect: surgical anatomy 215
Robert H. Anderson

Ventricular septal defect 222
Bruce A. Reitz

Tetralogy of Fallot: surgical anatomy 233
Robert H. Anderson

Tetralogy of Fallot: surgical treatment 239
Christopher Lincoln

Pulmonary atresia: surgical anatomy 252
Robert H. Anderson

Pulmonary atresia with ventricular septal defect 258
Marc de Leval

Right ventricular outflow tract obstruction with intact ventricular septum 267
Marc de Leval

Congenital aortic stenosis 275
Pietro A. Abbruzzese
Albert Starr

Rashkind procedures   **281**
William J. Rashkind

Complete transposition: surgical anatomy   **291**
Robert H. Anderson

Mustard's operation for transposition of the great arteries   **301**
J. Stark

The Senning operation for transposition of the great arteries   **312**
A. Gerard Brom
Jan M. Quaegebeur
John Rohmer

**Transposition of the great arteries with left ventricular outflow
tract obstruction**   **319**
J. Stark

Anatomical correction of transposition of the great arteries   **328**
Magdi H. Yacoub

Persistent truncus ateriosus: surgical anatomy   **341**
Robert H. Anderson
Benson R. Wilcox

Persistent truncus arteriosus   **346**
Marc de Leval

Persistent ductus arteriosus: surgical anatomy   **356**
Robert H. Anderson
Benson R. Wilcox

Surgery of persistent ductus arteriosus   **358**
J. D. Wisheart
J. P. Dhasmana

Coarctation of the aorta: surgical anatomy   **364**
Robert H. Anderson

Repair of coarctation of the aorta   **371**
John A. Waldhausen
David B. Campbell

Congenital abnormalities of the aortic arch   **381**
David I. Hamilton

Adult cardiac surgery

Pericardiectomy and pericardiotomy   **393**
Sir Keith Ross

Closed mitral commissurotomy   **399**
Avenilo P. Aventura

Mitral valve reconstructive surgery   **405**
Alain Carpentier

Valve prostheses   **415**
David J. Wheatley

Mitral valve replacement   **425**
Magdi H. Yacoub

Hypertrophic subaortic stenosis   **436**
Andrew G. Morrow

Surgical treatment of aortic valve disease   **446**
Denton A. Cooley

Aortocoronary saphenous vein bypass grafting   **454**
Stuart W. Jamieson

Internal mammary artery to coronary artery bypass grafting   **471**
Bruce W. Lytle
Floyd D. Loop

Surgery for the complications of myocardial infarction   **481**
Wayne M. Derkac
William M. Daggett

Trauma to the heart and great vessels   **497**
P. N. Symbas

Surgical treatment of thoracic aortic aneurysms   **509**
D. Craig Miller

Surgical treatment of aortic dissections   **526**
D. Craig Miller

Surgical treatment of aneurysms and dissections involving the transverse aortic arch   **538**
D. Craig Miller

Cardiac tumours   **550**
W. R. Eric Jamieson
Bonnie G. Massing
Noel F. Quenville

Surgical treatment of cardiac arrhythmias   **564**
Richard Cory-Pearce

Transplantation   **584**
Stuart W. Jamieson

Reoperation   **606**
William A. Baumgartner

Index   **613**

Preface

This edition has undergone profound changes. We decided that, since cardiac surgery has expanded so much over the last few years, it merited a separate volume and it has thus been separated from thoracic surgery.

The authorship of this volume has been expanded to reflect an international collection of surgeons who are the acknowledged experts in their field.

To avoid repitition that affected the previous edition separate chapters deal with anaesthesia, preoperative and postoperative care, surgical access, myocardial protection and cardiopulmonary bypass. Chapters have been added on many aspects of paediatric cardiac surgery as well as some important aspects of adult cardiac surgery, such as valve repair, internal mammary bypass grafting and transplantation.

This volume is the first to use one illustrator throughout. Though this obviously resulted in a heavy workload for Barbara Hyams the results speak for themselves.

Dr Andrew G. Morrow died during the writing of this book. his chapter was the first to be recieved and is the last of his many fine contributions to the medical literature. This edition is dedicated to his memory.

Stuart W. Jamieson
Norman E. Shumway

The assessment of cardiac disease

Robert E. Fowles MD, FACC
Adjunct Associate Professor of Medicine, Cardiology Division, University of Utah Medical Center and Salt Lake Clinic, Salt Lake City, Utah, USA

Introduction

Modern cardiac catheterization techniques have evolved into valuable, safe methods for the diagnosis and treatment of patients with all forms of cardiovascular disease. Newer invasive diagnostic techniques include electrophysiological mapping, endomyocardial biopsy and provocative pharmacological manoeuvres to detect coronary artery spasm. Recent therapeutic applications of cardiac catheterization include catheter retrieval of foreign bodies, intravascular placement of filters in venous thromboembolic disease, closure of congenital shunts with unfolding disc-like devices, percutaneous balloon angioplasty for proximal obstructive coronary arteriosclerosis and intracoronary infusion of thrombolytic agents during early or threatened myocardial infarction.

Non-invasive diagnostic techniques have proved highly valuable in many areas and, with their explosive development, promise to complement if not replace many invasive methods.

This chapter emphasizes the need for an integrated, rational approach to invasive techniques in the investigation of heart disease. The cardiovascular team – cardiologist, radiologist, surgeon, anaesthetist, intensive care specialist and others – must carefully select diagnostic procedures with specific questions in mind, using the most appropriate technique for a given query. For example, the best way to detect pericardial effusion is by echocardiography, but the way to diagnose constrictive pericarditis accurately is by invasive haemodynamic study.

Cardiac catheterization

INDICATIONS

There are several general indications for cardiac catheterization. Haemodynamic or angiographic data are used to: (1) reach a diagnosis, as in the patient with atypical but troublesome chest pain; (2) define anatomy, as in congenital heart disease; (3) assess the severity of a lesion, as in coronary or valvular disease; (4) evaluate an intervention – for example, administration of vasodilators; (5) determine prognosis, as in congestive cardio-myopathy; and (6) effect treatment, such as balloon coronary angioplasty.

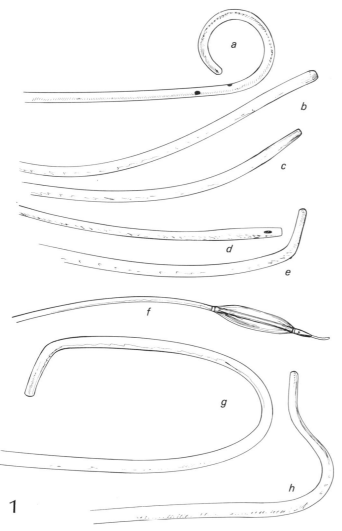

1

Range of cardiac catheters:
(a) Pigtail angiography catheter (end and side holes). (b) Cournand end-hole catheter. (c) Graft catheter (for aortocoronary grafts). (d) Sones coronary catheter. (e) Judkins right coronary catheter. (f) Balloon coronary angioplasty catheter with guide wire. (g) Judkins left coronary catheter. (h) Amplatz coronary catheter

INTERPRETATION OF CARDIAC CATHETERIZATION DATA

Haemodynamic and angiographic data must be critically reviewed since there are multiple sources of potential error. These include technical or mechanical factors such as wave-form distortion from fluid-filled catheters, damping of pressures due to faulty location of the catheter tip and inadequate radiographic exposure technique.

Any change in the patient's condition since cardiac catheterization must be considered. Altered fluid balance may greatly affect cardiac output, rendering a patient with normal haemodynamics at catheterization, if later fluid-depleted, dangerously unstable under cardiovascular stress. Interposed arrhythmias or fluctuating myocardial ischaemia can significantly alter cardiac performance.

Care and judgement must be exercised in drawing conclusions from catheterization data. To decide upon valve replacement solely on the basis of calculated orifice area or upon coronary artery bypass surgery only because of an abnormal angiogram may be erroneous without full consideration of the clinical circumstances.

BASIC CATHETERIZATION METHODS

Right heart catheterization

1

The techniques of right heart catheterization are relatively standard. The site and method of entry of the catheter will vary according to accessibility of vessels, the experience of the operator and the type of study to be performed. The Cournand (plain end-hole), balloon-tipped 'Swan Ganz' and Goodale-Lubin (end- and side-hole) catheters are most frequently used; their slight distal curve (or flow-directed balloon tip) permits directional guidance under fluoroscopic observation.

Once the catheter is in the pulmonary artery it can usually be advanced until it becomes 'wedged' or impacted in a tapering distal branch. At that point an end-hole catheter communicates directly with the capillary-venous compartment of the lung circulation, measuring what is termed the *pulmonary wedge, pulmonary artery wedge, pulmonary capillary wedge* or *pulmonary artery occlusive pressure*. In most cases the wedge pressure reflects left atrial pressure. The pulmonary artery diastolic pressure usually also gives a reasonable estimation of left heart filling pressure unless pulmonary vascular resistance is high or the patient is on mechanical ventilation.

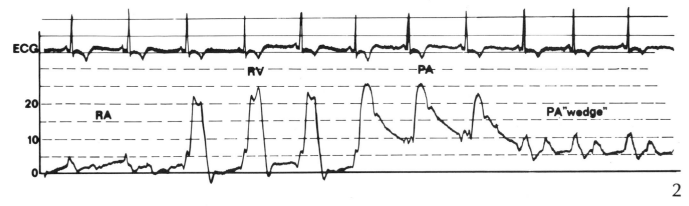

2

2

Normal pressure waveforms (in mmHg) obtained at right heart catheterization are illustrated here (RA = right atrium, RV = right ventricle, PA = pulmonary artery), with the surface electrocardiogram (ECG) above. The normal ranges are indicated in Table 1.

Table 1 Normal ranges for haemodynamic values in adults

Pressures (mmHg)	
Right atrium	
a wave	2–10
v wave	2–10
mean	1–8
Left atrium or pulmonary wedge	
a wave	4–16
v wave	4–18
mean	2–12
Pulmonary artery	
systolic	15–30
diastolic	4–12
mean	9–19
Systemic artery or aorta	
systolic	100–140
diastolic	60–90
mean	70–105
Right ventricle	
systolic	15–30
diastolic	0–8
end-diastolic	0–8
Left ventricle	
systolic	100–140
diastolic	0–10
end-diastolic	2–12

Oxygen saturation (per cent)	
Mixed venous	65–75
Arterial	94–100

Vascular resistance (dyne. sec/cm^5)	
Systemic	800–1200
Pulmonary	50–150

Cardiac index (ℓ/min/m^2)	2.8–4.2

Arterio-venous oxygen difference (ml/dl)	3–5

Left heart catheterization

There are several approaches to catheterization of the left ventricle, which is normally performed via a peripheral artery with retrograde passage across the aortic valve.

3

However, in cases of aortic stenosis, aortic valvular prosthesis or hypertrophic obstructive cardiomyopathy, transatrial puncture may be used. This technique is performed from the right femoral vein with a long, relatively rigid needle-catheter assembly, and is relatively safe in experienced hands. The distally curved flexible Brockenbrough-type catheter is placed high in the right atrium (RA) and then the long steel needle is introduced into the catheter just inside its tip. This assembly is then withdrawn over the bulge imposed by the ascending aorta while being rotated clockwise so that the curved needle points leftwards and posteriorly and into the fossa ovalis. The needle is gently advanced into the left atrium (LA), the catheter follows and the needle is removed. In rare instances transthoracic percutaneous puncture of the left ventricle through the apex is performed.

Normal values are shown in Table 1.

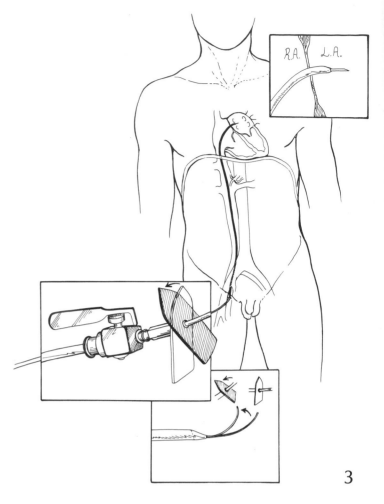

3

Measurement of blood flow

Accurate determination of cardiac output is essential in the complete haemodynamic study. Two methods are commonly used, the Fick principle and indicator dilution.

According to the Fick principle

$$\text{cardiac output } (\ell/\text{min}) = \frac{\text{O}_2 \text{ uptake (ml/min)}}{\text{(A–V)O}_2 \text{ difference (ml/}\ell\text{)}}$$

Oxygen uptake can be measured from exhaled air or approximated in the average resting patient as 130 ml per m^2 body surface area. Arteriovenous oxygen difference $((A–V)O_2)$ is determined from measured saturations in arterial and mixed venous (pulmonary arterial) blood:

$$(A–V)O_2 = 13.6 \times \text{(blood haemoglobin concentration)} \times$$
(ml/l)   (mg/100 ml)
(A–V)O$_2$ per cent saturation

It is clear from the Fick cardiac output equation above that small $(A–V)O_2$ differences will introduce more error; therefore, the Fick method is most accurate in patients with high $(A–V)O_2$ differences (that is, low cardiac output).

The other major method of cardiac output determination is indicator dilution, based on the principle that an unknown volume of fluid can be determined by adding a known quantity of an indicator and measuring its concentration. This is valid for fluids in motion and, if applied per unit time,

$$Q = \frac{A}{c \times t}$$

where Q is flow in ℓ/min, A is the amount of indicator added in milligrams, c is the average concentration of indicator in mg/ℓ during its appearance and t is the time in minutes over which the indicator's appearance is observed. In practice an indicator is injected into the pulmonary artery and its concentration curve is observed in a peripheral artery. This procedure is simplified by microprocessors that automatically compute cardiac output. Substances sufficiently inert and non-toxic to serve as indicators include indocyanine green dye and the gases nitrous oxide, krypton-85 and hydrogen.

A recent and very popular development is the use of cold fluid as indicator. In this thermodilution technique cooled physiological saline or dextrose solution is injected into the right atrium through the proximal port of a double-lumen balloon flotation catheter placed in the pulmonary artery. The resulting fall in temperature of the mixed blood is detected by a thermistor at the catheter tip. Again cardiac output is calculated automatically by microprocessor.

The indicator dilution method is least accurate in low-output states or in valvular regurgitation, in which non-exponential decay of indicator concentration may occur or in which the onset of recirculation may not be clear.

Detection and quantification of shunts

Intracardiac shunting commonly occurs in congenital malformations such as atrial or ventricular septal defects, persistent ductus arteriosus and anomalous pulmonary venous drainage. Shunting may also result from acquired abnormalities such as trauma or post-infarction interventricular septal defect formation. It is important not only to detect shunting but also to measure its magnitude.

Left-to-right shunts are usually detected by oximetry. Oxygen saturation is measured in a diagnostic run, samples being withdrawn at multiple sequential sites from pulmonary artery to vena cava. A significant step-up in oxygen saturation indicates shunting of blood from the left heart circulation. The significance of a step-up in saturation depends on the chamber from which the sample is taken, for the degree of mixing of venous blood increases from right atrium to right ventricle to pulmonary artery. Oximetry is only consistently able to detect shunts of greater than 25 per cent of the systemic blood flow.

During left heart catheterization angiocardiography may be useful in defining the anatomy of a shunting defect, but it cannot quantitate the shunt. It is currently popular to combine oximetry and angiocardiography in shunt detection because of their simplicity and ease of performance.

Right-to-left intracardiac shunting produces arterial hypoxaemia, but so may pulmonary disease. It is therefore important to locate and quantify any such shunt as accurately as possible in order to differentiate an anatomical cardiac defect from intrinsic lung disease.

Right-to-left shunts as small as 5 per cent of systemic flow can be detected by injecting into the right side of the heart indicators such as indocyanine green dye or ascorbic acid, which then appear prematurely in the left circulation. Dye is detected by a densitometer receiving blood from the catheter; ascorbic acid, a strong reducing agent, is sensed by a platinum electrode at the tip of the catheter. The ascorbate method is safe and avoids withdrawal of blood, which may be difficult in infants and small children. Substances normally cleared by the lungs after venous injection can also serve as indicators. Saline-dissolved hydrogen gas or krypton-85 introduced into the right heart circulation will reveal a right-to-left shunt if they appear in the systemic circuit.

Again, although angiography does not allow quantification it is a valuable technique for demonstrating right-to-left shunting. It is especially helpful in pulmonary arteriovenous fistulae, where the shunt is distal and close enough to the capillary bed to prevent detection of early appearance of indicator. Newly developed nuclear medicine techniques can identify and quantitate shunts non-invasively (see below).

Assessment of ventricular function

The continuing development of new therapeutic techniques for heart disease has intensified the need to assess ventricular performance accurately. Cardiac output is only the end result of a complex network of cardiovascular phenomena and cannot be equated with the contractile state of the heart, since even in the presence of advancing heart disease cardiac output is maintained by adaptive, compensatory mechanisms[1].

It is important to know the degree of myocardial dysfunction in treating the cardiac patient in order to answer the following questions: (1) To what extent are symptoms related to a mechanical problem (such as valvular stenosis) and therefore potentially reversible? (2) What are the patient's risks as reflected by intrinsic ventricular dysfunction? (3) How much myocardial reserve does the patient have to undergo anaesthetic induction and to withstand the stress of cardiac surgery? (4) In re-evaluating a patient, has a particular drug or operation improved cardiac function?

The output of the heartbeat, stroke volume, is determined by three factors: (1) *preload*, analogous to the stretching force upon the muscle in the relaxed state, determined in practice by end-diastolic pressure; (2) *afterload*, the force distributed in the ventricular wall during ejection, related to outflow impedance and instantaneous cardiac output as well as to ventricular volume and wall thickness according to the LaPlace relationship; and (3) *contractility*, analogous to shortening velocity of a muscle segment, the intensity of contraction.

Many indices of cardiac performance have been developed in an attempt to characterize basal myocardial contractility accurately. Measurements derived from the rate of change of left ventricular pressure during the pre-ejection phase of systole are termed isovolumic phase indices, including peak dP/dt. Values obtained during ventricular emptying are termed ejection phase indices and include ejection fraction, velocity of circumferential shortening, mean normalized systolic ejection rate and left ventricular stroke work index. The left ventricular end-diastolic pressure is often a useful diastolic phase index of cardiac performance.

Left ventriculography remains the standard method for the detection and measurement of segmental contraction abnormalities associated with infarcted or ischaemic zones in the hearts of patients with coronary artery disease. Angiographically determined cavity size allows the geometrical calculation of end-diastolic and end-systolic volumes. Mitral regurgitation caused by papillary muscle dysfunction is assessed most reliably by the ventriculogram, which can yield stroke volume and regurgitation fraction.

ANGIOGRAPHIC METHODS

Left ventriculography

Interpretation of the left ventriculogram is both descriptive and quantitative.

4a & b

The pattern of contraction is observed by comparing the diastolic (a) with the systolic shadow (b) on which the outline of the diastolic area is superimposed (dotted line). It is described according to standard nomenclature in which the left ventricular walls are divided into standard segments in both right anterior oblique (RAO) and left anterior oblique (LAO) views. These segments are: (1) anterobasal, (2) anteroapical, (3) apical, (4) inferior or diaphragmatic and (5) posterobasal. The aortic root (Ao), left atrium (LA) and mitral valve (MV) can be seen in the ventriculogram illustrated, which is a 30° RAO projection of a normal heart. Wall motion may be normal (concentric inward movement during systole), hypokinetic (velocity or amplitude or both diminished), akinetic (without movement) or dyskinetic (moving outward or paradoxically during systole). The left ventriculogram is also described according to the presence and degree of mitral regurgitation (best seen in the 30° RAO view), ventricular septal defect with left-to-right shunting (best seen in the 60° LAO view) and filling defects, obstruction or aneurysmal dilatation (either or both views).

Ejection fraction is calculated from the end-diastolic and end-systolic volumes. It is easily and reliably determined except in the presence of atrial fibrillation or a series of premature beats and must be measured after adequate hydration and with a heart rate between 60 and 100/min. The difference between end-diastolic and end-systolic volumes, the stroke volume, is divided by end-diastolic volume to yield the ejection fraction. It correlates with the prognosis of patients with coronary heart disease, valvular heart disease or myocardial disease and gauges the risk of cardiac surgery. An ejection fraction less than 0.55 is abnormal. Between 0.55 and 0.40 corresponds with mild left ventricular impairment, compensated function and no symptoms of heart failure; between 0.40 and 0.25 corresponds with moderate symptoms of heart failure (New York Heart Association Class III); and less than 0.25 with severe ventricular impairment or destruction with profound symptoms (New York Heart Association Class IV).

Selective coronary arteriography

Selective coronary arteriography may be performed by either of two main methods.

In the Sones technique a gently curved, thin-walled, woven catheter with tapering tip (see Illustration 1d) is introduced through a surgical cutdown and brachial arteriotomy; it may then be manipulated into the left and right coronary ostia and also into the left ventricle. Several injections of 2–5 ml of contrast fluid are made in multiple projections and recorded on 35-mm cineangiographic film, affording detailed visualization of the entire coronary arterial tree.

In the Judkins technique 'coronary seeking' catheters (see Illustrations 1e, g and h) are introduced percutaneously into the femoral artery and manipulated into the respective coronary ostia, separate catheters (Judkins or Amplatz) being required for the left and right coronary arteries.

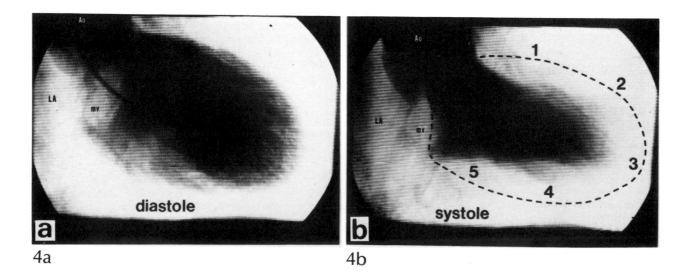

4a

4b

5

The interpretation of coronary arteriograms is currently a subjective matter, although automated, computer-assisted methods for exact measurement are under development. There are several sources of potential error in the evaluation of arteriograms. Multiple orthogonal views are mandatory, as vessels may cross over one another in some views but be shown clearly in others. Eccentric or asymmetric atherosclerotic narrowing may lead to entirely differing impressions of severity in opposite views, the constriction appearing minor in Plane A whereas in orthogonal Plane B it is revealed to be critically narrow.

Several special techniques have emerged that are useful in the evaluation of coronary disease. The selective visualization of aortocoronary bypass grafts and internal thoracic (mammary) artery implants has become increasingly important as reoperation for progressively occlusive coronary atherosclerosis is performed more frequently. Coronary vasospasm has become better recognized thanks to arteriography with provocative manoeuvres such as the infusion of low doses of ergometrine (ergonovine) maleate. Measurement of coronary blood flow with thermodilution catheters in the coronary sinus is also performed.

Interventive techniques include the infusion of thrombolytic agents such as streptokinase or tissue plasminogen activator during the first hours of myocardial infarction[2]. This is a novel method already achieving great popularity which is designed to lyse thrombi that have acutely precipitated early reversible ischaemia. Percutaneous transluminal angioplasty is mentioned below.

The potential complications of coronary arteriography[3] are presented in Table 2.

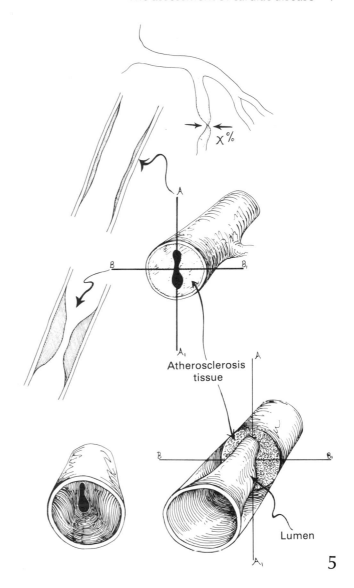

Atherosclerosis tissue

Lumen

5

Table 2 Potential complications of cardiac catheterization and angiography

Complication	Percentage
Allergic reactions to contrast material	0.1
Bronchospasm (pulmonary angiography)	0.6
Renal complications	<0.1
Pulmonary embolism	0.01
Arterial embolism	0.1–0.4
Cardiac or great vessel perforation	0.2–0.8
Serious arrhythmia	0.1
(asystole, heart block, supraventricular tachycardia, ventricular tachycardia or fibrillation)	
Myocardial infarction	0.25
Death	
high-risk patient	0.76
low-risk patient	0.05

Aortography

Aortic angiography is useful in the diagnosis of a wide variety of conditions. If mitral regurgitation is suspected as well as aortic, the 45° RAO projection is used. For visualization of the brachiocephalic vessels a steeper (45–60°) LAO view is employed to unfold the aorta. Shunting in persistent ductus arteriosus is best observed in the 45° LAO projection. Aortic coarctation is often studied in two planes, one being LAO 20–45°.

Dissection of the aorta is a dangerous condition which, despite the risks, requires aortography for diagnosis and definition of location and extent. Whether or not the ascending aorta is involved determines the operative approach, and additional information required is the extent of the dissection, the integrity of branching vessels and the status of the aortic valve and coronary arteries.

Pulmonary angiography

The chief indications for pulmonary angiography are: (1) suspicion of pulmonary thromboembolism; (2) elucidation of congenital malformations; and (3) anatomical visualization of the pulmonary artery or left atrium.

Certain patients, such as those with primary pulmonary hypertension, are at high risk in pulmonary arteriography. The risks and complications of this procedure are listed in Table 2.

Interpretation of the pulmonary angiogram in suspected pulmonary embolism involves inspection for intraluminal filling defects or abrupt cut-offs and also for areas of asymmetrical delayed filling or relative oligaemia. These latter findings may occur in chronic lung disease and are not in themselves diagnostic of pulmonary thromboembolism. Problem areas can be better delineated by specific local injection.

Pulmonary angiography for shunting (as in arteriovenous malformation or anomalous pulmonary venous return) or for left-heart visualization requires that films be taken throughout the course of travel of contrast into the left heart (laevo phase).

COMPLICATIONS ASSOCIATED WITH CARDIAC CATHETERIZATION

Certain subjects are especially vulnerable to potential complications, notably the elderly and very young (see Table 2). Patients in congestive heart failure or renal failure or with poor myocardial reserve may not tolerate the injection of large amounts of angiographic contrast material. Patients with critical aortic stenosis or hypertrophic obstructive cardiomyopathy may develop profound shock or dangerous arrhythmias during catheterization. Pulmonary angiography is extremely dangerous in the presence of marked pulmonary hypertension.

Special invasive methods

ELECTROPHYSIOLOGICAL STUDIES

Many rhythm and conduction disorders can now be effectively diagnosed by intracardiac electrocardiography. Information from these studies allows better understanding of cardiac electrophysiology and affords a rational approach to pharmacological, pacemaker or surgical treatment[4].

By appropriately positioning an electrode-tipped catheter within various cardiac chambers impulses can be recorded which are not detected on the usual 12-lead surface ECG. For example, with the electrodes along the right ventricular surface of the interventricular septum, depolarization of the right atrium, the bundle of His and the ventricles can be recorded, revealing the site of atrioventricular conduction delay.

More recently intracardiac records have been used to localize the site of anomalous atrioventricular pathways or bypass tracts in pre-excitation conditions such as the Wolff-Parkinson-White syndrome. This may guide pharmacological therapy or surgical ablation of the abnormal conducting tissue.

Electrode-catheter techniques may be used to initiate certain tachyarrhythmias. A programmable impulse generator allows stimulation of various intracardiac sites in a predetermined sequence. Induction of supraventricular or ventricular tachycardia in patients with these arrhythmias allows reliable selection and evaluation of drug treatment. This is important in patients with life-threatening arrhythmias, in whom clinical trial and error may be costly and perhaps risky.

The most recent application of electrophysiological techniques has been in the treatment of recurrent sustained ventricular tachycardia. This dangerous arrhythmia may occur in survivors of myocardial infarction, often in association with a ventricular scar or aneurysm. If antiarrhythmic drugs are not effective the abnormal tissue causing the tachycardia may be removed surgically. Routine or 'blind' ventricular aneurysmectomy appears less successful than specific endocardial resection guided by electrophysiological mapping to locate and remove the origin of the tachycardia.

CARDIAC BIOPSY

The transvascular endomyocardial biopsy technique was developed in the 1960s, allowing cardiac biopsy to be performed more safely and easily during routine cardiac catheterization without surgical assistance.

6

Endomyocardial biopsy[5] is performed with a catheter-mounted bioptome. For right ventricular biopsy this is introduced percutaneously into the right internal jugular or femoral vein and advanced under fluoroscopic control into the right ventricular apex, pointing towards the interventricular septum. The jaws of the bioptome are opened and gently advanced against the septal wall. They are then closed and a 2–3 mm diameter specimen of endomyocardium removed (see insert). This procedure has been performed at Stanford in over 5000 cases without any deaths and with a complication rate of less than 1 per cent. It can be performed repeatedly and yields enough tissue for adequate histological examination. Left ventricular percutaneous endomyocardial biopsy is performed via the femoral artery (direct transaortic method) or femoral vein (transatrial method) and is as safe as the right-sided procedure. The various routes are illustrated.

Catheter biopsy of the heart has been used for specific diagnosis in several diseases: cardiac allograft rejection, myocarditis, doxorubicin (Adriamycin) cardiac toxicity, cardiac amyloidosis, sarcoidosis and haemochromatosis, endocardial fibrosis and fibroelastosis, carcinoid disease, Fabry's disease of the heart, glycogen storage disease and others. Non-pathognomonic myocardial changes have been observed in idiopathic congestive cardiomyopathy, idiopathic hypertrophic subaortic stenosis, thyroid heart disease, myotonic dystrophy and mitral valve prolapse.

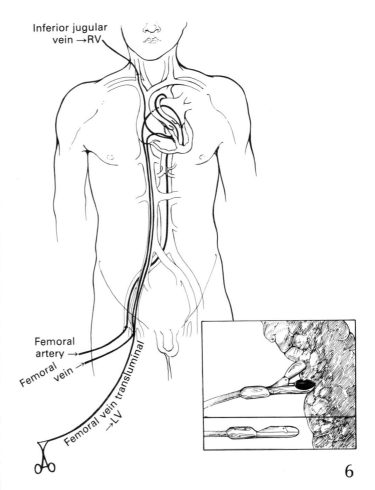

Inferior jugular vein →RV

Femoral artery →

Femoral vein →

Femoral vein transluminal →LV

6

PERCUTANEOUS TRANSLUMINAL CORONARY ANGIOPLASTY

A non-surgical treatment for obstructive coronary athero-sclerosis can have obvious advantages over the sometimes hazardous and clearly expensive operative procedures currently so extensively used[6]. In 1977 Dr Andreas Gruntzig in Zürich performed the first transluminal coronary angioplasty in humans, using a special balloon catheter.

7

A pre-shaped guiding catheter is first inserted percu-taneously into the region of the coronary ostium. A second catheter is then advanced through the guiding channel into the coronary artery. This dilatation catheter contains a thin guide wire which facilitates its advance across proximal coronary obstructions. A slender balloon is then inflated with contrast fluid to a pressure of 4–6 atmospheres for a few seconds, dilating the putty-like atheromatous narrowing as verified by pressure gradient measurements and subsequent angiography.

Percutaneous angioplasty is currently applicable to appro-ximately 20 per cent of all patients with coronary artery disease – those with proximal non-calcified lesions, usually in a single vessel patent enough to allow passage of the balloon catheter. Initial experience indicates that this is a very specialized technique best performed by highly experienced operators. Symptomatic and haemodynamic improvement occurs but is offset by an immediate mortality rate of 1 per cent, a need for early bypass surgery in nearly 10 per cent of patients and restenosis in another 10 per cent.

Further development of transluminal angioplasty may include refinement of equipment, improvement of technique, extension to a larger proportion of coronary patients and use in the operating theatre as an adjunct to bypass surgery.

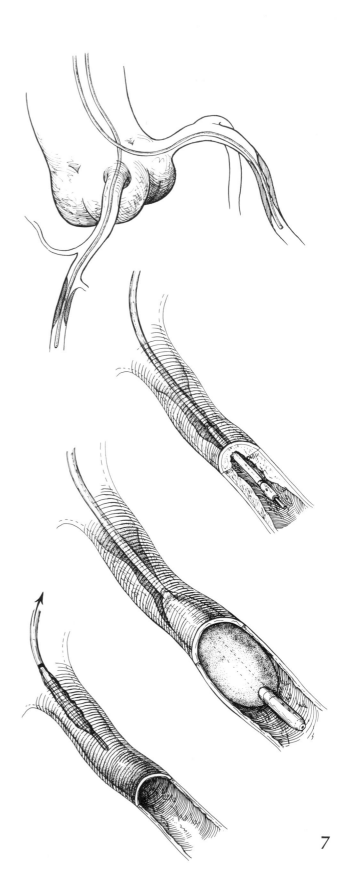

7

Non-invasive diagnostic methods complementing invasive studies

Non-invasive techniques have the virtues of safety, simplicity and economy and are now approaching the diagnostic accuracy of invasive methods, the 'gold standard' with which they have long been compared. Rather than replacing cardiac catheterization, non-invasive methods currently enhance invasive techniques: the non-invasive test is useful in screening patients and determining the appropriate time for catheterization and surgery. Non-invasive methods are particularly helpful in multiple serial studies and in the evaluation of critically ill, high-risk patients. This section will highlight the non-invasive methods which currently complement cardiac catheterization.

ECHOCARDIOGRAPHY

During the 1960s and 1970s echocardiography advanced from a new, relatively crude technique to its current position as a highly useful and reliable clinical tool involving increasingly sophisticated electronic equipment. Although definitely limited in its ability to diagnose cardiac disorders, echocardiography provides accurate, free-standing diagnosis of many conditions. This section will outline some of the clinical conditions in which echocardiography is most useful.

The echocardiograhic abnormalities of some cardiac conditions are specific enough to allow a positive diagnosis to be made solely by ultrasound. These include pericardial effusion and rheumatic mitral stenosis, two conditions in which the technique found early application. The echocardiographic findings in other heart disorders may not provide an absolute diagnosis but can confirm a clinical suspicion, localize an abnormality or indicate further diagnostic tests.

Conventional M-mode echocardiography has a limited diagnostic value in some conditions, such as mitral regurgitation. With the new technique of Doppler echocardiography the severity of mitral regurgitation may be estimated. Commercially available instruments employ circuitry using the ultrasound transducer as a receiver of reflected sound waves for graphic presentation (echo) as well as for electronic analysis of frequency shift (Doppler).

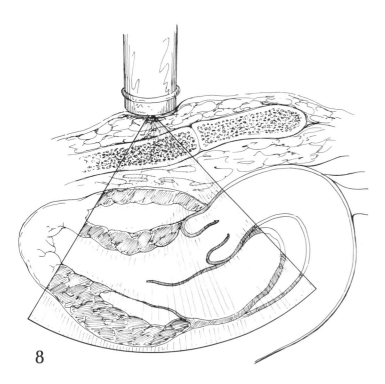

8

8

Two-dimensional cross-sectional echocardiography is a recent development which has greatly extended the diagnostic power of ultrasound. This technique, which is still undergoing rapid development, allows two-dimensional imaging of the heart in multiple planes from multiple angles. This spatial orientation proves valuable in estimating the severity of mitral and aortic stenosis, detecting intracardiac tumours and valvular vegetations, revealing the anatomy in congenital disease, assessing wall motion abnormalities and detecting ventricular aneurysms. Two-dimensional echocardiography has proved more sensitive than the M-mode technique in certain cases but is not necessarily wholly superior and is still a subject of active research. A two-dimensional echocardiographic view of the heart in long axis is illustrated, showing a cross-sectional image of the left ventricle posterior to the right ventricle, with the aortic and mitral valves, and the left atrium posterior to the aorta.

Echocardiography, especially two-dimensional cross-sectional sector scanning, can estimate ejection fraction and identify abnormal wall motion, may easily be performed in the coronary care unit in patients with acute myocardial infarction and allows serial study.

NUCLEAR CARDIOLOGY

Nuclear cardiology is a rapidly developing field which already has several clinical applications. Radioactive isotopes or radionuclides are injected intravenously and their activity recorded by complex scanners or cameras positioned over the heart. There are currently three main types of radionuclide scan: (1) perfusion imaging for evaluating myocardial blood flow; (2) infarction scintigraphy for detecting necrotic or injured myocardium; and (3) blood pool scanning for determining ventricular performance.

Myocardial perfusion imaging

This technique relies on uptake by normal cardiac cells of the potassium analogue ^{201}thallous chloride. Thallium accumulates rapidly and uniformly in normal myocardium within minutes after intravenous injection but unevenly or not at all in hypoperfused or infarcted tissue. The abnormal areas without thallium uptake produce 'cold spots' on the image; the size and severity of these defects depends on the ratio of blood flow in the abnormal area to that in the surrounding areas. Blood flow during exercise increases more in normal coronary arteries than in stenosed vessels and exercise may therefore intensify a resting thallium defect or produce a new one not observed at rest. For this reason ^{201}thallium perfusion imaging is most useful in conjunction with exercise electrocardiography; the combination of both techniques can detect coronary artery disease with greater sensitivity than either method alone. Thallium scanning is less likely to result in a false positive diagnosis of coronary artery disease than is exercise electrocardiography, especially in the setting of an abnormal ECG or digitalis effects. Other advantages of thallium imaging include its value in screening patients with atypical chest pain and an equivocal exercise ECG, assessing the physiological significance of a known coronary arterial lesion and determining coronary graft patency. The disadvantages of thallium imaging include its decreased sensitivity to the diffuse hypoperfusion abnormalities of multivessel coronary disease and its inability always to distinguish infarcted tissue from ischaemic myocardium.

Infarction scintigraphy

This technique depends on the increased uptake of ^{99m}technetium pyrophosphate by damaged myocardium. Thus areas of acute myocardial infarction will register a 'hot spot' on the image in contrast to unlabelled normal tissue. Technetium pyrophosphate scintigrams become positive 12–72 hours after infarction and usually revert to normal in about 10 days. They can be particularly useful in the diagnosis of myocardial infarction in several clinical settings, such as immediately after coronary artery bypass grafting. However, because it is a sensitive detector of all types of myocardial necrosis, technetium pyrophosphate scanning may also be positive in myocardial contusion, high-energy cardioversion, ventricular aneurysms or even old myocardial infarctions.

Blood pool scannning

This is the display and analysis of radioactivity remaining in the bloodstream after an intravenous injection. ^{99m}Technetium human serum albumin is the most common intravascular marker used. There are currently two blood pool scanning methods, *first-pass* radionuclide angiocardiography and *equilibrium-gated* blood pool imaging. The first-pass technique follows the marker as it moves through the cardiac chambers, allowing detection of shunts or valvular regurgitation. The equilibrium technique measures the marker after it has equilibrated within the vasculature, permitting repeated scans over several hours and during acute interventions. By 'triggering' or 'gating' the camera to the ECG the left ventricular image or representative counts can be recorded in end-diastole and end-systole, giving the ejection fraction. The main problem with radionuclide scanning as an angiocardiographic method is resolution. However, ejection fraction derived from gated imaging correlates well with that from contrast ventriculography.

Specific conditions

VALVULAR HEART DISEASE

Although many clinical signs and non-invasive investigations may enable the severity of valvular lesions to be estimated, cardiac catheterization is necessary for the full evaluation of stenosis or regurgitation or both. In addition, accurate assessment of ventricular function is important in determining the patient's ability to survive or benefit from cardiac surgery.

9 & 10

The grading of valvular stenosis requires measurement of both flow and pressure gradient across the valve in question. Normal flow across an unobstructed valve orifice requires a small (<5 mm/kg) pressure gradient. Gorlin established the following basic formula for valve orifice area:

$$\text{area (cm}^2) = \frac{\text{flow (cm}^3/\text{sec})}{\text{velocity (cm/sec)}} = \frac{\text{flow}}{k\sqrt{\Delta P}}$$

where ΔP is the main pressure gradient across the orifice and k is a constant for the valve in question (k = 31 for the mitral valve, 44.5 for the aortic valve). Of course, valve flow occurs only during the portion of the cardiac cycle in which the valve is open (the diastolic filling period for the mitral valve and the systolic ejection period for the aortic valve). Valve flow for the equation above is then calculated from cardiac output as follows:

$$\text{mitral flow (cm}^3/\text{sec}) = \frac{\text{cardiac output (cm}^3/\text{min})}{\text{diastolic filling period (sec/min)}}$$

$$\text{aortic flow (cm}^3/\text{sec}) = \frac{\text{cardiac output (cm}^3/\text{min})}{\text{systolic ejection period (sec/min)}}$$

From the equation giving valve orifice area the pressure gradient is inversely related to the square of the orifice area. Thus for a significant (that is, 20 mmHg or 4 × normal) detectable gradient, valve area must be diminished by one-half. As valve area is reduced further the gradient must increase as the square of that reduction to maintain the same flow. If increased flow is required (as in exercise) the gradient must increase. Eventually the necessary gradient cannot be maintained even at rest and cardiac output falls. For these reasons flow and gradient must be accurately measured in order to assess the severity of valve stenosis.

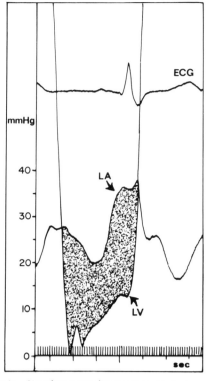

Mitral stenosis – Simultaneous direct pressure measurement in the left atrium (LA) and left ventricle (LV) reveals a persistent gradient (shaded area) through diastole. The mean gradient (ΔP) can be determined by measuring the total area and dividing by diastolic filling period

9

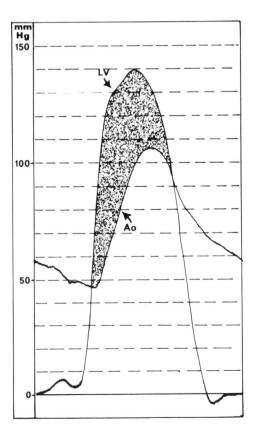

10

Aortic stenosis – Simultaneous direct pressure measurement in the left ventricle (LV) and aortal (Ao) shows a significant gradient (shaded area) systole. Mean gradient calculation is analogous to that described for Illustration 9

11a & b

Quantification of valvular regurgitation is more difficult than that of stenosis. It is common practice with both aortic and mitral valves to estimate qualitatively the severity of regurgitation by judging during angiography the amount of contrast material entering the upstream chamber from the downstream chamber. Thus for mitral regurgitation (a) contrast medium injected into the left ventricle (RAO projection) appears in the left atrium as well as being ejected into the aorta. For aortic regurgitation (b) supravalvular aortography is performed and contrast material appears in the left ventricle, severity being graded as follows: 1+ = small amount of contrast material entering left ventricle during diastole but clearing completely with each systole; 2+ = left ventricle faintly and incompletely opacified during diastole, contrast material not clearing with each systole; 3+ = left ventricle becoming progressively opacified during diastole and eventually completely opacified; and 4+ = left ventricle completed opacified after first diastole and remaining so for several cardiac cycles. The scale for mitral regurgitation is analogous.

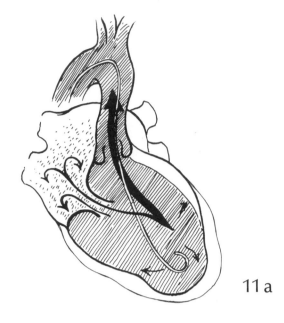

11 a

Large v waves in the left atrial or pulmonary artery wedge tracing may indicate the presence of mitral regurgitation.

A more quantitative approach to the estimation of valvular regurgitation is afforded by the use of indicator dilution curves. This requires an injecting catheter in the downstream chamber and a sampling catheter in the upstream chamber, so it is less popular in common clinical practice. With either the indicator method or cine-angiography the regurgitant fraction can be calculated and is the best indicator of severity. For the indicator method in aortic regurgitation:

$$\frac{\text{regurgitant}}{\text{fraction}} = \frac{\text{dye sampled in left ventricle (regurgitant volume)}}{\text{dye sampled in aorta (total sampled in aorta) (total volume forward plus regurgitant)}}$$

For the cineangiographic method:

regurgitant volume = total stroke volume
                    (from left ventriculogram)
                  − forward stroke volume
                    (cardiac output/heart rate)

$$\text{regurgitant fraction} = \frac{\text{regurgitant volume}}{\text{total stroke volume}}$$

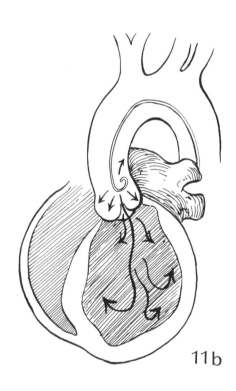

11b

Radionuclide angiography is a promising technique for the non-invasive estimation of regurgitant fractions in these lesions but does not stand alone as the definitive diagnostic approach.

CONGENITAL HEART DISEASE

Indications for cardiac catheterization in children vary according to age and nature of presentation. The neonate or infant presenting with cardiac symptoms or signs (cyanosis, congestive heart failure or respiratory problems) should undergo cardiac catheterization. These may occur in certain cases of transposition of the great vessels, total anomalous pulmonary venous return or tricuspid atresia, in which balloon septostomy may be life-saving. Any significant change in the course of a child's congenital heart disorder should prompt consideration of invasive study. Cardiac catheterization is performed before operation in all cases and often after the operation to assess results and to provide a postoperative baseline for future comparison.

The techniques of cardiac catheterization in children differ from those in adults in several ways. During the first week of life right-heart catheterization may be performed through the umbilical vein. Left-heart catheterization in many infants and children can be carried out through a patent foramen ovale.

There is a relatively increased frequency of complications of cardiac catheterization in children. Neonates undergoing invasive studies are at increased risk because they are usually severely ill; they are less tolerant of changes such as hypoxaemia or acidosis; they are subject to hypothermia, catheter perforation of heart chambers and vascular complications (because of vessel size); and they may not tolerate angiography or the removal of blood samples well because of their small blood volume.

Apart from the special problems of neonates, most children with congenital heart disease are vulnerable in three areas: (1) their small hearts are more likely to manifest ventricular ectopy; (2) cardiac output may be severely decreased by contrast injections (such as one into a reactive or resistive pulmonary vascular bed); and (3) arterial hypoxaemia can readily occur. This last may be due to sedation and may appear also with right-to-left shunting in conditions such as tetralogy of Fallot if systemic vascular resistance falls and pulmonary blood flow then decreases. Catheterization is performed under local anaesthesia with judicious sedation, usually with combinations of pethidine (meperidine) and hydroxyzine, droperidol or chlorpromazine. (Chlorpromazine, owing to its systemic vasodilator properties, is avoided in conditions such as tetralogy of Fallot where a fall in systemic resistance could significantly reduce pulmonary blood flow.)

Because of the preponderance of abnormal venous-arterial intracardiac communications the calculation of shunts is essential in the evaluation of congenital heart disease. Most commonly this relies on the measurement of oxygen saturation at various cardiovascular locations.

MYOCARDIAL DISEASE

Cardiac catheterization is valuable in answering many clinical questions regarding myocardial diseases. Thus a functional classification of these disorders is most helpful in describing their diagnostic approaches. In the temperate climates three main types of heart muscle disorder exist: hypertrophic, congestive and restrictive. (The term 'cardiomyopathy' has been applied to any heart muscle disorder but may be more appropriately reserved for those entities of unknown cause, the remainder being named according to the underlying disease affecting the myocardium.)

Hypertrophic cardiomyopathy

Because of the thick, inelastic ventricular wall, this condition is characterized by resistance to ventricular filling, usually reflected by elevated end-diastolic pressures. Systolic 'pump' function is preserved. In the obstructive form known as idiopathic hypertrophic subaortic stenosis or hypertrophic obstructive cardiomyopathy the outflow of blood is impeded by the disproportionately thickened interventricular septum producing an intracavitary gradient. This systolic pressure gradient can be extremely variable and during catheterization may be provoked by several manoeuvres, including infusion of an inotrope (isoprenaline (isoproterenol)), or induction of extrasystoles by catheter manoeuvre (in which the heightened contractility of the postextrasystolic beat produces a gradient across the left ventricular outflow tract). Cardiac catheterization is useful not only in diagnosing obstructive cardiomyopathy but may guide treatment; if the gradient is severe enough and not satisfactorily ameliorated with medical therapy, surgical intervention (septal myectomy) may be indicated.

Congestive cardiomyopathy

This is often diagnosed by non-invasive means; the clinical history, physical examination, chest film and echocardiogram are usually characteristic.

Cardiac catheterization is used to confirm the diagnosis, reveal the severity of the disorder, estimate myocardial reserve (after exercise or angiography), guide medical therapy (such as afterload reduction) and exclude certain conditions such as coronary artery disease or myocarditis. Left ventricular angiography reveals a diffusely enlarged chamber with overall hypokinesis and reduced ejection fraction and occasionally secondary mitral regurgitation and left ventricular filling defects caused by mural thrombi. The haemodynamics include a low cardiac index, although in mild or early forms of the condition ventricular dilatation may compensate for the myocardial insufficiency, which may be disclosed by resting or exercise-provoked increases in left ventricular end-diastolic pressure. The coronary arteries are usually patent despite occasional segmental wall motion abnormalities in congestive cardiomyopathy. In some instances a treatable condition such as myocarditis may be found and thus endomyocardial biopsy by catheter bioptome (see Illustration 6) has recently found limited usefulness when indicated by appropriate clinical circumstances.

Restrictive cardiomyopathy

This condition is typified by reduced ventricular filling due to diminished compliance. Restrictive features may be present in hypertrophic myocardial disease or caused by arterial hypertension or aortic stenosis. In its isolated form restrictive myocardial disease is usually caused by infiltrative disorders or extensive fibrosis. The main haemodynamic characteristics are: (1) elevated left- and right-sided venous pressures with large a and v waves: (2) ventricular diastolic dip and plateau (*square root sign*) pattern caused by late diastolic limitation of filling; and (3) left-sided filling pressures usually greater than with an intrinsic contraction defect.

Restrictive myocardial disease notoriously mimics constrictive pericarditis. The most reliable distinguishing feature is probably the fact that in restrictive disease left-sided filling pressures (left atrial or pulmonary artery wedge mean and left ventricular end-diastolic) usually exceed right-sided filling pressures by at least 10 mmHg. This differential may be latent until provoked by manoeuvres that preferentially stress the left side of the heart, such as exercise or afterload augmentation by isometric exertion (handgrip) or pharmacological means. Because cardiac amyloidosis usually presents with restrictive features endomyocardial biopsy may be helpful in achieving a diagnosis.

PERICARDIAL DISEASE

As noted above, this may be imitated by restrictive myocardial disease. Cardiac catheterization may distinguish between the two entities, usually by the different left- and right-sided filling pressures in constrictive disease. Venous pressure is elevated, but because the limit of ventricular filling is not reached until the latter portion of diastole a prominent right atrial y descent is usually recorded. If venous return is acutely augmented the limitation in flow through the encased ventricles will be exceeded and the venous pressure will rise. This is manifested in Kussmaul's sign (inspiratory rise in mean right atrial pressure) or after rapid infusion of crystalloid as a provocative manoeuvre.

Cardiac tamponade

Cardiac tamponade is due to compression of the heart by pericardial fluid, usually sufficient to cause circulatory compromise. Haemodynamically it may be detected by the presence of pulsus paradoxus and exaggeration of the physiological inspiratory fall in peak systolic arterial pressure. This sign may, however, be absent in several important conditions such as localized cardiac compression (often postoperative), aortic regurgitation, left ventricular hypertrophy or pre-existing elevated pulmonary artery wedge pressure. Kussmaul's sign is more suggestive of constrictive disease than of tamponade. Echocardiography can detect pericardial effusion but cannot reliably diagnose tamponade. Pericardiocentesis is often performed in the cardiac catheterization laboratory for therapeutic and diagnostic purposes as well as for optimal gathering of haemodynamic information in cases of mixed effusive (tamponade) and constrictive disease.

References

1. Sonnenblick, E. H., Strobeck, J. E. Derived indices of ventricular and myocardial function. New England Journal of Medicine 1977; 296: 978–982

2. Bergman, S. R. *et al.* Coronary thrombolysis achieved with human extrinsic plasminogen activator, a clot selective activator, administered intravenously. Journal of the American College of Cardiology 1983; 1: 615–000

3. Davis, K. *et al.* Complications of coronary arteriography from the Collaborative Study of Coronary Artery Surgery (CASS). Circulation 1979; 59: 1105–1112

4. Horowitz, L. N., Harken, A. H., Kaston, J. A., Josephson, M. E. Ventricular resection guided by epicardial and endocardial mapping for treatment of recurrent ventricular tachycardia. New England Journal of Medicine 1980; 302: 589–593

5. Mason, J. W. Techniques for right and left ventricular endomyocardial biopsy. American Journal of Cardiology 1978; 41: 887–892

6. Williams, D. O. *et al.* Guidelines for the performance of percutaneous transluminal coronary angioplasty. Circulation 1982; 66: 693–694

Surgical access to the heart and great vessels

Terence A. H. English, MB, BSc, MA, FRCS
Consultant Cardiothoracic Surgeon, Papworth and Addenbrooke's Hospitals, Cambridge, UK

Introduction

Satisfactory exposure of the operative field is the key to accurate anatomical dissection and safe surgical repair. Provision of optimum exposure is dependent on correct positioning of the patient on the operating table and on making the most appropriate incision for the operation to be performed.

Positioning the patient on the operating table

After induction of anaesthesia it is the responsibility of the surgeon to ensure that the patient is positioned correctly on the operating table. Different operations demand different routes of surgical access but the general principles relating to patient positioning are common to all situations and include the following:

1. All pressure areas, including the vertex of the head, must be adequately protected.
2. No metallic parts of the operating table, or its fixtures, should be in direct contact with the patient.
3. Electrical leads and catheters should not be kinked, nor allowed to cross under pressure areas.
4. The patient should be properly earthed. This is especially important in cardiac surgical patients who are often connected to a variety of electrical apparatus.
5. Unless a midline incision is used, the patient should be placed towards the edge of the operating table nearest the surgeon.
6. The patient's position must be stable on the table, thereby allowing the table to be rotated through its longitudinal or transverse axis if necessary. Such stability is achieved by a combination of pelvic and arm supports, supplemented by firm broad strapping.

Median sternotomy

Indications

This is the standard incision for most open intracardiac operations and is an excellent incision. It can be made rapidly through a relatively bloodless field and gives good exposure to all aspects of the heart. The aorta and right atrium are readily accessible so that, in an emergency, arterial and venous cannulation for bypass can be accomplished with the minimum of delay.

The incision is simple to make and close and, providing the divided edges of the sternum are securely approximated, it is relatively painless and heals well.

1

Position of patient and preparation

The patient is placed supine on the operating table, and after induction of anaesthesia ECG electrodes are applied, an electrocautery pad is placed beneath the buttocks and a urinary catheter is inserted and attached to a plastic measuring bag suspended from the operating table.

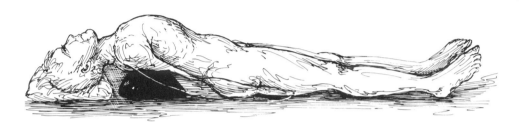

1

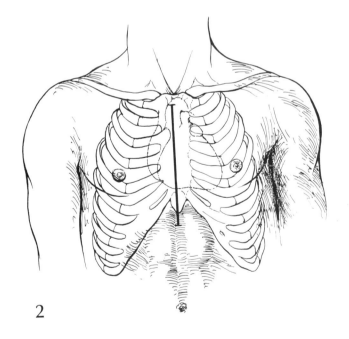

2

2

Incision

After preparation of the skin and the application of sterile drapes, a vertical skin incision is made from 2 cm below the suprasternal notch to 4 cm below the xiphisternum (Figure 1). It is important to divide the sternum precisely in the midline and this is facilitated by identifying the attachment of the linea alba to the xiphisternum below and the middle of the suprasternal notch above.

3

These two points are then joined by an electrocautery incision which is carried down to the sternal periosteum and acts as a marker for subsequent division of the sternum by the saw.

After gentle finger dissection deep to the upper manubrium between the two sternal heads of the sternomastoid muscle the suprasternal ligament is divided by electrocautery. Inferiorly the linea alba is incised throughout the length of the skin incision, taking care to preserve the underlying peritoneum, after which the xiphisternum is divided by scissors. A transverse vein running superficial to the sternoxiphisternal junction usually requires coagulation.

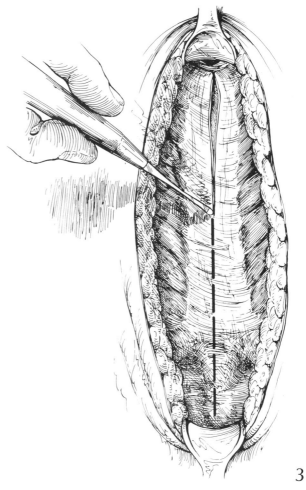

3

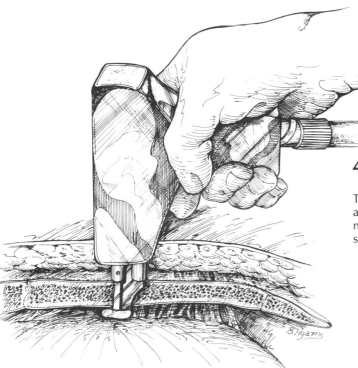

4

4

The sternum and manubrium are then divided cleanly with an oscillating saw. Various types of saws are available, the most suitable of which include a guard to protect structures deep to the sternum from damage.

5

The sternal edges are individually retracted and the periosteum cauterized on both sides from below upwards as far as the manubriosternal joint. A small retractor (Tuffier) is then inserted below and the suprasternal ligament divided with scissors. This allows haemostasis to be effected for the upper part of the incision; small amounts of bone wax are applied where necessary.

6

The left innominate vein is identified in the mediastinal fat in the upper part of the incision. This allows accurate definition of the thymus gland, or its remnant, which is separated into its two lobes. If an additional central venous line is required, the innominate vein may be cannulated via a small purse-string suture at this stage and the catheter advanced into the superior vena cava. One of the pleural reflections, usually the right, often extends across the midline and, if so, it is gently mobilized off the pericardium by a combination of blunt and sharp dissection.

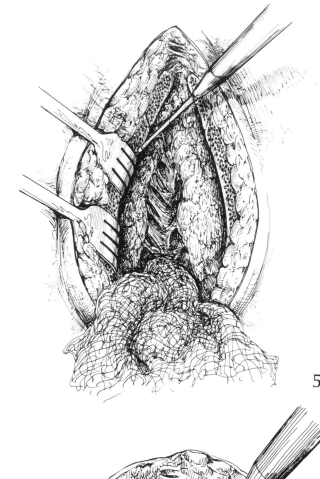

5

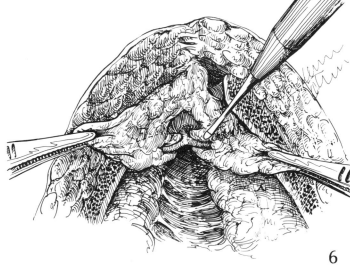

6

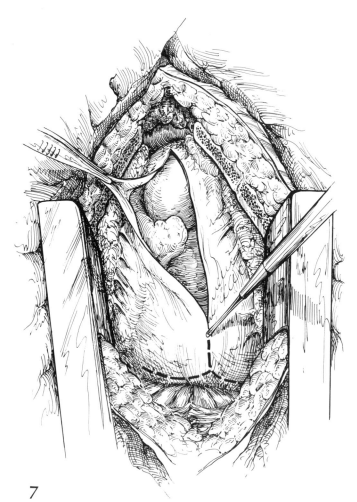

7

7

The pericardium is now exposed throughout its length and is divided by a gentle curved incision slightly to the left of the midline. The upper part of this incision extends as far as the pericardial reflection on to the aorta. The small retractor is removed and, after wound towels have been placed over the divided margins of the sternum, a large sternal retractor is introduced.

8

Increased mobilization is gained in the lower part of the wound by incising the pericardium laterally at its reflection with the diaphragm. The retractor may now be opened to the desired extent and the incision completed by suturing the upper cut edges of the pericardium to the wound towels.

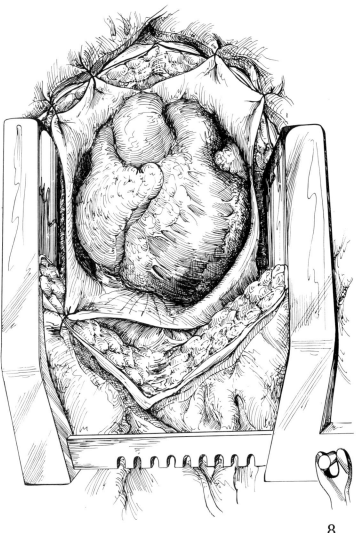

8

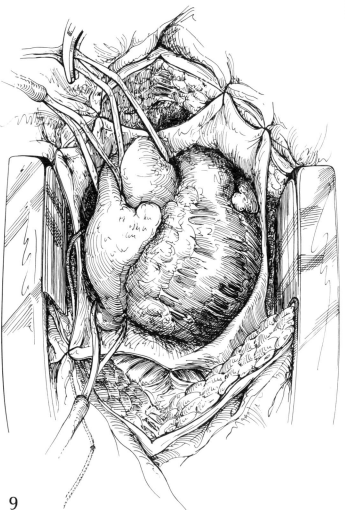

9

9

The heart having been exposed, preparations for cardiopulmonary bypass are completed by passing tapes around the aorta and, where relevant, both venae cavae. If the haemodynamic state is unstable, the latter is deferred until bypass has been commenced. A fine Teflon catheter may now be placed in the left atrium via the right superior pulmonary vein for pressure monitoring, and diagnostic pressures can be measured in the relevant cardiac chambers and great vessels. Further management, including heparinization and cannulation of the heart, is described in the chapter on 'Cardiopulmonary bypass and circulatory support', pp. 51–64.

10, 11 & 12

Closure of a median sternotomy incision is performed with interrupted wire sutures placed through the sternum. It is probably unnecessary to close the pericardium. Two drains are usually inserted.

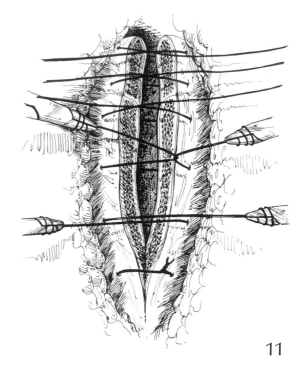

11

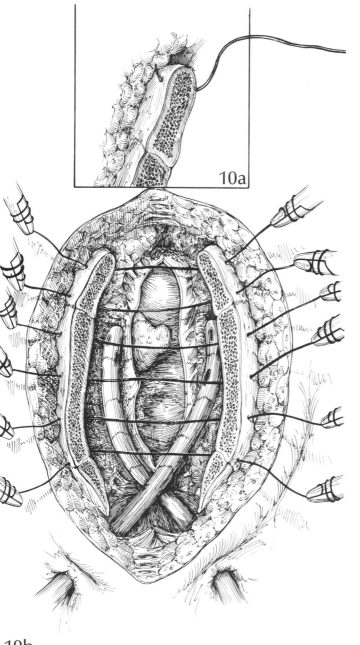

10a

10b

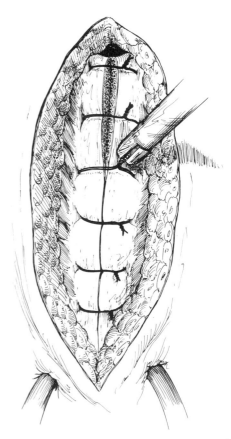

12

Posterolateral thoracotomy

Indications

This is the best incision for surgical procedures on structures in the central and posterior mediastinum. These include operations for:

1. Persistent ductus arteriosus;
2. Coarctation of the aorta;
3. Creation of systemic-pulmonary anastomoses;
4. Aneurysms and traumatic ruptures of the descending thoracic aorta.

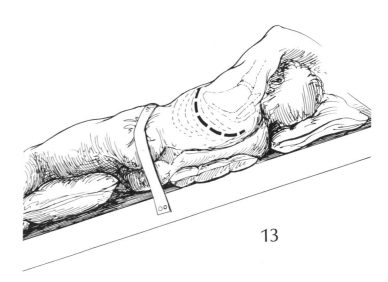

13

13

Position of patient

A stable full lateral position is required. This usually necessitates both a pelvic support and an anterior chest support. The back of the patient is placed adjacent to the edge of the operating table and the relevant scapula is elevated and abducted on the chest wall so as to give maximum access to the rib cage. This is obtained by holding the upper arm in abduction above the head and elevating the shoulder when positioning the patient on the table.

Skin incision

The skin incision is related to the extent and the level of thoracotomy that is planned. Most cardiac operations involving the arch and upper descending thoracic aorta are best performed through the lower border of the fourth rib. For closure of a persistent ductus arteriosus in an infant or child, a limited posterior thoracotomy will generally suffice, whereas a much fuller lateral incision is indicated for repair of coarctation of the aorta in an adult.

The incision commences anteriorly at the level of the mid-axillary (or mid-clavicular) line and extends posteriorly around the chest to a finger's breadth below the inferior angle of the scapula. From there it curves upwards to a point level with the spine of the scapula and midway between the spinous processes and the vertebral border of the scapula (see Illustration 13). The incision is then deepened vertically through the subcutaneous fat.

Muscle layer

For practical purposes two muscle layers are encountered:

1. Latissimus dorsi and trapezius;
2. Serratus and rhomboid major.

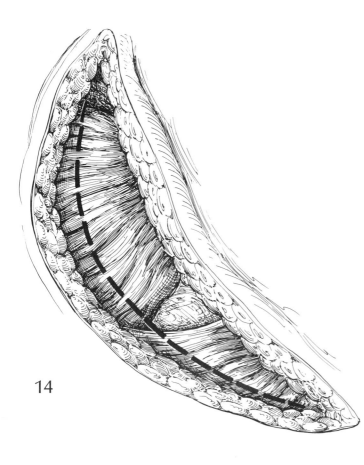

14

14

The anterior border of latissimus dorsi is located and the muscle divided throughout its length as low as possible, in the line of the skin incision. Electrocautery is used for this division. Posteriorly the muscular plane extends as a fascial layer to join the lower border of trapezius muscle, which itself is then divided as far as the upper margins of the skin incision.

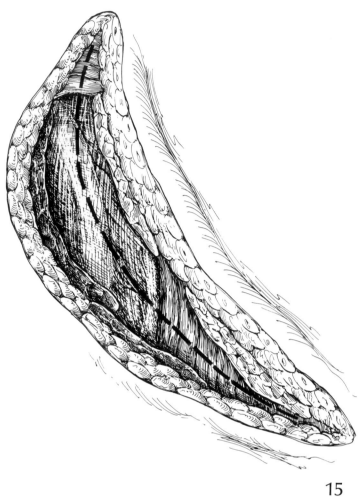

15

In the centre of the wound the ribs and intercostal layer are now only covered by a further fascial layer which is incised. Posterosuperiorly this fascia is continuous with rhomboid major, the lower part of which is divided.

15

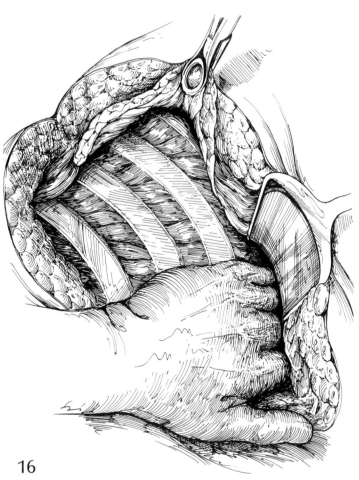

16

At this stage the selected rib should be identified by elevating the scapula with a retractor and introducing a hand into the avascular plane between it and the intercostal layer, keeping as close to the vertebral column as possible. The ribs can then be counted downwards, either from the first rib (which may be difficult to feel in adults), or from the third rib, which usually produces a natural step in the chest wall curvature, thereby allowing its identification.

16

17

The anterolateral part of the rib cage is covered by serratus anterior and, if additional exposure is required, the lower four digitations arising from the fifth, sixth, seventh and eighth ribs may be divided or detached from their costal origins. (These four digitations converge on the inferior angle of the scapula.) The incision on to the selected rib can then be continued anteriorly beneath skin and subcutaneous tissue, thereby exposing most of the length of the chosen rib, except posteriorly where it is covered by the erector spinae muscle mass.

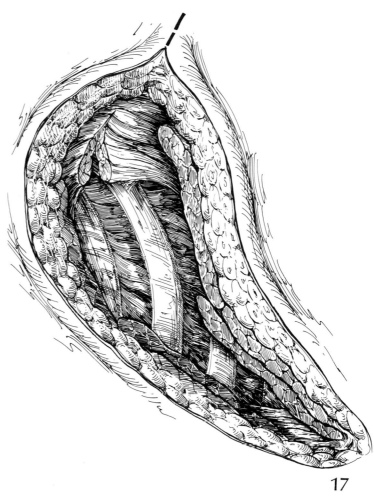

17

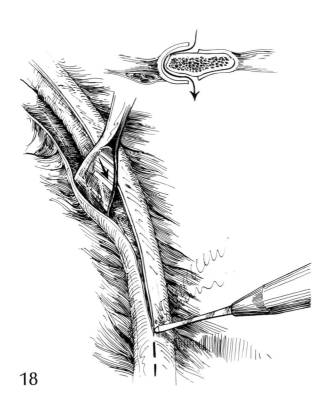

18

Intercostal layer

18

Entry into the chest cavity is gained by elevating the periosteum from the lower border of the rib and then incising the avascular plane forming the bed of the rib.

19a & b

Resection of a rib is now seldom necessary. Spreading the ribs for thoracotomy involves an extreme exaggeration of the natural rib movements and places an abnormal degree of strain on the anterior and posterior hinge mechanisms. It is important therefore to free the rib adequately so that its natural 'bucket-handle' movement can be made use of. Anteriorly this is accomplished by elevating the periosteum from the rib as far as possible and posteriorly by detaching and retracting the erector spinae muscles from the posterior end of the rib and then dividing the costotransverse ligament between it and the rib below with a Semb's chisel. (This may not be necessary in young children.) If proper mobility is ensured in this way and if the ribs are spread intermittently and progressively, it is rare to cause rib fractures.

If, however, access in the adult remains limited owing to increased ligamentous rigidity, resection of a short portion of the posterior part of the rib is sometimes necessary. This is performed by elevating the periosteum circumferentially from that part of the rib lying beneath the erector spinae muscles and then resecting a 2 cm length subperiosteally using a Tudor Edwards costotome.

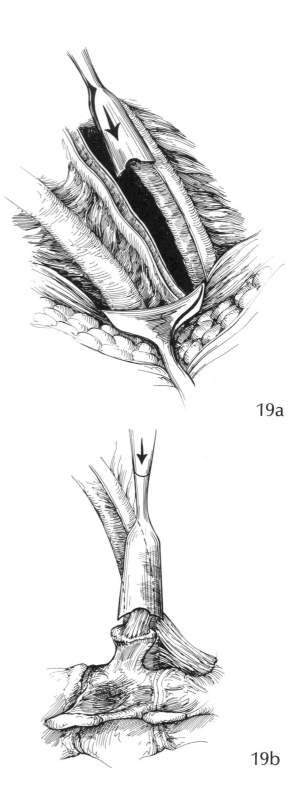

19a

19b

20 & 21

During closure, the muscles are approximated in the same three layers using continuous non-absorbable suture throughout.

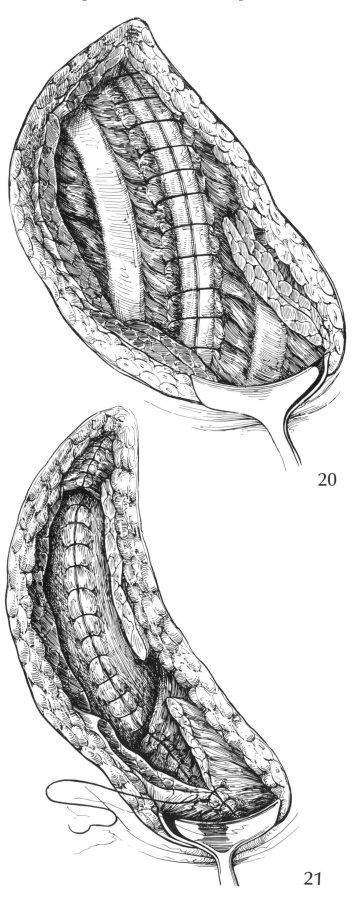

20

21

Anterolateral thoracotomy

22

Indications

On the left this incision gives satisfactory exposure of the left atrial appendage, pulmonary artery and left ventricular apex. It is therefore an appropriate incision for closed mitral valvotomy and for banding of the pulmonary artery. On the right it provides good access to the right atrium and both venae cavae and has been used for intra-atrial correction of transposition of the great arteries, and for closure of atrial septal defects. Right anterolateral thoracotomy has also been advocated by some for mitral valve repair but median sternotomy is now always preferable.

Position of patient

The patient is placed in an oblique lateral position on the operating table, incorporating a sandbag behind the sacrum and dispensing with the pelvic support. The arm that is uppermost is supported by appropriate strapping, thereby preventing the thorax from rotating too far posteriorly.

Skin incision

For closed mitral valvotomy it is important that the chest be entered via the lower border of the fifth rib. The fifth costal cartilage whould be identified by counting down from the second costal cartilage, which is identified by manubriosternal junction (angle of Louis), and clearly marked at its junction with the sternum. This is best done before the skin is prepared and drapes applied and allows the fifth rib to be identified with certainty during the subsequent procedures. The skin incision commences anteriorly over the previously marked costal cartilage and curves inferiorly along the inframammary skin crease and then posteriorly in a horizontal direction to end 2 cm below the inferior angle of the scapula. The incision is then deepened through the subcutaneous fat.

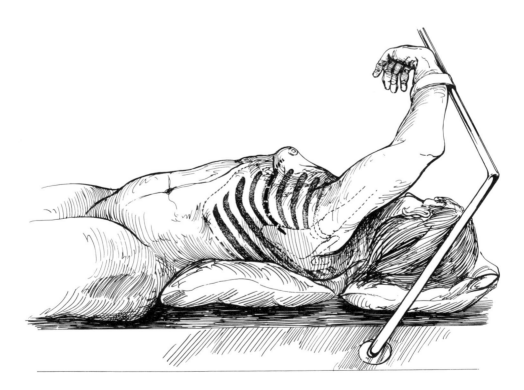

Muscles

23

The anterior border of latissimus dorsi is exposed posteriorly and in adult males this part of the muscle is divided in the line of the skin incision. Division of the muscle is usually not necessary in women and children.

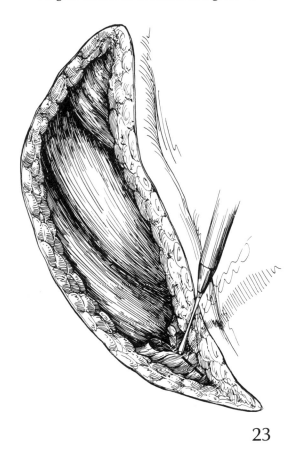

23

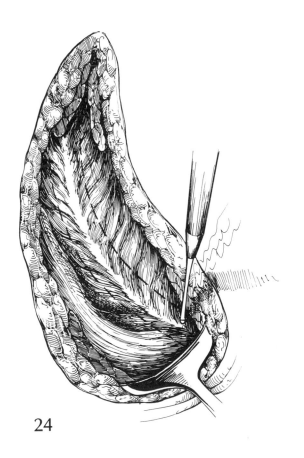

24

24

Anteriorly, fibres of the pectoralis major and rectus abdominis muscles are divided by electrocautery along the line of the fifth costal cartilage. In women that part of the breast overlying the fifth rib needs to be elevated as the dissection proceeds laterally. When the digitation of serratus anterior into the fifth rib is encountered, it is split longitudinally in the line of the muscle fibres, which coincides with the line of the rib.

This muscle split is extended posteriorly as far as the nerve to serratus anterior, which runs down on the external surface of the muscle and must be preserved. A hand is then inserted through this opening into the natural tissue plane deep to serratus anterior and the muscle split extended by manual separation of the fibres.

Intercostal layer

25

A scapula retractor is now inserted and the scapula elevated and retracted posteriorly. Division of the periosteum with electrocautery proceeds posteriorly as far as can be visualized and the periosteum is elevated from the inferior surface of the rib. The chest cavity is then entered through the exposed periosteal rib bed. Anteriorly the perichondrium is more difficult to elevate cleanly from the underlying cartilage but care here allows more satisfactory closure later.

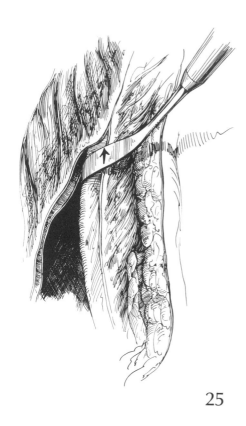

25

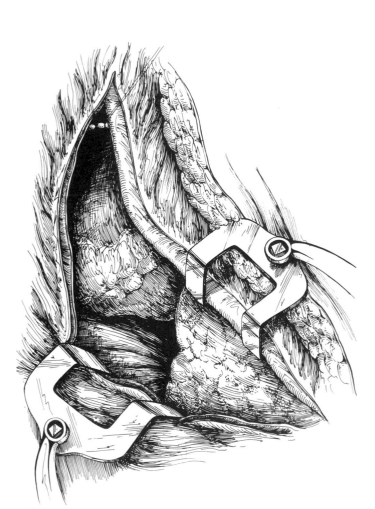

26

26

As the costal cartilage is retracted upwards, the internal mammary vessels are identified anteriorly and divided after suture-ligation. This allows free costosternal subluxation, which is preferable to fracture at the costosternal junction. A Price-Thomas rib-spreader is then introduced with the hinge mechanism posteriorly and the ribs gently spread apart. If access is adequate, this can usually be improved by extending the detachment of the intercostal layer from the lower border of the rib posteriorly, thereby increasing hinge mobilization.

27 & 28

Closure is effected by approximation of the intercostal and muscle layers with continuous monofilament sutures. It will be noted that the incision is a relatively avascular one compared with posterolateral thoracotomy. Other advantages include its stability and a reduced incidence of post-thoracotomy wound pain.

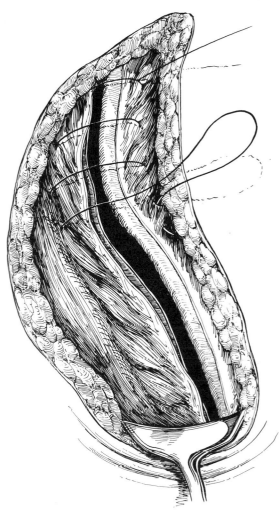

27

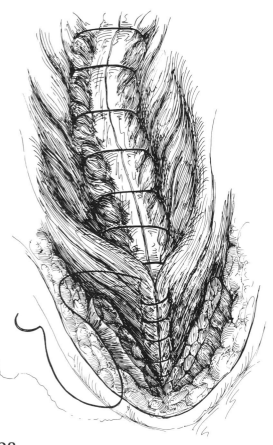

28

Anaesthesia for cardiac surgery

J. Kent Garman MD
Staff Anesthesiologist, Sequoia Hospital, Redwood City, California;
Clinical Associate Professor, Stanford University School of Medicine, Stanford, California, USA

Wayne H. Bellows MD
Staff Anesthesiologist, Cardiovascular Anesthesia, Permanente Medical Center, San Francisco, California, USA

Preoperative evaluation

The anaesthesiologist normally examines the patient the day before surgery, and a brief history is taken. Enquiries into a patient's exercise tolerance will provide information regarding cardiac reserve. The patient's prior anaesthetic experience may unmask problems concerning hypersensitivity or allergic reactions to previous techniques. An abbreviated, focused physical examination can also include the patient's response to mild exercise during the examination.

The chart is reviewed, including such items as referring letters, complete catheterization reports, old hospital records, history, physical examination and all laboratory reports (including electrocardiogram and chest X-ray). The usual laboratory studies should be available, including complete blood count, blood chemistry, urinalysis, coagulation studies and (if indicated) arterial blood gases and pulmonary function studies.

Cardiac catheterization data can help in planning the anaesthetic drug regimen. These data allow a decision to be made concerning cardiac reserve and the patient's response to stress. It is also helpful for the anaesthesiologist to study the patient's angiograms, either independently or with the surgical team, in order to have a stronger understanding of the severity of the patient's cardiac disease. The most important aspects of the cardiac catheterization report are the ejection fraction, the left ventricular filling pressures, and the presence or absence of abnormal ventricular wall motion on ventriculography. An ejection fraction of less than 0.5 and the presence of significant ventricular dysynergy are good predictors of preoperative ventricular dysfunction. Normal ventricular function can be inferred if no ventricular wall dysynergy is evident on the ventriculogram.

The electrocardiogram aids in planning for a safe intraoperative course. If an artificial pacemaker is present it is helpful to know if the patient is pacemaker dependent, since isoprenaline may have to be infused in case of pacemaker failure. If the pacemaker is programmable, a programming unit should be available for reprogramming of the pacemaker during surgery from a ventricular inhibited mode to a fixed rate mode in order to avoid problems with electrocautery interference.

The patient's response to a stress test can sometimes predict response to the stress of an anaesthetic induction and intubation. Exercise stress tests are evaluated by observing changes in ST segments in the electrocardiogram, changes in the heart rate and blood pressure, and the presence or absence of angina during the stress test. If the anaesthesiologist has some idea of blood pressure and heart rate limit at which the patient develops myocardial ischaemia then, hopefully, the induction and maintenance will be planned in order to avoid these limits.

The classification system most commonly used by anaesthesiologists is the American Society of Anesthesiologists physical status. This describes patient status on a 1–5 scale with 1 being normal and 5 being moribund. If an 'E' is added, the case is considered to be an emergency operation.

In general, all preoperative medication should be continued except for digitalis and diuretics. These two drugs are usually dose-reduced or discontinued several days before surgery. This allows the patient's serum potassium to become normalized and ensures that the patient will not be close to toxicity at time of surgery. Normal digitalis dosages may be necessary in a patient in atrial fibrillation in order to control heart rate. The continuation of beta-blocking agents, and perhaps calcium slow-channel blocking agents, is critical. The discontinuation of beta-blocking agents can lead to a hyperadrenergic state with angina, hypertension, arrhythmias and, on occasion, myocardial infarction.

Preoperative medications are usually given to decrease patient anxiety and to smooth out the anaesthetic induction. The anxious patient with coronary artery disease requires liberal amounts of preoperative medications whereas the sick patient with borderline cardiac failure should receive little or none. If the patient comes into the operating room in an anxious state, supplemental intravenous doses of sedative can be administered. We will not make specific recommendations for premedication because of the large number of drugs used.

Intraoperative management

This section covers the management of the patient during the perioperative phase. It concentrates on aspects of care that are common to cardiac surgical patients. Aspects of care that are specific to various disease states will be covered later in this chapter.

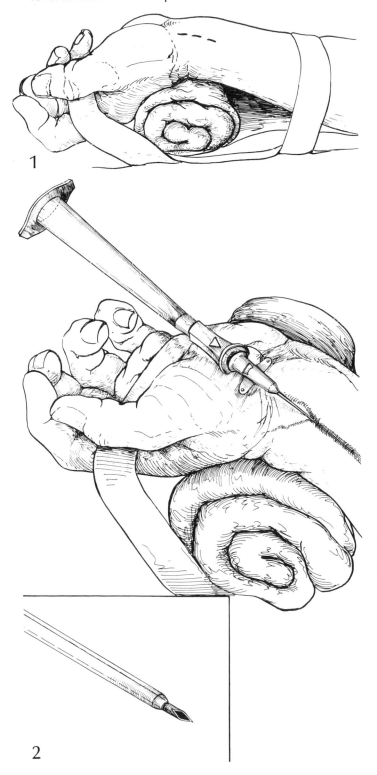

MONITORING AND LINE PLACEMENT

Every patient for cardiac surgery should have a large gauge (14 or 16) intravenous line placed. This line should be inserted just before surgery to ensure its adequate function. Patients in whom haemorrhage may be encountered (such as those having a second cardiac operation) should have two large-bore intravenous lines started. A liberal amount of local anaesthesia should be used for all line placements in order to decrease harmful pain reflexes in the pre-induction period. We feel strongly that, as far as possible, all monitoring lines should be placed in adults before anaesthetic induction is commenced. This markedly increases the safety of the anaesthetic induction and allows the anaesthesiologist to adjust drug dosages by using second-to-second feedback. It is no longer acceptable standard practice to induce sick cardiac surgery patients with a blood pressure cuff, electrocardiogram and one intravenous line.

The paediatric patient has to be approached somewhat differently. The administration of either rectal barbiturates, intramuscular barbiturates, inhalation anaesthesia or ketamine is then followed by line placement. All cannulae in children will obviously be of smaller gauge than those for adults.

1–3

Direct arterial blood pressure cannula

All cardiac surgery patients should be monitored with a direct arterial blood pressure cannula. Sites include radial, ulnar, dorsalis pedis, femoral, brachial and axillary arteries. *Illustrations 1–3* show details of radial artery line placement. This route is our most common approach for direct arterial monitoring. The wrist should be extended over a rolled towel and fixed in position with tape. The radial artery is then punctured with a suitable catheter, using a syringe without a plunger so that entry into the lumen of the vessel will be readily appreciated. The catheter is then connected to suitable tubing containing a stopcock.

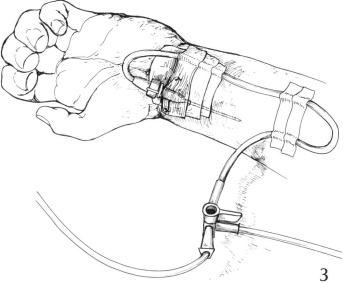

Central venous pressure cannula

All patients should also have a central venous pressure (CVP) cannula inserted, if possible, before the induction of anaesthesia. This cannula is used not only for monitoring purposes but also to draw blood for laboratory studies, to infuse potent drugs and occasionally to serve as an extra volume infusion port. The placement of several luer-locked stopcocks at the end of the CVP line allows easy blood drawing and drug infusion. The use of the modified Seldinger technique for central line placement has markedly increased the safety of this procedure.

4

The illustration shows the surface markings of the internal jugular vein.

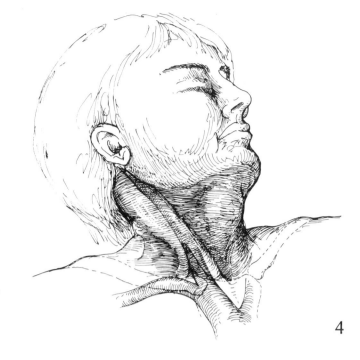

4

5, 6 & 7

The patient is placed in the Trendelberg position and the vein entered with a small gauge needle. When the position of the vein has been confirmed a larger needle is inserted and a guide-wire placed into the vein.

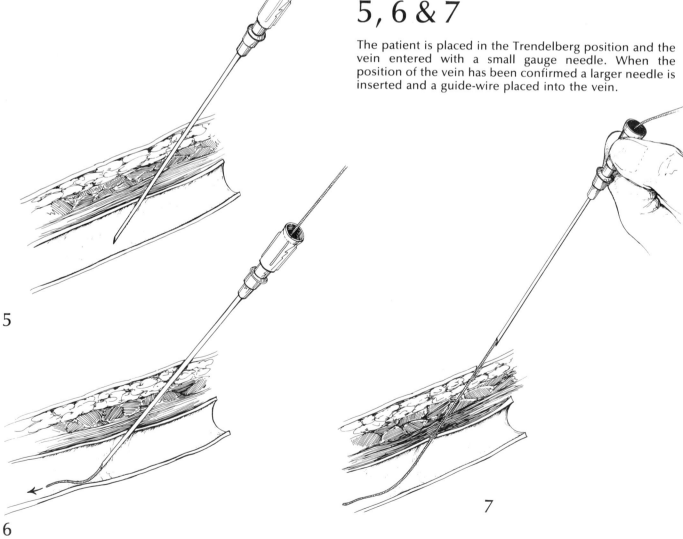

5

6

7

8 & 9

A No. 11 scalpel makes a small nick in the skin to allow passage of a trocar and sheath, which are inserted with a twisting motion.

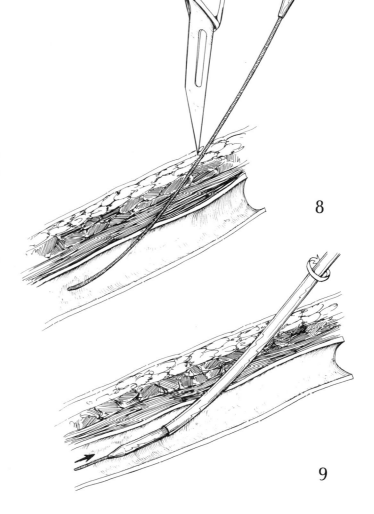

8

9

10

Removal of the wire and trocar leaves the sheath in place.

10

11

This is now connected to an intravenous line containing stopcocks for the infusion of addition fluids or drugs, and the sheath is sutured to the skin.

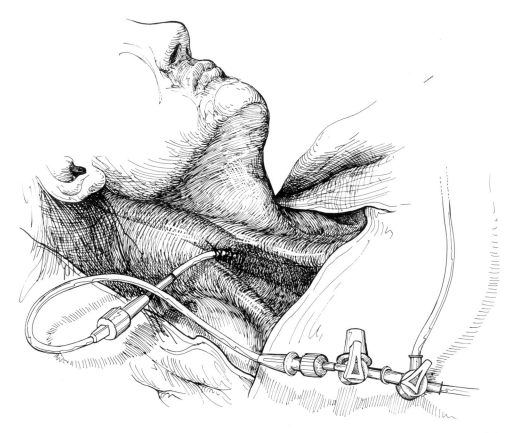

11

Pulmonary artery catheter

Institutional and local criteria generally determine whether a pulmonary artery catheter will be used in selected patients. In general, indications for pulmonary artery monitoring include poor left ventricular function, unstable angina, high grade coronary disease (especially left main disease), aortic aneurysm surgery associated with coronary disease, combined coronary artery and carotid artery disease, and the anticipation of large volume shifts in patients. Our most common route for pulmonary artery monitoring is the internal or external jugular vein. Other commonly used routes are the subclavian or brachial veins. Using the modified Seldinger technique, a large (8 Fr) introducer is placed under sterile conditions as previously described. Introducers are available with or without a side-arm adapter to be used as another infusion site. Care should be taken to avoid placing introducers into the carotid artery. If this occurs inadvertently, a vascular surgeon should be consulted regarding possible repair of the carotid laceration, since deaths have been reported after bleeding into the neck from such injuries.

Side-arm adapter

12

A side-arm adapter containing a one-way valve can now be placed on the outlet of the sheath. This contains a port for the administration of drugs, and allows the passage of a Swan-Ganz catheter through the main lumen. The pulmonary artery catheter should be attached to a transducer system. The electrocardiogram should be continuously monitored for arrhythmias.

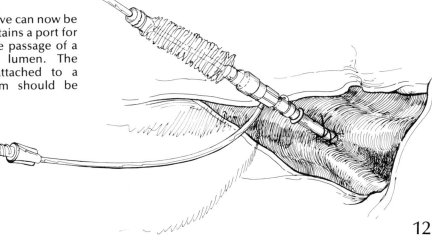

12

13

Once the catheter lumens have been flushed with heparinized saline and the balloon has been test inflated, the catheter should be inserted to 20 cm. At this point the balloon is inflated and the catheter is slowly advanced with continuous waveform observation. We have not found it necessary to use X-ray observation of catheter progress.

Figure 1 shows the typical waveforms seen when passing a flow-directed catheter through the right heart. Ventricular arrhythmias seen while passing through the right ventricle are usually transient. If they persist, the catheter should be withdrawn. Care should be taken to ensure that the catheter is always advanced with the balloon inflated and withdrawn with the balloon deflated.

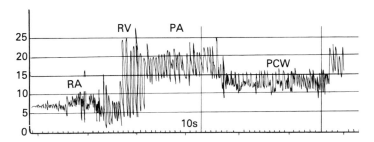

Figure 1 RA = right atrial; RV = right ventricular; PA = pulmonary artery; PCW = pulmonary capillary wedge pressure

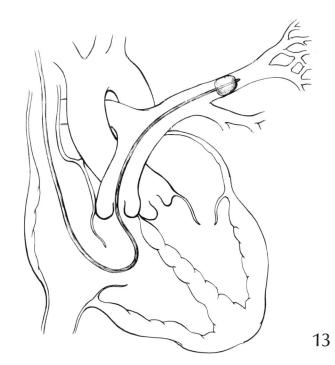

13

The electrocardiogram should be monitored with emphasis on a lead system sensitive to ischaemia. Either a unifocal V5 lead or a bifocal CS5 lead are the best leads to use. Both leads require lead placement at the cardiac apex or V5 position. This lead can be covered with a plastic steridrape and prepared over so it does not interfere with sterility.

The patient's temperature is monitored at two sites in order to follow both 'core' and blood temperatures. Rectal temperature is representative of the core temperature, while nasal or oesophageal represents blood temperature. Urine output should be followed during surgery. This requires urethral catheterization (performed after the patient is anaesthetized).

INTRODUCTION OF ANAESTHESIA

Preoperatively it is mandatory to check that the following equipment is available: a functioning anaesthetic machine, ventilator, full oxygen and N_2O tanks, suction apparatus, appropriate endotracheal tubes, laryngoscope and blades, electrocardiogram, blood pressure cuff and pressure transducers. In addition, drugs which should be drawn up or available include: thiopental, diazepam, succinylcholine, pancuronium and/or metocurine, calcium chloride, lignocaine (lidocaine; xylocaine), ephedrine, phenylephrine and a narcotic. The most commonly prepared drugs in 'drip' form are nitroprusside, dopamine, nitroglycerin and phenylephrine. Table 1 shows suggested dilutions and dosages for the most commonly used infusion drugs in the adult patient.

lines, is to be condemned. Modern cardiac anaesthesia practice requires second-to-second monitoring during all phases of the perioperative period, including induction of anaesthesia.

Administration of anaesthetic agents should be done in a graded, titrated manner. The induction should never be performed so rapidly that a large dose of any drug is administered without seeing the effect of a previous dose. Trends in haemodynamic status must be identified early and responded to in an appropriate fashion. In general, most patients are more stable if they are not hypovolaemic. A combination of volume challenges, inotropic drug administration and afterload reduction leads to haemodynamic improvement and stability. Patients with coronary artery disease present a special set of problems, requiring strict maintenance of perfusion pressure,

Table 1 Suggested dilutions and rate of administration for infusion drugs (adults only)

Drug	Dilution	Concentration	Dosage
Dopamine (Inotropin)	200 mg in 250 ml solution	800 µg/ml	1–10 µg/kg per min – beta effect 10–20 µg/kg per min – increasing alpha effect >20 µg/kg per min – alpha effect predominates
Isoprenaline (isoproterenol; Isoprel)	1 mg in 250 ml solution	4µg/ml	Start at 1–2 µg/min, titrate using heart rate effects (keep heart rate under 120/min)
Adrenaline (epinephrine)	1 mg in 250 ml solution	4 µg/ml	Start at 2–4 µg/min for average adult, titrate using blood pressure and heart rate effects
Nitroprusside (Nipride)	50 mg in 250 ml D5W	200 µg/ml	0.5–8 µg/kg per min, titrate using blood pressure. Usually start at 0.5 µg/kg per min. Toxicity may occur over 5 µ/kg per min
Lignocaine (lidocaine; xylocaine)	1000 mg in 250 ml solution	4 mg/ml	1–4 mg/min to control ventricular irritability
Trimetaphan (trimethaphan; Arfonad)	500 mg in 250 ml solution	2 mg/ml	Start with 50 µg/min in average adult, titrate using blood pressure effect
Metaraminol (Aramine)	100 mg in 250 ml solution	400 µg/ml	Start with 50 µg/min in average adult, titrate using blood pressure and heart rate effects
Noradrenaline (levarterenol; Levophal)	8 mg in 250 ml solution	32 µg/ml	5–50 µg/min. Start with 5 µg/min in average adult, titrate using blood pressure effects
Phenylephrine (neosynephrine)	20 mg in 250 ml solution	80 µg/ml	Start with 20 µg/min, titrate using blood pressure effects
Dobutamine (Dobutrex)	250 mg in 250 ml solution	1000 µg/ml	3–20 µg/kg per min. Start with 250 µg/min in average adult and titrate for effect
Nitroglycerin (Tridil)	50 mg in 250 ml solution	250 µ/ml	Start with 0.5 µg/kg per min, titrate using blood pressure and filling pressure effects

Note: Using the dilutions specified above, usual drip rates for all the drugs in this list are from 10 to 60 microdrops per minute in the average adult patient (60 microdrops = 1 ml). The importance of carefully titrating the drug to produce the desired effect cannot be over-emphasized.

After all monitoring (with the exception of temperature and urinary output) has been established, necessary infusion drugs connected to the CVP line and all anaesthesia equipment checked, the induction can commence. Except for paediatric patients and special situations, all intravascular monitoring lines should be placed before the induction begins since this period can be one of the most unstable. The common practice of the anaesthesiologist inducing and intubating the patient, followed by the surgeon placing all invasive monitoring

avoidance of high preload and avoidance of a hyperdynamic cardiac state. This is discussed in greater detail in the next section.

The choice of muscle relaxant varies. However, we prefer to use a long-acting non-depolarizing relaxant (usually pancuronium or dimethyltubocurarine) instead of succinylcholine. This allows more flexibility as to the time of intubation and ensures that the patient will not move during surgery.

14, 15 & 16

Oral intubation is generally preferred to nasal intubation because of the bacteraemia, bleeding and nasal trauma associated with the latter procedure. Intravenous and/or laryngotracheal lignocaine (lidocaine) given before intubation serves to attenuate the adverse blood pressure and heart rate changes associated with intubation.

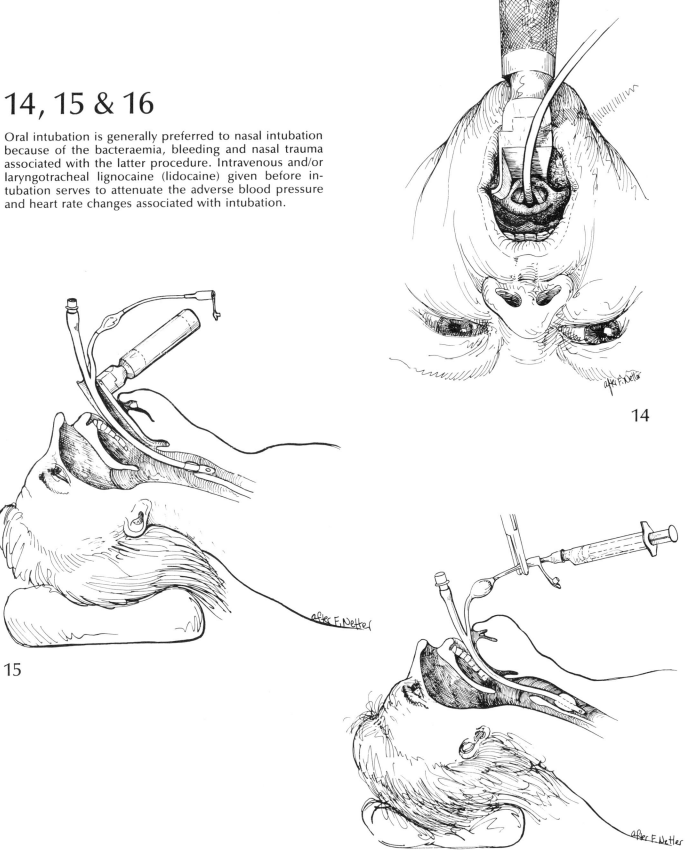

14

15

16

THE PREBYPASS PERIOD

Once the patient is safely induced and intubated, the surgical skin preparation begins. Very little anaesthesia is required during this phase owing to the lack of painful stimulus. However, the anaesthetist should anticipate the surgical incision and the resultant pain-induced haemodynamic changes by deepening the anaesthetic at the appropriate time. The patient's lungs should be disconnected from the ventilator during sternotomy to allow the anterior mediastinal contents to fall away from the sternum.

If the patient has a reasonable haematocrit, blood is not administered until after the bypass period, since a moderate amount of haemodilution (haematocrit of 20–25 per cent) is desirable during cardiopulmonary bypass. The adequacy of heparinization should be checked and confirmed by the use of an activated coagulation time or protamine titration before bypass commences. The surgeon and the anaesthesiologist are equally responsible for ensuring that heparin has been given before bypass. An activated coagulation time (ACT) of over 400 seconds should be maintained during bypass.

Prior to the institution of bypass the anaesthetist's role is to ensure adequate oxygenation (checked with blood gases), maintain adequate intravascular volume, regulate inotropic and vasodilator drugs to maintain haemodynamic stability, and keep an accurate record of the proceedings. The anaesthetist should be very aware of the progress of the surgery. Continuous communication between surgeon and anaesthetist enhances patient care.

Just before bypass commences, the following checklist should be considered to ensure a safe transition on to bypass:

1. All anaesthetic agents off.
2. All intravenous infusion agents off.
3. Heparinization confirmed by use of ACT.
4. Supplemental relaxant and sedative agents given.
5. Urimeter emptied.
6. Transducers checked for proper zero and calibration.
7. Cardioplegic solution prepared.
8. Pupils and skin colour checked for baseline.
9. All patient to equipment connections secured and bubble-free.

CARDIOPULMONARY BYPASS

A detailed discussion of cardiopulmonary of bypass is to be found in the chapter on 'Cardiopulmonary bypass and circulatory support', pp. 51–64. However, we will briefly discuss several points of patient management in this section. After going on bypass the following items should be checked (within the first 5 minutes of bypass time):

1. Ventilator turned off.
2. Proper bypass equipment function verified.

3. Venous drainage from head checked.
4. Head checked for possible arterial overperfusion (in case of an inadvertent carotid cannulation.)
5. Adequacy of heparinization rechecked with ACT.
6. Pupils and skin colour checked.
7. Vasoconstrictor or vasodilator drugs given to adjust blood pressure as necessary.
8. If used, electroencephalogram checked for abnormality.

During bypass frequent checks of blood gases and serum potassium are done to ensure normality. Additional potassium is usually required to avoid hypokalaemia after bypass. Additional intravenous sedative drugs or inhalation anaesthetics (into the bypass pump) may be given to avoid postoperative recall.

Local practice will dictate policy concerning blood pressure control. Hypertension during bypass can be treated by sedation, decreasing pump flow, vasodilator drugs or taking volume from the patient into the oxygenator. Hypotension during bypass is treated with alpha-adrenergic drugs, increasing pump flow and shifting volume from the oxygenator to the patient.

A moderate degree of hypothermia during bypass is commonly used. This reduces metabolic requirements. Rewarming should be started early enough to ensure normothermia at time of cessation of bypass.

Adequacy of heparinization must be ensured during bypass by the use of one of the available tests. Additional heparin should be administered to avoid a low-grade disseminated intravascular coagulation syndrome from developing during bypass. It is better to be over-heparinized rather than under-heparinized during bypass.

Preparations for coming off bypass include the following items:

1. Rewarming complete.
2. Inotropic infusion drugs started if the need is anticipated.
3. Stable cardiac rhythm established or pacemaker capability available (thresholds checked).
4. Ventilation restarted.
5. Transducers checked for proper zero and calibration.
6. Blood checked and hung.
7. Normal acid-base status established.
8. High normal serum potassium ensured.
9. Vasodilator infusion drugs available for afterload reduction.
10. Protamine available.
11. Fresh frozen plasma and platelets available if the need is anticipated.

Just before coming off bypass the patient's volume status is assessed, with pump blood being shifted to the patient to ensure normovolaemia. This can be assessed by direct observation of the heart, CVP, pulmonary artery wedge or diastolic pressures, or left atrial pressure. When the volume is correct and cardiac function is satisfactory, the venous line is clamped and the pump is turned off.

THE POSTBYPASS PERIOD

Concerns of the anaesthetist in the postbypass period include the adequacy of ventilation and oxygenation, achievement of haemodynamic stability, coagulation status and normality of laboratory studies.

Ventilation and oxygenation should be checked soon after cessation of bypass with arterial blood gases. After ruling out mechanical causes, relative hypoxia is usually treated with diuresis at this time since the administration of positive end-expiratory pressure (PEEP) tends to obscure the surgical field.

Reversal of heparin action is accomplished by the administration of protamine. This drug releases histamine and is a myocardial depressant. Protamine should be titrated carefully yet rapidly, both to hasten onset of clotting and to avoid hypotension due to too rapid injection. Simultaneous administration of calcium chloride can help to reverse the adverse effects of protamine. If the bypass time has been long or if bleeding is expected for any other reason, both fresh-frozen plasma and concentrated platelets should be given rapidly and as early as possible to avoid excessive blood loss.

The anaesthetist should be competent to choose and regulate the infusion of inotropic and vasodilator drugs as necessary. Intravenous calcium chloride is often an effective short-term inotropic agent. Volume must be administered rapidly enough to avoid the insidious onset of hypovolaemia. Familiarity with the fundamentals of the Frank-Starling mechanism allows the anaesthetist to determine the slope and intercepts of this curve by clinical titration of volume and observation of filling pressures and cardiac performance. The end point should be a patient who is well perfused peripherally. Representative curves illustrating ventricular function with normal, increased and decreased contractility are shown in *Figure 2*. An increase in preload will raise the mean arterial pressure, and this rise can be enhanced by the use of an inotropic agent. Cardiac output will increase with after-load reduction, e.g. by an infusion of nitroprusside, and increase even more with preload restoration (volume), with or without an inotropic agent. Representation of the increase of cardiac output with reduction of peripheral resistance (afterload) is seen in *Figure 3*.

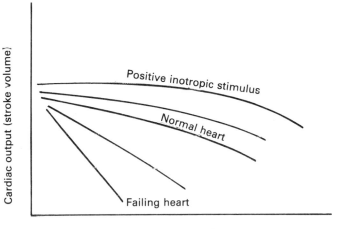

Figure 3 Output-resistance curve

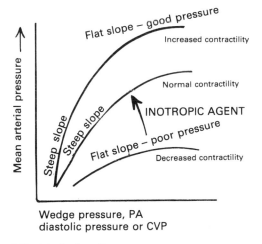

Figure 2 Ventricular function curves

Blood pressure control is important to avoid suture line disruption and bleeding. Pressure can be controlled with table tilt, vasodilator drugs and supplemental anaesthesia. Soon after all protamine and coagulation factors have been given and haemodynamic stability has been obtained, laboratory studies including haematocrit, a coagulation battery and serum potassium should be obtained to detect any abnormalities.

In the occasional instance where it is necessary to go back on bypass, the administration of heparin must not be neglected.

TRANSFER OF THE PATIENT TO THE INTENSIVE CARE UNIT

It is important to achieve haemodynamic stability by effectively regulating pharmacological therapy, epicardial pacing and mechanical assistance, if necessary, within the operating room prior to transferring the patient to the intensive care unit (ICU).

17

The degree to which the patient is monitored during transfer is to a great extent dependent upon how unstable he or she is. As a minimum standard, we directly measure mean arterial pressure while transferring the patient by connecting an anaeroid sphygmomanometer to the arterial cannula (as illustrated). However, in more unstable patients, continuous oscilloscopic display of ECG, arterial pressure and filling pressures is desirable.

In order to minimize changes in drug infusion rates, all potent inotropic and vasodilator drugs should be administered and regulated using a mechanical infusion pump or a calibrated microdrip device. The patient's volume status should be stable and additional volume taken with the patient to the ICU. An adequate tank of oxygen and a reliable means of deliverance to the patient should be checked and made available. If there is any reason to suspect instability, a defibrillator should accompany the patient. Laboratory studies such as arterial blood gases, haematocrit, potassium and coagulation studies should be sent before leaving the operating room so that this information will be available for analysis early in the postoperative period. The intensive care unit personnel should be given sufficient time and information to prepare adequately for the arrival of the patient.

Upon arrival in the ICU the anaesthetist must continue to treat any ongoing problems while the ICU personnel familiarize themselves with the patient. Early priorities upon arrival should include establishing adequate mechanical ventilation, clearing the chest tubes and regulation of drug infusions whilst monitoring the ECG, arterial pressure and filling pressures.

The following information should be given clearly and concisely to the ICU personnel

1. Procedure performed.
2. Complications.
3. Drugs currently infusing.
4. Pacing status and underlying rhythm.
5. Arterial pressure and filling pressures.
6. Urine output.
7. Last haematocrit, potassium and arterial blood gases.
8. Pertinent medical history including allergies.

Diligent attention to these details will make the transition from operating room to intensive care a smoother and safer one.

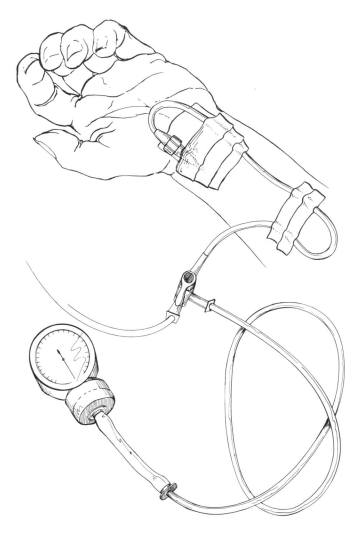

17

Special considerations

CONGENITAL HEART DISEASE

Recent advances in cardiac surgical technique, diagnosis and perioperative management of the critically ill neonate and child with congenital heart disease has led to a reduction in overall morbidity and mortality and a trend towards total correction at an earlier age. Since the majority of patients with congenital heart disease are being surgically corrected in infancy or childhood, this discussion of the anaesthetic management of congenital heart disease will deal exclusively with the paediatric patient.

A useful physiological classification in congenital heart disease is according to whether the predominant condition is cyanosis or congestive failure, though overlap certainly exists in complex cases. Surgically, either the patient will have to be treated as an emergency in the neonatal period or it may be possible to delay palliation or correction until the child is older.

Anaesthetic management of the neonate

The differential diagnosis of central cyanosis in the neonate includes pulmonary disease (airway obstruction, meconium aspiration, pneumothorax), central nervous system depression, methaemoglobinaemia and congenital heart disease. Cyanosis secondary to congenital heart disease is caused by right to left shunting with decreased pulmonary blood flow, or intracardiac admixture of systemic and pulmonary blood flow. The major cardiac causes of cyanosis are transposition of the great arteries, pulmonary stenosis or atresia, tricuspid atresia, tetralogy of Fallot, Ebstein's anomaly and anomalous pulmonary veins.

Congestive heart failure in the newborn is most commonly a result of underlying congenital heart disease although less common causes such as arrhythmias, pulmonary infection, myocarditis, arteriovenous fistulae and fluid overload should be excluded. Persistent ductus arteriosus is the most common cause of congestive heart failure in the newborn. Other less common cardiac causes are coarctation of the aorta, critical aortic stenosis, hypoplastic left heart syndrome and truncus arteriosus.

Assuming the infant has been adequately resuscitated at birth, neonates with either congestive heart failure or cyanosis should be transferred to the ICU for evaluation and care. If necessary, supplemental oxygen and artificial ventilation should be used to attempt to keep the PO_2 greater than 50 Torr (6650 Pa). Continuous arterial blood gas monitoring, generally through the umbilical artery, is preferable although some believe capillary blood gases or transcutaneous oxygen are satisfactory. Other areas of concern in the ill neonate are acid-base status, fluid and electrolyte balance, the level of haemoglobin, temperature regulation, hypoglycaemia and hypocalcaemia.

The cardiac evaluation, in addition to the physical examination, chest X-ray and electrocardiogram, may require an echocardiogram or cardiac catheterization for a complete diagnosis. This is frequently the point at which the anaesthesiologist becomes involved in the care of the patient. The anaesthetist should become familiar with the patient in order to provide a smooth transition from the ICU to the cardiac catheterization laboratory or the operating room.

No premedication should be given to the ill neonate, with the possible exception of atropine. A clear liquid feeding should be given approximately 3 hours prior to a surgical procedure. Generally, local anaesthesia and restraints are all that are necessary to perform a cardiac catheterization in the neonate. One must be especially aware of the catastrophic potential of hypovolaemia, arrhythmia, catheter occlusion of a critical pulmonary stenosis, or ductal closure in hypoplastic left heart syndrome secondary to a high inspired oxygen concentration. Haemodilution is usually accomplished by the cardiologist if there is severe polycythaemia.

Transfer of the neonate should always be in a device which provides a neutral thermal environment and continuous monitoring of the electrocardiogram and arterial pressure. The operating room should be warm (at least 24°C; 75°F) and a heating blanket and heating lamps used in order to prevent hypothermia with its resultant vasoconstriction and acidosis. The induction and maintenance of anaesthesia depends upon the underlying anatomy, pathophysiology and type of correction being planned. Generally, neonates require little more than nitrous oxide, muscle relaxants and perhaps small doses of narcotics. Special attention should be paid to regulation of inspired oxygen concentrations so that PaO_2 will not be high and perhaps exacerbate the tendency towards retrolental fibroplasia or ductal closure. Meticulous care should be taken to eliminate all air bubbles from intravenous lines to minimize the chance of systemic embolism.

If the patient has cyanotic congenital heart disease requiring either a palliative shunt procedure or attempted total correction, we feel that ketamine provides the smoothest induction. Maintenance anaesthesia will depend upon the type of surgical procedure and the response of the patient. Patients with left heart obstruction (e.g. aortic stenosis or coarctation) do not tolerate arrhythmias or myocardial depression. Therefore, anaesthesia is usually induced and maintained with a narcotic such as fentanyl rather than with halothane or ketamine. Neonates with persistent ductus arteriosus are usually given narcotics with supplemental inhalation anaesthesia.

Each procedure has its own potential hazards which the anaesthetist must be aware of. During systemic pulmonary artery anastomosis, when one pulmonary artery is partially or completely occluded, hypoxia and acidosis may occur, requiring atropine, calcium bicarbonate or inotropes. Pulmonary artery banding should result in a slight increase in systemic blood pressure; however, if the band is too tight, frequently there will be a bradycardia secondary to reduced pulmonary blood flow and hypoxia. The ligation of a ductus arteriosus will cause a haemodynamic deterioration rather than improvement if there is an underlying ductal dependency.

If total correction is attempted using cardiopulmonary bypass, the surgeon may elect to use deep hypothermia with circulatory arrest rather than moderate systemic hypothermia. Core cooling is generally easily accomplished using high flows and vasodilators. Haemodilution to the range of an haematocrit of 20–25 is desirable. We rarely use vasopressors to raise systemic pressure but find the perfusion pressure at flows of 75 ml/kg per min generally adequate. The usual parameters of systemic perfusion such as urine output, oxygenation and acid-base status are followed accordingly. We prefer to use uncorrected blood gas values for P_{CO_2} and pH, aiming for a mild alkalosis as an ideal condition.

Termination of cardiopulmonary bypass in infants involves the same considerations as with any patient. Indwelling catheters may have to be placed by the surgeon to measure filling pressures, either because the patient was too small to place them preoperatively or because of reorganization of intracardiac anatomy. The infant's cardiac output is rate dependent; therefore an inotrope with chronotropic tendencies such as isoprenaline (isoproterenol) or dopamine is desirable. In all except the most minor cases the patient should be left intubated. Transfer to the ICU should be accomplished in a warm incubator with complete monitoring capabilities. The anaesthetist should continue caring for the infant until the ICU personnel feel comfortable in assuming responsibility.

Anaesthetic management of the child

The preoperative evaluation of the older child admitted for elective cardiac surgery is different from the neonate, in that the trust and understanding developed between the anaesthetist, child and parents goes a long way towards converting an unfamiliar hostile environment into a more friendly one. A brief and positive explanation should be given to the child in terms appropriate for his or her age. In addition, a more detailed discussion should be conducted with the parents in the absence of the child.

Children older than 1 year of age should be heavily premedicated so that they will arrive asleep or sedated and cooperative. Patients with cyanosis should be continually observed for adequate respiratory effort following the administration of premedication. Routine feeding should be withheld 8 hours prior to induction, with clear liquids offered 3–4 hours prior to induction.

The ECG, blood pressure cuff and precordial stethoscope are always used during the induction of anaesthesia. We have found the following induction techniques useful. If the child arrives asleep or very sedated and does not have cyanotic heart disease a 'steal' induction using a lightly placed mask with halothane and nitrous oxide delivered by high flows is quite effective. Following loss of consciousness, intravenous cannulae can be placed, muscle relaxants administered and oral intubation accomplished. A 20 or 22 gauge catheter is then placed percutanously into a radial artery. Usually, a central venous catheter is placed into the right internal jugular vein using a Seldinger technique.

Cyanotic children are usually induced with ketamine and maintained with narcotics. Inhalation agents are to be avoided because of the potential of accentuating a right-to-left shunt. Many institutions prefer to use an intravenous induction technique. This is satisfactory if it is technically and psychologically possible to start an intravenous line on the awake child.

As in the infant, special attention should be directed towards maintaining thermal homeostasis. The operating room should remain a warm ambient temperature, heating blankets should be on the table for smaller children, and a heated humidifier should be available.

Because of the smaller blood volume and possible immaturity of renal excretory mechanisms, management of fluid and electrolyte balance tends to be more difficult than in the adult. All fluids should be administered using a calibrated administration device. The composition of the intravenous infusion rate depends upon the volume status of the patient. Blood is added, if necessary, to maintain the haematocrit in the range of 25 on cardiopulmonary bypass. The management of the child on bypass is similar to that of the infant as previously described. One must be aware that a pre-existing systemic-to-pulmonary anastomosis must be closed for adequate perfusion on bypass.

Prior to transfer to the ICU, the oral endotracheal tube is usually changed to a nasal tube because it is easier to care for and more comfortable for the paediatric patient. The infant or child will remain intubated until cardio-respiratory stability is established. Additional narcotics and sedative drugs may be necessary postoperatively to provide for a smoother course. Recommended doses of commonly used drugs for perioperative management are given in Table 2.

It should be kept in mind that these patients generally require very intensive management postoperatively and all persons involved should be skilful and comfortable with paediatric patients.

Table 2 Commonly used drugs for paediatric cardiac patients

Drug	Route	Dose/frequency
Atropine	i.v./i.m.	0.01–0.02 mg/kg per dose (max. 0.4 mg)
Calcium chloride	i.v.	10–20 mg/kg per dose
Calcium gluconate	i.v.	30–60 mg/kg per dose
Diazepam	i.v.	0.05–0.1 mg/kg per dose
	p.o.	0.1–0.3 mg/kg per dose
Dobutamine	i.v.	0–20 µg/kg per min constant infusion
Dopamine	i.v.	0–20 µg/kg per min constant infusion
Droperidol	i.v./i.m.	0.05–0.1 mg/kg
Adrenaline (epinephrine)	i.v.	5–10 µg/kg bolus 0.1–1.0 µg/kg per min constant infusion
Furosemide	i.v.	0.5–1.0 mg/kg per dose
	p.o.	1–4 mg/kg per day (1–2 doses)
Glucose	i.v.	0.5–2 ml of 50% solution (0.25–1.0 g)
Isoprenaline (isoproterenol)	i.v.	0.1–3.0 µg/kg per min constant infusion
Lignocaine (lidocaine)	i.v.	0.5–1.0 mg/kg per dose bolus 20–50 µg/kg per min constant infusion
Morphine	i.v.	0.05–0.1 µg/kg every 2–4 h
Nitroprusside	i.v.	0.5–10 µg/kg per min constant infusion
Pancuronium (Pavulon)	i.v.	0.05–0.1 mg/kg every 1–2 h
Sodium bicarbonate	i.v.	1–2 µg/kg per dose

i.v. = intravenous; i.m. = intramuscular; p.o. = per oral

CORONARY ARTERY DISEASE

The increasing popularity of aortocoronary bypass grafting challenges the anaesthetist to continue evolving an ever safer plan of anaesthetic management so that morbidity and mortality can be reduced to a minimum. Certainly the reduced mortality in recent years for this procedure is at least partly due to better anaesthetic care. The increasing awareness amongst anaesthetists of the importance of the degree of structural and functional impairment and the understanding of the pathophysiology of coronary artery disease provide a more rational approach for the administration of anaesthesia.

Maintenance of the proper balance of myocardial oxygen supply to oxygen demand is crucial to proper management of the patient with coronary artery disease. A thorough knowledge of the factors which determine myocardial oxygen consumption and myocardial oxygen supply is necessary to prevent and treat myocardial ischaemia (*Figure 4*).

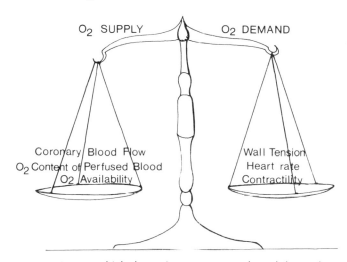

Figure 4 Factors which determine oxygen supply and demand

The major determinants of myocardial oxygen *supply* are coronary blood flow, oxygen content of the perfusing blood, and oxygen availability.

Coronary blood flow is coupled with myocardial oxygen demand and is proportional to the driving pressure across the coronary vascular bed divided by total coronary vascular resistance. The coronary perfusion pressure is often equated with aortic diastolic pressure minus left ventricular end-diastolic pressure (LVEDP). This is only a rough approximation since aortic diastolic pressure may not affect coronary artery pressure distal to an obstructive lesion and the pressure at which zero flow occurs through the coronary bed may be higher than LVEDP. However, the general concept is clinically useful. Coronary vascular resistance may play an even more important role in limiting coronary blood flow during periods of ischaemia. It appears that in classic exertion-induced angina, the coronary arteries, particularly in the subendocardium, have exhausted their coronary vascular reserve by vasodilating maximally, at which point coronary blood flow becomes 'pressure dependent'. However, recent evidence points to episodic increases in coronary vascular resistance or coronary artery spasm as playing an

important role in ischaemic syndromes. Therefore, modalities to decrease coronary vascular resistance such as calcium channel blockers are being investigated clinically.

The oxygen content of blood is the product of oxyhaemoglobin saturation and haemoglobin concentration plus a small contribution from dissolved oxygen. The oxygen availability is determined by the position of the oxyhaemoglobin dissociation curve which is shifted by temperature, pH and 2–3 DPG.

The major determinants of myocardial oxygen consumption (*demand*) are wall tension, heart rate and contractility. Wall tension, which is proportional to intraventricular pressure and internal radius and inversely proportional to wall thickness, can be lessened by manoeuvres which make the ventricle smaller (vasodilators, inotropic agents, positive airway pressure) or reduce intraventricular pressure (vasodilators, inhalation anaesthetics). The effect of an elevation of heart rate is disadvantageous for two reasons: the duration of diastole (during which the majority of coronary blood flow occurs) is decreased, and oxygen consumption is increased by the increased frequency of systole.

Increasing contractility by tachycardia, sympathetic outflow or inotropic agents increases myocardial oxygen consumption unless wall tension is decreased by reducing ventricular size, in which case oxygen consumption may fall. Conversely, agents which decrease contractility, such as volatile anaesthetics and beta-blockers, will decrease oxygen consumption unless ventricular size increases.

In addition to the usual concerns of the anaesthetist, what specific requirements should be met in the patient with coronary artery disease? Obviously, an imbalance between myocardial oxygen demand and supply caused by acute perioperative haemodynamic changes should be prevented if possible and, if they occur, diagnosed early and treated promptly. At the same time, myocardial contractility and oxygen delivery are sustained to meet the body's metabolic requirements.

Introduction of anaesthesia in a patient with coronary disease

The goals of monitoring in a patient with coronary disease are to avoid the precipitants of myocardial ischaemia, to detect early an unexpected ischaemic response and to obtain guidance for therapeutic manoeuvres.

There is no 'anaesthetic of choice' for patients with coronary artery disease. In the presence of poor ventricular contractility, a narcotic-based anaesthetic affords minimal myocardial depression and the margin of safety is probably larger than if an inhalation agent is used as the sole agent for induction and maintenance. In contrast, patients with relatively normal ventricular function probably benefit from a modest depression of contractility from volatile agents, with resultant lower oxygen demand if coronary perfusion pressure is not allowed to fall and ventricular dilatation does not occur. It has been our experience that even if large doses of narcotics are given to patients with coronary disease and normal ventricular function, frequently an inhalation agent will have to be added to the anaesthetic regimen because of hypertension or tachycardia secondary to inadequate suppression of the sympathetic nervous system.

If an inhalation agent is chosen as the major anaesthetic we generally start the induction with either small doses of thiopental or diazepam (0.2–0.4 mg/kg), then gradually increase the inspired concentration of inhalation agent while observing the effect on heart rate, blood pressure and pulmonary artery pressure. For intubation, a paralyzing dose of a non-depolarizing muscle relaxant, either pancuronium or metocurine, is slowly administered. In high doses pancuronium may cause hypertension or tachycardia and metocurine may cause hypotension from histamine release; usually these effects are negligible. A series of graded stimuli are given to the patient, for example, an oral airway, Foley catheter, then laryngoscopy and tracheal application of 4 per cent lignocaine (xylocaine) spray. If the level of anaesthesia appears adequate intubation is performed. Occasionally the blood pressure falls to a critical level such that coronary blood flow falls, causing myocardial ischaemia which may result in global ventricular dysfunction and aggravate the already existing hypotension and ischaemia.

The treatment of hypotension and ischaemia is predicated on the cause. Immediate causes to be excluded are hypovolaemia, rhythm change and myocardial depression. Unless the pulmonary capillary wedge pressure (PCW) or CVP is elevated, a volume challenge and Trendelenberg positioning are the appropriate initial manoeuvres. If the PCW is rising a modest dose of phenylephrine and nitroglycerin will usually raise the blood pressure and lower the PCW with little change in heart rate. This combination has proven efficacious in treating myocardial ischaemia. One can make an argument for the use of an inotropic drug such as Dopamine in the presence of global ventricular dysfunction rather than phenylephrine. To the extent that an inotrope may reduce ventricular size and myocardial oxygen demand, offsetting its effect on contractility, this argument may be valid; however tachycardia may limit its usefulness. Higher concentrations of inhalation anaesthetics may result in excessive depression of contractility, which can usually be reversed by decreasing the inspired concentration of anaesthetic but occasionally necessitates the use of short-term inotropic therapy.

The alternative method of induction of anaesthesia in patients with coronary disease involves the use of high doses of narcotics. Historically, morphine in doses of 1 mg/kg in combination with oxygen was the first high-dose narcotic technique. It had the advantages of minimal myocardial depression but the disadvantages of incomplete amnesia and unpredictable hypotension secondary to histamine release and vasodilatation. We still use high-dose morphine or hydromorphone (Dilaudid) but generally with the following modifications of the technique: the rate of administration is slow, volume loading is necessary to offset the decreasing preload secondary to venodilation, and diazepam is added during induction to facilitate amnesia. H_1 and H_2 receptor blockade by the prior administration of cimetidine (4 mg/kg) and diphenhydramine (1 mg/kg) may blunt the hypotensive response to histamine release.

Fentanyl (Sublimaze) has gained enormous popularity as an anaesthetic for open heart procedures. In high doses (50–100 µg/kg) in combination with oxygen it has shown little in the way of haemodynamic changes, no histamine release, and blunting of the release of stress hormones. Potential limitations include incomplete amnesia unless supplemental agents are added (such as diazepam), chest wall rigidity during induction unless muscle relaxants are started early, sinus bradycardia due to a parasympathomimetic effect, and 'breakthrough' hypertension and tachycardia requiring additional pharmacological therapy to prevent myocardial ischaemia. Overall, fentanyl has proved to be a relatively satisfactory anaesthetic for the induction and maintenance of anaesthesia in patients with coronary disease, particularly those with poor ventricular function. It is probable that as further clinical research is conducted with fentanyl analogues such as alfentanil and sufentanil an even more satisfactory narcotic will be available in the future.

In summary, the safe administration of anaesthesia to a patient with coronary disease requires a sophisticated knowledge of cardiovascular pharmacology, physiology and monitoring which, if used intelligently, cannot help but benefit the critically ill patient.

VALVULAR HEART DISEASE

The incidence of severe ventricular dysfunction as a result of long-standing valvular heart disease is decreasing as a result of prophylaxis for rheumatic fever and earlier surgical correction of valvular lesions. However, the challenge of anaesthetizing these patients remains formidable.

The goal in anaesthetizing a patient with valvular disease is to preserve or improve circulatory haemodynamics. In order to achieve this, one must have a thorough knowledge of the pathophysiology of each valvular lesion, the determinants of ventricular performance, and how each variable under the influence of the anaesthetist or surgeon affects circulatory homeostasis. Pressure-volume loops and their disturbance in disease are central to the understanding of the pathophysiology and management of patients with valvular disease (*Figure 5*). In the normal person, an increase in left ventricular volume occurs during ventricular filling with little change in pressure. During ventricular systole the pressure rises without change in volume (isovolumic contraction), until diastolic pressure is exceeded and the aortic valve opens. Volume then decreases whilst pressure rises (ejection phase). The end of systole is followed by a period of isovolumic relaxation until diastolic filling occurs once more. The loops in disease are shown. The area enclosed within the loop is the pressure-volume index, or a measurement of the work that the heart has to perform. As can be seen, this is greatest in combined aortic regurgitation and stenosis.

As a general rule, patients with valvular heart disease tend to have greater ventricular dysfunction than patients with coronary artery disease. This dictates a slightly different preoperative and intraoperative plan of management. Patients with congestive heart failure have traditionally been managed with digitalis and diuretics which have the potential for relative hypovolaemia, arrhythmias of digitalis intoxication, and hypokalaemia. As they become refractory to this form of therapy, other agents which reduce afterload or increase contractility may need to be added. In the very unstable patient use of invasive haemodynamic monitoring such as the pulmonary artery catheter is helpful in dictating response to therapeutic interventions prior to taking the patient to the operating room.

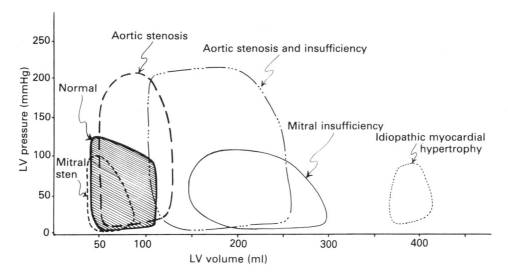

Figure 5 Pressure-volume loops

Narcotic techniques are usually the basis for the induction of anaesthesia since many patients will not tolerate further myocardial depression from inhalation anaesthetics. The sequence of induction is described earlier in the discussion of anaesthetic management of patients with coronary artery disease. We will now discuss the pathophysiology and anaesthetic management of specific valvular lesions.

Mitral stenosis

Pathophysiology

Progressive reduction in mitral orifice area results in reduction in left ventricular filling and alteration in left atrial and pulmonary artery haemodynamics. Left atrial pressure varies directly in proportion to flow and inversely to diastolic filling time and mitral valve area. A change from sinus rhythm to atrial fibrillation as the left atrium enlarges generally results in the initial episode of congestive heart failure. Once the ventricular response is controlled, the symptoms of congestive failure improve markedly. In a certain subset of patients, pulmonary hypertension develops as a result of pulmonary hypertension, reactive arteriolar constriction and obliterative vascular changes. This may eventually result in right heart failure, functional tricuspid regurgitation and a low cardiac output syndrome.

Anaesthetic considerations

The patient's ventricular rate should be controlled preoperatively with digitalis if the underlying rhythm is atrial fibrillation. Some centres routinely discontinue digitalis at least 48 hours preoperatively in order to minimize the risk of digitalis intoxication, though this may make the ventricular rate difficult to control intraoperatively.

Light premedication is given because of the increased sensitivity of these patients to premedicating drugs. Occasionally an extremely anxious patient will arrive tachycardic and in pulmonary oedema prior to induction, and will require intravenous sedatives, narcotics and supplemental oxygen for stabilization.

A pulmonary artery catheter is frequently inserted prior to induction in order to guide therapy, both intra-operatively and postoperatively. However, it has been increasingly realized that this subset of patients may be more susceptible to pulmonary artery haemorrhage. Care must be taken not to allow distal migration of the catheter, or persistent or over-inflation of the balloon.

Techniques which keep the heart rate slow, avoid decreasing preload, and minimize myocardial depression and elevation of pulmonary vascular resistance are desirable. This implies the use of narcotics, the avoidance of alpha agonists, N_2O, hypoxia and calcium chloride. Inotropic agents with beta activity such as isoprenaline (isoproterenol), dobutamine or dopamine may be useful in the presence of right heart failure associated with elevated pulmonary vascular resistance. Similarly, vaso-dilators such as phentolamine and nitroprusside may reduce pulmonary vascular resistance.

Mitral regurgitation

Pathophysiology

The pathophysiology of mitral regurgitation involves the preferential ejection of blood into the low-impedance left atrium rather than the aorta. The natural history depends on whether the process is acute (e.g. as a result of myocardial ischaemia or ruptured chordae tendinae), in which case there is fulminant pulmonary oedema and a rapid downhill course, or chronic, characterized by progressive dyspnoea and fatigue until congestive failure ensues. Compensatory changes, to increase forward stroke volume, occur by increasing rate and contractility through increased sympathetic nervous activity, use of the Starling mechanism by increasing end-diastolic volume, and eventually eccentric ventricular hypertrophy. Left atrial compliance is low in acute mitral regurgitation, resulting in elevated pulmonary artery pressures and large 'V' waves. The lower pulmonary artery pressures and V waves seen in chronic mitral regurgitation merely reflect a larger, more compliant left atrium and not necessarily a lower regurgitant fraction. It may be difficult to assess whether depressed ventricular contractility exists preoperatively since the ejection fraction will remain elevated even in the presence of decreased contractility because of the low afterload. Ventricular function after mitral valve replacement, as estimated by ejection fraction, declines at least transiently in most patients and may remain grossly abnormal in a small percentage.

Anaesthetic considerations

In order to maximize forward stroke volume and minimize regurgitant volume, systemic vascular resistance must be kept low, myocardial contractility maintained or augmented, and ventricular dilatation avoided. A pulmonary artery catheter is extremely useful in providing information such as thermodilution cardiac output, pulmonary artery pressures, height of the V waves, and systemic and pulmonary vascular resistance.

Induction is usually initiated with narcotics; occasionally an inhalation agent is added because of rising systemic vascular resistance and falling cardiac output as a result of inadequate blockade of the sympathetic nervous system. More commonly, nitroprusside is used to reduce systemic vascular resistance and improve forward flow. With severe ventricular dysfunction, inotropic drugs and vasodilators, or intra-aortic balloon pumping, is sometimes necessary to sustain an adequate cardiac output.

Aortic stenosis

Pathophysiology

As obstruction to left ventricular ejection increases, the work the left ventricle must do to maintain cardiac output increases. Ventricular hypertrophy occurs; this minimizes wall stress but results in several detrimental changes. Because of the increased size of the ventricle myocardial oxygen requirements increase, yet oxygen delivery decreases, making myocardial isachaemia more likely. Because of a decrease in ventricular compliance, stroke volume becomes more dependent upon the atrial contribution and a loss of sinus rhythm may result in hypotension.

Unlike patients with mitral regurgitation in whom the ejection fraction may remain normal in the face of poor contractility, patients with aortic stenosis may have a low ejection fraction, yet have normal contractility solely on the basis of the 'afterload mismatch' caused by the stenotic valve. Hence, patients with aortic stenosis generally improve their contractility postoperatively.

Anaesthetic considerations

Premedication is light in order to minimize the chance of hypotension prior to the induction of anaesthesia. Unless there is very poor ventricular function or coexisting coronary artery disease, a pulmonary artery catheter is not necessary. Care should be taken to maintain an adequate preload, sinus rhythm, normal heart rate, contractility and systemic vascular resistance in order to avoid hypotension which may be irreversible. Narcotics are generally the anaesthetic of choice because of the lack of myocardial depression. Supplemental inhalation anaesthesia is added if sympathetic responses are not blunted.

If the patient becomes hypotensive a diagnosis must be made quickly and therapy started without delay in order to avoid further hypotension and cardiac arrest. Hypovolaemia, changes in heart rate and rhythm, and changes in systemic vascular resistance or contractility should be excluded. Usually volume infusion and temporary administration of drugs with alpha-agonist or inotropic potential will be sufficient to restore the blood pressure to a normal level, unless a change in rate or rhythm has occurred. Nodal rhythms or atrial fibrillation may respond to drug therapy but if there is serious haemodynamic compromise direct current cardioversion is necessary. Likewise, sinus bradycardia and tachycardia may be poorly tolerated and should be treated with atropine or atrial pacing and propranolol respectively.

Aortic regurgitation

Pathophysiology

Patients with aortic regurgitation, as with mitral regurgitation, should be separated into categories of acute onset (which usually leads to fulminant congestive heart failure) and chronic onset (which follows a slow insidious course of ventricular enlargement until congestive heart failure ensues). As in chronic mitral regurgitation, the compensatory mechanisms to maintain forward output are sympathetic nervous system discharge, ventricular dilation and ventricular hypertrophy.

The determinants of regurgitant volume are the duration of diastole, the aortic valve area, and the aortic to left ventricle pressure gradient. The low diastolic blood pressure does not necessarily correlate with the severity of aortic regurgitation but probably does impair coronary blood flow. Likewise, a low left ventricular end-diastolic pressure or pulmonary capillary wedge pressure does not necessarily imply a normal left ventricular end-diastolic volume since, typically, left ventricular compliance is generally increased.

Anaesthetic considerations

Patients with chronic aortic regurgitation without significant ventricular dysfunction do very well with narcotic anaesthesia. The heart rate is kept normal or slightly higher than normal in order to maximize coronary perfusion pressure by elevating aortic diastolic pressure and lowering left ventricular end-diastolic pressure. The use of vasodilators or inotropes is rarely necessary.

In contrast, patients with severe acute aortic regurgitation may require inotropic and vasodilator support which can only be safely managed using a pulmonary artery catheter.

CARDIAC TAMPONADE

Cardiac tamponade is a life-threatening situation which requires some form of surgical intervention for improvement. The management of tamponade is dependent upon its aetiology and rate of development of the pericardial effusion. The most commonly encountered situations are postoperative bleeding in open heart patients, trauma, dissecting aortic aneurysm, uraemia and malignancy.

The pathophysiology of tamponade involves elevation of pericardial pressure which results in diminished venous return, equalization of end diastolic pressure in all four chambers, and eventually diminished cardiac output as stroke volume becomes fixed. Pulsus paradoxus, an enlarging cardiac silhouette, low cardiac output and the echocardiogram are aids in diagnosis. Clinical experience dictates aggressive therapy if a high degree of suspicion of tamponade exists in the postoperative open heart patient.

Anaesthetic considerations depend upon the urgency of the situation. If tamponade is severe, either pericardiocentesis, subxiphoid exploration or reopening of the chest in a postoperative patient is necessary. If there is time to take the patient to the operating room, we generally insert an arterial line, central venous catheter and a large-bore peripheral intravenous line. The patient is placed in a semi-Fowler position and supplemental oxygen is given by mask.

At the same time we attempt to maintain an adequate cardiac output by volume loading, maintaining a fast heart rate, and administering an inotropic agent. If the surgery cannot be done under local anaesthesia we will induce anaesthesia with ketamine and intubate with either pancuronium or gallamine. These agents generally will not depress systemic vascular resistance or myocardial contractility and will tend to maintain an elevated heart rate. Once the patient is intubated and placed on positive ventilation, the blood pressure and cardiac output may fall even further owing to reduced venous return. The surgeon should therefore be in the operating room with the patient prepared and draped prior to the induction of anaesthesia.

IDIOPATHIC HYPERTROPHIC SUBAORTIC STENOSIS

Idiopathic hypertrophic subaortic stenosis (IHSS) may be a disease process with multiple expressivity or a spectrum of pathological processes, making the clinical course unpredictable. Generally, there is a variable and labile dynamic obstruction of left ventricular outflow resulting from apposition of the anterior leaflet of the mitral valve to the hypertrophied interventricular septum. Three conditions may worsen the degree of obstruction: increased myocardial contractility, decreased aortic pressure and decreased left ventricular volume. In addition to decreased systolic performance there is usually decreased diastolic compliance and, occasionally, mitral regurgitation.

Premedication of the patient should be adequate to suppress anxiety and sympathetic output. Beta blockers and calcium channel blockers should be continued. A pulmonary artery catheter is helpful to assess left ventricular volume. Anaesthetic techniques which maintain aortic pressure and left ventricular volume and which decrease myocardial contractility are preferable. It is common to base the anaesthetic technique on an inhalation anaesthetic such as halothane. Hypotension should be treated with volume and an alpha agonist (such as phenlyephrine) rather than an inotrope which will worsen the outflow tract obstruction.

CARDIAC TRANSPLANTATION

The recent advances in immunosuppressive therapy and earlier diagnosis of acute rejection have substantially increased the survival of cardiac transplant patients. This makes it likely that the number of patients with end-stage cardiac disease who will be successfully transplanted in the future will increase.

Contraindications to cardiac transplantation include age of more than 55 years, active infection, significant multi-organ failure at time of transplantation, insulin-dependent diabetes mellitus, pulmonary vascular resistance greater than 8 Wood units and a positive lymphocyte crossmatch.

Since the patient is immunosuppressed and has end-stage cardiac disease with severe ventricular dysfunction, the two main anaesthetic concerns are the strict adherence to sterile technique and the maintenance of adequate systemic output.

Skin preparation and draping are done in a sterile manner before inserting indwelling cannulae. The central venous catheter is usually placed in the left internal jugular vein, reserving the right internal jugular vein for subsequent endomyocardial biopsies. Even though it would be useful, a pulmonary artery catheter is not inserted because of an increased risk of infection and the need to remove it with the excision of the recipient heart. All of the equipment for airway management is kept in a sterilized pack until the induction of anaesthesia. A urinary catheter and nasal intubation are avoided because of the potential bacteraemia. Instead, a suprapubic catheter is placed following bypass.

The induction of anaesthesia in these patients requires techniques which will not depress ventricular function. Frequently, in addition to narcotic anaesthesia, concomitant inotropic and vasodilator drugs will be given to maximize cardiac output.

Isoproterenol is used to increase the cardiac output in the denervated donor heart after separation from cardiopulmonary bypass. The dosage is titrated to keep the heart rate around 90–110. Nitroprusside is used if the patient becomes hypertensive.

As the life expectancy of cardiac transplant patients increases, more are presenting after transplantation for surgery unrelated to their heart. Sterility remains the primary concern because of the immunosuppressed state. Several physiological characteristics should be kept in mind when formulating an anaesthetic plan.

Filling pressures are normal at rest in the denervated heart but the cardiac index is lower. With exercise, the cardiac index increases by changes in stroke volume with the heart rate increasing only slightly by circulating catecholamines. There is no change in heart rate from changes in vagal tone since there is no reinnervation in the donor heart. If the patient is in a period of acute rejection inotropic support may be necessary.

Except for consideration of the above-mentioned characteristics, the anaesthetic management of the transplanted patient should not differ markedly from that of the normal patient.

Further reading

Branthwaite, M. A. Anaesthesia for cardiac surgery and allied procedures, 2nd ed. Oxford: Blackwell, 1980

Braunwald, E. ed. Heart disease. Philadelphia: Saunders, 1980

Brown, B. R. Jr, ed. Anaesthesia and the patient with heart disease. Philadelphia: F. A. Davis, 1980

Conahan, J. T. ed. Cardiac anesthesia. Menlo Park: Addison-Wesley, 1982

Hillis, L. D., Braunwald, E. Myocardial ischaemia. New England Journal of Medicine 1977; 296: 971, 1034–1093

Kaplan, J. A. ed. Cardiac anesthesia. New York: Grune & Stratton, 1979

Lappas, D. G., Powell, W. M. J., Dagget, W. M. Cardiac dysfunction in the perioperative. Period pathophysiology, diagnosis and treatment. Anesthesiology 1977; 47: 117–137

Laver, M. B., Lowenstein, E. Anesthesia and the patient with heart disease. In: Johnson, R. A., Harber, E., Austen, W. G. eds. The practice of cardiology. Boston: Little-Brown, 1980

Philbin, D. Anesthetic management of the patient with cardiovascular disease. International Anesthesiology 1979; 17(1):

Radney, P. A. ed. Anesthetic considerations for pediatric cardiac surgery. International Anesthesiology Clinics 1980; 18(1): 1–231

Ream, A. K., Fogdall, R. P., eds. Acute cardiovascular management: anaesthesia and intensive care. Philadelphia: Lippincott, 1982

Rogers, M. C., Smith, R. M. Anesthesia for intrathoracic and cardiac surgery. In: Smith, R. M. ed. Anesthesia for infants and children 4th edn. St. Louis, Mosby, 1980

Tarhan, S., ed. Cardiovascular anesthesia and postoperative care. Chichago: Yearbook Medical Publishers, 1982

Cardiopulmonary bypass and circulatory support

Allen K. Ream MS, MS, MD, FACA
Associate Professor of Anesthesia; Director, Institute of Engineering Design in Medicine
Stanford University School of Medicine, Palo Alto, California, USA

Apparatus

Cardiac surgery is dependent on a number of special techniques, but the most significant is cardiopulmonary bypass. Bypass serves a number of purposes: control of body temperature, gas exchange with the blood and transport of nutrients via blood to tissue. This is done in a way which bypasses the surgical field. This chapter is concerned with the most practical aspects; a more detailed discussion of history and principles is provided elsewhere[1].

Bubble oxygenator

Although the physical appearance of a bubble oxygenator varies markedly from one commercial product to another, the elements of its design are consistent.

1

Venous blood from the patient is brought to a chamber which admits gas through ports at the bottom. The rising gas mixes with the blood, adding oxygen and removing carbon dioxide. The oxygenated blood is then passed through a filter with a large surface area, treated with a defoaming agent and held in a reservoir until returned to the patient. Because heat is lost during bubbling and transport of the blood a heat exchanger is necessary to secure the desired blood temperature. Heat exchange is performed before defoaming to ensure that all bubbles formed during warming are removed before the blood is returned to the patient.

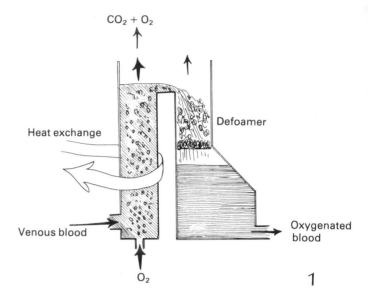

2

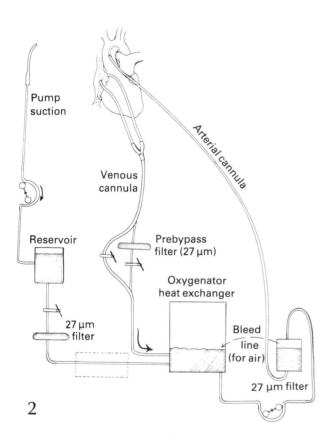

A typical arrangement of the bypass apparatus using a bubble oxygenator is illustrated diagrammatically. In the main circuit blood is withdrawn from the patient via the venous line, passed through the oxygenator/heat exchanger using gravity and the flow of oxygenator gases and then returned to the patient via a pump and filter.

A second circuit (shown on the left of the diagram) is the 'coronary' or 'pump' suction. Originally a return for blood from the coronary sinus, it is used for blood removed from the operative field which is suitable for reinfusion. The blood is passed via a pump to a reservoir and electively returned to the oxygenator through a filter.

Despite careful precautions during construction of these disposable oxygenators shed particles appear when the system is primed. In order to remove these particles the bypass system is operated before connection to the patient with the arterial and venous lines connected and the return to the oxygenator passing through the prebypass filter.

During clinical use the blood is filtered just before returning to the patient to remove emboli. The filter is inverted and a bleed line from the top of it to the oxygenator is maintained to remove any gas which may accumulate. The system is surprisingly effective; gas has lower viscosity than blood and a significant quantity of gas can be quickly removed once the fluid has passed through the bleed line.

3

Membrane oxygenator

A membrane oxygenator does not require a direct gas-blood surface. Blood is distributed to a very thin passage between semipermeable membranes exposed to the oxygenator gas mixture. The thin passage reduces the minimum channel length necessary for oxygenation at a given flow and thereby reduces the priming volume. The inlet must also be carefully designed to minimize priming volume while uniformly distributing blood to the oxygenator. Because of these constraints a large surface area for gas exchange is needed and the surface material must be unusually compatible with blood. This usually requires that the heat exchanger shall not be integral with the oxygenator mechanism.

Because of the higher flow resistance associated with this design a pump is usually required before the oxygenator. The large surface area, small passages and the need for efficient gas exchange usually mean that the blood passage dimensions change with transmembrane pressure. Since the pressure on the blood side is controlled by perfusion requirements it is common practice to control the gas pressure to ensure the proper spacing and thereby the gas exchange efficiency.

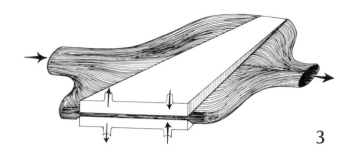

3

Heat exchanger

A heat exchanger is an essential element, even when modest hypothermia is used, because of the heat loss through the oxygenator. A bubble oxygenator has higher losses than a membrane oxygenator owing to increased loss of water vapour. Most disposable bubble oxygenators include an exchanger; if significant hypothermia is contemplated an external unit is also necessary.

4

Heat exchange is conceptually similar to gas exchange. Blood and heated water must be brought into close proximity, without mixing, long enough for exchange to occur. Theoretically heat exchange can be carried out with the fluids either in parallel or in 'countercurrent' flow.

In parallel current flow the blood and water exit with a common temperature between their two entering values. In the plot of temperature illustrated the average value across the flow channel is presented. The blood closest to the exchange surface will be warmer (closer to the water temperature) than the value shown. Note that in parallel flow the temperature of the blood at the exchange surface at the inlet will exceed the mixed blood outlet temperature.

In the example of countercurrent flow (heat exchange fluid running in the opposite direction to bloodflow) illustrated, it is assumed that the flow of water is greater than the flow of blood. In this instance the exit temperature of the blood is very close to the highest temperature it has encountered.

For the same water inlet temperature blood warming is faster and more efficient when countercurrent flow is employed. This mode is also safer than parallel flow because none of the blood is exposed to a temperature higher than that desired. An external heat exchanger should therefore always be connected in countercurrent fashion to minimize the maximum blood temperature. As already pointed out, an external heat exchanger should never be used between the oxygenator and the patient since warming of the blood can result in air embolism.

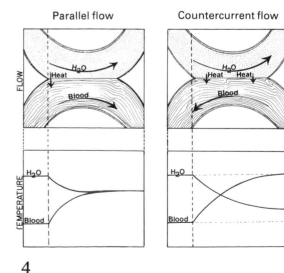

4

5

Heat exchanger design must provide the large surface area between the blood and the water which is necessary for efficiency. This may be accomplished by carrying one medium in multiple small tubes surrounded by the other medium, as in the design illustrated. When this design is incorporated in a bubble oxygenator orientation of the tubes so that the blood flows upwards permits gas bubbles to assist blood flow.

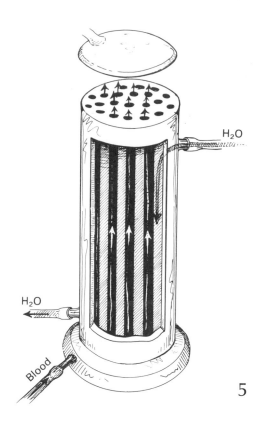

5

Techniques

Hypothermia

If low flow (40 ml/min per kg body weight) and local (cardiac) cooling are used the patient may be cooled to 31°C. With higher flow (55–70 ml/min per kg) it is preferable to cool to approximately 28°C. For circulatory arrest corporeal temperature should ordinarily be less than 20°C (profound hypothermia).

For profound hypothermia externally assisted cooling is desirable, with a cooling blanket, vasodilators, dry respiratory gases, chilled intravenous solutions and other adjuvants. Blood viscosity increases with falling temperature and haemodilution is usually essential.

Pump prime

A satisfactory priming solution is normal (physiological) saline with added sodium bicarbonate and mannitol. Protein-containing solutions are not necessary and blood need only be added to maintain the packed cell volume (haematocrit value) above 0.20–0.25 (20–25 per cent) during bypass. Lactate is often used but may be undesirable because of impaired metabolism at lower temperatures. Calcium should be added with blood to balance the citrate and anticoagulation is maintained with heparin.

Anticoagulation

The patient is given an initial heparinizing dose, typically 300 U/kg, and heparin is also added to the perfusate. Anticoagulation is monitored with the activated coagulation time (measured in the operating theatre) and additional heparin given as necessary to ensure a value exceeding 400 seconds.

Cannulation

Cannulation is performed after anticoagulation. Femoral cannulation was the most popular early technique and is preferable if closed chest arrest for hypothermia is planned, for partial bypass during operations on the descending aorta or when cannulation of the ascending aorta is not possible.

6

Femoral cannulation

For femoral cannulation a cannula is placed in one of the
femoral arteries. One or both femoral veins are cannulated, one cannula being passed to the level of the heart
and the other to the junction of the iliac veins. One
femoral venous catheter is sufficient for partial bypass.

Atrial cannulation

The usual site for venous cannulation is through the right
atrium after sternotomy, cannulae being threaded into the
superior and inferior venae cavae. Tapes are not placed
around the venae cavae over the cannulae unless the right
heart will be entered. The absence of caval snares permits
blood entering the right heart by other routes to be drawn
off. Improving drainage improves the rate of cooling and
avoids cardiac distension.

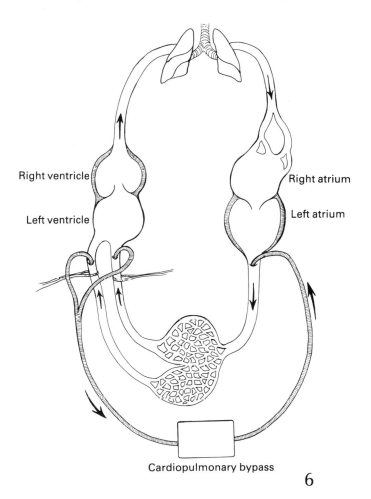

Right ventricle

Left ventricle

Right atrium

Left atrium

Cardiopulmonary bypass

6

7 & 8

Atrial cannulation is accomplished by placing a purse-string suture around the atrial appendage, occluding the base with a vascular clamp, removing the tip and releasing any internal adhesions which would interfere with passage of the cannula. The cannula is then placed through the opened clamp, inserted into the orifice of the inferior vena cava to a depth previously marked and fixed with the purse-string suture.

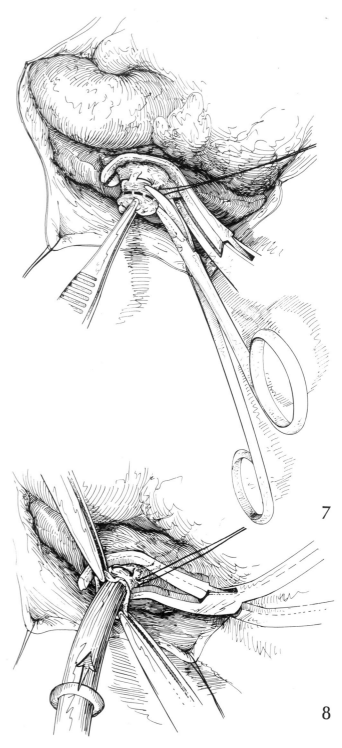

7

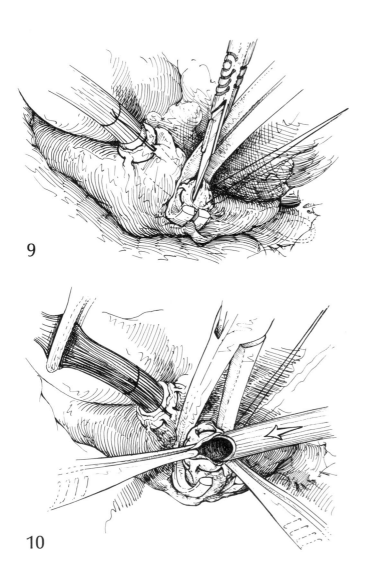

9

10

8

9 & 10

To place the superior vena cava cannula a purse-string suture is placed on the midlateral margin of the atrium, the area is occluded with a vascular clamp and a scalpel is used to open the wall. The cannula is placed through the released clamp, threaded into the orifice of the superior vena cava to the marker and fixed with the purse-string.

Aortic cannulation

11, 12 & 13

Aortic cannulation begins with removal of overlying loose tissue at the site and placement of a purse-string suture. For most operations the optimal site is just below the origin of the innominate artery. A stab wound is made with a No. 11 blade (care being taken not to injure the posterior aortic wall) and held closed by the application of forceps. The wound is just small enough to ensure a snug fit with the cannula. The occluded aortic cannula is then placed through the wound to the marker and the purse-string tightened and tied to the cannula.

The cannula is then connected to the return line from the pump so that no air is introduced. This may be accomplished by releasing the clamp long enough for the cannula to fill with blood, filling the return line with saline and squeezing both lines at the moment of connection to expel fluid, the lines being held so that the last point where fluid may escape as the connection is made is the highest (so that gas escapes first). After the connection has been made it should be carefully inspected and the procedure repeated if any bubbles are visible.

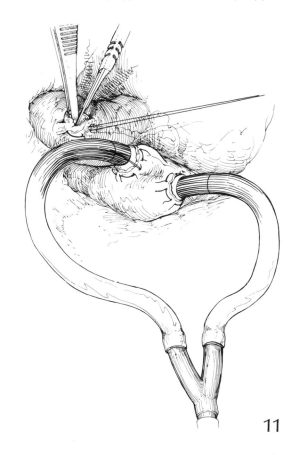

11

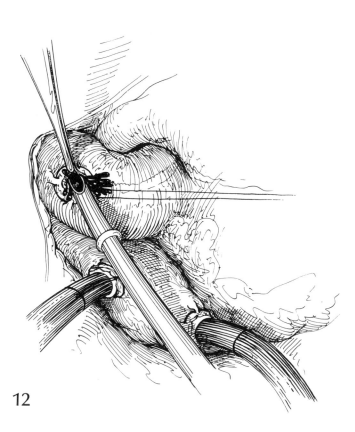

12

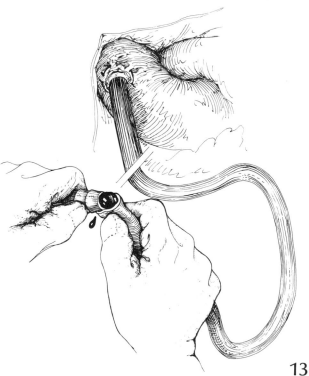

13

Bypass

Bypass can be begun rapidly if adequate venous drainage to the bypass system is assured. Ventilation may be stopped when the aortic valve is no longer opening. Bypass pressure is initially quite low because of the low viscosity of the perfusate in the oxygenator. A vasopressor is usually not necessary; if it is, a short-acting drug such as ephedrine should be employed. Because of the low perfusion pressures vascular resistance changes with static pressures are significant and the legs should not be below heart level.

14

Coronary artery bypass grafting is an example of typical perfusion. After bypass has been started the aortic cross-clamp is placed between the heart and the aortic cannula. If topical hypothermia is employed it may be started first. For cardioplegia a small cannula is placed in the aortic root so that it is proximal to the aortic cross-clamp. After the clamp has been placed perfusion is begun (see chapter on 'Myocardial protection', pp. 65–70).

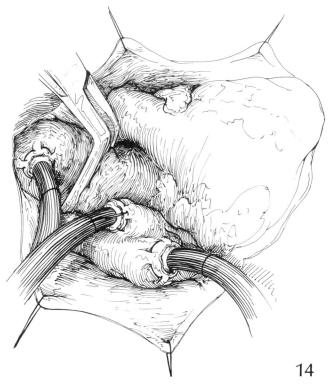

14

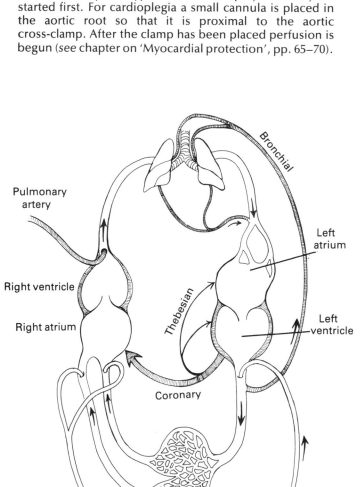

15

15

Venting

During bypass blood may return to the right heart via the coronary circulation and to the left heart via the venae cordis minimae (Thebesius' veins) and bronchial veins or by aortic regurgitation after the cross-clamp has been removed. Certain congenital lesions also cause increased return. It is desirable to remove this blood to avoid cardiac distention and warming. A loose fit between the venae cavae and the venous cannulae provides significant drainage to the bypass system. If blood return is sufficiently large venting the pulmonary artery is helpful. This is the preferred approach because it is easy to reach, flow from the right heart is interrupted, the left ventricle is drained by retrograde flow, septal warming is minimal and removal of the cannula is safe and simple.

It is also possible to vent via the cardioplegia cannula inserted in the aortic root. However, this approach vents the right heart via flow through the left ventricle, may permit the entry of air into the aortic root by leakage around the cannula and cannot vent the heart after the aortic clamp has been removed.

A vent placed directly into the left ventricle permits venting of the left heart after the aortic clamp has been removed but shares the other deficiencies of an aortic root vent. In addition there is the possibility of myocardial injury, with cannulation or repair and distortion of the heart, which reduces the efficiency of contraction. It cannot be safely removed after termination of bypass.

Pressure and flow

Controversy exists regarding adequate perfusion pressure and flow. The practice at Stanford is to use 'low flow' (approximately 1.5 l/min per square metre of body surface); this works well with adequate local cooling of the heart and has the advantage of reduced blood trauma. Low flow should not be coupled with significant use of vasopressors; there is no evidence that the resulting changes in distribution of blood flow are beneficial. While most other centres have used higher flows (up to 3.5 l/min per m^2) it appears that this is becoming less common.

There is considerable evidence to suggest that pulsatile flow is advantageous; however, it is technically difficult and the advantages may be quite small. Most centres use non-pulsatile flow; pulsatile flow is likely to become more common when it is easier to employ.

Humoral factors

Potassium

The serum potassium concentration decreases during bypass and is usually supplemented. A typical adult dose is 20–60 mEq. Hypokalaemia predisposes to arrhythmias, while hyperkalaemia may cause cardiac depression.

Magnesium

The serum magnesium level is depleted by dilution and possibly by diuretic therapy. Hypomagnesaemia is associated with arrhythmias and difficulty in defibrillation. A typical dose is 8–16 mEq.

Calcium

Calcium is part of the common pathway for inotropic effects on the heart. Depletion may be caused by haemodilution and the administration of blood and blood products. Up to 2 g of calcium chloride may be given near the end of bypass to enhance inotropic effects but should not be given automatically. The effects may be undesirable in the hyperdynamic or ischaemic patient.

Acid-base balance

It is essential that the patient's pH be maintained at the normal level. Acidosis is particularly dangerous; it not only impairs the inotropic response but also increases obligatory perfusion requirements by causing vasodilation in healthy tissue. The optimum pH changes with the temperature of the patient. It is convenient to use the pH measured in the laboratory at 37°C (the 'uncorrected' value) and to maintain this value at approximately 7.42 rather than memorize the proper value as a function of patient temperature[2]. An older practice is to maintain the pH at 7.42 *at the patient temperature* (corrected value). This approach produces acidosis and should be avoided.

Ventilation

It is most common to stop ventilation during the bypass period when the heart is not ejecting. Minimal positive end-expiratory pressure (about 1 cmH$_2$O) appears to protect pulmonary function and is not usually obtrusive for the surgeon. A modest oxygen flow of about 1 l/min is usually maintained to preserve apnoeic oxygenation. Ventilation is helpful during manoeuvres to remove air from vascular spaces associated with the heart both to provide bloodflow and to eliminate gases directly. Ventilation should be restarted with the resumption of cardiac ejection.

Cardiac resuscitation

Rewarming is begun shortly before the restoration of cardiac perfusion. The maintenance of pump flow and the use of vasodilators will assist rewarming[3].

After the aortic cross-clamp has been removed the heart is passively perfused until it is warm enough to support coordinated contraction. A period of active contraction with low peak systolic ventricular pressure is essential to ensure washout of accumulated anaerobic metabolites. This is called the idling time. With the newer techniques of myocardial preservation spontaneous defibrillation is more common, but direct current shock may be necessary to prevent the heart continuing in fibrillation when warm.

If coronary air embolism occurs it may be necessary to permit a relatively high aortic root pressure to facilitate washout. The continuous use of vasopressors at this stage is contraindicated[4]. Pulsatile flow (by allowing the heart to eject) appears to be beneficial in the rapid elimination of air within the coronary arteries.

Terminating cardiopulmonary bypass

It is essential to terminate bypass smoothly so as to transfer the work to the heart slowly enough to avoid unnecessary stress and to permit precise adjustment of preload and afterload. The idling time should be adequate for warming and washout, coronary air embolism should be corrected if it has occurred and an adequate heart rate should be established (80–100/min is best).

Bypass flow is decreased from maintenance levels over 1–2 minutes, the filling pressure is increased until the heart appears 'full' (effective ventricular contraction without failure to fill completely during diastole) and mean aortic root pressure is maintained at approximately 75 mmHg, a rapid-acting vasodilator (sodium nitroprusside) being used if necessary.

Proper adjustment of filling pressure before the termination of bypass requires observation of the heart. Starling's law applies but refers to end-diastolic volume. Because of the insult of bypass, cardioplegia and circulatory arrest of the heart, cardiac compliance, and thereby the proper filling pressure, may be altered. Reference to pressure alone, including pulmonary artery pressure, will not adequately define this change. When the proper pressure is reached the heart will be full at the beginning of systole but will contract significantly. The associated pressures may then be noted.

When the patient is stable one venous cannula and the aortic cannula are removed.

16, 17 & 18

Removal of the aortic cannula begins with placement of a purse-string suture. The previous purse-string is then released, the cannula is removed and the wound is occluded by the assistant. The purse-string is then gently tightened and held by the assistant. A second purse-string is placed and tied. It is helpful during this stage if the arterial pressure is kept low to reduce wall stress while the suture is being tightened.

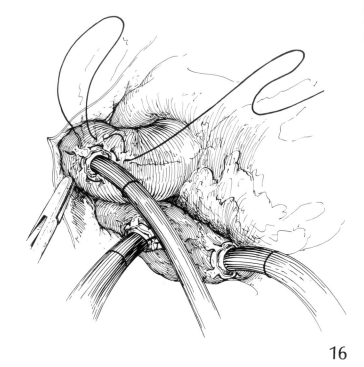

16

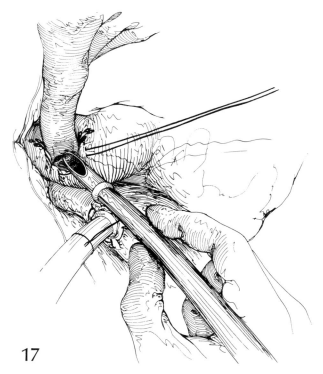

17

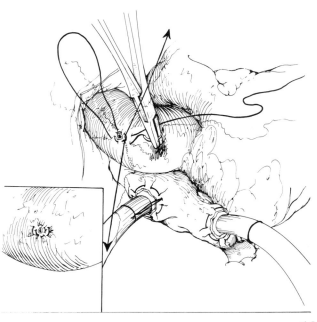

18

19

After this procedure has been completed the remaining perfusate in the bypass system is returned to the patient. A convenient technique is to connect the arterial cannula to the venous cannula previously placed in the inferior vena cava and clamp the venous line returning blood to the oxygenator. This allows the return of 'pump blood' to the patient without the risk of air embolism or of clotting in the aortic cannula after the administration of protamine. Blood is then slowly pumped into the patient via the inferior vena cava while aortic pressure is held constant with a fast-acting vasodilator (usually sodium nitroprusside). Occasionally a ganglionic dilator such as hydralazine or chlorpromazine may also be required.

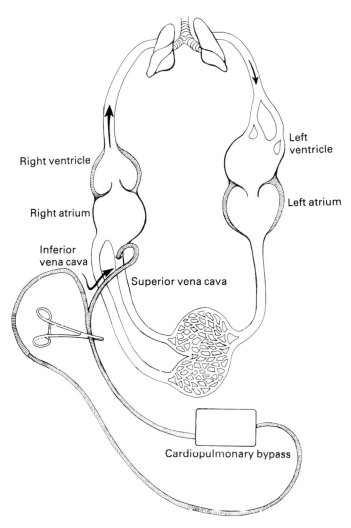

19

Special devices

Successful weaning of a patient from cardiopulmonary bypass requires adjustment of filling pressures, control of afterload and titration of inotropic agents (usually in that order). The adjustment of electrolytes, control of the pH, use of vasodilators and judicious use of inotropic agents are frequently appropriate.

If the heart first appears able to function after termination of bypass and then begins to fail rapidly it is better to return to bypass than to increase the dosage of inotropic agents. The most common cause of this state is ischaemia. Because inotropic agents increase myocardial oxygen consumption they should not be aggressively administered without evidence of benefit[5].

On occasion it may prove impossible to wean a patient from cardiopulmonary bypass because the heart is not able to support the circulation without assistance. Several alternatives are available or are being developed. The choice depends on the degree and nature of cardiac impairment and the probability of return to adequate function without support.

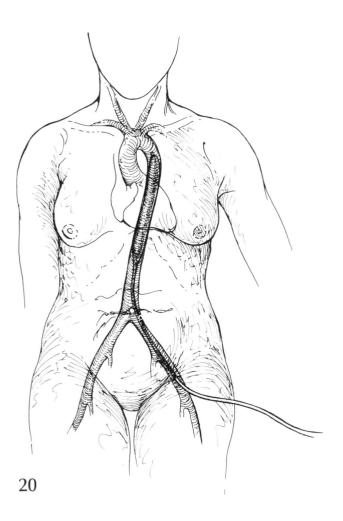

20

20

Intra-aortic balloon assistance

Often a patient has a modest deficit (below the minimum necessary flow) and can be presumed likely to return to adequate function after recovering from the acute insults associated with surgery. Most often failure is reversible with augmentation of left heart function.

The intra-aortic balloon is generally used to provide circulatory assistance after bypass but it may also be inserted early to augment perfusion during bypass. It is customarily inserted through a femoral artery and placed just below the aortic arch. The balloon is cyclically inflated and deflated in the counterpulsation mode, to raise pressure during the diastolic phase and to decrease it during the systolic phase. This has three beneficial effects: (1) diastolic pressure is elevated, improving coronary perfusion, (2) systolic pressure is decreased, reducing myocardial oxygen demand and (3) cardiac output is increased by reducing afterload, improving systemic perfusion.

The balloon may be inflated with helium to decrease the inflation and deflation times, but carbon dioxide is more common because it is thought to be safer should a gas embolus be released, is less expensive and is less difficult to obtain.

21

Left ventricular assist devices

Left ventricular assist devices offer a greater degree of augmentation and the possibility of chronic use. They are currently under development, with trials in several centres, and the design is still evolving[6]. An example is the Novacor/Stanford left heart assist device. The unit pumps from the apex of the left ventricle to the abdominal aorta. At present the system is powered by externally supplied electrical power; eventually it may be powered by implanted batteries inductively charged in a diurnal cycle.

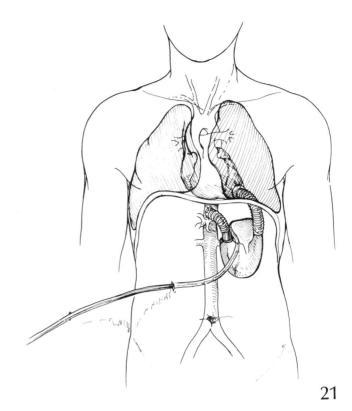

21

Extracorporeal membrane oxygenation

The primary application of membrane oxygenators in bypass procedures of normal duration is in infants and young children, in whom blood trauma is greater because of the greater ratio of priming blood volume to patient blood volume and a higher cardiac index. For the same flow and duration a membrane oxygenator offers less trauma than a bubble oxygenator.

Studies of support of patients with traumatic lesions have indicated that extended use of an extracorporeal membrane oxygenator is possible. Pulmonary function is often impaired, usually through fat embolism secondary to the fracture of large bones. If oxygenation can be sustained for a period of days the lung may recover function. Careful examination of available reports suggests that survivors are rare with extended support when flow through the extracorporeal oxygenator exceeds 70 per cent of cardiac output. This is, however, notably better than the bubble oxygenator permits[7].

Complications

The complications of cardiopulmonary bypass are bewildering in their extent[8]. However, several patterns may be noted.

Simple approaches are the best. There is less opportunity for error and it is easier to identify problems and often easier to correct them than with more elaborate techniques. This is particularly helpful in avoiding failure and operator misuse of equipment. Specific problems include leaks, gas embolism, pump or oxygenator failure and contamination.

Blood trauma is a major concern. Coagulation is impaired because of cooling and exposure to gas and material interfaces. Red cell damage results from contact with foreign surfaces and may present either as haemolysis or increased clearance. Emboli form and may be found in the tissues of the patient, particularly the lung. Inadequate heparin administration will exacerbate these effects; some reports suggest that excessive heparinization is also dangerous. Variables which influence the degree of blood trauma include the perfusion time, blood flow rate, gas flow rate, temperature, blood glucose concentration, clotting time, perfusion pressure and gas line pressure.

After the blood the most sensitive target organ is the kidney. The mechanisms are poorly understood but appear to be related to perfusion pressure and the degree of pulsatile flow. There appears to be no evidence that the use of vasopressors is helpful and these agents appear likely to act preferentially on the kidney.

Other significant target organs are the lungs, which may be injured by both emboli and humoral agents, and the brain, which appears primarily vulnerable to microemboli. As noted above, the issue of low-flow low-pressure perfusion remains unsettled with reference to cerebral preservation; the best centres using each technique appear to achieve similar results.

Conclusion

Without cardiopulmonary bypass many techniques of modern cardiovascular surgery would not be possible. Effective use of the approach demands a knowledge of patient physiology and device technology, the ability to monitor the patient closely, the dexterity to accomplish the physical tasks and a sense of the time-dependent factors in the procedure.

The early concepts concerning cardiopulmonary bypass have proved largely correct, but recent work has extended the reliability, safety and reproducibility of the technique.

References

1. Ream, A. K. Cardiopulmonary bypass. In: Ream, A. K., Fogdall, R. P., eds. Acute Cardiovascular Management: Anesthesia and Intensive Care. 1st edn. 420–455. Philadelphia and Toronto: Lippincott, 1982

2. Ream, A. K., Reitz, B. A., Silverberg, G. D. Temperature correction of P_{CO_2} and pH in estimating acid-base status: an example of the emperor's new clothes? Anesthesiology 1982; 56: 41–44

3. Noback, C. R., Tinker, J. H. Hypothermia after cardiopulmonary bypass in man: amelioration by nitroprusside-induced vasodilation during rewarming. Anesthesiology 1980; 53: 277–280

4. Sink, J. D., Hill, R. C., Chitwood, W. R., Jr., Abriss, R., Wechsler, A. S. Effects of phenylephrine on transmural distribution of myocardial blood flow in regions supplied by normal and collateral arteries during cardiopulmonary bypass. Journal of Thoracic and Cardiovascular Surgery 1979; 78: 236–243

5. Lazar, H. L., Buckberg, G. D., Foglia, R. P., Manganaro, A. J., Maloney J. V., Jr. Detrimental effects of premature use of inotropic drugs to discontinue cardiopulmonary bypass. Journal of Thoracic and Cardiovascular Surgery 1981; 82: 18–25

6. Pae, W. E. Jr., Pierce, W. S. Temporary left ventricular assistance in acute myocardial infarction and cardiogenic shock: rationale and criteria for utilization. Chest 1981; 79: 662–695

7. Bregman, D., ed. Mechanical Support of the Failing Heart and Lungs. 1st edn. New York: Appleton-Century Crofts, 1977

8. Mortensen, J. D. Safety and efficacy of extracorporeal blood oxygenators: a review. Medical Instrumentation 1978; 12: 128–132

Myocardial protection for cardiac surgery

Stuart W. Jamieson MB, FRCS, FACS
Professor and Head, Cardiothoracic Surgery, University of Minnesota, Minneapolis, Minnesota, USA

Introduction

Adequate protection of the myocardium whilst performing heart surgery involves a compromise between progressive cardiac injury and optimal operating conditions. The following techniques have been advocated over the years for myocardial protection during surgery:

Without the aorta cross-clamped:

1. Ventricular fibrillation;
2. Surgery on the empty beating heart.

With the aorta cross-clamped:

3. Continuous coronary perfusion;
4. Topical (local) hypothermia;
5. Infusion of cardioplegic solutions;
6. A combination of (4) and (5).

Almost all cardiac surgery is now performed during cardiac arrest, though there are still exceptions to this. The alternative is to maintain a continuous blood supply to the heart by not clamping the aorta, or by individual perfusion of the coronary arteries with blood. This results in continuous ventricular fibrillation or a beating heart that does not eject.

Although surgery on the empty beating heart may be performed for certain right-sided conditions if intracardiac shunts are not present, the heart must be either arrested or in ventricular fibrillation if the left-sided chambers of the heart are to be opened, so as to avoid air embolism. An exception to this occurs when the aorta is cross-clamped and the aorta opened for aortic valve surgery. In this case separate cannulation of the coronary ostia is required.

Some degree of cardiac injury always occurs during cardiac arrest or ventricular fibrillation, and may also occur with perfusion of the empty beating heart and coronary perfusion techniques. Injury during coronary perfusion arises because of the fixed, non-pulsatile perfusion pressure; coronary anatomy that may make it difficult or impossible to perfuse the myocardium adequately; or obstructive coronary lesions.

Preferred methods

Myocardial protection during cardiac surgery is the central feature of all operations and should be carried out methodically and meticulously. We prefer the method of initial cardiac arrest by cardioplegic solution, followed by profound topical hypothermia. Cold cardiac arrest facilitates cardiac surgery by providing a still and flaccid myocardium without blood flow through vessels, thus allowing operation to be performed more precisely and more rapidly. An additional benefit is better exposure and a minimum amount of trauma as a result of retraction. Local hypothermia reduces metabolic rate, and by the law of Van't Hoff the logarithm of the rate of oxygen consumption is proportional to the logarithm of the absolute temperature (for each 10°C drop in temperature, the arrested heart requires two to three times less oxygen per gram of heart muscle). Thus the cooler the myocardium, the less the oxygen requirement.

Infusion of cardioplegic solution achieves instant arrest of the heart and rapid local cooling, and since cold is the essential factor in myocardial protection it is important to maintain profound local hypothermia. This is achieved by:

1. Low-flow techniques on cardiopulmonary bypass;
2. Two caval cannulae;
3. A vent (both (2) and (3) aid in cooling by removal of bronchial flow or right ventricular blood, thus decreasing temperature)
4. Initial infusion of cardioplegic solution followed by continuous topical lavage; and
5. A perfusion temperature that is initially cold.

Two caval cannulae are inserted into the right atrium, with their tips at the orifices of the great vessels. Bypass is then instituted and the heart emptied. A vent is inserted.

Bypass

On bypass, low-flow techniques are used, with a flow rate of 30–50 ml/kg per minute, maintaining a systolic pressure between 30 and 60 mmHg mercury. It is advisable deliberately to maintain the pressure below 60 mmHg; this reduces coronary circulation, and since the perfusion temperature will inevitably be greater than the temperature in the myocardium, less local rewarming will result. Moderate systemic hypothermia (28–30°C) is used for this reason during the cross-clamp interval. We do not believe it is necessary or advisable to use greater degrees of systemic hypothermia.

After the aorta is cross-clamped, the cardioplegic solution is run into the aortic root through a small catheter. The volume of cardioplegic solution is 500 or 1000 ml, and in our institution no further cardioplegic solution is administered subsequent to this. Cardioplegic solution should be infused at a maximal pressure of 150 mmHg. Direct endothelial injury may be caused at higher pressures. For coronary artery surgery this catheter is removed and the needle hole sutured before commencing the operation. The hole may be left for other operations, such as valve replacement, for subsequent removal of air from the ventricular cavities. During infusion of cardioplegic solution cold saline is poured on to the heart for additional topical hypothermia. The left ventricle should be periodically checked for distension.

Vent

A pulmonary artery vent is preferable and has the following advantages:

1. Complete emptying of the heart is achieved even on the left side (by reversed flow through the pulmonary vasculature).
2. A pulmonary artery vent is easily inserted and removed without distortion of the heart, and no left ventricular muscle is placed in jeopardy.
3. There is no risk of air embolization.
4. By removing any right ventricular blood, exposure is improved, maximum immersion of the heart in cold saline is achieved and rewarming of the septum after initial cooling by cardioplegic solution is minimized.

The one disadvantage of a pulmonary artery vent is that after removing the aortic crossclamp, if the heart does not resume ventricular beating, left ventricular distension is a possibility if there is aortic regurgitation. This can usually be dealt with by manual decompression until the heart commences beating.

1

Topical hypothermia

Continuous lavage is carried out with cold saline once the aorta is cross-clamped. This is effected with a line placed into the pericardial cavity, and is run at about 150 ml/minute. The saline should be at 4°C. In order to maintain an effective level of saline in the pericardial cavity the operating table is placed with 30° of head tilt and 15° of left bank. Flexion of the table at its midpoint will keep the legs horizontal. The saline is removed by suction tubing wrapped in a gauze sponge at the bottom of the wound. Where possible, intracardiac lavage is carried out with additional cold saline. This has the effect of reducing temperature, and also removes debris after valve or aneurysm resection.

The level of cold saline is maintained just below the heart incision or the area being revascularized, by constant infusion. Topical hypothermia is important, since in a technique that uses cardioplegia alone areas of myocardium supplied by critically stenotic vessels do not become significantly cooled. These areas require myocardial protection most since they will continue to be deprived of an adequate blood supply after the aortic cross-clamp is removed but before the proximal anastomoses are performed.

Cardioplegia

The fact that almost every centre uses its own cardioplegic solution probably indicates that there is no clear advantage to any one formula. The principles of cardioplegia are the rapid induction of cardiac arrest at the onset of interruption of blood supply, and rapid cooling of the myocardium. These both reduce myocardial oxygen demand.

Although there are many recipes for cardioplegic solutions, the essentials probably include:

1. A high potassium concentration to achieve immediate arrest;
2. Dextrose as a substrate for anaerobic metabolism;
3. A buffer to reduce the deleterious effects of local acidosis;
4. Hyperosmolarity in order to reduce myocardial and interstitial oedema (dextrose, mannitol or albumin are commonly added to achieve this).

Some solutions include local anaesthetics or steroids in order to stabilize cell membranes, and calcium antagonists to block abnormal calcium fluxes. The composition of the cardioplegic solution used at our centre is shown in *Table 1*. This solution has a pH of 8.1–8.4 at 4°C, with a molality of 440 mmol.

Cold cardioplegic solution may be administered at the beginning of the aortic cross-clamp period, with hypothermia subsequently maintained by topical application of cold saline. An alternative may be to reinfuse the cardioplegic solution at 20-minute intervals. The former approach is preferred since it does not interrupt the flow of the operation, and maintains continuous hypothermia.

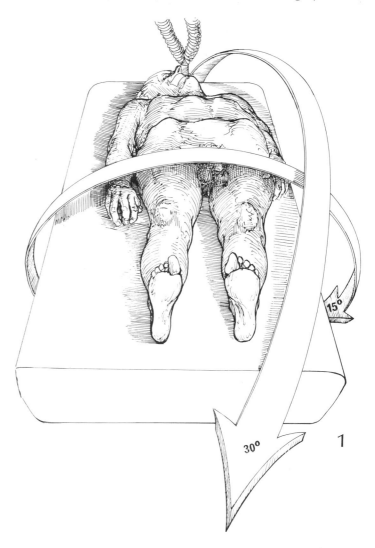

1

After the cross-clamp has been removed topical application of cold saline is discontinued. It is important to let the pressure rise to at least 60 mmHg. This is especially necessary in coronary artery surgery, when the proximal anastomoses have not been performed and important coronary stenoses will still be present. Venting of the heart should be continued until the operation has neared its end. It is important to allow the heart to beat with an empty ventricle during recovery. Since the coronary artery supply is predominantly in diastole the lower the end-diastolic pressure maintained the greater the myocardial perfusion.

Table 1 Composition of 'Stanford' cardioplegia solution

Ingredient	Concentration per litre
Potassium	30 mmol
Sodium	25 mmol
Chloride	30 mmol
Bicarbonate	25 mmol
Dextrose	50 g
Mannitol	12.5 g

Myocardial protection during specific operations

2

Coronary artery surgery

Cardioplegic solution is instilled initially, and the grafts are performed beginning on the front of the heart. This enables the entire heart with the exception of the area being operated upon to be cooled with the cold topical saline. The grafts on the right side are performed next, so that when the heart has to be lifted from the topical saline for performance of obtuse marginal grafts it is thoroughly cold.

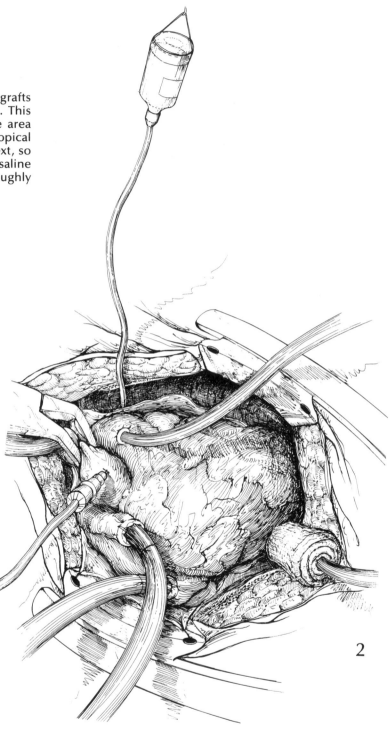

2

3

Aortic valve replacement

Cardioplegic solution should not be infused into the aortic root if aortic regurgitation is present. Since some degree of regurgitation is present in most cases of aortic stenosis, and it is difficult to judge left ventricular distension in the face of severe left ventricular hypertrophy, it is probably best to avoid aortic root perfusion whenever aortic valve disease is suspected. After the aorta has been cross-clamped, the aortic root is opened and cardioplegic solution is infused directly into each coronary ostium. Care must be taken not to cause dissection of the coronary ostia, or dislodgement of debris or calcific material into the coronary arteries.

Hypertrophy of the left ventricle with aortic valve disease mandates thorough and careful myocardial protection. When the cardioplegic solution has been inserted, the aortic valve is removed and additional myocardial protection is obtained by thorough lavage of the left ventricle with cold saline. This can be repeated at intervals throughout the operation and has the additional advantage of removing any particulate matter from the left ventricular cavity. Suitable tilt of the table will allow the heart to be covered with cold saline whilst the valve is being replaced. The suction for the topical cold solution is placed to the right of the aorta.

When aortic valve replacement is combined with coronary artery surgery, it is most convenient to do the distal coronary anastomoses after removing the valve and irrigating the left ventricle, but before placing the valve sutures. The cold infusion line may be placed directly into the left ventricular cavity when performing the distal anastomoses. The endocardial cooling thus obtained is highly effective and also has the advantage of cooling the septum.

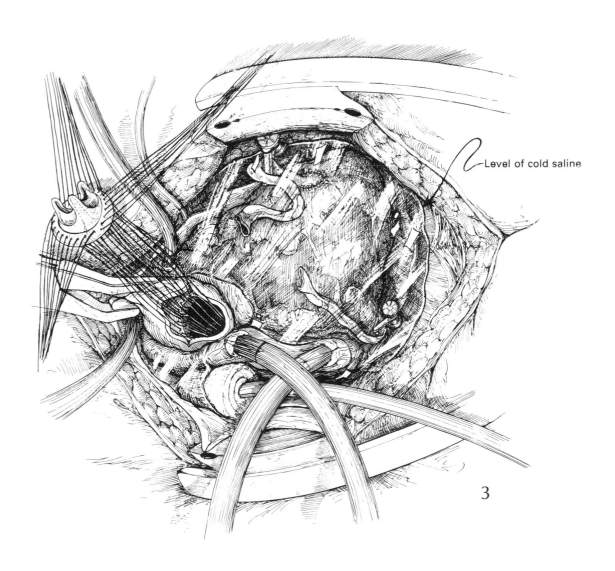

Level of cold saline

3

4

Mitral valve replacement

A similar sequence is carried out in mitral valve surgery, with initial infusion of cardioplegic solution. This may be performed through the aortic root in the normal way, provided there is no aortic regurgitation. After the mitral valve is removed thorough lavage of the left ventricular cavity is carried out.

Again, suitable tilt of the operating table will allow the heart to be covered with cold saline during the performance of valve replacement. Care should be taken not to penetrate the pericardial reflection beneath the inferior vena cava, as this will prevent the maintenance of an adequate level of cold solution over the anterior aspect of the heart. Good ventricular cooling can be carried out with a continuous infusion of topical cold saline during mitral valve surgery, provided the right ventricle is collapsed with a pulmonary artery vent and low flow on bypass. The suction for the topical cold solution is placed directly over the inferior vena cava.

When mitral valve replacement is combined with coronary artery grafting the distal anastomoses are again performed first.

Reoperation

It is important to achieve complete mobilization of the heart prior to aortic cross-clamping when reoperating. Effective topical hypothermia is not possible unless the heart is completely free. The remainder of the operation proceeds normally.

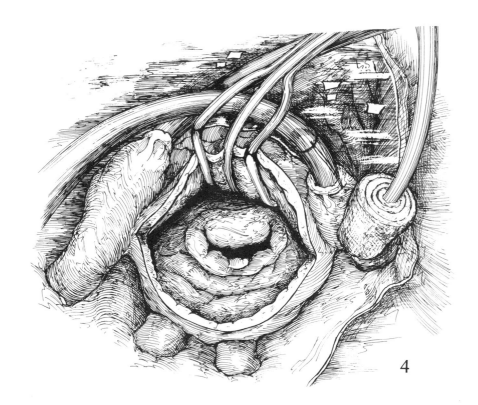

4

Postoperative care

John A. Macoviak MD
Chief Resident in Cardiac Surgery, Stanford University Medical Center, Stanford, California, USA

Optimal postoperative care is based upon continuous monitoring and frequent reassessment of each patient. The prompt recognition of incipient problems will simplify subsequent management. The postoperative intensive care unit (ICU) management of cardiac surigcal patients, including paediatric and transplant patients, is presented in this chapter.

Monitoring

Well-trained ICU nurses caring for the immediate postoperative patient on a one-to-one basis provide the most important aspect of monitoring. Upon arrival of the patient in the ICU, observation and recording of electrocardiogram (ECG), mean arterial pressure (MAP), central venous pressure (CVP), urine output and chest tube output are begun. A pulmonary arterial catheter will allow continuous monitoring of pulmonary artery diastolic pressure (PAD) and frequent measurement of pulmonary capillary wedge pressure (PCWP) or thermodilution cardiac output. These catheters are useful in selected patients with low cardiac output, but are unnecessary in most cardiac surgical patients. Direct left atrial pressure monitoring only rarely yields information significant enough to justify the risk of left-sided air embolism.

Respiratory care

The patient arrives in the ICU intubated; muscle relaxants and additional narcotics are given just before leaving the operating room. In routine cases, extubation is planned for 8–12 hours later, with sedation and ventilator settings gradually changed to meet this goal. Certain patients, such as those having a simple ASD repair, will be extubated in 4–5 hours, when the ventilatory depressant effects of the intial narcotic anaesthetic have dissipated.

The relatively prolonged period of ICU intubation in the routine patient following cardiac surgery allows for adequate rewarming, assurance of haemodynamic stability, and the intiation of spontaneous diuresis, before full awakening and extubation. In the occasional patient who requires re-exploration for bleeding or tamponade, transfer to the operating room can be rapid and smooth, thus avoiding the stress and delay of induction of anaesthesia for reintubation.

Rewarming, aided by vasodilation and volume expansion in the first 4–6 hours following surgery, results in increasing CO_2 production. Ventilatory rate must be adjusted to maintain normocarbia. Arterial blood gas (ABG) measurements are obtained immediately after arrival in the ICU and 15 minutes after each ventilator adjustment, or at least every 2 hours until the patient's temperature has stabilized. After the rewarming period, arterial blood gas measurements are rarely required more frequently than every 4 hours.

The inspired oxygen concentration is gradually reduced, allowing the patient to maintain a PO_2 of at least 80 mmHg. Hyperthermia increases oxygen consumption, so aggressive reduction in delivered oxygen concentration is best deferred until the patient's temperature stabilizes. Ventilator rate (IMV) is gradually decreased as the patient awakens. Extubation is usually performed in the awake, non-acidotic patient with a PO_2 of at least 80 mmHg on an FIO_2 of 40% and a PCO_2 of 35–45 on continuous positive airway pressure (CPAP). In equivocal cases, determination of the maximal insipiratory force (at least −25 cm water) and vital capacity (at least 15 ml/kg) can be helpful.

After extubation, most patients can cooperate with respiratory exercises to prevent atelectasis. Occasionally, chest physiotherapy with percussion, vibration, and postural drainage is ordered in those with heavy secretions or persistent atelectasis. Bronchodilator inhalants or aminophylline infusions are necessary in those with bronchospasm. When arrhythmias prevent continuation of bronchodilation, a short course of low dose steroids can abate bronchospasm in most cases.

Rarely is intermittent positive pressure breathing or a continuous positive airway pressure mask indicated; the problems of air swallowing and aspiration mitigate against these therapies, especially in the patient with dulled senses. When stridor occurs following extubation, reintubation can often be avoided by the administration of parenteral steriods or racemic epinephrine inhalants.

Diuresis is initiated in most patients 12–24 hours postoperatively. Prolonged intubation may be indicated in those with pulmonary oedema, low cardiac output, acute renal failure, or dulled sensation.

Cricothyroidotomy or a highly placed tracheostomy is performed in those requiring prolonged ventilatory support. This is usually done 7–10 days following surgery, but may be deferred for up to 3 weeks in equivocal cases. High placement of a soft-cuffed tracheal tube reduces the risk of sternal and mediastinal wound infection as well as the risk of innominate artery erosion. These patients require frequent high volume sighs, bagging, and suctioning to prevent atelectasis. Tracheal aspirates are routinely cultured to allow the prompt treatment of infection.

Acid base balance

Normal acid base balance is necessary for the optimal function of the myocardium and its appropriate response to inotropic agents. Disorders of acid base balance are frequent in the postoperative patient; attention should be directed toward treatment of the cause of the disorder and not simply correction of the pH.

Respiratory acidosis is treated with increased minute ventilation, which may require reintubation. PCO_2 is kept at 35–45 mmHg unless preoperative CO_2 retention as a result of chronic obstructive pulmonary disease is documented. An occasional patient will develop respiratory acidosis after extubation as a result of residual narcosis. A naloxone infusion (0.4 mg in 100 ml D5W) can be slowly titrated until the patient becomes alert.

Respiratory alkalosis only rarely occurs as primary, central hyperventilation; most often, it is secondary to metabolic acidosis, pulmonary oedema, or mechanical hyperventilation.

Metabolic alkalosis is usually a result of depletion of intravascular volume from diuresis or chloride ion loss from gastric suctioning. Other causes are excessive administration of bicarbonate or acetate. Chloride repletion as KCl or NaCl is performed with concommitant volume expansion. Acetazolamide 250 mg every 12 hours may be a useful diuretic adjunct in those with excess total body water. Occasionally, a dilute HCl infusion is carefully run with frequent blood pH determinations in severely alkalotic patients or those with fluid overload. This infusion must be given slowly and only through a central venous line.

Metabolic acidosis is usually secondary to low cardiac output, renal failure, or sepsis. As the underlying disorder is treated, sodium bicarbonate is titrated to keep the pH normal.

Fluids and electrolytes

In the early postoperative period, the central venous pressure (preload) is frequently adjusted to maximize cardiac output. Blood components are given as needed. Once bleeding is controlled and coagulation factors are repleted, isotonic crystalloid solutions (normal saline or Ringer's lactate) are used for volume expansion. Serum sodium concentration is monitored and delivered sodium altered accordingly. Five per cent albumin or 25% albumin (less sodium for equivalent volume expansion effect) is administered to those whose net fluid intake exceeds 25 ml/kg/day of crystalloid (up to 100 ml/kg/day in children less than 20 kg), or in those who are hypoalbuminaemic.

Normal serum potassium concentration is essential for the prevention of arrhythmias. In the early postoperative period and during diuresis, the serum potassium is monitored every 4 hours. In adults, potassium is replaced intravenously by administering 1 mEq for every 0.1 mEq less than 5.0 mEq/l serum concentration. The rate should not exceed 0.3 mEq/kg/hour and must be administered through a central vein with continuous ECG monitoring. Transient hyperkalaemia may result in severe bradyarrhythmias or asystole. In cases of hyperkalaemia, treatment varies with the urgency required to reverse effects. Acute hyperkalaemia causing arrhythmias is treated with intravenous calcium chloride, sodium bicarbonate, and 50 per cent dextrose with insulin. Less urgent hyperkalaemia will respond to diuretics, enteral polystyrene resin, or dialysis.

Cardiac output

Cardiac output is determined by heart rate and stroke volume, the latter being affected by preload, afterload, and cardiac contractility. Each of these factors may be affected by the patient's disease or surgery, and careful attention to optimizing each component in the postoperative patient is essential.

A heart rate of 80–100/min in adults and 100–160/min in children is optimal. Sinus rhythm allows the highest cardiac output for a given rate; A-V sequential pacing may therefore be useful in the patient with A-V block and a low cardiac output. Ventricular or atrial pacing wires are usually sutured to the epicardium at surgery, and are useful in the patient with bradycardia or heart block. In patients without pacing wires, isoproterenol (10–100 ng/kg/min) may be used to increase heart rate, but tachyarrythmias may occur.

Sinus tachycardia is most commonly caused by volume depletion, and should be treated with fluids. Pain, CO_2 retention, hypoxia, and sepsis must also be considered as potential causes of sinus tachycardia. (For discussion of other arrhythmias, see p. 74).

Management of optimal preload is based on consideration of preoperative filling pressures. A central venous pressure (CVP) of 8–16 cmH$_2$O is usually adequate for most patients. Blood components are given to replace ongoing blood loss. Red cell transfusion is most efficient in expanding intravascular volume. Controversy continues as to the benefits of colloid versus crystalloid in the fluid therapy of the patient who is not anaemic. In general, if the haematocrit remains between 30 and 35 per cent, isotonic crystalloids are used as maintenance fluids unless their net input exceeds 20–30 ml/kg/day in adults. Colloids such as albumin or synthetic plasma expanders are then used to supplement crystalloid therapy or to replace it in the severely hypoalbuminaemic patient.

Systemic vascular resistance (afterload) is frequently increased in the early postoperative patient because of hypothermic vasoconstriction and systemic hypertension. Nitroprusside (0.5–5.0 μg/kg/min) is routinely infused until the patient warms to 37°C and is continued in those with persistent hypertension or poor left ventricular function. Mean arterial pressure is usually maintained at 65–85 mmHg. Nitroprusside assists rewarming by vasodilation, and increases the cardiac output by decreasing afterload. Fluid administration to restore preload will then further increase cardiac output. Patients with chronic mitral regurgitation are especially benefitted by afterload reduction in the postoperative period.

Myocardial contractility may be depressed by acidosis, ischaemia, prior infarction, myocardial oedema following cardiopulmonary bypass, or cardiomyopathy. When heart rate, preload, and afterload have been optimized and cardiac output is still inadequate, efforts must be made to improve contractility. Of course, increased contractility occurs at the expense of increased myocardial oxygen demands, and drugs which augment contractility may worsen ischaemia. Dopamine is the most commonly used inotropic agent in the postoperative period. Doses up to 8 μg/kg/min will usually increase cardiac output without renal and splanchnic vasoconstriction, although undesirable tachycardia may occur at lower doses. Digoxin is rarely useful as an inotrope in the acute setting.

Low cardiac output

The presence of normal mentation, adequate urine output, and warm distal extremities indicates a normal cardiac output in the postoperative patient. A transient low output state may occur in patients between 4 and 16 hours postoperatively and is thought to be secondary to myocardial oedema. By 24 hours after operation, this oedema usually resolves. In the patient with hypotension and a high CVP, poor urine output, or signs of hypoperfusion, a pulmonary artery catheter may be placed to measure thermodilution cardiac output. Patients with normal preoperative cardiac output and bypass times less than 2 hours rarely have low cardiac output problems postoperatively.

In the patient with obvious low cardiac output, manifest by acidosis, hypotension, oliguria, and cool distal extremities, prompt evaluation and correction of arterial blood gases is imperative. Once heart rate, preload and afterload are optimal, attention is turned to increasing contractility. Treatment usually begins with an infusion of dopamine (3–5 μ/kg/min). Should a rapid improvement not be apparent, epinephrine (up to 100 ng/kg/min) may be substituted or added to the other agents if tachycardia or dysrhythmia do not occur. The addition of inotropes may allow more aggressive afterload reduction with nitroprusside or nitroglycerin. Acidosis will decrease the effectiveness of inotropes, and high doses of alpha-agonists, which may worsen acidosis by peripheral vasoconstriction in the patient with pulmonary hypertension and low cardiac output, should be avoided.

Intra-aortic balloon pump (IABP)

In some patients, drug treatment is inadequate to maintain an acceptable cardiac output. In these patients, use of intra-aortic balloon pumping may be indicated, and up to 15 per cent augmentation of cardiac output may be obtained from the IABP in suitable patients. The most common reason for insertion of the IABP is failure to wean from cardiopulmonary bypass despite moderate dosages of inotropes. The principal mechanism of action is systolic afterload reduction induced by balloon deflation and diastolic coronary and systemic blood flow augmentation induced by balloon inflation.

The intra-aortic balloon pump used for adults is usually 9.5 French diameter with a 40 cm^3 balloon pumped with CO$_2$ or helium. Triggering can be set from the R wave of the ECG or the dicrotic notch of the arterial wave form.

In patients with adequate femoral arteries, percutaneous IABP insertion is attempted. The common femoral artery just distal to the inguinal ligament is the best site for insertion, avoiding selective cannulation of the superficial or deep femoral arteries. Percutaneous insertion of the balloon while on cardiopulmonary bypass will succeed in most cases; cutdown is necessary in the remainder, with insertion under direct vision. A purse-string suture prevents leakage around the catheter. Occasionally, even with a guide wire placed, the balloon catheter cannot be threaded past occlusive lesions in the iliac artery. In these cases, ascending aortic balloon insertion is performed. This can be accomplished by placing the catheter through a purse-string suture and passing it just past the left subclavian artery. Repeat sternotomy is then required for balloon removal.

Careful monitoring of distal pedal pulses is necessary to avoid ischaemia of the lower leg. Heparin in therapeutic doses or dextran is recommended as soon as mediastinal bleeding has been controlled.

Balloon augmentation is continued until haemodynamic stability occurs, and then is weaned from the one-to-one mode to two-to-one, and finally three-to-one. Generally, the IABP is removed in the operating room, with thrombectomy and repair of the artery performed under direct vision.

Left ventricular assist systems

The current protocol at Stanford for the use of the left ventricular assist device calls for selected patients who have potentially reversible acute myocardial failure or who are transplant candidates who would not otherwise survive. Stanford, in conjunction with Navocor Medical Corporation, has been developing this system since 1972.

The two-component system consists of the implanted electromechanical energy convertor/blood pump and an external microprocessor control console. It is designed to assume total cardiac output function (up to 7.8 l/min). It is implanted in the left upper abdominal wall anterior to the abdominal fascia with inflow from the apex of the left ventricle and outflow to the ascending aorta. Severe pulmonary hypertension can lead to failure of this system due to lack of adequate blood flow to the left atrium.

Arrhythmias

The therapy of ventricular dysrhythmias first requires attention to normal acid base balance, oxygenation, potassium levels, magnesium levels, and the avoidance of arrhythmogenic drugs. In those patients with sustained ventricular tachycardia, lignocaine should be administered as a bolus and electrical cardioversion (usually 400 watt seconds) performed. Bretyllium or amiodarone (300 mg i.v.) may also be useful.

Chronic suppression of ventricular arrhythmias is achieved by slow taper of lignocaine infusion and concommitant treatment with procainamide or quinidine. Occasionally, other antiarrhythmics such as amiodarone, mexilitene, or lorcanide will be required. In those with refractory ventricular dysrhythmias, electrophysiological mapping and arrhythmia focus ablation or implantation of an automatic implantable defibrillator may become necessary.

Supraventricular tachyarrhythmias will usually respond to electrical cardioversion. Atrial flutter will convert with 50–100 watt second external synchronous cardioversion in most cases; occasionally, rapid atrial pacing can convert flutter to normal sinus rhythm. Up to 400 watt seconds synchronized cardioversion is necessary for the treatment of atrial fibrillation, usually starting with 100 watt seconds.

In haemodynamically stable patients, intravenous verapamil can slow or occasionally convert supraventricular tachyarrhythmias. It is administered in 2.5 mg doses every 15 min for heart rates of more than 130 up to a maximum of 10 mg in one hour. It is not administered if the MAP is less than 60, and should never be administered with an intravenous beta blocker. Intravenous beta blockade is reserved for the treatment of hypertension with tachycardia in those with normal hearts having undergone aortic surgery.

Digoxin is useful in most patients with supraventricular tachycardia for its effect on atrioventricular nodal conduction. High normal digoxin levels are mandatory for adequate control of recurrent supraventricular tachycardia with rapid ventricular response.

Quinidine is administered to haemodynamically stable patients to induce chemical cardioversion. If conversion has not occurred within several days despite therapeutic levels of digoxin, quinidine and potassium, then elective electrical cardioversion should be considered. Procainamide or amiodarone may be useful in selected patients in whom quinidine is ineffective.

Haemorrhage and coagulation management

Intraoperative haemostasis following protamine reversal of heparin effect is the first essential to the management of postoperative bleeding. Adequate heparin reversal is assured in the operating room with the activated clotting time (ACT).

Prolonged bypass periods may cause platelet dysfunction, which can be treated with platelet infusion. Massive blood replacement causes a dilutional thrombocytopenia; 6–8 units of platelets are routinely given for each 6–8 units of blood transfused. Preoperative hepatic congestion or coumadin administration will necessitate the administration of fresh frozen plasma for haemostasis. Further procoagulant therapy should be guided by tests of coagulation sent after protamine administration: platelet count, prothrombin time, partial thromboplastin time, thrombin time, fibrinogen, and possibly euglobulin lysis time. Epsilon aminocaproic acid may be useful in some patients with fibrinolysis following bypass, indicated by a prolonged euglobulin lysis time. Factor IX concentrates have occasionally been useful in the treatment of uncontrollable haemorrhage after bypass.

Positive and expiratory pressure (PEEP) is controversial in the treatment of postoperative mediastinal bleeding. PEEP up to 15 cmH$_2$O may be used in patients who are actively bleeding, although hypotension may occur. This level of PEEP probably does not significantly tamponade 'surgical' bleeding; however, it may slow bleeding from sites of lesser importance and provide time for repletion of deficient clotting factors.

Continued bleeding at rates exceeding 3 ml/kg/hour for several hours is an indication for surgical re-exploration. A continuing coagulopathy is not always a contraindication to re-exploration.

Cardiac tamponade

A low cardiac output associated with high preload and normal afterload and contractility in a patient with a recent history of mediastinal bleeding should prompt consideration of cardiac tamponade. Clinically, the diagnosis is made by the onset of low cardiac output and rapid diminution of chest tube drainage. A pulmonary artery catheter will demonstrate equalization of right atrial, right ventricular diastolic and pulmonary artery diastolic pressures. An echocardiogram will indicate fluid accumulation and the cardiac silhouette will be enlarged on chest X-ray. In the immediate postoperative period, surgical exploration is necessary.

Relative tamponade may occur in those with massive cardomegaly and myocardial oedema, and require reopening of the sternum. Temporary closure of the skin only or placement of an occlusive silastic sheet sewn to the skin may be necessary. In these patients, a constant irrigation of povidone iodine solution may help avoid mediastinitis prior to chest reclosure.

Delayed tamponade may be seen 5–10 days postoperatively as thrombus lyses and osmotic fluid influx occurs.

Drainage can sometimes be achieved with percutaneous needle catheter insertion or subxiphoid chest tube placement. Occasionally, severe pericarditis may result in tamponade.

Cardiac arrest

Cardiac arrest in the ICU cardiac surgical patient is managed by endotracheal intubation and ventilation with 100 per cent oxygen and closed chest massage. Sodium bicarbonate is administered. If the arrest is caused by ventricular tachycardia or fibrillation, lignocaine (1 mg/kg) is given. DC countershock cardioversion (300–400 watt seconds) is attempted. Bretyllium or procainamide may also be used. Epinephrine (1 mg) or isoproterenol may convert fine ventricular fibrillation to coarse fibrillation, which is more amenable to defibrillation.

If the arrest is asystolic, epinephrine and isoproterenol may induce ventricular fibrillation, which can then be cardioverted to an acceptable rhythm. Ventricular pacing may be effective in asystole. If tamponade is suspected, the chest must be opened at the bedside; internal cardiac massage may be more effective in producing an adequate cardiac output in some patients. All patients should receive NaHCO$_3$ every 10 min and calcium chloride (1 g) every 15 min, and arterial blood gases should be monitored frequently. Once resuscitated, infusions of inotroper should be very slowly tapered.

Sepsis

Systemic hypotension which occurs more than 48 hours postoperatively may be due to sepsis. Fever, leucocytosis, peripheral vasodilation, oliguria, gastritis, lung infiltrate, and signs of wound infection all indicate this diagnosis.

Blood, urine, and tracheal aspirates for culture and gram stain are immediately obtained. Broad spectrum antibiotics chosen to cover potential nosocomial infection are instituted. All indwelling lines are removed or changed.

Pulmonary artery catheterization may be performed for determination of cardiac output in the hemodynamically unstable patient. High outputs are usually seen in sepsis, indicating a need for volume repletion. Vasoconstricting agents such as neosynephrine or norepinephrine are occasionally useful in septic patients with extremely low systemic vascular resistance.

Endocarditis and medastinitis must be suspected in postoperative cardiac surgery patients without apparent focus for continuing sepsis. A white blood cell scan may be useful. In patients who are immunocompromised or have been on long-term antibiotics, a pointed search for opportunistic infection is made, especially fungaemia.

Pericarditis

Postcardiotomy pericarditis is heralded by the development of positional anterior chest pain, a friction rub, pericardial effusion, and fever or leucocytosis. Infection must be excluded.

Most patients will repond to an anti-inflammatory agent such as indomethacin (150–300 mg/day) in divided doses. In those who are anticoagulated or have a gastritic problems, low-dose steroids in conjunction with antacids may be beneficial. The majority of patients will respond to these manoeuvres. Postcardiotomy pericarditis rarely causes a significant pericardial effusion requiring drainage.

Renal failure

Renal failure may occur following cardiac surgery, especially in patients with pre-existing renal dysfunction or low output state. In the patient with postoperative renal failure, adequate renal perfusion must be maintained.

Diuretics are used sparingly, but may help to avoid oliguric renal failure. Nephrotoxic drugs are avoided. Those drugs excreted by the kidney are adjusted to appropriate dosages.

Daily determinations of creatinine clearance, fractional excretion of sodium, serum and urine osmolality, serum potassium, magnesium, calcium, and phosphorus are obtained. Metabolic encephalopathy, acidosis, hyperkalaemia, hypercalcaemia, hypermagnesia, hypernatraemia, and hyperphosphataemia are indications for dialysis. Oliguria with fluid overload is treated by plasma ultrafiltration. In the haemodynamically stable patient, haemodialysis is preferred; peritoneal dialysis may be better tolerated in the unstable patient.

Anticoagulation

Following coronary artery bypass surgery, all patients are treated with aspirin 80 mg/day and dipyridamole 75 mg three times daily. These are continued to prevent platelet aggregation-induced graft occlusion. On empirical grounds, any patient requiring more than a single endarterectomy is given coumadin to keep the prothrombin time 15–17 seconds for 3 months; aspirin and dipyridamole are then substituted.

Most patients at Stanford receive porcine valve replacements. In those with aortic valve replacement, coumadin is recommended for 6 weeks postoperatvely. In those with mitral valve replacement, coumadin is recommended for 12 weeks if sinus rhythm is present; in those with atrial fibrillation, coumadin is continued. Any patient with a thromboembolic episode also should remain on coumadin. In general, a prothrombin time of 16–19 seconds is sought. Patients receiving mechanical valves are heparinized postoperatively and placed on coumadin for life.

Care for the paediatric patient

Surgical repair of congenital cardiac anomalies often results in a paediatric patient who arrives in the ICU cold, vasoconstricted, and tachycardic. A warming blanket and external heating device are useful. Cold infants can rapidly become acidotic; pulmonary hypertension, if present, will worsen. Neonates do not shiver, but shivering in older children can markedly increase oxygen consumption and demand for cardiac output. Warming and adequate volume expansion (usually with blood) is carried out. Heart rates of 120–160 are optimal. A mean arterial pressure of 55–70 mmHg is maintained. Hypotension may be caused by hypoglycaemia or hypocalcaemia, in addition to the usual causes.

Long bypass runs or myocardial oedema may result in decreased contractility in spite of adequate preload. Dopamine up to 8 mg/kg/min may be useful. Isoproterenol may result in the salutary combination of increased contractility and heart rate, pulmonary vasodilation, and systemic afterload reduction. Prostaglandin E₁ has been effective in some paediatric patients with a high pulmonary vascular resistance. Nitroprusside, nitroglycerine, and epinephrine are all occasionally useful.

In general, more frequent monitoring and smaller incremental changes are safer in paediatric patients. Serum glucose and calcium should be checked and replaced regularly. Extubation should not be attempted until temperature and haemodynamics are stable, even if the child must receive additional sedation. A small endotracheal tube can easily become blocked by secretions; frequent suctioning is essential. Nurses experienced in the postoperative care of paediatric patients must be available.

Care of the heart transplant patient

Isoproterenol is usually begun following cardiopulmonary bypass for heart transplantation, and titrated to keep the heart rate at 90–100. The denervated heart cannot respond with reflex tachycardia to augment cardiac output if systemic vascular resistance or preload suddenly falls. Dopamine is usually added (3–5 μg/kg/min) to improve renal perfusion. Isoproterenol and dopamine can be discontinued after the immediate postoperative period, when temperature, volume shifts, and haemodynamics have stabilized. The transplanted heart will usually continue to have a mild tachycardia because of the absence of resting cholinergic tone. Evidence of reduced cardiac output in this period may indicate rejection, which must be aggressively diagnosed and treated.

Immunosuppression is currently maintained with cyclosporine, steroids, azathioprine, and anit-thymocyte globulin. Other immunosuppressive protocols are constantly undergoing evaluation. Treatment is begun preoperatively with an oral dose of cyclosporine adjusted for renal and hepatic dysfunction (10–18 mg/kg). Immediately following cardiopulmonary bypass, methylprednisoline 500 mg is given intravenously. Methylprednisolone is continued at 125 mg every 12 hours for three more doses. Prednisone is given by mouth twice daily. It is begun at 1 mg/kg/day and tapered to 0.5 mg/kg/day by one month, and to 0.2 mg/kg/day by 2 months following surgery.

Cyclosporine is administered enterally in the range of 5–10 mg/kg/day in two divided doses and adjusted to achieve trough serum levels of 200–250 ng/ml. After one month, most patients will require doses that achieve levels of 100–150 ng/ml.

Meticulous attention to the prevention and detection of infection is essential in these immunocompromised patients. In general, reverse isolation procedures are used until the first negative cardiac biopsy is obtained and continued in those with ongoing rejection or infection. All indwelling lines are rotated and cultured at least every 5 days. Transtracheal or endotracheal aspirates are performed when signs of fever or leucocytosis occur. Blood cultures, urine cultures, and occasionally needle aspiration or open lung biopsy and culture of infiltrates may be necessary. Rejection must be ruled out (by cardiac biopsy) in those with persistent fever. Early extubation and aggressive chest physiotherapy help to prevent tracheobronchial superinfection.

Cardiac biopsies are performed transvenously 6 days following surgery when rejection is suspected, 3 days after treatment of a rejection episode, and routinely every week for the first 6 weeks. Thereafter, they are performed every 2 weeks for 6 weeks, then every 3 months for life.

Myocyte necrosis on the cardiac biopsy requires treatment with methylprednisolone 1 g intravenously each day for 3 days. Another positive biopsy 3 days later is treated with another 3-day course of methylprednisolone; intramuscular rabbit anti-thymocyte globulin is added if the first check biopsy shows worsening rejection or rejection persists on the second check biopsy. Diastolic function, as measured by the isovolumic relaxation period calculated from the M-mode echocardiogram, appears to be a useful adjunct in the diagnosis of acute rejection.

Cardiac pacemaker implantation

Vincent A. Gaudiani MD
Sequoia Hospital, Redwood City, California, USA

Introduction

As the indications for temporary and permanent pacing have increased in the past decade techniques and equipment have also improved. We can now provide safe and efficient pacing for nearly all patients who require it.

This chapter concentrates on the techniques of placing pacing devices and summarizes some of the advances in equipment design which facilitate these techniques.

The operations

TEMPORARY PACING

Temporary pacing is now used as a routine to optimize haemodynamics in the postoperative period. The need for it is enhanced by the preoperative use of beta blockers and calcium channel agents in patients with coronary artery disease. The technique for placing temporary postoperative pacing wires is simple.

Placement of temporary wires

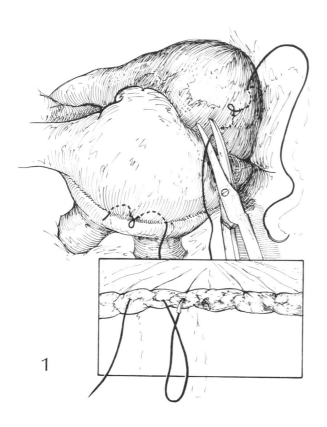

1

Nearly all patients after open heart surgery, except those in chronic atrial fibrillation, have both atrial and ventricular pacing wires placed. Two atrial wires are placed in Sondergard's groove along the atrial septum, just above the area where the incision is usually made in the left atrium for mitral valve replacement. The wires should be buried entirely in the atrial myocardium up to the insulated portion and the needle with its excess wire cut flush with the atrium. This prevents activation of the phrenic nerve during pacing. Only one atrial pacing wire is shown in the illustration, but two are always placed. Bipolar temporary pacing is uniformly more successful and simplifies reading the cardiac monitor. The second wire is also placed in the atrial septum or occasionally in the rosette of tissue formed by the removal of the atrial cannula. The exact location of the wires with respect to each other is not important so long as they do not touch. We prefer the atrial septum because there is more atrial myocardium to contact the wires.

Besides providing the opportunity for 'physiological pacing', temporary atrial wires facilitate the diagnosis and treatment of atrial arrhythmias. An atrial electrogram can be obtained by attaching one or both of the wires to the monitoring system. This permits accurate differentiation of supraventricular arrhythmias. Atrial tachycardia and flutter may be converted to sinus rhythm by rapid atrial pacing, thus overdriving the atrial rate above that of the arrhythmia. Sinus rhythm is then restored either by sudden termination of pacing or by gradual reduction of the atrially paced rate to the normal range.

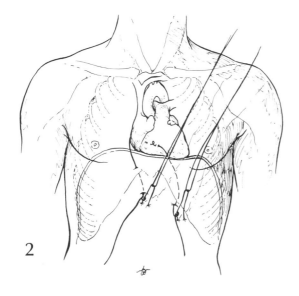

2

Atrial wires are always brought out on to the skin under the right costal margin and securely fastened with a non-absorbable suture. Temporary ventricular wires are placed in the anterior right ventricular muscle and fixed to the epicardial fat with a fine-grain gut suture. Exact location is unimportant so long as good contact is made with the myocardium. The wire is always brought out beneath the left costal margin. We generally place only one ventricular wire and use a subcutaneous earth (ground) to complete the circuit. A second ventricular wire is not usually necessary but is often helpful as a trigger for the intra-aortic balloon when this is required.

PERMANENT PACING

Pacing generators, leads, and insertion techniques have all improved in the past few years. Two improvements in lead design are passive and active fixation for endocardial leads and polyurethane insulation.

3

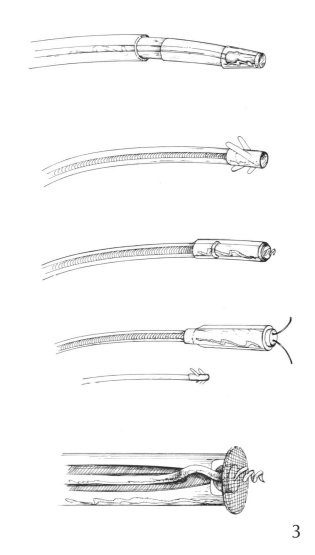

The leads illustrated show the standard type of electrode tip, the 'tined' tip which passively engages endocardial trabeculae and two 'active' fixation leads which the operator may insert in the subendocardial muscle. The final lead shown is a typical screw-in epicardial lead mounted on its inserter. With tined electrodes lead displacement occurs only rarely. Active fixation leads are usually reserved for special anatomical conditions, such as an unusually smooth, untrabeculated right ventricle, or for atrial placement in previously operated patients whose atrial appendage has been foreshortened.

Polyurethane insulation permits manufacture of a thinner lead which exposes less surface area to the bloodstream, reducing the potential for thrombosis. This is particularly useful for patients in whom two leads are required for the function of a 'dual chamber' pacemaker.

Our preferred technique for inserting endocardial leads into the central circulation is by cannulation of the patient's left side with placement of the generator in the left infraclavicular space. The location of the generator depends on the patient's handedness, activities and special circumstances. Generally, right-handed patients prefer a left-sided pacemaker generator. It is important, however, to inquire about specific activities such as bowling and shooting to prevent impairment by generator location. In special circumstances, such as in young women with cosmetic concerns, the generator may be positioned behind the breast.

3

Preoperative preparation

Preparation for pacer insertion should include a thorough explanation of the type of generator chosen, agreement on its location, explanation of the procedure, careful skin preparation and preoperative intravenous administration of antibiotics. At present we use a single intravenous dose of cephalosporin begun in the operating theatre. Skin preparation should extend from the angle of the jaw to the costal margin and from the axilla to beyond the midline. This permits cannulation of the subclavian, internal or external jugular veins or isolation of the cephalic vein.

Several aspects of preoperative preparation deserve special attention. First, we prefer to do all pacemaker implantations with standby general anaesthesia. Although this increases the cost of the procedure we believe the price is well paid for by the additional control available when a trained anaesthetist is monitoring the patient.

Secondly, if the patient has a high degree of atrioventricular (A-V) block a temporary transvenous pacer should be placed in advance. Manipulation of a pacing catheter within the heart often produces complete heart block with profound bradycardia; this can be controlled if a temporary pacer is in place.

As the vast majority of patients will have pacers inserted under local anaesthesia their arms should be well secured on the operating table so that they cannot inadvertently bring their hands into the operative field. A finger pulse plethysmograph is often a useful adjunct. The reassuring bleep of the electrocardiographic monitor is no substitute for pulse wave-form, and an occasional disaster from mistaking a pacing spike for a QRS complex will be averted.

Insertion of the catheter

4 & 5

Our preferred approach to the placement of the pacing catheter is through an infraclavicular incision. The incision should be 3–4 cm below the clavicle and extend from the deltopectoral groove medially for 5 or 6 cm. This is deepened to the pectoralis fascia. A subcutaneous pocket is then formed superiorly towards the calvicle, and inferiorly for 3–4 cm. With the patient placed in the Trendelenberg position the subclavian vein is punctured and a guide wire placed in the central circulation. Its position in the superior vena cava should be confirmed fluoroscopically. If A-V pacing is required a second wire is introduced through a separate puncture. Although the thinner polyurethane leads can be introduced through a single introducer, we have had less interference between the catheters during placement by using two separate entries.

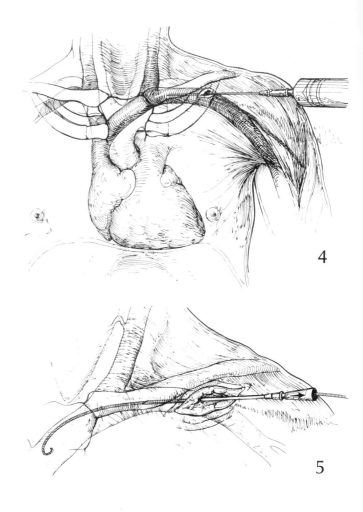

4

5

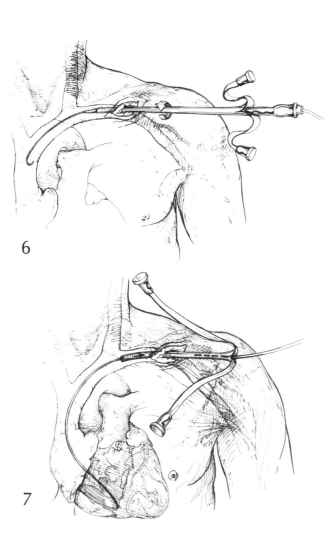

6

7

6 & 7

Insertion of a peel-away catheter introduced over the guide wire is illustrated here. The peel-away introducer is stiff and can perforate a central vein; therefore it must be inserted with a gentle twisting motion and the location of the guide wire must be known. Removal of the guide wire and dilator permits introduction of the permanent pacing catheter as shown in the lower illustration.

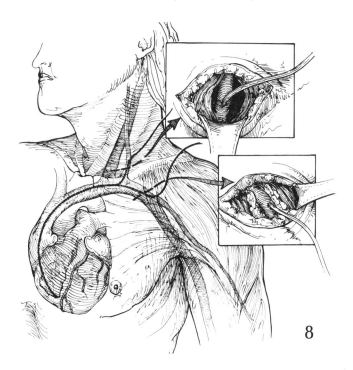

8

8

The internal jugular, external jugular or cephalic vein may be used instead of the subclavian vein as sites for entering the central circulation. If the internal jugular vein is selected the pacing catheter may be introduced directly through a purse-string suture in the vein, the lead positioned in the right ventricular apex and the lead connector tunnelled to the subclavicular pocket either over or under the clavicle. Alternatively, the external jugular or cephalic vein may be isolated and cannulated. Both of these veins may, of course, be tied off distally.

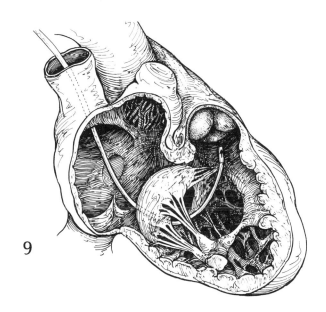

9

9

Ventricular lead placement

The stilette of the placing catheter should be so formed as to facilitate entry into the right ventricle. When the lead is inserted with a gentle 'J' shape in the stilette, it frequently crosses the tricuspid valve spontaneously. Therefore changes in rhythm, particularly higher degrees of A-V block, premature ventricular beats or ventricular tachycardia, should be anticipated.

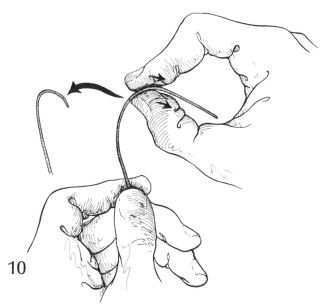

10

10

The lead and curved stilette are now advanced into the pulmonary artery. Seeing the tip of the lead in the proximal pulmonary artery on the fluoroscope is certain proof that it has not coiled in a large right atrium, crossed a patent foramen ovale or entered the coronary sinus.

11

In order to position the pacing catheter in the right ventricular apex the pacing catheter and curved stilette are withdrawn from the pulmonary outflow tract, the catheter flopping down towards the right ventricular apex when no longer constrained by the outflow tract.

12

The curved stilette is now carefully removed and replaced with a straight stilette. This assembly is then advanced to the right ventricular apex. Although stilettes are now being manufactured to be more flexible, this assembly can perforate the thin apical muscle. The key, therefore, is gently to engage the trabeculae at the apex without undue force.

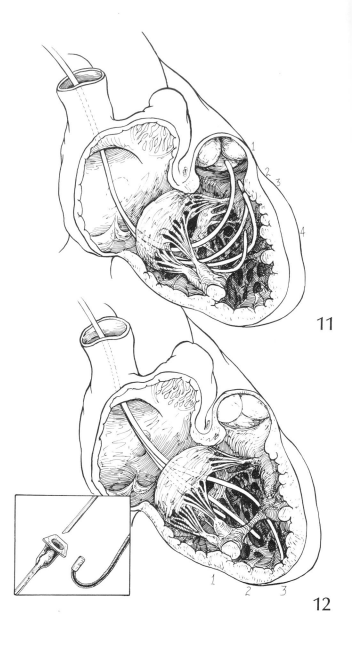

11

12

13

The final position of the catheter and its tip are illustrated here. The body of the catheter within the heart should be slack enough to permit a 'windscreen wiper' motion similar to that seen in a right coronary arteriogram. The patient should be asked to breathe deeply and cough while being paced by the catheter. Pacing should remain perfect and the catheter on fluoroscopy should continue to move rhythmically with the heart.

Testing the pacing catheter for sensing and threshold functions is described on p. 87. When the position is judged satisfactory the catheter should be fixed to the pectoralis fascia with a non-absorbable suture.

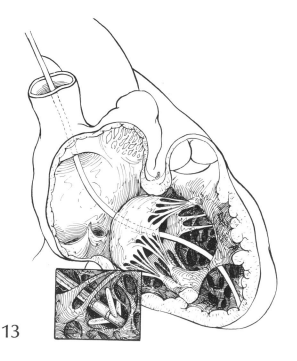

13

Atrial lead placement

Both active and passive fixation leads may be used. Passive fixation leads 'remember' their original form, and therefore assume a satisfactory 'J' shape when the straight stilette has been removed. Active fixation leads are straight, but to ease catheter manipulation within the atrium they are packaged with a 'J'-shaped stilette which is removed after fixation of the lead in the atrial wall. At present we recommend using the simplest, sturdiest endocardial 'screw-in' lead available. Those with moving parts, retractable engaging devices or electrodes which are separate from the screw are difficult to manipulate or fail more frequently during insertion.

14 & 15

Both active and passive fixation leads should be placed in the central circulation using a straight stilette and a technique identical to that used for ventricular catheters. The lead should be finally positioned low in the right atrium just above the diaphragm, slightly to the right of the spine fluoroscopically. Thus if the catheter passes through the tricuspid valve its position is incorrect for atrial placement and it is withdrawn into the atrium above the valve. When the stilette is removed from a passive fixation lead the 'J' shape naturally re-forms. If an active fixation lead is used the preformed 'J' stilette is inserted.

16

In either case it is important to know the exact orientation of the 'J' within the atrium. This is easily done by manipulating the catheter so that the tip of the 'J' points medially and somewhat anteriorly inside the atrium. This position places the 'J' close to the opening of the atrial appendage. The catheter is then withdrawn gently and the tip of the catheter engages the orifice of the atrial appendage like a grappling hook.

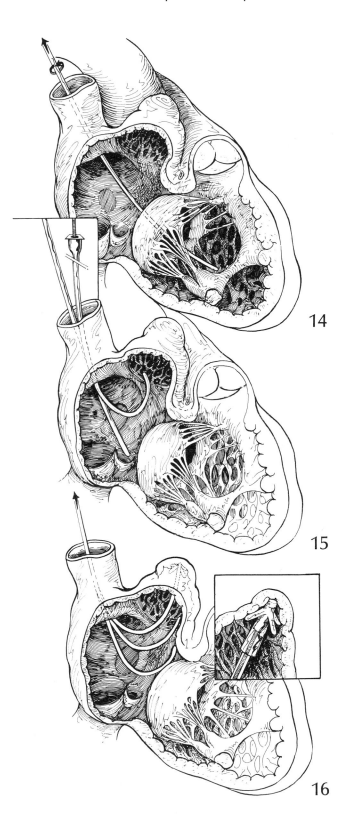

14

15

16

17

When this occurs the operator can recognize it on the fluoroscope by two means. First, the tip of the 'J' stops moving and further catheter withdrawal bends the 'J' open. Second, the tip of the 'J' wags rhythmically with the motion of the atrial appendage. If preliminary threshold and sensing values are satisfactory the final adjustment of lead position is made. At full inspiration the 'J' should be bent open by the downward movement of the heart so that it forms a 90° angle with regard to the body of the catheter. At full expiration the 'J' should close to a point just short of its relaxed shape. Such a position maintains tension at the tip of the 'J' at all times and reduces the likelihood of dislodgement. Repeat electrophysiological measurements are performed and the catheter is fixed to the pectoralis fascia.

If an active fixation lead is used the 'J' stilette is used to grapple the catheter along the atrial wall. In general, manipulation of endocardial screw-in electrodes is easier if all movements are accompanied by a gentle counter-clockwise twist. This prevents a screw from engaging endocardium prematurely. When the catheter tip engages in the required position the 'J' stilette is held still while the catheter is twisted clockwise a few times on the axis of the stilette. This preliminary engagement by the screw permits electrophysiological testing. If the results are satisfactory six to ten full twists are applied, the 'J' stilette withdrawn and the catheter retested.

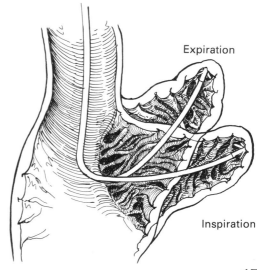

Expiration

Inspiration

17

Epicardial lead placement

The need for thoracotomy to achieve satisfactory permanent pacing has lessened as endocardial techniques have improved. The main indication for transthoracic pacing is the presence of a tricuspid prosthesis. Only rarely will a transvenous technique fail with the active fixation endocardial leads now available. Epicardial pacing is secure but it is more traumatic and expensive than the transvenous techniques and more difficult to revise if complications occur.

18 & 19

The patient is prepared for a major thoracotomy and placed on the table with a small roll under the left chest. A left inframammary incision is made. If possible the pectoralis muscle is retracted rather than cut. The chest is entered in the fifth or sixth intercostal space without rib resection. The pericardium is opened and a site is selected free of epicardial coronary vessels. Two screw-in electrodes are placed 1–2 cm apart. Three and a half turns are usually sufficient to engage the electrode.

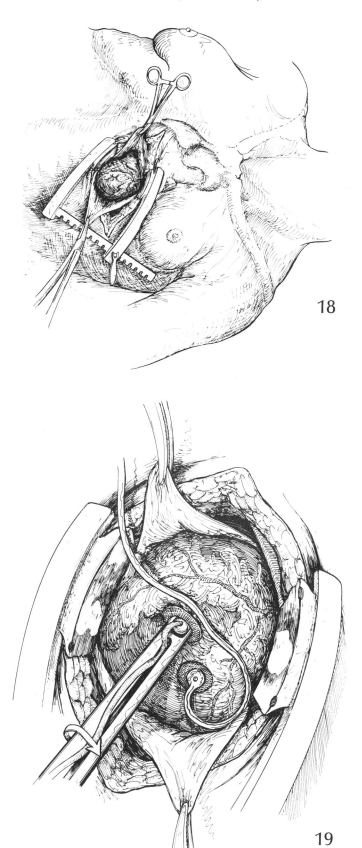

18

19

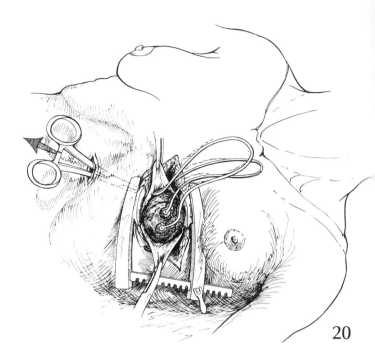

20

20 & 21

The leads are brought to a subcutaneous site. The pacemaker generator site should be where movements and articles of clothing, especially belts, will not interfere with comfort.

Although subxyphoid approaches for the insertion of a permanent right ventricular wire are well described, they do bear the risk of fatal haemorrhage from the right ventricular wall if the procedure is not performed with care.

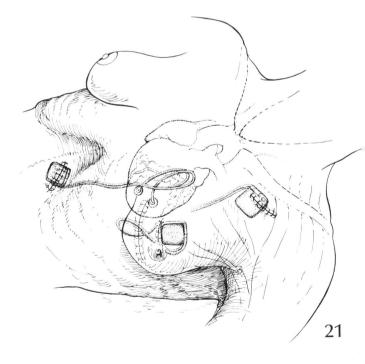

21

22

The skin incision is made in the mid-line, its upper limit being the lower part of the sternum (a). The xiphisternum is excised. The incision is deepened until the diaphragm is reached (b). A self-retaining retractor will expose the inferior surface of the right ventricle.

23

Two screw-in electrodes are placed, care again being taken to avoid coronary branches. The electrodes used for right ventricular placement should have two turns only in their screws and the screw-in portion may be flattened before insertion to avoid penetration into the right ventricular cavity.

22

23

Testing

The purpose of testing pacing leads is to assure a low pacing threshold and adequate sensing in order to permit accurate and economic pacer function. An increasing variety of devices is available for this purpose, and each operator should become familiar with one of them.

To test threshold, the pulse width of the testing device is set to match that of the chosen generator. The pacing rate is set above the patient's intrinsic rate, and millivolt output is gradually decreased until capture is lost. The procedure is then repeated, starting with low millivolt output and increasing this until the threshold is regained. For a newly placed lead, threshold should be less than 1 mV. For an endocardial lead, the chronic threshold should be less than 1.5 mV. This results in a resistance of about 400–800 Ω. Epicardial leads usually have somewhat higher thresholds. A very low resistance (less than 250 Ω) suggests a lead fracture with leakage of current. Atrial thresholds are measured in the same manner, but an acceptable threshold is 2–2.5 mV.

Sensing can only be tested if the patient has an intrinsic rhythm. Most modern generators can sense ventricular signals of less than 2 mV, but we prefer signals higer than 4 mV to assure an adequate signal-to-noise ratio. Many testing devices stop pacing when testing sensing. Therefore, care must be taken to prevent prolonged bradycardia. The usual range of sensed ventricular signals is 4–20 mV.

P wave signals are generally much smaller, and an adequate P wave signal is 2–4 mV. The exact method of determining R wave or P wave size depends on the design of the testing device. Because dual chambered pacing has become so popular, it is important to test for the presence and size of retrograde P waves conducted back to the atrium during the ventricular pacing phase. This permits appropriate programming of the AV pacer to 'blank' this signal and prevent endless loop tachycardias.

The anatomy of congenital heart disease

Robert H. Anderson BSc, MD, MRCPath
Joseph Levy Professor of Paediatric Cardiac Morphology, Cardiothoracic Institute, Brompton Hospital, London, UK

Benson R. Wilcox MD
Professor and Chief of Cardiothoracic Surgery, University of North Carolina, Chapel Hill, North Carolina, USA

Introduction

Knowledge of detailed cardiac anatomy is a prerequisite for successful surgery. Nowhere is this more important than in the setting of congenital cardiac malformations. Although the anatomy displayed in these anomalies is often complex, it is not necessarily difficult to understand. This introductory chapter describes the basic rules of cardiac anatomy which permit the surgeon to diagnose and recognize the arrangement of the cardiac chambers at surgery, at the same time providing guidelines to the position of the vital conduction tissues. The basic layout of the heart should, of course, be established prior to commencement of intracardiac procedures. The diagnosis of even the most complex cases demands in the first instance only the distinction of a right atrium from a left atrium, a right ventricle from a left ventricle and an aorta from a pulmonary trunk. After describing the anatomy which permits distinction of these various chambers and vessels, therefore, we will outline an approach for simple sequential segmental analysis[1]. Obviously, the anatomy of 'holes' and 'stenoses', etc. are of equal or even greater significance, but they will be described briefly in an introduction to the appropriate chapter. Here we are concerned specifically with setting the 'ground rules' for a systematic approach to cardiac anatomy.

Approaches to the heart

In the usual arrangement the heart lies in the mediastinum with its apex pointing to the left and two-thirds of its bulk to the left of the midline. An unusual location of the heart should alert the surgeon to the possibility of complex malformations, although these are not always present. When the heart is abnormally located, our preference is to describe this finding in simple terms, e.g. heart mostly in the right chest with the apex pointing to the left or as appropriate. Whatever its position, the heart and great vessels can be approached either through the midline anteriorly or via the thoracic cavities.

A median sternotomy is used most frequently. The anterior mediastinum immediately behind the sternum is devoid of vital structures. This tissue plane is reached through separate incisions in the suprasternal notch and beneath the xiphoid process, the two being joined by blunt dissection. Splitting the sternum will then expose the pericardial sac between the pleural cavities. An important structure in this region in the infant is the thymus gland. This wraps itself over the anterolateral aspects of the pericardium in the area of the arterial pole. The gland itself is made up of two lateral lobes joined by a midline isthmus which sometimes must be divided or partially excised to provide adequate exposure. Care must be taken with its arterial supply from the internal thoracic and inferior thyroid arteries. If divided, these arteries may retract beneath the sternum and produce troublesome bleeding. The thymic veins are also a potential problem, being fragile structures which often empty via a common trunk to the left brachiocephalic vein. This may be inadvertently damaged by undue traction.

Once the pericardium is exposed via a median sternotomy, access to the heart poses few problems. The vagus and phrenic nerves traverse the length of the pericardium well clear of the operative field, the phrenic nerves anterior and the vagi posterior to the lung hila respectively. The phrenic nerves may be vulnerable when the pericardium is harvested for use as an intracardiac patch or baffle. Again, excessive traction on the pericardial cavity is to be avoided, since this can avulse the origin of the pericardiaco-phrenic arteries which accompany the phrenic nerves. The internal thoracic arteries themselves should not be at risk during exposure of the heart via a median sternotomy but may be damaged when the incision is closed.

Lateral thoracotomies provide exposure either to the heart or great vessels via the pleural spaces. Most frequently these incisions are made in the fourth intercostal space, using the posterior bloodless triangle between the edges of the latissimus dorsi, trapezius and the teres major muscles. The floor of this triangle is the sixth space, but division of the latissimus posteriorly, together with serratus anteriorly, frees the scapula and provides access to the fourth space which is identified by counting from above. An incision midway between the ribs avoids the intercostal neurovascular bundle which is protected beneath the lower margin of the fourth rib. Having entered the pleural space on the left side, retraction of the lung posteriorly exposes the middle mediastinum with the left thymic lobe overlying the pericardium and the aortic arch with its associated nerves and vessels. If access is needed to the heart, this is usually done anterior to the phrenic nerve. More frequently the aortic isthmus and descending aorta are approached and then the lung is retracted anteriorly and the parietal pleura divided on its medial aspect posterior to the vagus nerve. An important structure in this area is the left recurrent laryngeal nerve (*Figure 1*) which takes origin from the vagus and passes round the inferior border of the ligamentum arteriosum (or ductus). Excessive traction to the vagus can cause injury to this structure just as readily as direct trauma in the environs of the ligamentum. The thoracic duct ascends through this area to drain into the left jugular vein at its junction with the internal jugular. Accessory lymph channels draining into the duct can be troublesome when dissecting the origin of the left subclavian artery.

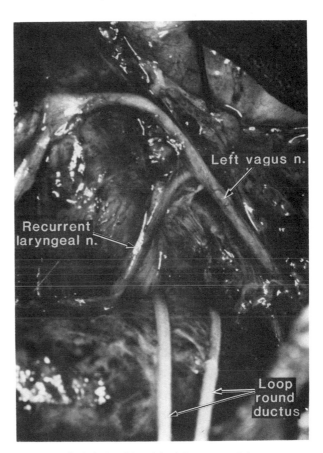

Figure 1. The relationship of the left vagus and the recurrent laryngeal nerve to the aortic arch as seen through a left thoracotomy

A right thoracotomy is performed in similar fashion and then the heart can be reached via the fifth interspace or the right-sided great vessels can be reached via the fourth interspace. When approaching the right pulmonary artery it is sometimes useful to divide the azygos vein near its junction with the superior vena cava. On the right side the recurrent laryngeal nerve passes round the subclavian artery as it courses medially from the vagus towards the larynx. Also encircling the artery on this side is the ansa subclavia, a loop from the sympathetic trunk. Damage to this structure can result in Horner's syndrome.

Surface anatomy of the heart

Opening the pericardial cavity reveals the surface of the heart, which almost always is mostly in the left hemithorax with its apex pointing to the left. Important and readily recognizable landmarks enable the nature of the cardiac chambers to be determined with considerable accuracy by external inspection. Attention should first be directed to the atrial appendages (*Figure 2*). These outpouchings from

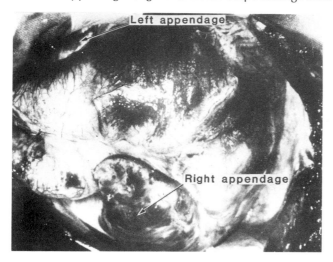

Figure 2. The usual arrangement of the atrial appendages as seen through a medial sternotomy

the venous atrial components usually clasp the arterial pedicle. The finding of both appendages on the same side of the pedicle is itself an anomaly – so-called juxtaposition of the atrial appendages. Left-sided juxtaposition (*Figure 3*) is almost always associated with abnormal chamber connections[2], but right-sided juxtaposition (*Figure 4*) tends to be found with relatively simple malformations

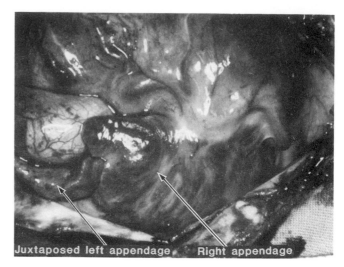

Figure 3. A morphological specimen with left juxtaposition of the atrial appendages

such as atrial septal defect[3]. Juxtaposition in itself is a nuisance to the surgeon since it will necessitate alterations in planning the cannulation, etc. It can also give rise to difficulty in atrial surgery for complete transposition. However, once recognized, the problems produced are readily surmountable.

Having established the position of the appendages, the next step is to establish their morphological nature. The shape and arrangement of the appendage is by far the most reliable means of distinguishing the morphologically right from the morphologically left atrium*. The right appendage has a triangular shape with a broad base at its junction with the atrial venous component. The left appendage is much narrower and crenellated with a

* When we use the terms 'right' and 'left' we will use them to indicate morphology. Where position is abnormal, this will be indicated separately.

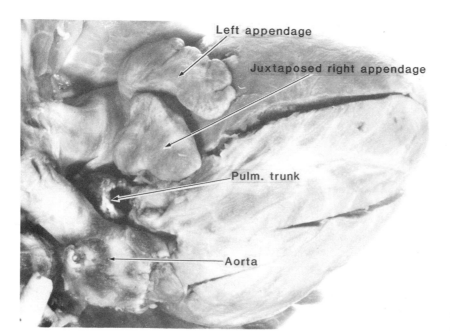

Figure 4. Right juxtaposition of the atrial appendages as seen through a median sternotomy

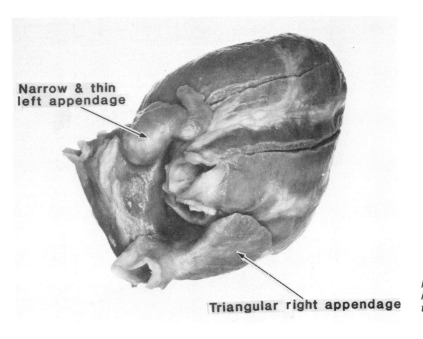

Narrow & thin
left appendage

Triangular right appendage

Figure 5. The anatomy of the atrial appendages as seen in an autopsy heart placed in surgical orientation with the great arteries removed

narrow atrial junction. These differences are best appreciated by inspection of the isolated heart (*Figure 5*) but can be easily seen at straightforward surgical inspection (see *Figure 2*). In most instances the triangular appendage is right-sided and the narrow, hooked appendage is left-sided (usual atrial arrangement – so-called 'situs solitus'). Rarely the hooked appendage is right-sided and the triangular one is left-sided; the mirror-image or 'inverted' arrangement. Mirror-image is a better term than 'inversus' because the atria are not turned upside down. More frequently in congenitally malformed hearts an arrangement will be found in which the appendages have the same morphology (isomeric). Then, either both are broad and triangular or both are hooked and narrow[4]. The syndromes associated with the presence of isomeric atrial appendages are known as the 'splenic syndromes' or visceral heterotaxy. Interest in these constellations has been largely the province of the pathologist, but by the simple expedient of inspecting the appendages the surgeon has the means of diagnosing these entities during life and drawing the inferences which go with the recognition of right atrial isomerism ('asplenia') or left atrial isomerism ('polysplenia').

While inspecting the appendages the surgeon will at the same time examine their atrial junctions. Here again there is a vital difference between morphologically right and left sides. The right junction is the extensive terminal sulcus, marking the site of the internal terminal crest. Lying in the terminal sulcus, in an immediate subendocardial position and lateral to the crest of the atrial appendage, is the sinus node (*Figure 6*). The left junction is not marked by any such prominent sulcus and no conduction tissue is present at this junction. These findings complement the information gained from appendage position. Thus, with the usual atrial arrangement the sinus node is right-sided, whereas with mirror-image atria it is a left-sided structure. In right atrial isomerism there are bilateral sinus nodes, but in left atrial isomerism the sinus node is hypoplastic and abnormally positioned, being variously located in the posterior atrial wall[5].

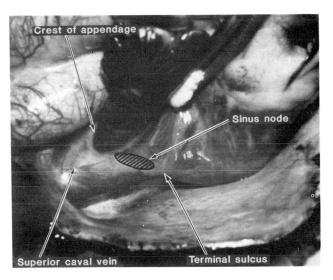

Crest of appendage

Sinus node

Superior caval vein

Terminal sulcus

Figure 6. The crest of the right atrial appendage, the terminal sulcus and the site of the sinus node as seen by the surgeon through a median sternotomy

Inspection of the appendages should lead attention directly to the venoatrial connections. Here the important features to note are abnormal connections of either the pulmonary veins or the venae cava. A persistent left superior vena cava should be searched for between the left appendage and the left pulmonary veins, while the finding of left atrial isomerism should always alert the surgeon to the likelihood that the inferior caval vein is interrupted and continued via the azygos or hemiazygos veins, which would be correspondingly enlarged.

Considerable information can be derived from external inspection concerning the ventricular arrangement. Here it is the descending branches of the coronary arteries which are the guide[6]. In the usual situation the anterior descending coronary artery arises from the left coronary artery and descends close to the obtuse margin of the ventricular mass (*Figure 5*). When the anterior descending artery arises from the right-sided coronary artery then almost always there is a mirror-image ventricular arrangement with the left ventricle on the right side. The precise chamber connections present will depend upon the atrial arrangement, but this arterial arrangement should immediately suggest the presence of corrected transposition, which should be readily identified from the arterial relationship (*see below*). The other abnormal arterial arrangement to be sought by inspection is the presence of two 'delimiting' arteries on the anterior surface of the ventricular mass, rather than one prominent descending artery. This indicates a disproportion between the size of the ventricular chambers. Usually it suggests the presence of a dominant left ventricle and a rudimentary right ventricle, such as is found in 'single ventricle' or tricuspid atresia. Alternatively, the finding of no descending arteries on the anterior ventricular surface should raise the suspicion of a solitary indeterminate ventricular chamber or else a dominant right ventricle with a posterior rudimentary left ventricle.

The final feature to be inspected, which will usually be studied at the same time as the ventricular mass, is the relationship of the arterial trunks. The first step is to confirm the presence of separate aortic and pulmonary trunks as opposed to a common truncus. When separate trunks are found then almost always the aortic trunk is posterior and right-sided and the pulmonary trunk spirals around it as it divides. Abnormal relationships of the great arteries always indicate intracardiac malformations, but the connections of the cardiac chambers cannot be inferred from an abnormal relation. At best the anomalous arterial positions raise the suspicion of a given lesion. Thus, most frequently an anterior and right-sided aorta is found with complete transposition but this can be seen with double outlet right ventricle. An anterior and left-sided aorta suggests corrected transposition but it, too, can be found with double outlet right ventricle or rarely with usual atrioventricular and ventriculoarterial connections – so-called 'anatomically corrected malposition'. In similar fashion it cannot be presumed that the ventriculoarterial connections are normal simply because the arterial trunks are 'normally related'. Often there are 'normal' arterial relationships in the presence of double outlet right ventricle and rarely this arrangement can be found with complete transposition.

Anatomy of the cardiac chambers

In the previous section we have described how it is possible to recognize the morphology of the different chambers, but at the same time we have alluded to the possibility that these chambers are not always in their usual position, nor connected to their usual neighbours. However, each chamber has a relatively constant anatomy irrespective of its position or its connections, although subtle changes in morphology are found in the presence of abnormal chamber connections. In this section we will describe the anticipated morphology for the normal cardiac chambers, adding remarks concerning abnormal chambers where pertinent.

The right atrium

The right atrium has the extensive triangular appendage separated from the venous sinus by the terminal sulcus (*Figure 7*). As usually seen by the surgeon, the superior caval vein enters the left-hand side and the inferior caval vein the right-hand side of the sleeve-like sinus, which is separated inferiorly by Waterston's groove from the right pulmonary veins. Waterston's groove marks the site of the interatrial septum, and is the surface of a considerable infolding of the right and left atrial walls. As discussed above, the terminal sulcus is a vital surgical landmark since immediately beneath its epicardial surface lies the sinus node.

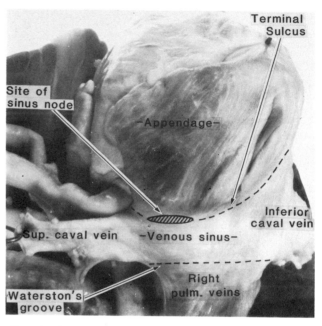

Figure 7. An anatomical specimen arranged to show the terminal sulcus and Waterston's groove

Opening the right atrium with the freedom permitted the morphologist reveals the extensive terminal crest which underlies the terminal sulcus (*Figure 8*). This swings round the orifices of both the superior and inferior caval veins. An extension from the terminal crest then runs into the atrial septum and, as seen by the surgeon, strikes towards the vestibule of the tricuspid valve. This is the sinus septum which separates the orifices of the inferior caval vein and the coronary sinus. Extending as opposing sickle-shaped folds from this septum are the Eustachian and Thebesian valves, guarding the inferior caval and coronary sinus orifices respectively. The commissure of these two valves buries itself in the sinus septum and runs toward the left-hand margin of the tricuspid vestibule. This important fibrous structure, which becomes buried in the muscular atrial septum, is the tendon of Todaro. As seen by the surgeon there is then an extensive pouch above the coronary sinus orifice between it, the tricuspid valve attachment and the extension of the terminal crest. This is the post-Eustachian sinus (of Keith). A triangular area is thus formed with the post-Eustachian sinus as its

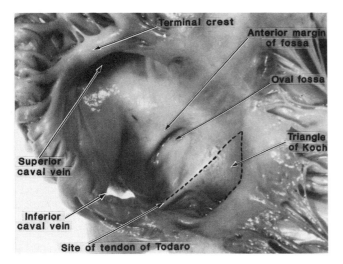

Figure 8. The right atrium opened by the morphologist to illustrate the salient anatomical features

base. Its inferior border (as viewed operatively) is the site of the tendon of Todaro, and its superior border is the site of annular attachment of the septal leaflet of the tricuspid valve. This vital area is the triangle of Koch. The atrioventricular node is entirely contained within its confines and the atrioventricular bundle penetrates towards the left ventricular outflow tract at its apex (Figure 9).

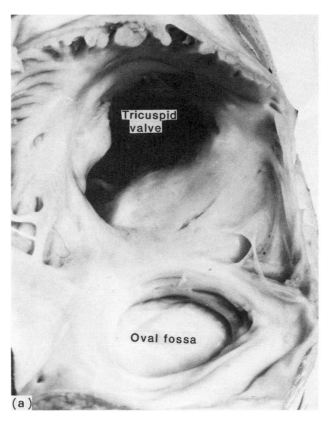

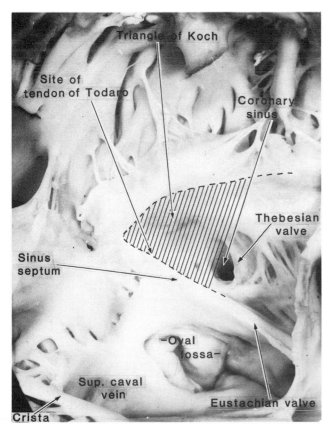

Figure 9. The triangle of Koch as seen by the surgeon through a right atriotomy

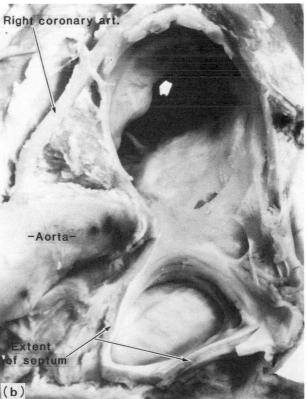

Figure 10. An anatomical specimen orientated in surgical fashion to illustrate the true extent of the atrial septum. The subject is shown before (a) and after (b) dissection of the non-septal structures

Between the triangle of Koch and the orifice of the superior caval vein is the right atrial surface of the oval fossa. At first sight this entire surface gives the impression of being a septal structure (*Figure 10*). Dissection shows that this is not the case (*Figure 10b*). The septal area is confined to the floor of the fossa and its immediate surrounds[7]. The extensive mound to the left-hand side of the fossa is the atrial wall overlying the aortic root. The so-called superior limbus between the fossa and the superior caval orifice (seen in inferior position by the surgeon) is simply the infolded walls of the interatrial sulcus (Waterston's groove). The right-hand margin is the wall of the inferior caval vein. Finally, the 'inferior' limbus (seen superiorly by the surgeon) is the sinus septum and most of this is an atrioventricular septal structure (*see below*).

The left atrium

The proportions of the left atrium formed by appendage and venous component are reversed compared to the right atrium, and overall the left atrium has a much simpler structure. The venous component receives the four pulmonary veins, one at each corner. This leads directly into the mitral vestibule. As seen by the surgeon entering through the atrial roof (*Figure 11*) the narrow junction with the hooked appendage is in the left-hand position while the septal surface is to the right. The sweep of muscular tissue above the mitral vestibule is the extensive anterior atrial wall related to the aortic root. The inferior margin of the mitral vestibule overlies the coronary sinus as it runs round from the obtuse margin of the ventricular mass. The septal surface of the left atrium is much simpler than the right and is the flap valve of the oval fossa

The atrioventricular junction

The surgeon will never see the entirety of the atrioventricular junction although at different times he will be concerned with its various parts. However, a knowledge of the junction in its entirety is fundamental to the proper understanding of several congenital anomalies (e.g. atrioventricular septal defects)[8]. In this section, therefore, we will detail the anatomy of the entire region.

The best appreciation of the junction (*Figure 12*) is obtained by removing the atrial chambers and great arteries and viewing it from the superior aspect. The dominant feature is the 'wedge' position of the aortic valve. Equally significant is the oblique orientation of the mitral and tricuspid valve rings relative to the aortic root. Although we usually speak of the valve annuli, none of the four cardiac valves has a true and complete fibrous ring which supports its leaflets. The mitral annulus approximates most closely to the concept of a valve ring, but in its parietal parts there is very little collagenous tissue supporting the valve mural leaflet and separating the atrial and ventricular myocardial masses. In the tricuspid ring it is very rare to find a collagenous annulus and usually it is the fibro-fatty atrioventricular sulcus which separates atrial muscle from the ventricular mass. When the arterial valves are considered, then the concept of a 'ring' becomes totally deficient. Rather, each of the semilunar valve leaflets is attached to the underlying ventricular structures. The subarterial roots are therefore coronet-like structures, tenting up in the areas of the commissures and sweeping down to the nadir of the leaflet attachments. These attachments in the pulmonary 'ring' are exclusively to muscular structures. However, in the case of the aortic valve a good half of the circumference is supported by and attached to fibrous and collagenous tissues. This is because, as a consequence of its wedge position, the aortic valve is in extensive fibrous continuity with both the mitral and tricuspid valves. The entire 'anterior' leaflet of the mitral valve has fibrous continuity with two of the aortic leaflets. For this reason, this leaflet of the mitral valve is more accurately termed the aortic leaflet, differentiating it in this way from the mural leaflet. The two ends of the region of aortic-mitral valvar continuity are thickened to form the fibrous trigones (*Figure 13*). The

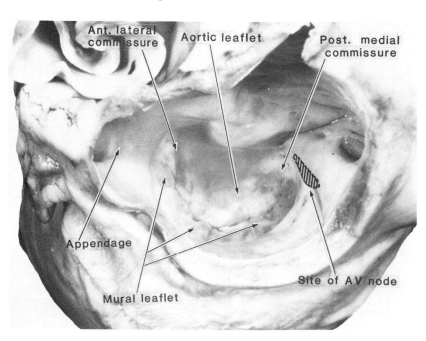

Figure 11. The morphologist's view of the left atrium orientated in surgical fashion

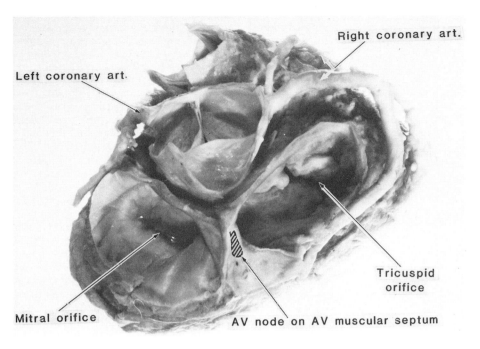

Right coronary art.

Left coronary art.

Tricuspid
orifice

Mitral orifice

AV node on AV muscular septum

Figure 12. An anatomical dissection of the atrioventricular junction viewed from the atrial aspect after removal of the atrial chambers and the arterial trunks. Note the arrangement of the coronary arteries and the site of the atrioventricular node

right fibrous trigone is an integral part of the fibrous mass where the aortic root is continuous with the tricuspid annulus, and this whole area is usually called the central fibrous body. The part between the aortic root and the right side of the heart is the so-called membranous septum, and this forms the medial wall of the subaortic outflow tract immediately beneath the commissure between the right coronary and non-coronary aortic valve leaflets. Long axis section taken at right angles to the septum through this region (*Figure 14*) shows that the tricuspid valve septal leaflet is attached to the right-sided aspect of this area. It is this tricuspid valve attachment

which divides the membranous septum into its atrioventricular and interventricular components.

The obliquity of the mitral and tricuspid valve rings relative to each other is responsible for the unusual morphology of the septum immediately behind the central fibrous body. A dissection of the region shows how the wedged aortic outflow tract 'lifts' the aortic leaflet of the mitral valve away from the inlet part of the ventricular septum. Because of this it is over only a short distance that the two atrioventricular valves are attached to opposite sides of the septum, or in other words 'face' each other (*Figure 15*). But in this facing area the tricuspid

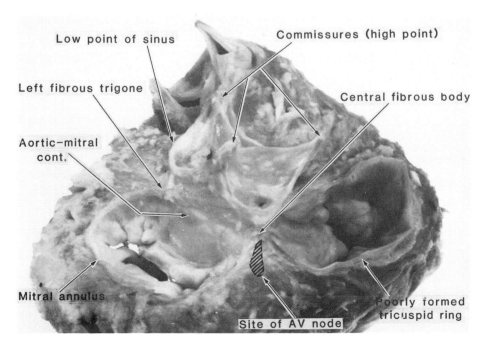

Low point of sinus   Commissures (high point)

Left fibrous trigone

Central fibrous body

Aortic–mitral
cont.

Mitral annulus

Site of AV node

Poorly formed
tricuspid ring

Figure 13. Further dissection of the atrioventricular junction illustrating the site of the fibrous trigones and morphology of the aortic valve

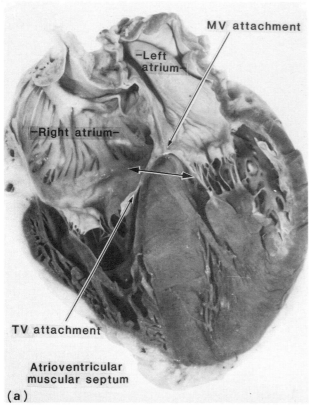

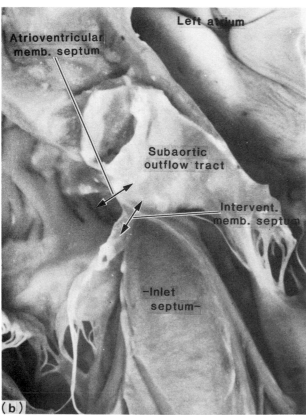

(a)

(b)

Figure 14. Cross-sections through the heart at right-angles to the inlet septum showing (a) the atrioventricular muscular septum and (b) the components of the membranous septum. MV = mitral valve; TV = tricuspid valve

valve is attached to the septum more towards the ventricular apex than is the mitral valve. By virtue of these differential levels of attachment, part of the septum interposes between the left ventricle and the right atrium (*Figure 14b*). This is the atrioventricular *muscular* septum. It is a very short and shallow part of the septum because almost immediately posterior to the aortic root the two atrioventricular valve annuli diverge away from each other, the posterior 'swing' of the tricuspid orifice being more marked than that of the mitral valve (*Figure 15*). It is into this posterior bay that the coronary sinus opens, having traversed the posterior aspect of the left atrioventricular junction.

The atrioventricular muscular septum is important also because its atrial component contains the atrioventricular node. The cross-sectional cut (*Figure 14b*) shows the oblique nature of the atrioventricular junction at this site. The atrioventricular node lies on the sloping atrial aspect of this junction. Examination of *Figure 15* shows that from the left atrial aspect this point is marked by the posteromedial commissure of the mitral valve. By virtue of the extensive posterior diverticulum of the aortic root, the atrioventricular bundle, having penetrated through the central fibrous body, passes directly into the left ventricular outflow tract. From the standpoint of the subaortic

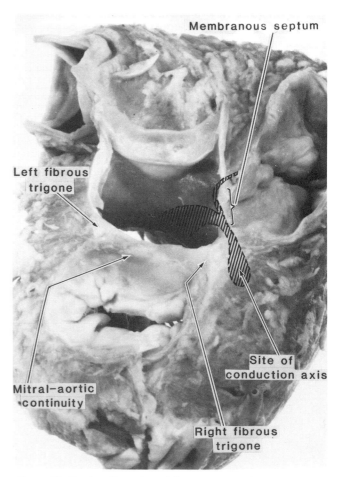

Figure 15. Further dissection of the atrioventricular junction showing the relationship of the left ventricular outflow tract to the right atrioventricular junction and the atrioventricular conduction tissues.

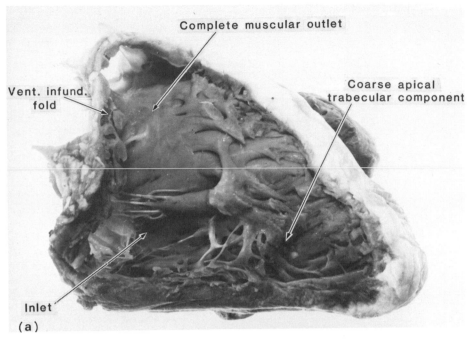

Complete muscular outlet

Vent. infund. fold

Coarse apical trabecular component

Inlet

(a)

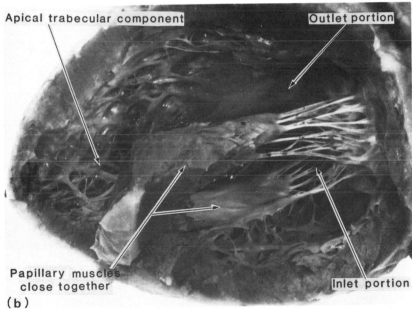

Apical trabecular component

Outlet portion

Papillary muscles close together

Inlet portion

(b)

Figure 16. Window dissections illustrating the component parts of (a) the right ventricle; and (b) the left ventricle

root, the landmark to the point of penetration is the commissure between the right and non-coronary aortic valve leaflets. Thus, the landmarks of the triangle of Koch delineate the site of the specialized atrioventricular junction as seen from the right atrium. Seen from the left atrium it is the posteromedial mitral commissure which points to the danger area. From the aorta, the non-coronary–right coronary valve commissure indicates the danger area. Finally, when seen from the right ventricle it is the area backwards from the medial papillary muscle and anteroseptal commissure which must be avoided (*Figure 15*).

Examination of the dissected atrioventricular junction (*see Figure 12*) reveals other features of note. The encircling branches of the coronary arteries are an integral part of the junction. The right coronary has an extensive

junctional course. In its first few centimetres or so it lies directly within the inner curvature of the heart. This is the right margin of the ventriculoinfundibular fold which, when viewed from the right ventricle, presents as the enigmatic supraventricular crest. The left coronary artery emerges into the inner curvature immediately above the left-sided counterpart of the 'crista' and then immediately branches into its anterior descending and circumflex branches. The anterior descending branch immediately moves out of the junction. The circumflex artery, in contrast, becomes an integral part. The extent of its intimate relationship to the junction varies markedly from heart to heart. Most frequently it fades out at the obtuse margin and the right coronary artery extends across the crux to supply the diaphragmatic surface of the left ventricle. In other cases, the right coronary turns down at the crux to become the posterior descending artery while the circumflex artery supplies the diaphragmatic left ventricle. Least frequently the circumflex supplies the diaphragmatic region and continues to become the posterior descending artery. This highly significant variability cannot be expressed simply in terms of right and left 'dominance' of the coronary arteries. Instead it is necessary to specify separately the origins of the posterior descending coronary artery and the arteries which supply the diaphragmatic surface of the left ventricle.

The right ventricle

Before going into specifics of ventricular morphology, a few remarks concerning ventricular division and valve morphology are appropriate. Traditionally ventricles have been divided simply into inlet and outlet parts, or sinus and conus respectively. For the normal heart this convention is adequate. However, when abnormal hearts are considered, its deficiencies are soon evident. The rudimentary right ventricle in tricuspid atresia, for example, lacks an inlet component. Nevertheless, it is unequivocally recognized as a right ventricle, this usually being attributed to the presence of the sinus component[9]. Thus, at least in tricuspid atresia, the 'sinus' is not synonymous with the ventricular inlet. This whole problematic area is circumvented by looking at the ventricle from a different viewpoint. In terms of descriptive morphology, each ventricle can be considered to possess three rather than two components, namely the inlet, apical trabecular and outlet portions (*Figure 16*). In our experience all ventricular chambers, no matter how deformed, are readily described using this tripartite convention. For instance, the problematic rudimentary right ventricle in tricuspid atresia has outlet and apical trabecular components; it lacks its inlet portion. In this and subsequent chapters, therefore, we will describe ventricular anatomy in terms of these three descriptive components.

When considering valve morphology then, in both normal and abnormal hearts it is important to have a convention which enables leaflets to be distinguished from one another and from so-called valve 'scallops'. We take as our criterion of the division between two leaflets the presence of a commissural chord arising from a prominent and easily recognized papillary muscle. In the left ventricle we recognize two such papillary muscles and therefore distinguish two leaflets. In the right ventricle it is not so easy, but usually it is possible to find a relatively constant but small medial muscle, a large anterior muscle and an intermediate-sized inferior muscle. In this way we nominate anteroseptal, anterior and inferoseptal commissures, and by this means distinguish the septal, anterosuperior and inferior leaflets of the tricuspid valve.

Returning now to the right ventricle, this chamber when normally constituted possesses the tricuspid valve in its inlet portion. Its three leaflets are readily seen by the surgeon from the right atrium (*Figure 17*). The anteroseptal commissure, supported by the medial papillary muscle, is 'round the corner' from the area of the membranous septum. Often the septal leaflet is itself cloven to the level of the membranous septum. This area is not the commissure, but is intimately related to the site of

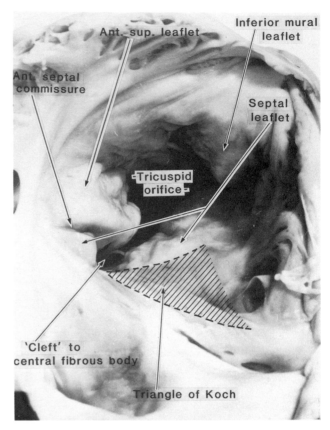

Figure 17. An anatomical dissection showing the leaflets of the tricuspid valve orientated as they would be seen by the surgeon

penetration of the atrioventricular bundle. The apical trabecular component of the right ventricle has typically coarse trabeculations. Indeed, it is from this morphology that the ventricle is most reliably differentiated from a left ventricle (*see Figure 16*). Extending upwards and leftwards from the trabecular component is the outlet portion supporting the pulmonary valve. In the normal right ventricle this outlet part is a complete muscular structure. The presence of the full infundibulum provides another very characteristic feature of the right ventricle, namely, the supraventricular crest which separates the tricuspid and pulmonary valves. As can be appreciated from study of the atrioventricular junction (*see Figure 15*), this apparently extensive muscle bundle seen from inside the ventricle (*see Figure 16a*) is no more than the inner aspect of the parietal ventricular wall. In other words it is the ventriculoinfundibular fold[10]. This is readily confirmed by simple dissection (*Figure 18*), which at the same time shows the important relationship of the right coronary artery to the muscular fold. One further very characteristic anatomical feature of the right ventricle is the extensive septal muscle bundle which runs down into the apical trabecular component and splits up into various trabeculae including the moderator band, the anterior papillary muscle and various septoparietal trabeculae. The basal part of this prominent bundle itself divides into two limbs which embrace the supraventricular crest. The posterior of these two limbs gives rise to the medial papillary muscle while the anterior limb runs up to the pulmonary valve. It

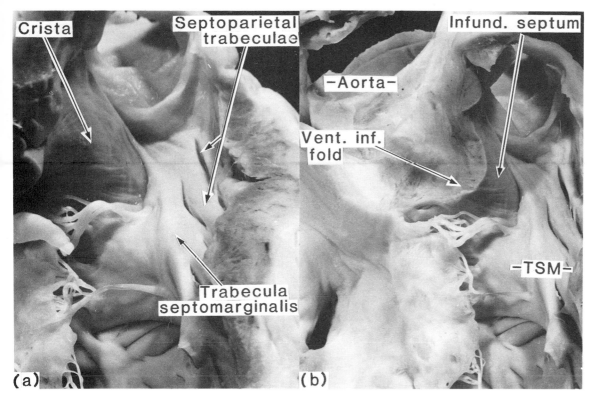

Figure 18. An anatomical dissection of the supraventricular crest of the right ventricle (a) showing how it is mostly composed of the heart inner curvature, the ventriculoinfundibular fold (b) (Reproduced from The Morphology of Congenital Heart Disease *by Anderson et al. 0000 by courtesy of Prof. A. E. Becker and Castle House Publications)*

has been common practice to consider this extensive bundle as part of the supraventricular crest; hence its designation as the 'septal band'[11]. However, even the most cursory examination shows that this structure cannot at the same time be both septal and supraventricular. Our practice is therefore to distinguish this important structure as the septomarginal trabecula, separating it in this way from both the ventriculoinfundibular fold (the normal supraventricular crest) and from the outlet component of the ventricular septum[10]. In addition to its role in giving origin to tricuspid valve tension apparatus, the surgical significance of the septomarginal trabecula is that in relation to its posterior limb the atrioventricular conduction axis branches on the left ventricular aspect of the septum. The right bundle branch then penetrates through the septum and surfaces beneath the medial papillary muscle before running down towards the apex either on the surface of, or embedded within, the body of the septomarginal trabecula.

The left ventricle

As with the right ventricle, the left ventricle can readily be divided into inlet, apical trabecular and outlet components (*see Figure 16b*). The inlet component contains the mitral valve. When viewed from the atrial aspect, the commissures between the leaflets are in anterolateral and posteromedial position (*Figure 19*). By virtue of this, the two mitral leaflets have grossly dissimilar annular attachments. The aortic leaflet has a relatively short attachment: only about one-third of the circumference. However, opening the valve shows that this leaflet has considerable depth and is a well-defined sail-like structure (*Figure 20*). In contrast, the mural leaflet, although having a much more extensive annular attachment, has much less depth and is more curtain-like. Indeed, in many hearts this mural leaflet is further divided into a series of 'scallops'. Usually there are three such scallops, but five or even six may be seen on occasion. The overall result of these dissimilar arrangements is that the two valve leaflets have more or less equal surface area. As discussed in the section on the atrioventricular junction, it is the area around the posteromedial commissure which is related to the site of the penetrating atrioventricular bundle.

The apical trabecular component of the left ventricle is characterized by particularly fine trabeculations. The apex of the ventricle itself is remarkably thin, there often being no more than 1 mm between the epicardial and endocardial surfaces at this point[12]. Unlike the right ventricle, the trabecular component of the left ventricle has a smooth septal surface down which cascades the fan-like left bundle branch. The initial portion of the fan is an undivided fascicle, but having descended about one-third of the septum the bundle divides into its interconnected anterior, septal and posterior divisions.

Although not a completely muscular structure as in the right ventricle, the outlet portion is well-formed in the left ventricle and has a particularly prominent posterior

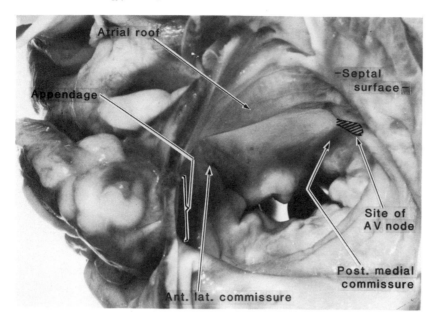

Figure 19. *An anatomical section showing the leaflets of the mitral valve viewed from the atrial aspect*

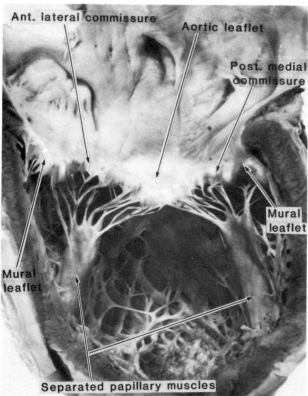

Figure 20. *The mitral valve opened by an incision through its posterior annulus and illustrating the different morphology of its leaflets*

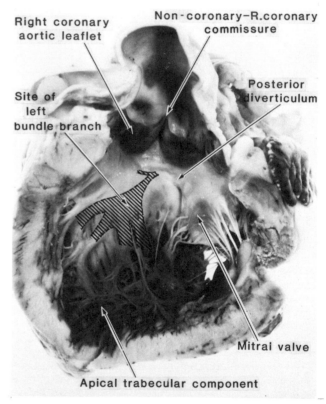

Figure 21. *A dissection illustrating the outflow tract of the left ventricle*

diverticulum (*Figure 21*). The outlet does not have completely muscular walls because of the fibrous continuity between the aortic and mitral valves, the ventriculoinfundibular fold being eradicated in this area (*see Figure 15*). The significant surgical feature of this area, in addition to the fact that the posterior diverticulum is related to a considerable area of the right atrium, is the coronet-like attachment of the aortic valve leaflets. Thus,

at the heights of the commissures the aortic outflow tract is directly related to such structures as the anterior wall of the left atrium and the transverse sinus. Further important features are the descent over the midseptal surface of the outflow tract of the left bundle branch and the origin of the coronary arteries from two of the aortic sinuses. All of these are highly significant when planning operations to enlarge the aortic root.

Sequential segmental analysis of congenital heart disease

In the preceding paragraphs we described the basic morphology of the cardiac chambers and indicated how they may be recognized by the surgeon. At the same time, we showed how the basic disposition of the conduction tissues is dictated by this morphology. However, we considered this mostly in the setting of the normal heart. Almost all patients operated upon will have congenital cardiac lesions in the setting of the normal heart. For example, persistent patency of the ductus or a simple coarctation in no way alters the basic cardiac morphology. Similarly the presence of a simple atrial or ventricular septal defect, or even an atrioventricular septal defect, does not distort the basic arrangement to such an extent that it is not readily recognized as being normal. However, in a few cases the anatomy can be exceedingly bizarre, often with the heart itself abnormally positioned, but even in these complex cases understanding can be simply achieved if attention is paid to the principles established in our previous paragraphs. This is because the ways in which the atrial chambers themselves can be arranged are strictly limited, as are the ways in which the atrial chambers can connect to the ventricles and the ventricles in turn connect to the great arteries. We will therefore conclude this chapter with a brief description of the principles and philosophy of sequential segmental analysis[1], concentrating once more on the vital information these principles can give to the distribution of the atrioventricular conduction tissues.

Philosophy of sequential segmental analysis

When describing any given congenital cardiac malformation it is necessary to account separately for the features of the morphology of the individual cardiac segments, the connections of the segments to each other and the interrelationships of the chambers within each segment[13]. It does not particularly matter how each of these features is described, provided that each is accounted for using mutually exclusive terms. We ourselves have used a variety of terms for this purpose during the evolution of our approach, but we are now convinced of the value of simple everyday words in description rather than having a vocabulary deeply rooted in classical etymology. We have already described the essential morphological features of each of the cardiac chambers, but it is necessary to decide which of these features we take as the final arbiter for identification of a given chamber. In this respect, we follow the so-called 'morphological method', which argues that chambers, however deformed or abnormal, should always be identifiable in terms of their own intrinsic characteristics[14,15]. This means, for example, that venous connections cannot be used to identify an atrium, since the veins themselves may connect anomalously. An atrioventricular valve cannot be used as the final arbiter of the nature of a ventricle because some ventricles do not possess atrioventricular valves. And so on. Thus, the morphology of the atrial appendages turns out to be the most reliable feature for atrial recognition. For the

ventricles it is the nature of the apical trabecular component which is most useful. Unfortunately the great arteries have no intrinsic features which permit their recognition, but almost always their branching pattern is sufficiently discrete to permit distinction of an aorta from a pulmonary trunk from a truncus. For full description it is necessary to account for connections and relations, and ideally each should have equal weight in description. Practically, there is little doubt that the surgeon is most concerned with connections, and therefore this account places connections in a pre-eminent position and relegates relationships to a secondary role.

Atrial arrangement

We have already referred to the importance of inspecting the atrial appendage morphology and have described the possible variations. For sequential analysis the recognition of atrial arrangement is doubly important, since the remainder of the heart cannot be analyzed adequately without knowledge of the morphology of the atrial segment. There are only four ways in which the atrial chambers can be arranged (*Figure 22*). In the first two

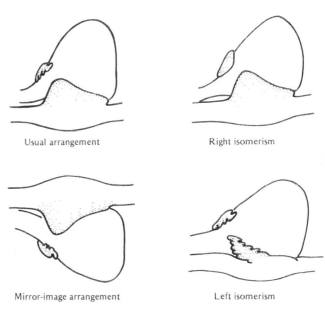

Usual arrangement　　　Right isomerism

Mirror-image arrangement　　　Left isomerism

Figure 22. The four basic arrangements in which the atrial appendages can be disposed. This is the basis of so-called 'atrial situs'

patterns both a morphologically right and a morphologically left atrial chamber are present (lateralized atria). When the right atrium is right-sided this is the usual arrangement (so-called solitus). When the right atrium is left-sided then there is a mirror-image arrangement (so-called inversus). The other two patterns exist when both appendages have comparable morphology, or in other words are isomeric. Right atrial isomerism then describes the existence of two appendages both having right morphology, while left atrial isomerism exists when both appendages have left morphology. As described above, the disposition of the sinus node is dictated by the atrial morphology.

Atrioventricular junction

Analysis of the atrioventricular junction demands knowledge of the nature of both the atrial and ventricular chambers. Then it is necessary to determine how the atria are connected to the ventricles (the type of connection) and the morphology of the atrioventricular valves which guard the junction (the mode of connection). When each atrium connects to its own separate ventricle then there is a biventricular atrioventricular connection. This can occur either with lateralized or isomeric atrial chambers. With lateralized atria there are then two possibilities which can exist either with usually arranged or mirror-image atria (*Figure 23*). The first is when the right atrium connects to the right ventricle and the left atrium to the left ventricle. This is atrioventricular concordance. The second is when the right atrium connects to the left ventricle and the left atrium to the right ventricle. This gives a discordant

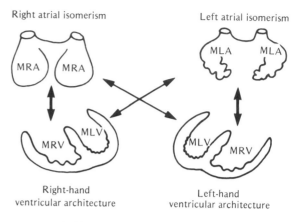

Ambiguous atrioventricular connection

Figure 24. The ambiguous atrioventricular connection which is found when isomeric atrial chambers each connect to their own ventricle

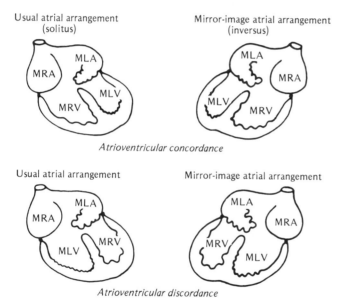

Atrioventricular concordance

Atrioventricular discordance

Figure 23. The two ways in which lateralized atria may be connected to their own ventricular chambers

atrioventricular connection. When there are isomeric atrial chambers, then whatever the arrangement of the ventricles the atrioventricular connection must perforce be ambiguous (*Figure 24*). In this situation the ventricular architecture is of vital importance. There are only two basic patterns of ventricular architecture (*Figure 25*). The usual pattern is seen in the normal heart with usual atrial arrangement and atrioventricular concordance. The right ventricle more or less wraps itself round the left ventricle in such a way that, figuratively speaking, the palmar surface of only the observer's right hand can be placed on the septal surface with the thumb in the inlet, the wrist in the apex and fingers in the outlet (*Figure 25*). This arrangement can therefore be considered a right-hand pattern of architecture. The second basic pattern is typically seen in the heart with usually arranged atrial chambers but with atrioventricular discordance. With this architecture it is only the left hand which can be placed upon the right ventricular septal surface, hence a left-hand pattern (*Figure 25b*). Either of these two architectural arrangements can exist with either right or

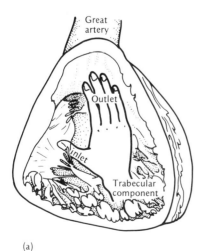

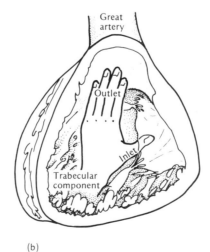

(a)   (b)

Figure 25. The two basic patterns of architecture of the ventricular mass. They can be likened to the way in which the observer's hand can be placed upon the septal surface of the right ventricle (see text for discussion)

left atrial isomerism (*Figure 26*) and must be described for full categorization. This is important because the architecture dictates the conduction tissue disposition when there is an ambiguous connection (*see below*). Almost without exception the ventricular architecture is harmonious with the atrioventricular connection in patients with lateralized atria. Usually the ventricular relationships are also as expected, i.e. right ventricle to right with right-hand pattern and right ventricle to left with left-hand pattern. However, sometimes the ventricular relationships may be unexpected because of either rotation or tilting of the ventricular mass around its long axis. Such rotation or tilting produces the so-called 'criss-cross'[16] or 'upstairs-downstairs'[17] hearts. Providing that relations are described and identified separately from connections and architecture these should not give problems either in diagnosis or description.

There is a second group of hearts in which the atrial chambers connect only to one ventricle, or in other words hearts which have a univentricular atrioventricular connection. These can exist with either lateralized or isomeric atrial chambers. The connections making up this group are double inlet ventricle, together with absence of either the right or the left atrioventricular connection (*Figure 26*). These univentricular connections can be found when the atria connect to a left ventricle, a right ventricle or a solitary indeterminate ventricle. Almost always when

there is a univentricular connection to either a left or a right ventricle the complementary ventricle is present in hypoplastic and rudimentary form because it lacks at least its inlet portion. Rudimentary right ventricles, found with univentricular connection to a left ventricle, are always in anterosuperior position although they may either be right-sided or left-sided. Rudimentary left ventricles, found with univentricular connection to a left ventricle, are always posteroinferior but again may be either right- or left-sided. By arguing from developmental principles it is possible to account for rudimentary chamber position in terms of right-hand and left-hand architectural patterns, but we find it simpler just to describe the position of the rudimentary ventricle using anterior/posterior, superior/inferior and right/left coordinates. Solitary indeterminate ventricles do not possess second rudimentary ventricles.

The mode of atrioventricular connection simply describes the arrangement of the atrioventricular valves. When there are concordant, discordant, ambiguous and double inlet connections then both atria connect with the ventricular mass. The dual atrioventricular junctions can therefore be guarded by two separate valves or a common atrioventricular valve. One of two valves, or rarely both, may straddle the interventricular septum when the tension apparatus is attached on both sides of the septum. Usually when a valve straddles, its annulus also over-rides the septum. The degree of this over-ride determines the commitment of the valve to the two ventricles. It is well known that there are spectra of degrees of over-ride with different segmental combinations which extend from the hearts having an effectively biventricular to an effectively univentricular atrioventricular connection[18]. For the purposes of categorization of the precise connection present in such hearts, i.e. double inlet versus biventricular connection, we assign the over-riding valve to the ventricle connected to its greater part (the 50 per cent law)[13]. Common valves usually straddle, but not always. For instance, a common valve in the presence of a double inlet connection can be exclusively connected to one ventricle. However, a common valve guards two atrioventricular junctions (the right and the left) so this fact must be taken into account when assessing the degree of over-ride. A further mode of connection when there are two valves is for one of the valves to be imperforate. This is quite different from an absent atrioventricular connection. Imperforate valves and absent connections both produce atrioventricular valve atresia, but it is not generally appreciated that absent connection is probably the commonest cause (*see* chapter on 'Single ventricle', pp. 000–000). When one atrioventricular connection is absent, then the modes of connection of the persisting junction are strictly limited. The atrioventricular valve may either be exclusively connected to one ventricle or alternatively may straddle or over-ride.

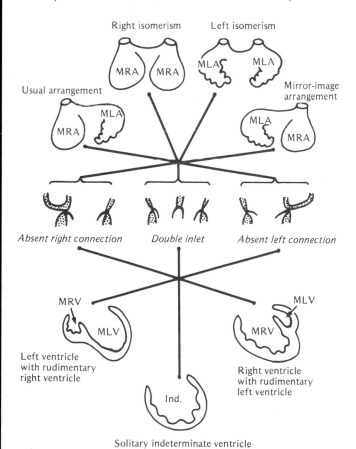

Figure 26. The combinations which produce a univentricular atrioventricular connection. This exists when the atrial chambers connect to only one ventricular chamber which may be of right, left or indeterminate pattern

Influence of ventricular architecture on conduction tissues

In the section on normal atrioventricular junction we described how the triangle of Koch provided the landmarks to the atrioventricular junctional area. However, in hearts with abnormal atrioventricular connections the regular atrioventricular node is not always the one which gives rise to the penetrating atrioventricular bundle. It is known that during fetal life a complete ring of potential conduction tissue surrounds the atrioventricular junction[19]. Remnants of this ring often persist into adult life, but then they are sequestrated on the atrial aspect of the fibrous annulus and do not give rise to atrioventricular conduction bundles. In the presence of abnormal chamber connections, however, parts of this atrioventricular ring tissue can take over the role of the atrioventricular node[20]. The rules which determine whether there is to be a regular or an anomalous node, or rarely both, are governed by several factors. The most important is whether there is good alignment between the atrial septum and the inlet part of the ventricular septum. Almost always in hearts with atrioventricular concordance this alignment is found and there is a regular conduction system. The exception is when the tricuspid valve straddles. Then an anomalous node is formed at the point at which the septum makes contact with the atrioventricular junction[19]. In hearts with usual atrial arrangement and atrioventricular discordance this septal alignment is lacking. In these hearts, therefore, there is an anomalous anterior atrioventricular node[21]. This arrangement is also seen in hearts with univentricular connection to a left ventricle[22]. Here the anterior position of the septum means that there cannot be alignment with the atrial septum, so that again an anterior node is the rule. However, with univentricular connection to a right ventricle then there is septal alignment so that regular conduction systems are found. Similarly, when atrioventricular discordance is found with mirror-image atrial chambers there is again usually good septal alignment and a regular conduction system[23]. However, the ventricular architecture is also significant. Thus, abnormal systems are found most frequently when there is a left-handed pattern of ventricular architecture. This holds good also when there is univentricular connection to a right ventricle[24] and when there is an ambiguous atrioventricular connection[5]. The exception to this is found when left-handed architecture coexists with mirror-image atrial chambers, because almost always this means that there will be atrioventricular concordance. Thus, the atrioventricular connection is the best guide to disposition of the atrioventricular conduction axis but the ventricular architecture present is also highly significant.

The ventriculoarterial junction

At this junction it is again necessary to take account of the type and mode of connection. Additionally, attention should be paid to arterial relationships. Outflow tract morphology (infundibular or conal anatomy) is also variable but is rarely of surgical significance.

The ventriculoarterial connection is said to be concordant when the aorta is connected to the left ventricle and the pulmonary trunk to the right ventricle. An aorta connected to a right ventricle and a pulmonary trunk to a left ventricle produces a discordant connection. Both arteries connected to the same ventricle are described as double outlet, whereas single outlet of the heart is used for the situation in which only one patent arterial trunk can be traced to make contact with a ventricular chamber. The latter may be a truncus or alternatively an aortic trunk with pulmonary atresia, or a pulmonary trunk with aortic atresia. The modes of connection are more limited at the ventriculoarterial junction. A common valve only exists with truncus. When there are two valves, then both may be patent. One or both may then over-ride the septum. As with the over-riding atrioventricular valves, the precise connection is determined by the 50 per cent law. Finally, one valve may be imperforate. In this situation rarely either the imperforate valve or the patent valve may over-ride.

All of the above connections are determined irrespective of the arterial interrelationships. It is not possible to infer with complete accuracy the connection of the great arteries from their relationships. This is not to say that relationships give no help in diagnosing connections. There are certain basic arrangements which are seen more frequently with one given connection, for example a right-sided and anterior aorta with ventriculoarterial discordance. These are not, however, immutable laws, and should be treated as a guide to abnormal connections. When describing such abnormal relationships it is necessary to account for both the positions of the arterial valves and the orientation of the ascending portions of the arterial trunks. We prefer to describe valvar relationships by describing the position of the aortic valve in comparison to the pulmonary valve in right/left and anterior/posterior coordinates. When describing the orientation of the arterial trunks there are two basic patterns: either the

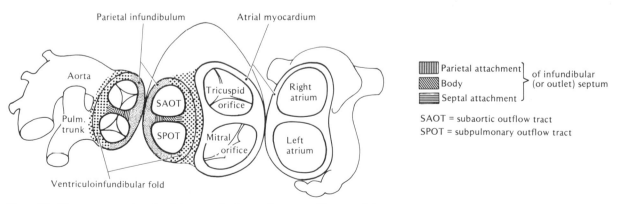

Figure 27. The component parts of the ventricular outflow tracts illustrated diagrammatically by 'unfolding' a hypothetical heart with a bilateral infundibulum, the great arteries being side-by-side with the aorta to the right

pulmonary trunk spirals round the aorta towards its bifurcation or else the trunks ascend in parallel fashion. By combining these two variables we have found it an easy matter to describe all patterns of arterial inter-relationship that we have encountered.

Although outflow tract morphology in itself is rarely of surgical significance, great emphasis has been placed in the past on the role of the 'bilateral conus' or infundibulum. Each arterial valve is potentially capable of being supported by a complete muscular infundibulum with any ventriculoarterial connection. These infundibula have three basic components. One component separates the arterial valves and their subvalvar outflow tracts from each other. This is the outlet septum. The second part is simply the free parietal ventricular wall. It is the third part which has given most problems in comprehension. This part represents the inner heart curvature between the anterior wall of the atrium and the posterior wall of the great artery. It separates the arterial valve from the atrioventricular valve and is the ventriculoinfundibular fold (*Figure 27*). The variability in outlet morphology usually depends on the integrity of this fold. When it is intact then there is atrioventricular-arterial valve discontinuity and usually there is a complete muscular infundibulum. When the fold is deficient then there is atrioventricular-arterial continuity and a deficient infundibulum. The term 'usually' is used above purposely, since it is possible for the ventriculoinfundibular fold to be intact, producing arterial-atrioventricular discontinuity, and yet for the outlet septum to be deficient, with aortic-pulmonary valvar continuity, so that there is not a complete muscular infundibulum. Obviously, therefore, the integrity of the ventricular outflow tracts depends on the morphology of both the ventriculoinfundibular fold and the outlet septum. It should also be noted that this discussion has made no mention of the septomarginal trabecula. This is an integral part of the right ventricle and is not part of the subvalvar outflow tracts.

Subsequent steps in sequential analysis

The analysis described thus far accounts only for the segmental combination of the heart. In most instances this will be normal. But it will have cost the surgeon nothing to prove this normality, and indeed, it is essential to do so. Having established the segmental pattern, analysis is concluded by assessing all the associated defects present. This is best done also, we believe, in segmental fashion. We therefore start by confirming that the venoatrial connections are appropriate. We then study the atrial segment, the ventricular segment and the aterial segment in turn, at the same time looking for any junctional malformations which may not have been accounted for during the analysis of the connections. Finally we study the anatomy of the aortic and pulmonary pathways. In this way any congenital heart lesion, or combination of lesions, however simple or complex, is accounted for and understood in the segmental setting of the heart itself. Thus far we have been able to cater for all anomalies we have encountered.

References

1. Anderson, R. H., Ho, S. Y. The pathology of congenital heart disease. In: Barson, A. J., ed. Fetal and neonatal pathology: perspectives for the general pathologists. Eastbourne and New York: Praeger Publishers, 1982: 213–238

2. Melhuish, B. P. P., Van Praagh, R. Juxtaposition of the atrial appendages. A sign of severe cyanotic congenital heart disease. British Heart Journal 1968; 30: 269–284

3. Anderson, R. H., Smith, A., Wilkinson, J. L. Right juxtaposition of the auricular appendages. European Journal of Cardiology 1976; 4: 495–503

4. Macartney, F. J., Zuberbuhler, J. R., Anderson, R. H. Morphological considerations pertaining to recognition of atrial isomerism. Consequences for sequential chamber localisation. British Heart Journal 1980; 44: 657–667

5. Dickinson, D. F., Wilkinson, J. L., Anderson, K. R., Smith, A., Ho, S. Y., Anderson, R. H. The cardiac conduction system in situs ambiguus. Circulation 1979; 59: 879–885

6. Anderson, R. H., Becker, A. E. Coronary arterial patterns: a guide to identification of congenital heart disease. In: Becker, A. E., Losekoot, T. G., Marcelletti, C., Anderson, R. H., eds. Paediatric cardiology, Vol. 3. Edinburgh: Churchill Livingstone, 1981: 251–262

7. Sweeney, L. J., Rosenquist, G. C. The normal anatomy of the atrial septum in the human heart. American Heart Journal 1979; 98: 194–199

8. Becker, A. E., Anderson, R. H. Atrioventricular septal defects. What's in a name? Journal of Thoracic and Cardiovascular Surgery 1982; 83: 461–469

9. Bharati, S., McAllister, H. A., Tatooles, C. J. et al. Anatomic variations in underdeveloped right ventricle related to tricuspid atresia and stenosis. Journal of Thoracic and Cardiovascular Surgery 1976; 72: 383–400

10. Anderson, R. H., Becker, A. E., Van Mierop, L. H. S. What should we call the 'crista'? British Heart Journal 1977; 39: 856–859

11. Van Praagh, R. What is the Taussig-Bing malformation? Circulation 1968; 38: 445–449

12. Bradfield, J. W. B., Beck, G., Vecht, R. J. Left ventricular apical thin point. British Heart Journal 1977; 39: 806–809

13. Tynan, M. J., Becker, A. E., Macartney, F. J., Quero-Jimenez, M., Shinebourne, E. A., Anderson, R. H. Nomenclature and classification of congenital heart disease. British Heart Journal 1979; 41: 544–553

14. Lev, M. Pathologic diagnosis of positional variations in cardiac chambers in congenital heart disease. Laboratory Investigation 1954; 3: 71–82

15. Van Praagh, R., David, I., Van Praagh, S. What is a ventricle? The single ventricle trap. Pediatric Cardiology 1982; 2: 79–84

16. Anderson, R. H. Criss-cross hearts revisited. Pediatric Cardiology 1982; 3: 305–313

17. Van Praagh, S., LaCorte, M., Fellows, K. E. et al. Superoinferior ventricles: anatomic and angiocardiographic findings in ten postmortem cases. In: Van Praagh, R., Takao, A., eds. Etiology and morphogenesis of congenital heart disease. Mount Kisco, New York: Future Publishing Company, 1980: 317–378

18. Milo, S., Ho, S. Y., Macartney, F. J. *et al*. Straddling and overriding atrioventricular valves morphology and classification. American Journal of Cardiology 1979; 44: 1122–1134

19. Anderson, R. H., Davies, M. J., Becker, A. E. Atrioventricular ring specialized tissue in the normal heart. European Journal of Cardiology 1974; 2: 219–230

20. Becker, A. E., Wilkinson, J. L., Anderson, R. H., Atrioventricular conduction tissues: a guide in understanding the morphogenesis of the univentricular heart. In: Van Praagh, R., Takao, A., eds. Etiology and morphogenesis of congenital heart disease. Mount Kisco, New York: Futura Publishing Company, 1980: 489–514

21. Anderson, R. H., Becker, A. E., Arnold, R., Wilkinson, J. L. The conducting tissues in congenitally corrected transposition. Circulation 1974; 50: 911–923

22. Anderson, R. H., Arnold, R., Thaper, M. K., Jones, R. S., Hamilton, D. I. Cardiac specialized tissue in hearts with an apparently single ventricular chamber (double inlet left ventricle). American Journal of Cardiology 1974; 33: 95–106

23. Wilkinson, J. L., Smith, A., Lincoln, C., Anderson, R. H. Conducting tissues in congenitally corrected transposition with situs inversus. British Heart Journal 1978; 40: 41–48

24. Essed, C. E., Ho, S. Y., Hunter, S., Anderson, R. H. Atrioventricular conduction system in univentricular heart of right ventricular type with right-sided rudimentary chamber. Thorax 1980; 35: 123–127

Shunt procedures

Hillel Laks
Professor and Chief, Division of Cardiothoracic Surgery, UCLA School of Medicine, Los Angeles, California, USA

Introduction

Shunts are performed between the systemic and pulmonary circulations to provide improved systemic oxygenation where the underlying condition is unsuitable for complete repair because of age, size, anatomy or other considerations.

The most commonly used shunts are placed between the subclavian artery and the pulmonary artery or between the central aorta and the main pulmonary artery, either directly or by interposition of synthetic material.

The operations

BLALOCK-TAUSSIG SHUNT

1

The Blalock-Taussig shunt is generally performed on the side opposite the aortic arch and on the side of the innominate artery. The patient is positioned on the table with his back at about 80° to the table with the hips taped and a small roll under the left shoulder. The incision is made starting in the submammary crease about one finger breadth lateral to the nipple line and about one and a half finger breadths below the nipple; it extends to a point below the tip of the scapula, ending midway between the tip of the scapula and the spine. The latissimus dorsi and serratus anterior muscles are divided. The chest is entered through the third or fourth intercostal space.

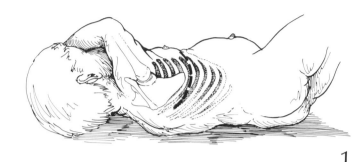

1

2

2

The lung is retracted with two malleable retractors. The phrenic nerve is seen running along the superior vena cava and then on the pericardium anterior to the origin of the azygos vein. The vagus nerve is shown giving off the recurrent laryngeal nerve, which runs underneath the innominate artery. Great care must be taken not to injure the phrenic nerve either by cautery in this vicinity or by blunt trauma from retraction.

3

The azygos vein is divided between ligatures, leaving a long stump on the proximal end, the ligature on this end being then used for retraction. In addition, retraction sutures are placed in the adventitia and pericardium over the superior vena cava to retract it away from the pulmonary artery and vein. The pleura overlying the subclavian artery is divided, care being taken not to injure the vagus and recurrent laryngeal nerves.

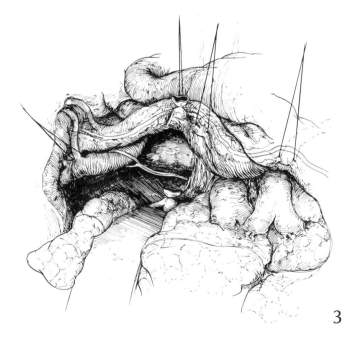

3

4a & b

The branches of the subclavian artery are divided between 4/0 silk ligatures (a) and, before the last branch is divided, heparin 1 mg/kg body weight is administered intravenously. The subclavian artery is then withdrawn through the sling formed by the vagus and recurrent laryngeal nerves and clamped close to its origin. The distal end of the artery is then divided, removing the ligated branches, and an incision is made through the stump of its branches to give the distal anastomotic suture line maximum length (b).

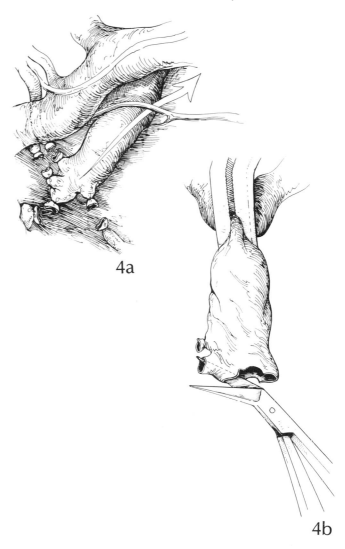

4a

4b

5

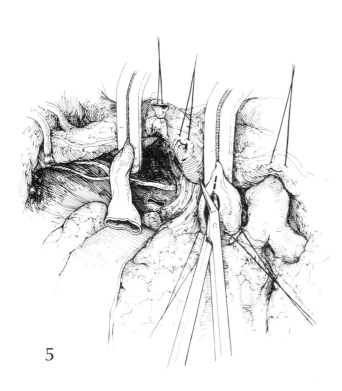

5

Traction is then placed on the subclavian artery to expose the innominate and carotid arteries, which are freed of their adventitial attachments to facilitate movement of the subclavian artery down towards the pulmonary artery. The proximal pulmonary artery is then clamped with an angled vascular clamp and its distal branches are snared. An incision is then made on the upper aspect of the pulmonary artery. The lateral extent of the incision is kept away from the upper lobe branch, which may become obstructed by the suture line.

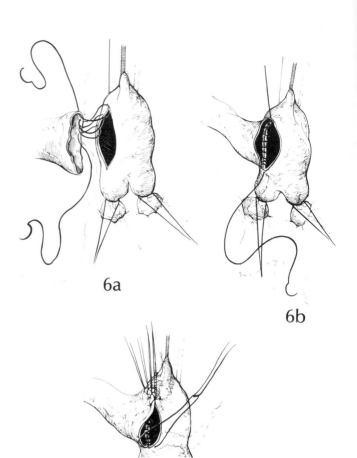

6a

6b

6c

6a-c

A suture line is begun with 6/0 or 7/0 polypropylene, the suture being passed through the medial corner of the subclavian artery from outside in and then through the pulmonary artery from inside out (a). After two bites have been taken the subclavian artery is lowered down to the pulmonary artery by traction on the sutures. A running suture is used for the posterior layers of the anastomosis (b). Interrupted corner sutures are placed to which the running suture is tied. Then, starting from either end, interrupted simple sutures of 6/0 polypropylene are used to complete the anastomosis (c).

7

The clamps and snares are then removed and the completed shunt is shown here.

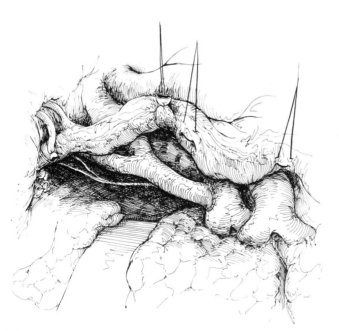

7

SUBCLAVIAN TO PULMONARY ARTERY GORETEX GRAFT

Two types of subclavian to pulmonary artery Goretex shunt may be used: (1) the interposition graft consists of a graft between the end of the subclavian artery and the side of the pulmonary artery; (2) the H-type shunt involves placement of a graft between the side of the subclavian artery and the side of the pulmonary artery, leaving the distal subclavian artery in continuity.

Interposition graft

This shunt is frequently useful on the side opposite the innominate artery to avoid the kinking which otherwise occurs in bringing down the subclavian artery. With the inability of the Goretex to grow this shunt is generally used where palliation is desired for 1–2 years. Although the proximal subclavian artery does control the amount of flow to some extent, an excessively large Goretex graft on the subclavian artery may result in excessive circulation to the lungs.

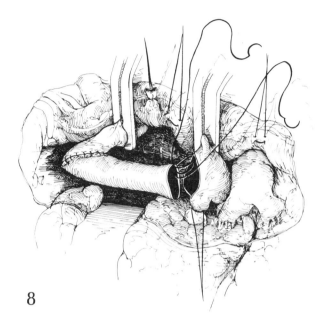

8

8

The Goretex graft anastomosed to the bevelled end of the subclavian artery followed by its anastomosis to the pulmonary artery is shown. Both anastomoses are formed with a running stuture both anteriorly and posteriorly. Heparin 1 mg/kg is given before the clamping of the arteries and is usually not reversed at the end of the procedure.

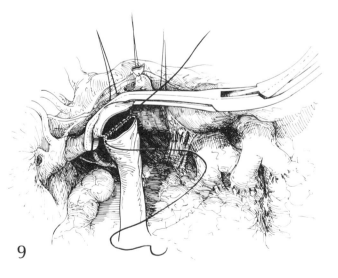

9

9

H-type shunt

In this procedure a Goretex graft is placed directly between the main subclavian artery and the ipsilateral pulmonary artery. An end-to-side anastomosis is made to the subclavian artery as shown and the pulmonary artery anastomosis is performed as described above. Provided that an appropriate-sized shunt is used this has not resulted in a problem with subclavian steal.

10

Use of silicone rubber to facilitate shunt take-down

We have found it useful to place a strip of silicone rubber around the Goretex shunt and leave the ends attached to the anterior mediastinum to facilitate shunt take-down at the corrective procedure.

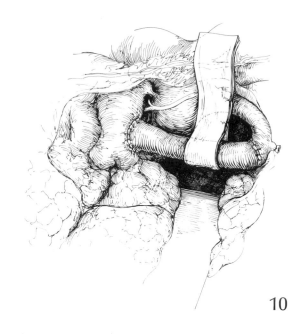

10

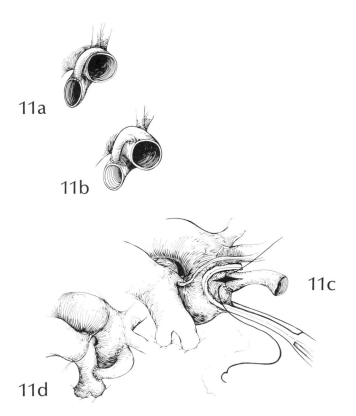

11a

11b

11c

11d

11

SUBCLAVIAN ARTERIOPLASTY FOR THE IPSILATERAL BLALOCK-TAUSSIG SHUNT

If a Blalock-Taussig shunt has to be perfomed on the same side as the aortic arch there is a tendency for it to kink. This can be overcome by performing a subclavian angioplasty. A vertical incision is made through the base of the subclavian artery and extended on to the aorta. This incision is then closed transversely. This provides a more anterior take-off of the subclavian artery and reduces the tendency for the subclavian artery to kink at its origin.

WATERSTON SHUNT

We generally avoid the Waterston shunt because of its two major problems. These are: (1) excessive circulation to the lungs, which may cause cardiac failure, and also makes subsequent repair more difficult owing to the development of pulmonary vascular disease; and (2) the development of a stricture on the medial aspect of the shunt. The shunt is performed between the right pulmonary artery and the ascending aorta through a right lateral thoracotomy through the fourth interspace.

12

The pulmonary artery is exposed and snares passed around its distal branches. The artery is freed up posteriorly as far medially as possible and the superior vena cava is mobilized, exposing the anterior aspect of the pulmonary artery as far medially as possible. The superior vena cava is retracted anteriorly, exposing the ascending aorta.

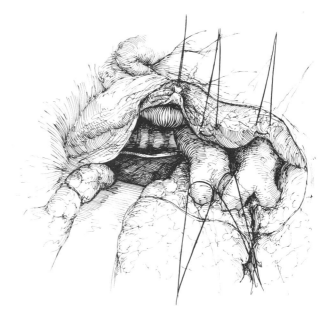

13

The place chosen for the anastomosis should be on the posterior aspect of the aorta and not on the lateral aspect in order to avoid kinking of the pulmonary artery. A side-biting clamp is placed with the posterior blade behind the right pulmonary artery and the anterior blade excluding a portion of the ascending aorta, including the site for the anastomosis.

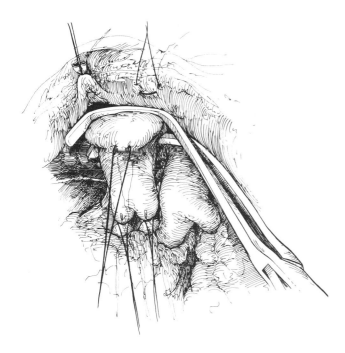

14a-d

A longitudinal incision is then made in the pulmonary artery and in the aorta approximately 3 mm in width. A running suture of 6/0 polypropylene is then used for the posterior layer of the suture line (a) and interrupted sutures of 6/0 polypropylene are used for the anterior suture line (b). The correct placement of the anastomosis on the posterior aspect of the aorta should avoid kinking of the right pulmonary artery (c). When the anastomosis is made more laterally on the aorta (d) it results in kinking of the right pulmonary artery medially, with most of the flow going to the right pulmonary artery.

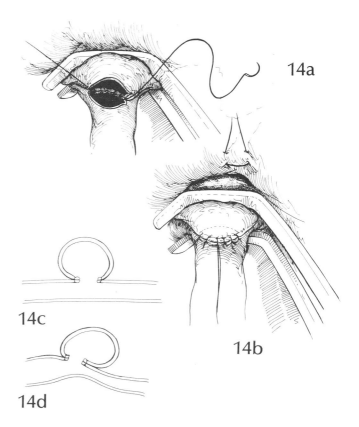

14a

14b

14c

14d

CENTRAL AORTA TO PULMONARY ARTERY GRAFT

This shunt is performed through a median sternotomy. This has the disadvantage of causing adhesions, which make the subsequent definitive repair somewhat more difficult. We generally only use it where other shunts have failed, but we use it as the shunt of choice for patients with pulmonary atresia and an intact ventricular septum who are undergoing a pulmonary valvotomy at the same time.

15

Some surgeons prefer to place a short segment of Goretex between the ascending aorta and the main pulmonary artery as shown in the illustration. This has a tendency to become kinked and some have experienced a fairly high occlusion rate. For this reason we prefer to use a longer segment of Goretex placed with its convexity inferiorly. The reinforced Goretex graft reduces the risk of kinking.

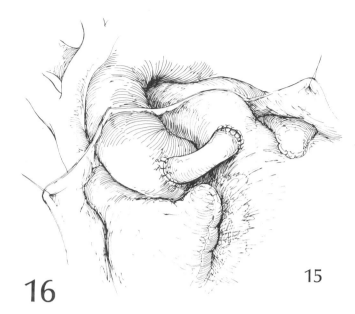

15

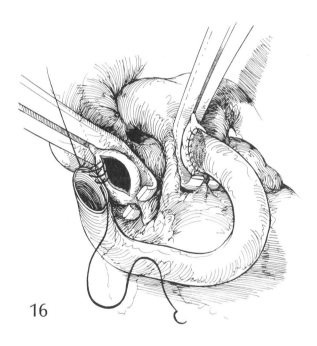

16

16

A side-biting clamp is placed on the anterior aspect of the pulmonary artery, a vertical incision is made and the 4 mm Goretex graft which is generally used in the neonate is anastomosed to the main pulmonary artery with a running suture of 6/0 polypropylene. The clamp is left on the pulmonary artery to avoid blood entering the graft and a side-biting clamp is placed on the ascending aorta. Care must be taken to avoid obstructing the flow of blood through the aorta to prevent instability while the anastomosis is being performed. A longitudinal incision is then made in the aorta and the proximal portion of the graft is anastomosed to it with a running suture of 6/0 polypropylene. The clamp on the pulmonary artery is then released and a small hole is made in the Goretex with a 6/0 needle to allow the air to escape. The clamp on the aorta is then released.

17

A snare may be left on the graft, a 0 polypropylene thread being used, the ends of which are passed through a polyethylene catheter which is then clipped using a silver hemaclip. The snare is left behind the linea alba to facilitate reducing the flow through the shunt should this be necessary or occluding it if the pulmonary valvotomy proves adequate. This can be performed using local anaesthesia without reopening the chest.

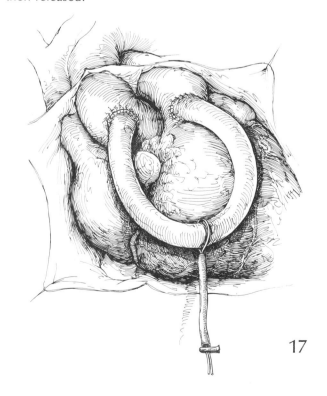

17

GLENN SHUNT

18

The Glenn shunt has the advantage of oxygenating systemic venous blood without causing an additional volume load on the heart. Preoperatively an anomalous left superior vena cava must be excluded. The procedure is performed using a right lateral thoracotomy. The pulmonary artery is dissected out anteriorly and posteriorly on the right side. The superior vena cava is mobilized, giving maximum exposure to the orgin of the right pulmonary artery. The azygos vein is divided, leaving a long stump on the superior vena cava, particularly if the vein is large and is located close to the pulmonary artery. This is so that the stump of the azygos vein can be incorporated in and enlarge the anastomosis. The branches of the pulmonary artery are then snared and a side-biting clamp is placed on the right pulmonary artery behind the superior vena cava. The artery is then divided as shown by the dotted line.

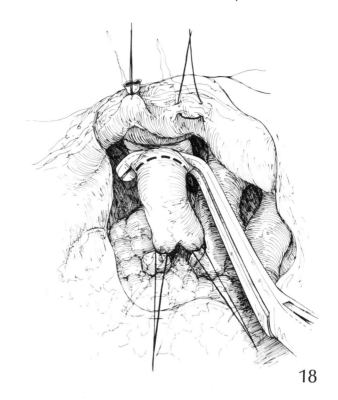

18

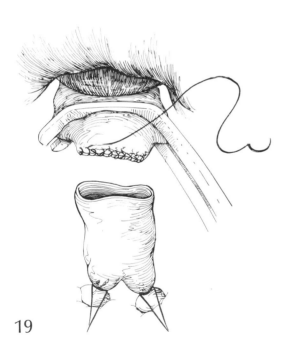

19

19

The stump of the pulmonary artery having been oversewn with a double suture line of 5/0 polypropylene, the side-biting clamp is placed on the superior vena cava. The stump of the azygos vein may be included in the clamp if it is close to the pulmonary artery. Care must be taken in applying the side-biting clamp to avoid total occlusion of the superior vena cava, which could result in cerebral oedema, and it is useful to monitor the venous pressure above the clamp.

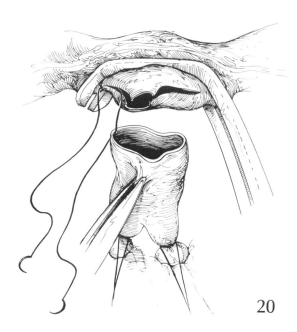

20

20 & 21

The incision in the superior vena cava (and in the stump of the azygos vein if available) is then made and the anastomosis performed with a running suture of 6/0 polypropylene posteriorly, starting in the superior corner, and with interrupted sutures for the anterior layer. The superior vena cava is occluded below the anastomosis, thus directing superior vena caval flow into the right pulmonary artery. We now use very large hemaclips to occlude the cava. We have found that when these are removed continuity between the superior vena cava and the right atrium can quite easily be restored for a Fontan procedure.

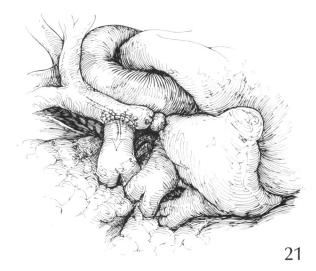

21

Pulmonary artery banding

Charles H. Moore MD
Humana Hospital, San Antonio, Texas, USA

Introduction

Because the prognosis of patients with tetralogy of Fallot is so much better than that of patients with large ventricular septal defects (VSDs) without pulmonary outflow tract obstruction it seemed a logical step to constrict the pulmonary artery in these patients in an effort to help them recover from the effects of large left-to-right shunts and pulmonary vascular congestion. Muller and Dammann[1] performed the first pulmonary artery constriction in 1952 and Albert et al. first reported banding of the pulmonary artery in 1958[2].

Constriction of the pulmonary artery decreases the volume of the left-to-right shunt and thus the work of the left ventricle, and minimizes pulmonary vascular engorgement. The indications for pulmonary artery banding have included large VSDs in infants, single ventricle, double-outlet right ventricle, complete atrioventricular canal, transposition of the great arteries with VSD, truncus arteriosus and coarctation of the aorta with VSD or large persistent ductus arteriosus.

The mortality for this procedure has ranged from 2 to 11 per cent in simple VSD banding to over 50 per cent for banding in complex lesions[3-5]. Since improved operative methods and postoperative care has provided improved results with primary correction, pulmonary artery banding is generally restricted at present to sick infants less than 6 months of age with large VSDs and intractable congestive failure and failure to grow, or with those complex lesions, unsuitable for primary repair in infancy. It is also a preferred procedure initially with the multiple muscular septal defects of the 'Swiss cheese' variety.

The operation

1

The operative technique requires an anterolateral left thoracotomy through the third intercostal space, with the incision under the breast in female patients. If a persistent ductus arteriosus is not present a simple small anterior incision will suffice.

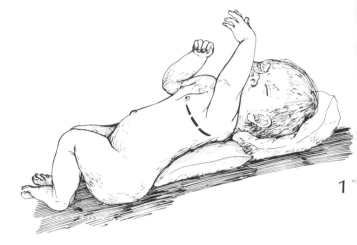

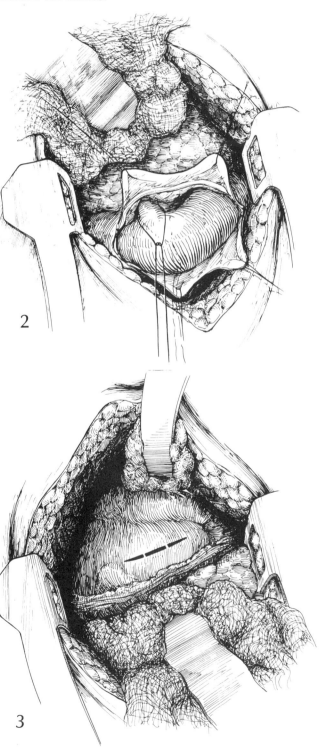

2 & 3

Dissection of the ductus is performed first by either an intra- or an extrapericardial approach. Closure of the ductus by ligation or division or by simple suture ligation for ligamentum arteriosum is performed. The lung is now retracted posteriorly and the pericardium incised anterior to the phrenic nerve.

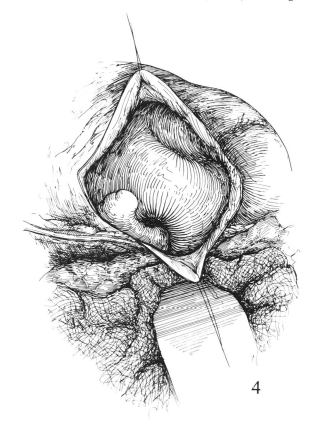

4

4, 5 & 6

Pericardial fluid is aspirated and sutures placed in the pericardial edges for retraction. Dissection of the visceral pericardium between the aorta and the pulmonary artery is performed anteriorly with sharp dissection and electrocautery. A right-angle clamp is gently placed around the pulmonary artery, special care being taken not to perforate the posterior aspect of the right pulmonary artery. A cotton umbilical tape is grasped in the clamp and passed around the pulmonary artery. An alternative suitable band is one of Teflon tape, which has the slight advantage of ease of removal at the time of debanding.

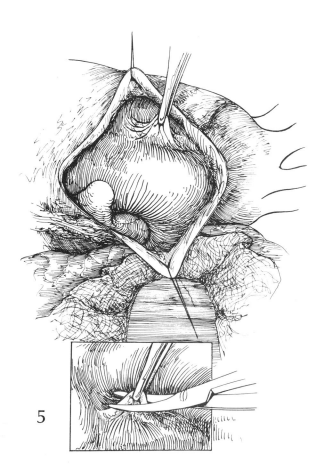

5

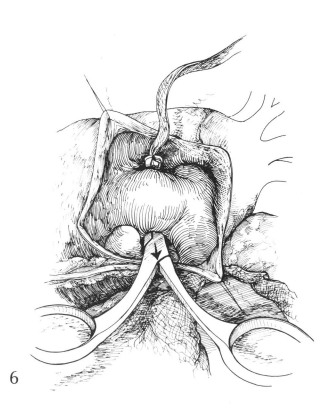

6

7

The cotton umbilical tape is initially marked for 25 mm so that this banding will leave an approximate diameter of 8 mm, the ideal measurement for successful constriction of the pulmonary artery[6]. The objective of banding is to decrease intra-arterial pressure distal to the band to a level approximately half the proximal pulmonary artery pressure, or 30–40 mmHg. A 2/0 silk ligature is tied beneath the right-angle clamp constricting the cotton umbilical tape.

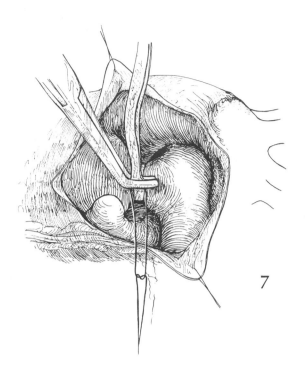

7

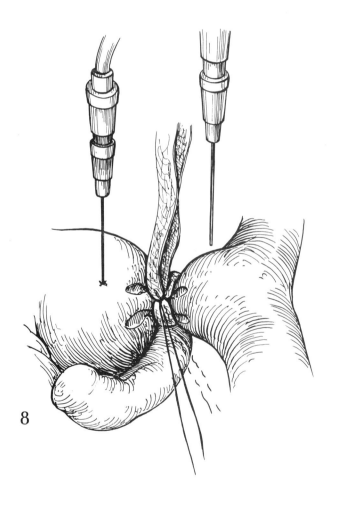

8

8

Pressure measurements are made in the proximal pulmonary artery and then distal to the pulmonary artery band to confirm satisfactory reduction of pulmonary artery pressure by one half.

9 & 10

Occasionally low cardiac output during the operation makes these pressure measurements unreliable. Some authorities therefore advocate simply making the pulmonary band tight enough to result in an equal diameter of both aorta and pulmonary artery. Observation of cardiac function should indicate a rise in systemic arterial pressure with a decrease in left-to-right shunting. When satisfactory constriction of the pulmonary artery is obtained a second mattress suture is placed through the umbilical tape for security and the excess tape is removed. The pericardium is closed loosely, the lung is inflated and a chest tube may be inserted. This is not generally necessary in most neonates and infants.

When a band is placed around the pulmonary artery in transposition of the great arteries with VSD, dissection around the posterior pulmonary artery may be difficult. It is a simple matter to dissect around the posterior aspect of the aorta (i.e. the anterior great artery), and when the band has been placed between the aorta and pulmonary arteries one end of the band should be passed through the transverse sinus so that the band then lies around the pulmonary artery and can readily be narrowed from that position.

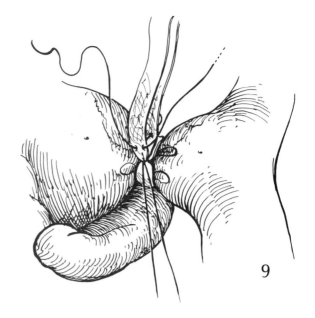

9

Complications

Complications of pulmonary artery banding include too tight a band, resulting in inadequate pulmonary blood flow and cyanosis, or too loose a band, this not preventing progressive pulmonary vascular obstructive changes. The band may migrate distally or may cause pulmonary infundibular stenosis.

At the time of removal of the band it can often be simply divided, followed by gentle dilatation of the pulmonary artery. Occasionally angioplasty by longitudinal incision with transverse closure or, rarely, patch angioplasty may be required to relieve stenosis.

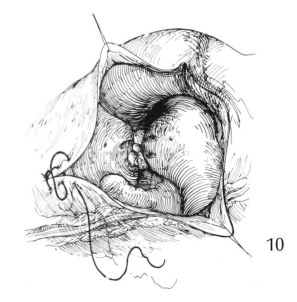

10

References

1. Muller, W. H. Jr., Dammann, J. F. Jr. The treatment of certain congenital malformations of the heart by the creation of pulmonic stenosis to reduce pulmonary hypertension and excessive pulmonary blood flow: a preliminary report. Surgery, Gynecology and Obstetrics 1952; 95: 213–219

2. Albert, H. M., Atik, M., Fowler, R. Production and release of pulmonary stenosis in dogs. Surgery 1958; 44: 904–909

3. Stark, J., Aberdeen, E., Waterston, D. J., Bonham-Carter, R. E., Tynan, M. Pulmonary artery constriction (banding): a report of 146 cases. Surgery 1965; 69: 808–818

4. Blackstone, E. H., Kirklin, J. W., Bradley, E. L., DuShane, J. W., Appelbaum, A. Optimal age and results in repair of large ventricular septal defects. Journal of Thoracic and Cardiovascular Surgery 1976; 72: 661–679

5. Hunt, C. E., Formanek, G., Levine, M. A., Castenada, A., Moller, J. H. Banding of the pulmonary artery: results in 111 children. Circulation 1971; 43: 395

6. Subramanian, S., Wagner, H. R. Pulmonary artery banding and debanding in patients with ventricular septal defect. In: Barratt-Boyes, B. G., Neutze, J. M., Harris, E. A., eds. Heart Disease in Infancy. Edinburgh and London, Churchill Livingstone 1973; 127

Total anomalous pulmonary venous connection: surgical anatomy

Robert H. Anderson BSc, MD, MRCPath
Joseph Levy Professor of Paediatric Cardiac Morphology, Cardiothoracic Institute, Brompton Hospital, London, UK

Introduction

Total anomalous pulmonary venous connection is a lesion in which all the pulmonary veins are connected to a site other than the morphologically left atrium. Although anomalous pulmonary venous connection is often considered to be the same as total anomalous pulmonary venous drainage, this is not strictly the case since in rare cases the pulmonary veins may be normally connected to the left atrium yet drain anomalously because of associated lesions such as the combination of mitral atresia, intact atrial septum and either a fenestrated coronary sinus or a laevoatrial cardinal vein. The term 'anomalous connection' is therefore preferable.

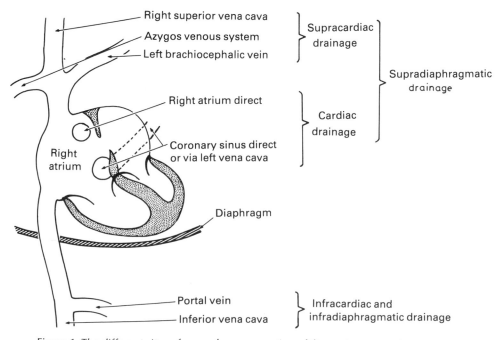

Figure 1 *The different sites of anomalous connection of the pulmonary veins.*

For there to be a totally anomalous connection all the pulmonary veins must join to a site other than the left atrium, either separately or, as is more usual, collectively via a common venous channel which may be termed the confluence. Partial anomalous pulmonary venous connections may also be found. Indeed, in isolation these may be one of the commonest congenital lesions, but their incidence is very difficult to estimate. Hughes and Rumore[1], when making this comment on incidence, did so on the basis of finding two cases in a routine study of 280 cadavers (0.7 per cent). What is certain is that in isolation they rarely produce problems.

Partial anomalous connection of the pulmonary venous bed is much more significant when associated with certain lesions. For instance, the combinations stand out with both sinus venosus atrial septal defects (see chapter on 'Atrial septal defect: surgical anatomy', pp. 138–142) and bilateral atrial connections with left atrial isomerism ('polysplenia'). Also noteworthy is the anomalous connection which forms part of the 'scimitar syndrome'. However, the topic dealt with in this section is the variant in which the entirety of the pulmonary venous bed is anomalously connected.

The salient anatomical features to be considered in each case are firstly whether the veins connect separately (mixed drainage) or via a confluence, and secondly the site of anomalous connection. The site of connection of individual veins in mixed drainage can be any of the sites to which a confluence, when present, may connect. The site of anomalous connection is certainly the most important feature, but also the presence of obstructive lesions along the anomalously connecting pulmonary venous pathway is significant. Last but not least, the presence of associated intracardiac malformations is important.

The site of anomalous connection is always to a systemic venous channel. This may be: to a vein draining into the superior vena cava or directly to the superior vena cava (supracardiac drainage); to the morphologically right atrium directly or via the coronary sinus or the left superior vena cava (cardiac drainage); or to the portal vein or inferior vena cava (infracardiac drainage) (see Figure 1). Since the supracardiac and cardiac types connect to systemic veins within the thoracic cavity while the infracardiac variant pierces the diaphragm to connect with abdominal veins another division is into supra- and infradiaphragmatic categories of anomalous connection. There are many subtle variations in the exact route taken by the anomalous venous channel [2–4], but certain types are sufficiently constant to stand out.

Supracardiac drainage

Supracardiac drainage is most frequently via an ascending vertical vein which connects to the left brachiocephalic vein, which then runs horizontally to the superior vena cava, which in turn returns vertically to the right atrium *(see Figure 2)*. It is this circuitous course which under-scores the characteristic 'snowman' or 'cottage loaf' chest radiograph. The confluence is almost always immediately posterior to the rudimentary left atrium; it is usually of good size so that surgical anastomosis of the two is rarely a problem. Of note is the course of the vertical vein relative to the pulmonary hilum. Usually the venous channel passes anterior to the arterial and bronchial structures and is generally not obstructed, but it may pass between the bronchus and pulmonary artery and then obstruction is to be expected ('the pulmonary vice'[4] – *see Figure 3*). Sometimes it may pass behind the hilum and then obstruction is again a possibility *(see Figure 2)*. The possible presence of an obstructed venous pathway should be catered for when designing the appropriate surgical repair.

More rarely a pathway connecting in supracardiac fashion may take a different route to the superior vena cava. Instead of ascending vertically it courses horizontally to the right side of the spine and then ascends vertically, picking up the right pulmonary veins, to connect either, directly to the superior vena cava or indirectly via the azygos vein *(see Figure 4)*. Despite the different pathway the left-sided component of this confluence remains adjacent to the left atrium and surgical management

follows the principles for the more usual supracardiac variant[5]. In the few cases seen of this type the site of connection of the anomalous pathway to the vena cava has often been described as abnormal, being aneurysmal in some cases. More rarely supracardiac drainage can be directly to the superior vena cava. This type is seen with mixed drainage.

Cardiac drainage

Cardiac drainage is most usually via the coronary sinus, when then achieves considerable size. The pulmonary veins may connect separately and directly to the sinus or else there may be a short confluence which represents a persistent left superior vena cava *(see Figure 5)*. In either event the surgical problems are the same. Since the coronary sinus is immediately adjacent to the rudimentary left atrium there is extensive 'party wall' between these structures. Thus there are two anatomical options for repair. It is feasible to make an extensive window between sinus and left atrium and simply close the orifice of the sinus *(see Figures 5b and 6)*. Alternatively the coronary sinus roof can be cut back to become confluent with the atrial septal defect or oval fossa and a large patch placed around both he confines of the fossa and the orifice of the sinus. In either event care must be taken not to damage the atrioventricular node (in its usual position in the triangle of Koch) or to produce residual obstruction at the patch. Naturally occurring obstruction of connection to

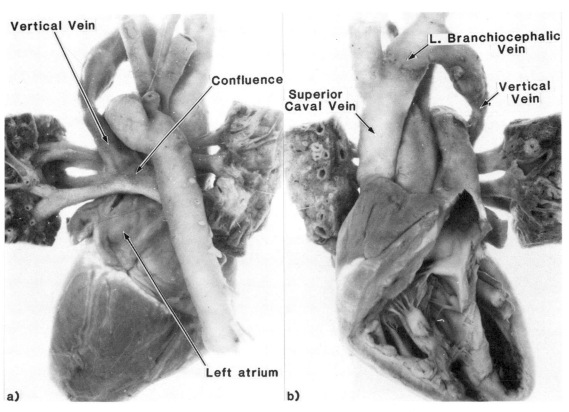

a)   b)

Figure 2 *The typical supracardiac 'cottage loaf' configuration, seen (a) from behind and (b) from in front. In this case the anomalous channel passes behind the bronchopulmonary hilum and is narrowed at this point. Photographed by kind permission of Dr L.M. Gerlis, Killingbeck Hospital, Leeds.*

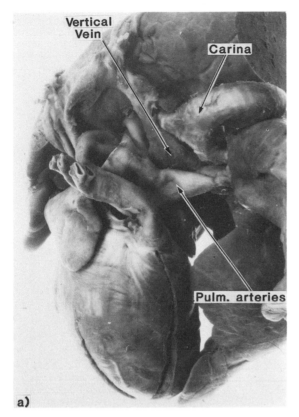

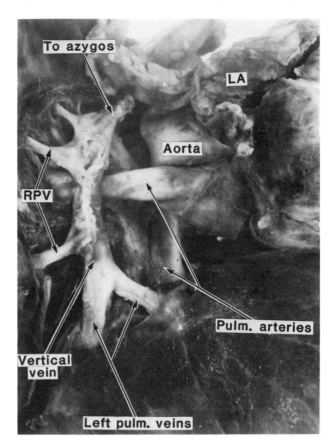

Figure 4 *The variant of supracardiac connection with a right-sided vertical vein. Photographed by kind permission of Dr L.M. Gerlis, Leeds.*

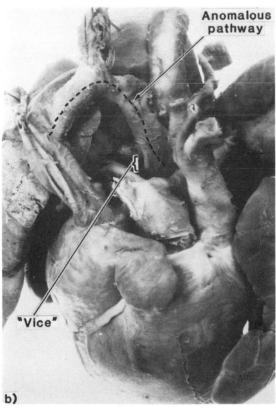

Figure 3 *A 'cottage loaf' drainage pattern associated with a bronchopulmonary vice seen (a) from the left and (b) from the right. Photographed by kind permission of Dr J.L. Wilkinson and Mrs Audrey Smith, University of Liverpool.*

the coronary sinus is rare but may occur because of stenosis at the opening of the sinus to the right atrium.

Direct connection to the right atrium is rarer and almost always occurs with significant associated malformations (*see Figure 6*). In this context right atrial isomerism ('asplenia') is the outstanding lesion. Hearts in this situation always have two atrial chambers of morphologically right type so that even when the pulmonary veins connect to the atrial chambers they do so in anomalous fashion. Usually they are crowded into a small aera of atrial roof (*see Figure 7*). With cardiac drainage, be there normal or abnormal atrial arrangement, the surgery will be designed to correct the anomalous connection by means of an interatrial patch joining the pulmonary venous orifices to the oval fossa (if present). Each case must be treated on its own merits, taking into account the other associated atrial lesions and noting the site of the sinus node and its blood supply (which will be bilateral in the presence of right atrial isomerism). Fortunately obstruction is exceedingly rare with direct atrial pulmonary venous connections.

Infracardiac and infradiaphragmatic drainage

Infracardiac and infradiaphragmatic anomalous venous connection is almost exclusively confined to the portal venous system but may occur via the inferior vena cava.

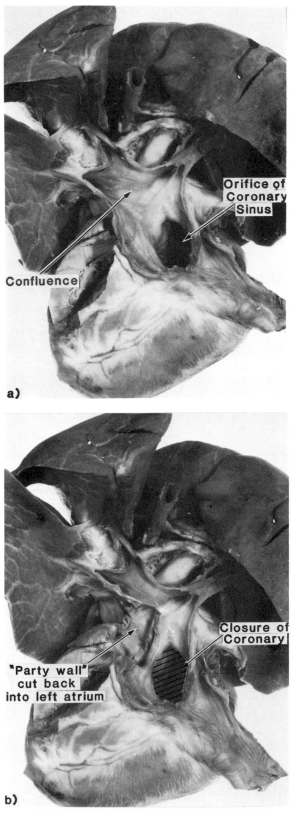

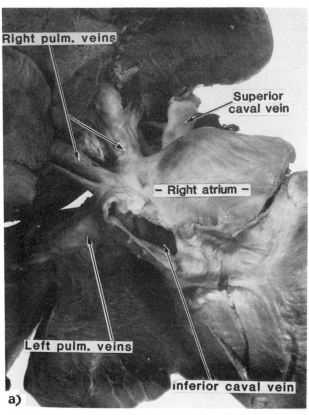

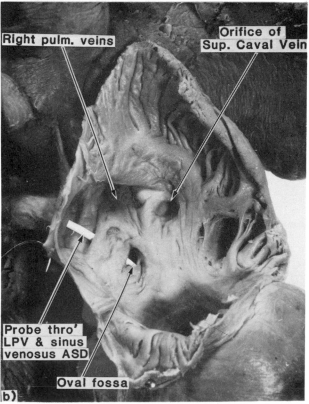

Figure 5 *Cardiac anomalous connection via the coronary sinus vein seen from behind* (a). *In* (b) *the 'party wall' has been cut away. Closure of the coronary sinus orifice then corrects the flow pathway. Photographed by kind permission of Dr J.L. Wilkinson and Dr Audrey Smith, Liverpool.*

Figure 6 *Anamolous connection directly to the right atrium seen* (a) *externally and* (b) *with the atrium opened. Photographed by kind permission of Dr J.L. Wilkinson and Dr Audrey Smith, Liverpool.*

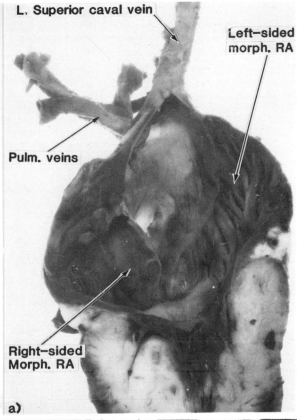

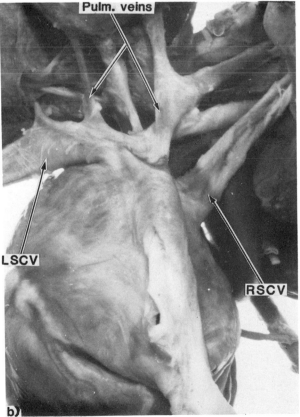

Figure 7 *The anomalous connection of the pulmonary vein to the atrial roof in right atrial isomerism seen (a) in 'four chamber' section and (b) from behind.*

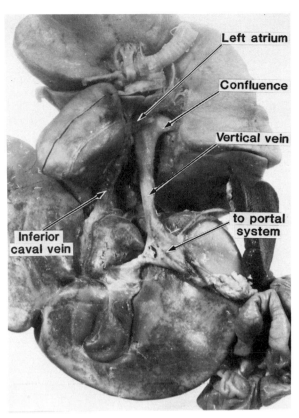

Figure 8 *Intradiaphragmatic connection to the portal vein. Photographed by kind permission of Dr L.M. Gerlis, Leeds.*

When the connection is to the portal system obstruction is to be expected within the hepatic sinusoids. This may be bypassed via the ductus venosus, so closure of this channel may produce rapid deterioration in the patient's condition. In any form of infradiaphragmatic drainage obstruction may also occur at the point where the venous channel crosses the diaphragm. The confluence remains adjacent to the left atrium in most cases and the potential site for obstruction is where the vertical vein passes through the oesophageal orifice of the diaphragm *(see Figure 8)*. Usually, as stated above, it then connects to the portal vein, but in one case studied recently obstruction was produced by the vertical vein, having penetrated the diaphragm, breaking up into a leash of small veins which terminated in the walls of the stomach.

Obstructive lesions

From the descriptions given above it will be noted that in general terms most obstructive lesions exist between the confluence and the termination of the anomalous pulmonary venous pathway. If, therefore, a good anastomosis can be made between the confluence and the left atrium the obstructive lesions will no longer present a problem. One worry in trying to create such an anastomosis is the size of the remnants of the left atrium and the left ventricle. Although these structures often seem small in autopsy specimens and have been reported to be so by some authors[7,8], part of the smallness is because the right-sided structures are enlarged. Measurements made in a recent study[9] indicated that left-sided dimensions were usually within normal limits and our observations support this finding. Only in the presence of severe associated lesions, such as univentricular atrioventricular connection to the right ventricle, is the left ventricle grossly hypoplastic. In the absence of such lesions artificial enlargement of the left atrium[10] has not improved surgical results. However, a more recent echocardiographic study has suggested that the left ventricle is significantly smaller in children not surviving operation[11]. Notwithstanding this, the main extraneous feature that will limit surgical success is the presence of associated lesions. The significance of right atrial isomerism in this respect cannot be overemphasized since the most anomalous pulmonary venous connection is but one of many complex lesions.

References

1. Hughes, C. W., Rumore, P. C. Anomalous pulmonary veins. Archives of Pathology 1944; 37: 364-366

2. Snellen, H. A., Dekker, A. Anomalous pulmonary venous drainage in relation to left superior vena cava and coronary sinus. American Heart Journal 1963; 66: 184-196

3. Bharati, S., Lev, M. Congenital anomalies of the pulmonary veins. Cardiovascular Clinics 1973; 5: 23-41

4. Delisle, G., Ando, M., Calder, A. L. et al. Total anomalous pulmonary venous connection; report of 93 autopsied cases with emphasis on diagnostic and surgical considerations. American Heart Journal 1976; 91: 99-122

5. Stark, J. Anomalies of the pulmonary venous return. In: Stark, J., de Leval, M., eds., Surgery for congenital heart defects. London: Grune and Stratton, 1983: 235-251

6. Van Praagh, R., Harken, A. H., Delisle, G., Ando, M., Gross, R. E. Total anomalous pulmonary venous drainage to the coronary sinus: a revised procedure for its correction. Journal of Thoracic and Cardiovascular Surgery 1972; 64: 132-135

7. Burroughs, J. T., Edwards, J. E. Total anomalous pulmonary venous connection (a review). American Heart Journal 1960; 59: 913-931

8. Mathew, R., Thilenius, O. G., Replogle, R. L., Arcilla, R. A. Cardiac function in total anomalous pulmonary venous return before and after surgery. Circulation 1977; 55: 361-370

9. Haworth, S. G., Reid, L. Structural study of pulmonary circulation and of heart in total anomalous pulmonary venous return in early infancy. British Heart Journal 1977; 39: 80-92

10. Katz, N. M., Kirklin, J. W., Pacifico, A. D. Concepts and practices in surgery for total anomalous pulmonary venous connection. Annals of Thoracic Surgery 1978; 25: 479-487

11. Lima, C. O., Valdes-Cruz, L. M., Allen, H. D. et al. Prognostic value of left ventricular size measured by echocardiography in infants with total anomalous pulmonary venous drainage. American Journal of Cardiology 1983; 51: 1155-1159

Total anomalous pulmonary venous drainage: surgical repair

J. Stark MD, FRCS, FACS
Consultant Cardiothoracic Surgeon, Thoracic Unit, The Hospital for Sick Children, Great Ormond Street, London, UK

Total anomalous pulmonary venous drainage occurs in about 1.5 per cent of children born with congenital heart disease. Most patients become symptomatic within the first months of life. Without treatment 80 per cent of the symptomatic infants die before they reach their first birthday[1].

Preoperative

Diagnosis

Infants with total anomalous pulmonary venous drainage usually present with heart failure and/or cyanosis. Pulmonary oedema is common. An electrocardiogram shows right axis deviation and right atrial and right ventricular hypertrophy. A heart that is not enlarged but is associated with pulmonary oedema and hepatomegaly is almost diagnostic of obstructive total anomalous pulmonary venous drainage. Accurate diagnosis can be established by real time echocardiography[2]. To exclude additional cardiac lesions and ascertain exactly the site of drainage from all parts of the lungs cardiac catheterization with angiocardiography is performed on some infants. Many can, however, be operated upon on the basis of echocardiographic examination alone.

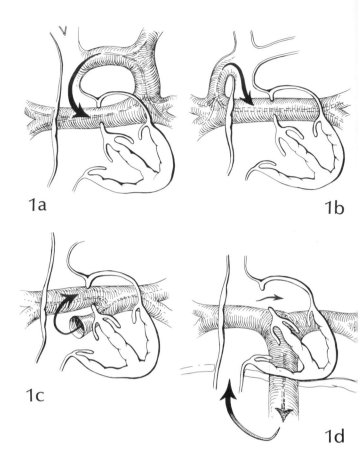

1a   1b

1c

1d

1a–d

The basic types of total anomalous pulmonary venous connection are fully described in the chapter on surgical anatomy, pp. 00–00 and are illustrated here. They are termed supracardiac (a,b), cardiac (c) and infracardiac (d) respectively.

Indications for operation

All infants with total anomalous pulmonary venous drainage and pulmonary hypertension should be operated upon immediately. In the absence of pulmonary hypertension and/or pulmonary venous obstruction surgery can be delayed, but patients in the latter category usually do not have symptoms in infancy. If they do, an early operation is preferred.

Anaesthesia

The patients are often severely ill on admission. They may require insertion of arterial and central venous lines for pressure and blood gas monitoring. If they hypoventilate or are suffering from pulmonary oedema they should be intubated and ventilated. A catecholamine drip is often helpful to treat severe heart failure. Premedication and anaesthesia are the same as for other open heart procedures in infants. For sick infants with total anomalous pulmonary venous drainage the technique of circulatory arrest under deep hypothermia is preferred.

The operation

Surface cooling

The use of surface cooling is somewhat controversial. Surface cooling is preferable for very young and sick infants. If cardiac arrest or ventricular fibrillation occurs in the initial stages of the operation the lower temperatures provide protection of the vital organs before cardiopulmonary bypass can be established. Surface cooling is achieved with ice packs. The extremities, the area of the skin incision and the lumbar region (kidneys) are not cooled. During surface cooling serum potassium levels should be monitored carefully and if necessary potassium supplements given intravenously.

Incision and cannulation

A midline sternotomy is performed when the nasopharyngeal temperature reaches 26–28°C. These infants are often dystrophic and a further fall of approximately 2°C in nasopharyngeal temperature can be expected. The pericardium is opened in the midline. The aorta and the right atrium are cannulated. All dissection is then carried out on cardiopulmonary bypass while the infant is further cooled to 19°C.

Perfusion

As soon as the perfusion is started a small incision is made in the confluence of the pulmonary veins and a small sucker tip is inserted. This decompresses the pulmonary veins and avoids damage to the pulmonary capillaries.

It is important to check for a persistent ductus arteriosus for, apart from the haemodynamic consequences, a persistent ductus might allow air embolization when circulatory arrest is begun and the systemic pressure falls to zero.

When the desired temperature is reached perfusion is stopped, the patient's blood is drained into the oxygenator, the aorta is cross-clamped, the superior and inferior venae cavae are snared and the venous cannula is removed from the right atrium.

In older children the operation can be performed using standard cardiopulmonary bypass with moderate hypothermia and cardioplegic arrest. Care should be taken to open the common pulmonary vein as soon as the ascending vein is ligated so as to avoid obstruction of pulmonary venous drainage resulting in distension and damage to the pulmonary capillaries.

The surgical technique depends on the anatomical type of total anomalous pulmonary venous drainage present.

SUPRACARDIAC TYPE

Surface cooling is used in small and sick neonates. A midline sternotomy is then performed and cardiopulmonary bypass instituted, cooling the patient to 19°C.

2

The vein connecting the pulmonary vein to the innominate vein is dissected outside the pericardium. Care must be taken not to damage the phrenic nerve and to pass the ligature above the entry of the left upper pulmonary vein. This may be rather high. When the circulation is stopped the vein is doubly ligated. Premature ligation of this vein would completely obstruct pulmonary venous drainage and damage the lungs. The aorta is cross-clamped and cardioplegic solution infused into the ascending aorta.

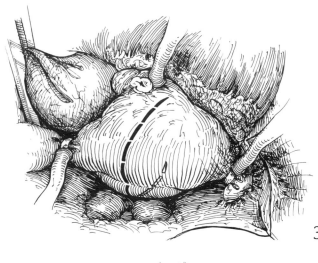

3

3 & 4

The right atrium is opened transversely from the atrioventricular groove across the crista terminalis and across the septum. The incision continues through the foramen ovale to the posterior wall of the left atrium down to the base of the left atrial appendage.

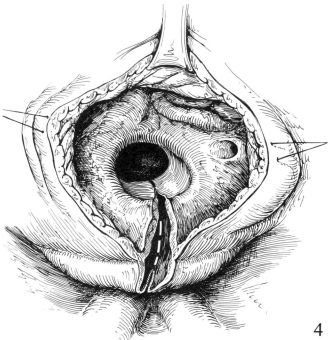

4

5

The horizontal confluence of the pulmonary veins lies just beneath this incision and is now incised. A ligature is placed on the tip of the left atrial appendage, which is retracted to the left. This prevents the appendage from invaginating into the left atrium and obscuring the surgeon's view when the anastomosis is being constructed.

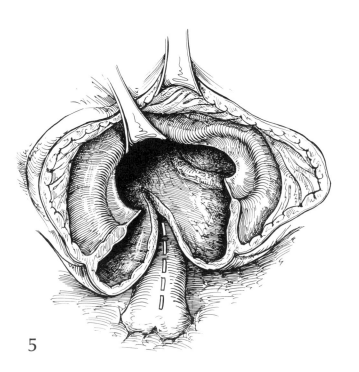

5

6, 7, 8 & 9

The posterior wall of the left atrium and the common pulmonary veins are joined by a suture of 6/0 polypropylene. As long an anastomosis as possible is created. Care must be taken when both sides of the posterior left atrial wall and the septum are joined to the right side of the common pulmonary vein since it is of great importance to avoid constriction of the vein. The atrial septal defect can be closed directly or with a patch.

The left atrium and left ventricle have been reported to be small in patients with total anomalous pulmonary venous drainage[3]. Recent experience[4] has failed to show any difference in the survival rate whether or not the left atrium was enlarged with a patch. Before the atrial septum is closed the left ventricle and the left atrium are filled with saline.

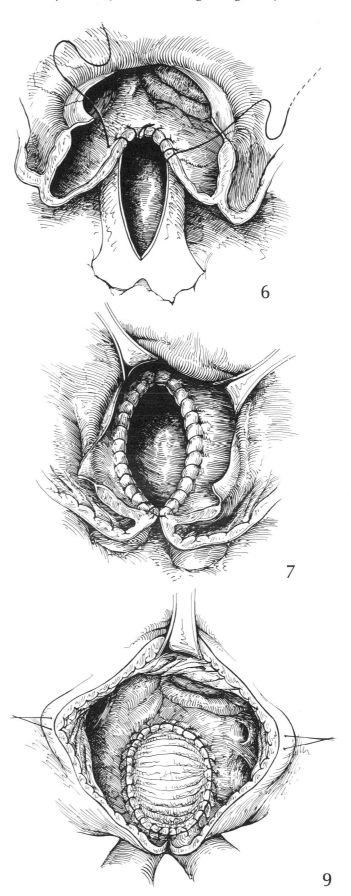

6

7

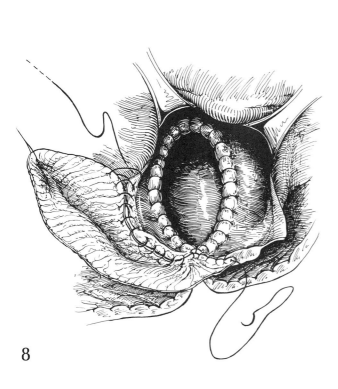

8

9

10

The atriotomy is closed with a running polypropylene stitch, the venous cannula is replaced into the right atrium and perfusion is restarted and the patient rewarmed. Air must be evacuated meticulously from the left side of the heart, usually via an aortic needle vent.

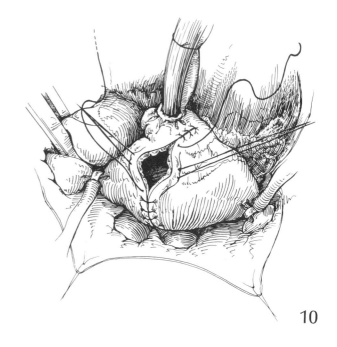

10

CARDIAC TYPE

11

The right atrium is opened and the anatomy inspected. The most common site of intracardiac drainage is the coronary sinus, although separate entry of the pulmonary veins into the right atrium is possible.

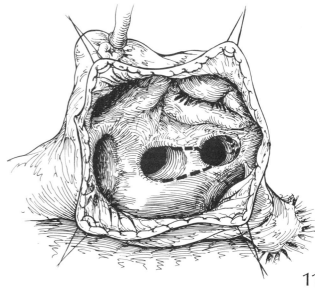

11

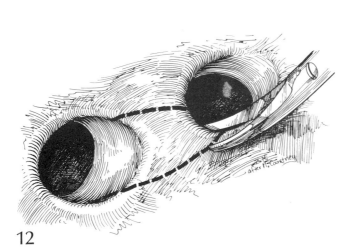

12

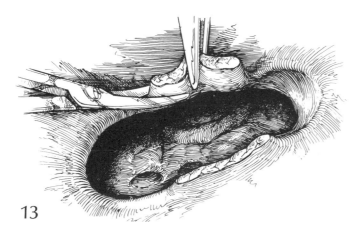

13

12 & 13

The septum between the coronary sinus and patent foramen ovale is excised. This creates a large communication between the coronary sinus and the left atrium.

14 & 15

A patch of pericardium or thin Dacron is used to divert all pulmonary venous blood, together with the coronary sinus blood, to the left atrium. Anteriorly the suture line runs through the floor of the coronary sinus away from its anterior rim so as to avoid any damage to the tail of the atrioventricular node. The small right-to-left shunt resulting from the coronary sinus blood admixture is not significant and is usually not detected by oximetry at postoperative cardiac catheterization.

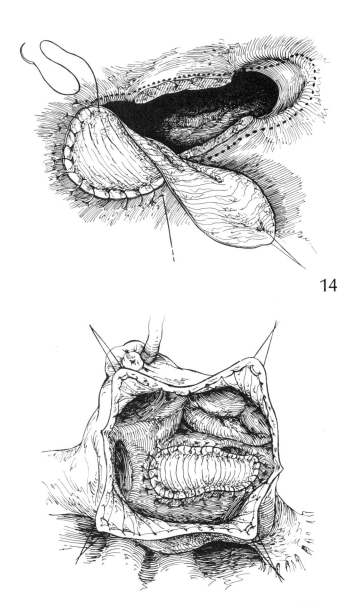

14

15

INFRACARDIAC TYPE

For the repair of this type a retrocardiac approach is preferred, again using the technique of deep hypothermia and circulatory arrest. This allows better exposure of the common vein which is usually orientated vertically. As soon as perfusion is started the confluence of the pulmonary veins is opened and a sucker tip inserted to decompress the pulmonary veins.

16, 17 & 18

In patients in whom there is a long distance between the confluence of the pulmonary veins and the left atrium the descending vein can be doubly ligated and divided. This allows the site of the anastomosis to come into closer apposition with the left atrium. (Following a report of liver necrosis after ligation of the descending vein in infra-diaphragmatic total anomalous pulmonary venous drainage[5] some surgeons prefer not to ligate this vein.) Oblique parallel incisions are then made in the confluences of the pulmonary veins and in the posterior wall of the left atrium. The incision starts from the origin of the left upper pulmonary vein and extends into the upper portion of the dilated descending vein, allowing a large anastomosis to be created. The atrial septal defect or patent foramen ovale is closed through a separate right atriotomy.

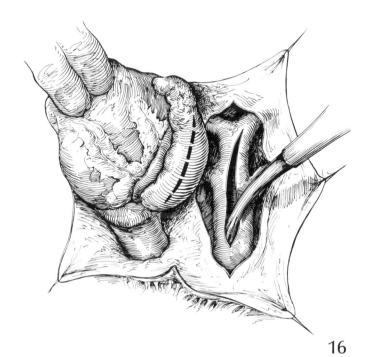

16

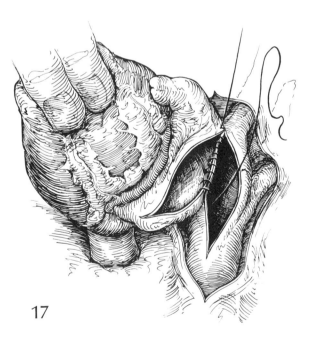

17

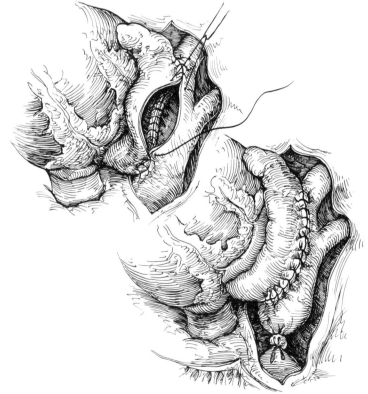

18

MIXED TYPE TOTAL ANOMALOUS PULMONARY VENOUS DRAINAGE

Almost any combination of the types of drainage described, may exist. If one lobe drains differently from the rest of the lungs it can be left uncorrected without great physiological consequences. Commonly the left upper lobe drains to the innominate vein while the remaining drainage is intracardiac.

Postoperative care

Rewarming and terminating perfusion

When the repair is completed the heart is filled with saline. The venous cannula is replaced into the right atrium and the patient slowly transfused from the oxygenator. When the superior vena caval pressure reaches 12–15 mmHg the caval snares are loosened and air is aspirated from the venous line. The left ventricle and ascending aorta are aspirated of air, bypass is restarted and the aortic clamp released.

During rewarming the venous pressure is kept at 6–8 mmHg, thus allowing the heart to eject. It is believed that pulsatile flow at this stage is beneficial. When the temperature reaches 36°C bypass is discontinued and the venous cannula removed. Occasionally it is necessary to remove the aortic cannula quickly as the aorta is usually small and can be partly obstructed. Because of the tendency of patients with total anomalous pulmonary venous drainage to develop pulmonary oedema the central venous pressure or left atrial pressure is kept lower than with other lesions. Usually 8–10 mmHg is sufficient for adequate cardiac output.

Complications

Pulmonary oedema is common, even if a large anastomosis has been constructed. Segmental or lobar atelectasis is treated with intensive physiotherapy; occasionally deep suction is required.

Late deaths due to stenosis of the anastomosis or stenosis of pulmonary veins have been described[6,7,8]. Progression of pulmonary vascular obstructive disease has also been observed.

Results

The operative mortality depends on the anatomical type of total anomalous pulmonary venous drainage and on the condition of the patient on admission to the hospital[4,9,10]. It is lowest in patients with cardiac drainage and highest in those with infracardiac drainage. Our recent results are most encouraging; during 1979–1982 we operated on 28 infants with 4 deaths (16 per cent). Among 55 survivors of the operation from the years 1971–1977 there was only one late death, due to pulmonary obstructive disease.

Acknowledgement

Illustrations 6, 7, 9, 11, 12 and 13 have been modified from illustrations by M. Courtney in J. Stark, Anomalies of the Pulmonary Venous Return, In: Stark, J., de Leval, M. R., eds. Surgery for Congenital Heart Defects pp. 235–251. London and New York: Academic Press, 1983 with kind permission of the publisher.

References

1. Bonham-Carter, R. E., Capriles, M., Noe, Y. Total anomalous pulmonary venous drainage: a clinical and anatomical study of 75 children. British Heart Journal 1969; 31: 45–51

2. Smallhorn, J. F., Sutherland, G. R., Tommasini, G., Hunter, S., Anderson, R. H., Macartney, F. J. Assessment of total anomalous pulmonary venous connection by two-dimensional echocardiography. British Heart Journal 1981; 46: 613–623

3. Burroughs, J. T., Edwards, J. E. Total anomalous pulmonary venous connection (a review). American Heart Journal 1960; 59: 913–931

4. Katz, N. M., Kirklin, J. W., Pacifico, A. D. Concepts and practices in surgery for total anomalous pulmonary venous connection. Annals of Thoracic Surgery 1978; 25: 479–487

5. Appelbaum, A., Kirklin, J. W., Pacifico, A. D., Bargeron, L. M., Jr. The surgical treatment of total anomalous pulmonary venous connection. Israeli Journal of Medical Sciences 1975; 11: 89–96

6. Friedli, B., Davignon, A., Stanley, P. Infradiaphragmatic total anomalous pulmonary venous return: surgical correction in a newborn infant. Journal of Thoracic and Cardiovascular Surgery 1971; 62: 301–306

7. Whight, C. M., Barratt-Boyes, B. G., Calder, A. L., Neutze, J. M., Brandt, P. W. T. Total anomalous pulmonary venous connection: long-term results following repair in infancy. Journal of Thoracic and Cardiovascular Surgery 1978; 75: 52–63

8. Clarke, D. R., Stark, J., de Leval, M., Pincott, J. R., Taylor, J. F. N. Total anomalous pulmonary venous drainage in infancy. British Heart Journal 1977; 39: 436–444

9. Stark, J. Anomalies of pulmonary venous return. In: Stark, J., de Leval, M. R., eds. Surgery for Congenital Heart Defects 1983; 235–251. London: Academic Press

10. Stark, J. Analysis of the factors which might improve the survival rate of infants with congenital heart disease. In: Rickham, P. P., Hecker, W. C. H., Prevot, J., eds. Causes of Postoperative Death in Children. Baltimore: Urban and Schwarzenber 1979; 109–114

Illustrations in this chapter by Siew Yen Ho

Atrial septal defect: surgical anatomy

Robert H. Anderson   BSc, MD, MRCPath
Joseph Levy Professor of Paediatric Cardiac Morphology, Cardiothoracic Institute, Brompton Hospital, London, UK

Introduction

Provided the surgeon is aware of the confines of the atrial septum[1,2] and the disposition of the sinus and atrioventricular nodes, little difficulty should be found in completing uneventful repair of the defects which may permit interatrial shunting of blood. The phrase 'interatrial shunting of blood' is used advisedly, since various types of so-called 'atrial septal defect' are outside the confines of the interatrial septum and so, strictly speaking, are not *septal* defects. Although this may seem an unnecessarily pedantic point, it is these variants outside the normal confines of the septum which are most likely to present problems, so it is well to be fully conversant with their anatomy. This in turn can only be achieved when their true position is appreciated relative to the extent of the septum.

1

Thus, true atrial septal defects are all found within the confines of the oval septum. Of the variants which, although outside the septum, permit interatrial communication, the so-called ostium primum atrial septal defect is an atrioventricular septal defect[3] and is described elsewhere. The sinus venosus defects are in the mouths of either the superior or inferior caval veins and exist because either the caval veins or the right pulmonary veins have a biatrial attachment (see below). Finally, the so-called coronary sinus defect is the opening of the coronary sinus. It permits interatrial communication because of unroofing of the coronary sinus[4]. The illustration is a drawing of the opened right atrium in surgical orientation showing the sites of the different types of interatrial communication.

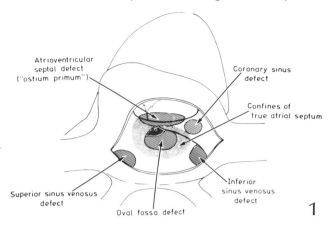

1

The defects

2

DEFECTS WITHIN THE OVAL FOSSA

These are by far the commonest type of interatrial communication[5]. Although frequently termed secundum defects, they rarely result from a deficiency of the so-called septum secundum. This secondary septum forms the margins of the oval fossa and only rarely do the rims become so stretched that shunting can occur across a normally formed floor of the fossa. Defects within the fossa almost without exception result from deficiencies of the floor, which is derived from the embryonic primary septum. The size of the defect depends upon the degree of deficiency of the floor. If the flap valve is minimally deficient or perforate, then the defect will be small (a). If the flap valve is almost totally eroded the defect will be large (b) and its size often increased because of stretching of the margins. The larger the defect, the closer to the edge is the site of the atrioventricular node (AVN).

With considerable dilatation of the atria a defect at the oval fossa can effectively produce a common atrium, but the latter is more usually seen with atrioventricular septal defects. In equivocal cases the distinction between the two is readily made from the morphology of the atrioventricular valves. Simple patency of the oval fossa occurs when the flap valve overlaps the margins but is not adherent to them.

When left atrial pressure is higher than right a patent fossa does not permit shunting of blood. When defects within the oval fossa are being repaired the sinus node is unlikely to give problems since it is separated from the defect by the orifice of the superior caval vein. The major danger is the AVN lying in the triangle of Koch. As indicated above, if the fossa is stretched the superior border of the nodal triangle may be a direct margin of the defect (b). Attention to the landmarks of the triangle will enable this possibility to be assessed and, when encountered, the necessary steps can be taken to avoid nodal damage. In this context it is worth re-emphasizing that there are no specialized tracts of internodal conduction tissue in the margins of the fossa (or elsewhere). The preferential routes for internodal conduction[6] are composed of ordinary 'working' atrial myocardium[7].

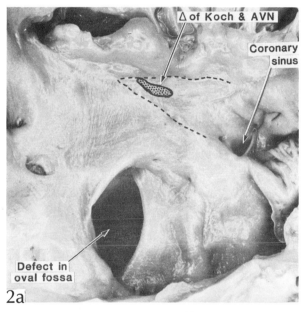

2a

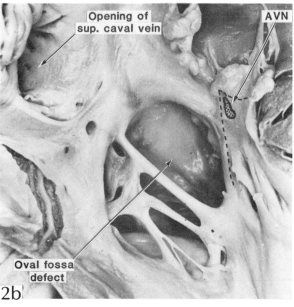

2b

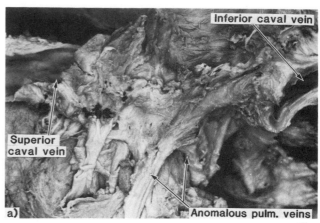

3a

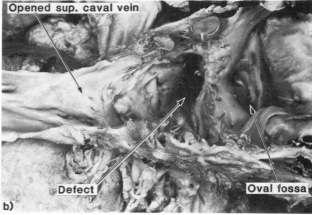

3b

SINUS VENOSUS DEFECTS

3a & 3b

These communications are found usually in the mouth of the superior caval vein, the illustration showing the external appearance of a superior sinus venosus defect with anomalous connections of the right pulmonary veins (a) and the overriding superior caval vein (b).

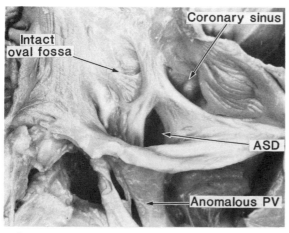

4

4

Much more rarely there is an inferior sinus venosus defect in the orifice of the inferior caval vein with an intact oval fossa.

5

Since the defects are outside the confines of the normal atrial septum they can only exist if a venous structure has a connection to both right and left atrial chambers. The apparent 'atrial septal defect' in actuality occurs through the lumen of anomalously connected veins. In the case of the superior defect there is usually a biatrial connection of the superior caval vein, which overrides the upper rim of the oval fossa, together with anomalous connection of the right pulmonary veins into the caval channel (see *Illustration 3*).

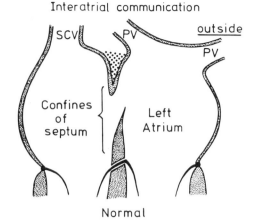

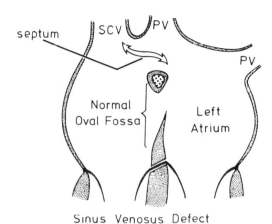

Sinus Venosus Defect

5

Anomalous pulm. veins   Site of sinus node

6

6

It is these anomalous venous connections which produce the difficulty in surgical repair of a superior sinus venous defect. Often it is difficult to close the defect in such a way as to redirect pulmonary venous drainage to the left atrium without at the same time obstructing the superior caval pathway. In these circumstances it is necessary to widen the vena cava with a gusset[8]. Then the position of the sinus node is a vital consideration. This usually lies lateral to the cavoatrial junction and the incision for widening the pathway must be made to avoid this area. It is still possible that an incision placed anywhere round the caval circumference could divide the sinus node artery because of its variable course. Even if the possibility of arterial damage exists, however, it is more vital to avoid the node itself and this can certainly be accomplished.

An inferior sinus venosus defect is much rarer and may coexist with anomalous connection of the right lower pulmonary vein. Because the defect is more distant from the sinus node the problems in repair are not nearly as great.

7

CORONARY SINUS DEFECT

This is the rarest type of interatrial communication. The defect is in the right atrial orifice of the coronary sinus and permits interatrial communication only because the left superior caval vein connects to the left atrial roof with unroofing of its intermediate portion. It has been argued[4] that the type of bilateral drainage of the superior caval veins found in the presence of atrial isomerism is the extreme form of unroofed coronary sinus. Because of this it is important to distinguish both the unroofed sinus and the interatrial communication at the atrial orifice of the sinus. In atrial isomerism when the caval veins connect bilaterally to the atrial roof then there is usually no coronary sinus orifice. Only when the orifice is formed is there a discrete interatrial communication. Repair then depends upon the interconnections between the caval veins. If there is a free communication, then the left caval vein can be ligated and the coronary sinus orifice closed, care being taken to avoid the atrioventricular node. If the left caval vein has no alternative route of drainage, however, it must be channelled in suitable fashion to the sinus orifice, which will then be left open.

(Illustrations 2, 3, 4 and 7 are reproduced by kind permission of Dr. J. R. Zuberbuhler, of the Children's Hospital of Pittsburg. Illustration 6 is reproduced by kind permission of Dr. B. R. Wilcox, of the University of North Carolina).

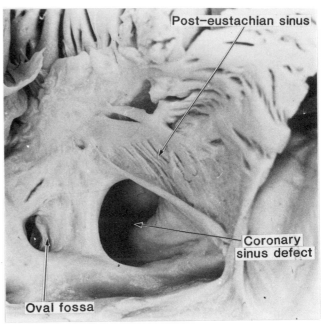

7

References

1. Sweeney, L. J., Rosenquist, G. C. The normal anatomy of the atrial septum in the human heart. American Heart Journal 1979; 98: 194–199

2. Anderson, R. H., Becker, A. E. The interatrial septum. In: Anderson, R. H., Becker, A. E. Cardiac anatomy – an integrated text and colour atlas. London: Gower, Edinburgh: Churchill Livingstone, 1980: 2.18–2.22

3. Becker, A. E., Anderson, R. H. Atrioventricular septal defects: what's in a name? Journal of Thoracic and Cardiovascular Surgery 1982; 83: 461–469

4. Quaegebeur, J., Kirklin, J. W., Pacifico, A. D., Bargeron, L. M. jr. Surgical experience with unroofed coronary sinus. Annals of Thoracic Surgery 1979; 27: 418–425

5. Bedford, D. E. The anatomical types of atrial septal defect, their incidence and clinical diagnosis. American Journal of Cardiology 1960; 6: 568–574

6. Spach, M. S., Miller, W. T. III, Geselowitz, D. B., Barr, R. C., Kootsey, J. M., Johnson, E. A. The discontinuous nature of propagation in normal canine cardiac muscle: evidence for recurrent discontinuities of intracellular resistance that affect the membrane currents. Circulation Research 1981; 48: 39–54

7. Anderson, R. H., Ho, S. Y., Smith, A., Becker, A. E. The internodal artrial myocardium. Anatomical Record 1981; 201: 75–82

8. Kyger, E. R., Frazier, O. H., Codey, D. A., Gillette, P. C., Reul, G. J., Sandiford, F. M., Wukasch, D. C. Sinus venosus atrial septal defect: early and late results following closure in 109 patients. Annals of Thoracic Surgery 1978; 25: 44–50

Atrial septal defect

John R. W. Keates MB, BChir, FRCS
Consultant Cardiothoracic Surgeon, King's College Hospital, London, UK

Preoperative

INDICATIONS

The presence of an atrial septal defect with a significant left-to-right shunt (more than 1.5 to 1) at cardiac catheterization is an indication for surgical closure. Ideally, the operation would be carried out before puberty, but there is no contraindication to operation in older age groups.

CONTRAINDICATIONS

The relatively rare presence of increased pulmonary vascular resistance[1] increases the risk of closure. Where this is responsible for a balanced or reversed shunt closure is contraindicated.

The operations

Incision: external appearance of the heart

A vertical sternotomy gives the best exposure and is most usual. Occasionally a right anterolateral thoracotomy through the fourth rib bed is used for the so-called 'secundum defect'. It gives adequate exposure and a less prominent scar, which may be important in some cases.

The right atrium, right ventricle and pulmonary artery are enlarged, while the aorta is small, reflecting the right-to-left shunt. A search is made for anomalies of pulmonary venous drainage at and around the termination of the superior vena cava. There is often only one right superior pulmonary vein in these cases, entering at the junction of the superior vena cava and the right atrium immediately in front of the interatrial groove. However, there may be small vessels entering the posterior aspect of the superior vena cava at a higher level.

The presence of a left-sided superior vena cava should be suspected if the brachiocephalic vein is either very small or absent and the superior vena cava (right) is smaller than normal.

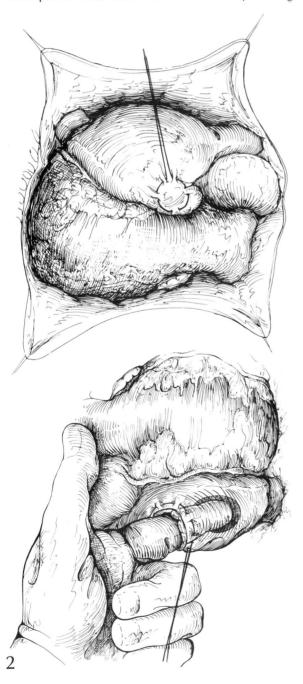

2

1 & 2

Digital exploration of the right atrium

While this is not an essential part of the procedure when the clinical and laboratory data point to a simple pathological condition, it is useful in the complicated case. It is particularly useful in assessing the severity and anatomical cause of mitral valve regurgitation.

3a & b

Preparation for exposure of the defect

An arterial cannula is introduced into the ascending aorta through a purse-string suture (a). Two vena caval cannulae are inserted via purse-string sutures in the right atrium. The purse-string sutures should be sited to allow optimum exposure of the defect with the smallest incision necessary. This will vary, for example, with the sinus venosus defect, which is high up in the septum. In the occasional case where a left-sided vena cava is present this is best cannulated via the coronary sinus through a separate purse-string suture at this stage (b). Alternative techniques are to remove the blood draining from it by direct suction when the atrium is opened or simply to clamp it as it enters the heart.

Cardiopulmonary bypass is instituted.

Myocardial protection

In order to produce a clear operating field a vent is placed and the ascending aorta is cross-clamped before the atrium is opened. Myocardial protection is gained by the use of cardioplegic solution and topical hypothermia. In view of the relatively short time involved it is not necessary to use systemic hypothermia in addition.

Defects within the dual fossa (septum secundum defects)

The septum secundum defect is the one most often encountered surgically, while the persistent foramen ovale is a normal finding in 10–20 per cent of the population[2]. The latter only becomes surgically important in relation to other lesions obstructing the right heart, such as pulmonary valve stenosis when, in the presence of decreased right ventricular compliance, it may be responsible for allowing a right-to-left shunt and cyanosis.

4

Atrial incision

The atrial incision should be made with care to avoid the area of the sinoatrial node around the insertion of the superior vena cava. This incision should not be unnecessarily large if postoperative problems in transatrial conduction are to be avoided. A stay suture placed in the posterior lip of the incision and a small retractor anteriorly should provide an excellent view.

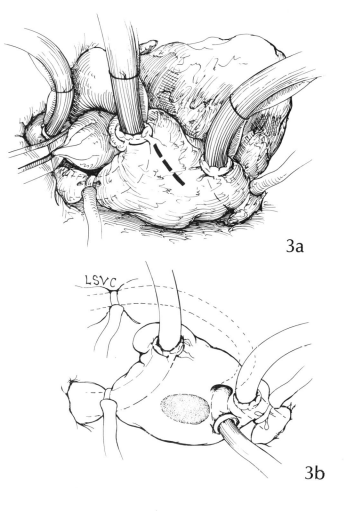

3a

LSVC

3b

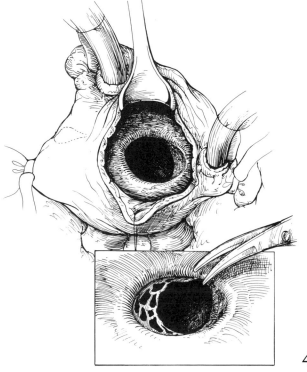

4

Closure of the defect

5

When the atrium is opened the defect is inspected, as is the mitral valve if necessary. The thin fenestrated tissue sometimes seen in the vicinity of the defect is not suitable to hold sutures and may be excised if redundant. A double-armed 3/0 polypropylene (or other synthetic) suture is placed across the lower margin of the defect, thus defining it, avoiding the Eustachian valve.

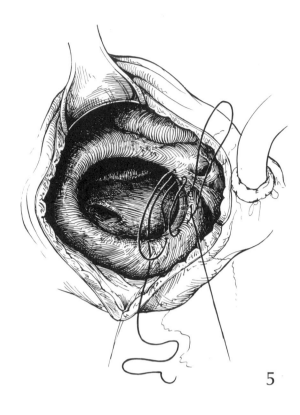

5

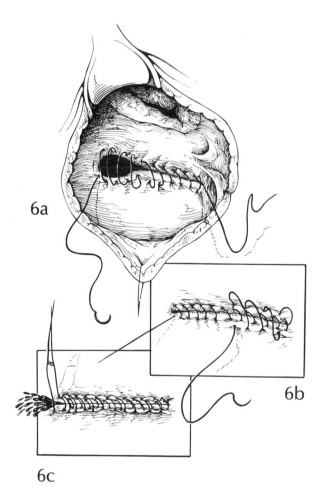

6a

6b

6c

6a, b & c

The suture starts at the lower margin and is carried up as a continuous whip stitch incorporating the thick muscular margins of the defect (a). The other end of the suture is used to oversew the repair (b) and the two ends are tied together at the end of the row (c) after the left atrium has been filled with blood by stopping the vent and gently inflating the lungs.

7

The larger defects seen in older patients[3] where there is a deficiency of tissue may be closed with a patch of pericardium or two-way stretch fabric. This should be cut to a size a little smaller than the defect as seen in the relaxed heart and sutured in place with a fine suture such as 4/0 polypropylene.

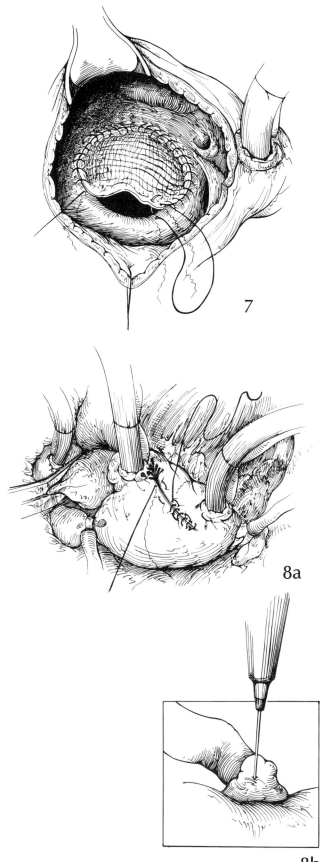

7

8a & b

Closure of the right atrium

This is performed with an everting suture of double-armed 3/0 polypropylene starting from the inferior limit. Again before completion of the suture the right atrium is allowed to fill with blood by releasing one of the caval snares and gently restricting the venous return. The suture line is reinforced with a whip stitch (a). In the trabeculated part of the atrium anterior to the crista terminalis care should be taken to place the needle through and not between the trabeculae to avoid tearing the atrial wall with subsequent troublesome bleeding.

8a

The elimination of air

Air ejected from the left heart into the systemic circulation is a serious hazard of this operation and all efforts should be made to avoid it. Residual air in the atrium is expelled as detailed above immediately before completion of the repair, air trapped in the left atrial appendage is evacuated with a syringe and needle (b) and air in the ascending aorta is evacuated in the same way as the aortic clamp is being released.

After the aortic clamp has been removed the heart is electrically fibrillated until all air in the left ventricle has been expressed via the vent hole. After defibrillation of the ventricle the ascending aorta is allowed to vent freely with a suitable needle while the heart action is recovering and for the first few minutes as the heart takes over the circulation.

8b

SINUS VENOSUS DEFECTS

In this condition there are always one or more anomalous pulmonary veins entering the terminal superior vena cava[4]. They can easily be seen externally and palpated through the atrial wall, but if necessary a finger in the right atrium will confirm and identify the defect, which is normally small and lies within the entrance of the superior vena cava. It has a sharp crescentic inferior margin. A number of sinus venosus defects have an associated left superior vena cava.

9 & 10

Exposure and cannulation

The preparation of the patient is as before but the incision in the atrium will be higher and more posterior. Special care must be taken to avoid damage to the sinus node and in the placement of the superior vena caval snare to allow safe and adequate exposure of the defect.

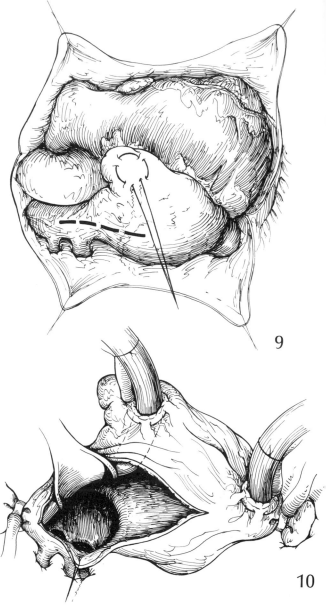

9

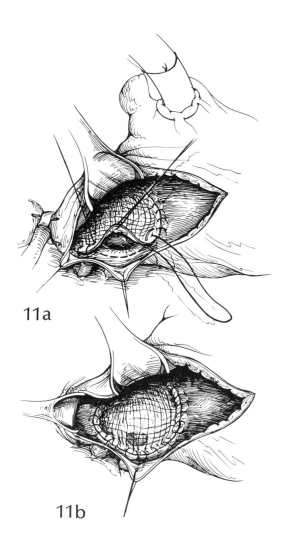

11a

11b

10

Closure

11a & b

The defect is closed with a patch which also covers the anomalous vein(s), deflecting the pulmonary venous blood into the left atrium. The patch may be of pericardium or of prosthetic material and is sutured into place with continuous 4/0 polypropylene or equivalent sutures, reinforced if desired with interrupted sutures[5,6].

Attempts to mobilize the veins and apply a direct suture to the defect are not recommended owing to the risk of occlusion and thrombosis of the pulmonary veins[7]. When a small pulmonary vein enters high on the superior vena cava it is best ignored as the corresponding shunt will be haemodynamically unimportant.

12 & 13

PRIMUM DEFECTS

Defects of the septum primum represent one end of the spectrum of atrioventricular canal anomalies more fully described elsewhere (*see* chapter on 'Atrioventricular septal defect' pp. 151–159). In the absence of deficiencies of the atrioventricular valves the repair of these defects is similar to that of septum secundum defects. However, the one important difference is that the defect is low and the inferior edge of it lies close to the conduction tissue. In order to avoid distortion of the atrioventricular valve a patch is used and the lower lip attached to the margin of the mitral valve until the area of conducting tissue is cleared. Temporary pacing wires are left in situ as a precaution. However, permanent atrioventricular dissociation is uncommon if care is taken in the placing of sutures.

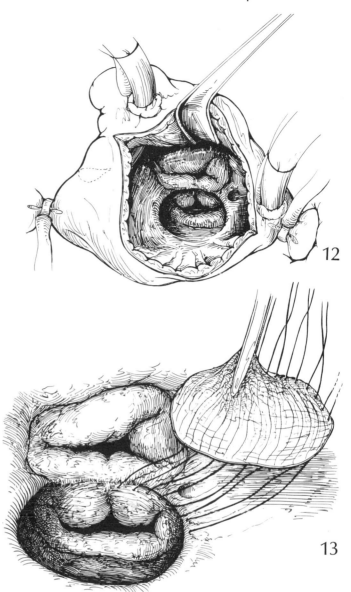

12

13

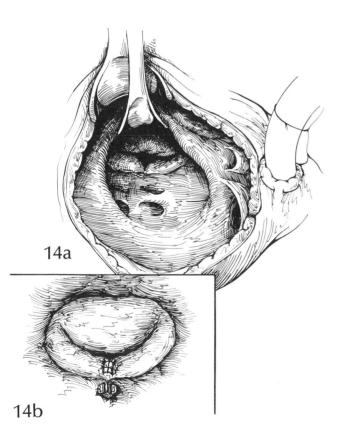

14a

14b

14a & b

MITRAL REGURGITATION

Although atrioventricular canal anomalies are more commonly the cause of mitral regurgitation due to cleft anterior cusps in the presence of a septum primum defect, clefts and prolapse of the posterior cusp are occasionally seen in conjunction with secundum defects[8–11].

If small, clefts may be closed by direct suture with or without an imbricating suture of the mitral valve annulus. Assessment of the status of the valve may be made digitally via the defect before the institution of bypass. Prolapse of either cusp may be repaired by conventional means. If simple repair is not feasible and the leak is serious, then replacement of the mitral valve may be achieved through the same incision, although an interrupted suture technique is advisable owing to the constrained exposure.

Postoperative care

Cases of atrial septal defect repair usually run an uncomplicated postoperative course.

Overtransfusion should be avoided and any residual pump prime given slowly. At the end of a short bypass, and particularly in small patients, the clear pump prime has not been fully distributed or excreted and it is very easy to overtransfuse the patient even to the point of pulmonary oedema[12]. This has given rise to the concept that the left ventricle is 'inadequate'. This is highly unlikely to be a serious problem as these patients are usually asymptomatic and have a normal cardiac output before the operation. Careful monitoring of the left atrial pressure while they are coming off bypass and during equilibration over the first few postoperative hours will enable this complication to be avoided.

Arrhythmias may occur. These usually take the form of supraventricular tachycardias and are treated by digitalization. Exceptionally resistant cases will usually respond to amiodarone.

If the atrium or sinus node has been damaged a slow junctional rhythm may supervene. Temporary pacing or a small dose of isoprenaline may be indicated if the rate is slow enough to compromise the cardiac output.

After a patch of prosthetic material has been used it is probably wise to anticoagulate the patient for 2–3 months as, very occasionally, embolism has been reported in such cases.

References

1. Craig, R. J., Selzer, A. Natural history and prognosis of atrial septal defect. Circulation 1968; 37: 805–815

2. Hudson, R. The normal and abnormal interatrial septum. British Heart Journal 1955; 17: 489–495

3. Sutton, M. G., St J., Tajik, A. J., McGoon, D. C. Atrial septal defect in patients aged 60 years or older: operative results and long term postoperative follow up. Circulation 1981; 64: 402–408

4. Davia, J. E., Cheitlin, M. D., Bedynek, J. L. Sinus venosus atrial septal defect: analysis of 50 cases. American Heart Journal 1973; 85: 177–185

5. Ross, D. N. Atrial septal defect: surgical anatomy and technique. Guy's Hospital Reports 1957; 106: 205–214

6. Lewis, F. J. High defects of the atrial septum. Journal of Thoracic and Cardiovascular Surgery 1958; 36: 1–11

7. Long, D. M., Rois, M. V., Elias, D. O., Meir, M. A., Dubrow, T. W. Parietal and septal atrioplasty for total correction of anomalous pulmonary venous connection with the superior vena cava. Annals of Thoracic Surgery 1974; 18: 466–471

8. Goodman, D. J., Hancock, E. W. Secundum atrial septal defect associated with a cleft mitral valve. British Heart Journal 1973; 35: 1315–1320

9. Leachman, R. D., Cokkinos, D. V., Cooley, D. A. Association of ostium secundum atrial septal defect with mitral valve prolapse. American Journal of Cardiology 1976; 38: 167–169

10. Nagata, S. et al. Mitral valve lesion associated with secundum atrial septal defect. British Heart Journal 1983; 49: 51–58

11. Davies, M. J. Mitral valve in secundum atrial septal defects. British Heart Journal 1981; 46: 126–128

12. Beyer, J. Atrial septal defect: acute left heart failure after surgical closure. Annals of Thoracic Surgery 1978; 25: 36–43

Atrioventricular septal defect: surgical anatomy

Robert H. Anderson   BSc, MD, MRCPath
Joseph Levy Professor of Paediatric Cardiac Morphology, Cardiothoracic Institute, Brompton Hospital, London, UK

Introduction

The group of anomalies to be discussed in this chapter are well known and recognized under various names – for example, endocardial cushion defects, persistent atrioventricular canal malformations or simply atrioventricular defects. The knowledge needed by the surgeon to produce optimal repair of the lesions is, however, provided only by full understanding of what they really are, atrioventricular septal defects[1]. The basic anatomy of the group is fundamentally different from that of the normal heart. Perhaps of most significance is the major difference between the left atrioventricular valve in the anomalies to be discussed and the normal mitral valve. Satisfactory repair will best be achieved when this difference is appreciated together with the markedly dissimilar appearance of the atrioventricular junction compared with the normal heart.

Basic anatomy of atrioventricular septal defects as compared with the normal

1

The major feature of the normal heart is the 'wedged' position of the aortic valve between the mitral and tricuspid valves. The three valves together present a clover-leaf appearance when seen from above (*Figure 1*). The stem of this clover is the area of juxtaposition of the atrial (AV) and ventricular muscular (MV) septa. These two septa do not meet edge to edge. Instead there is an oblique atrioventricular junction, the tricuspid valve (TV) being attached more towards the ventricular apex than the mitral valve. Because of this the overlapping septa produce a muscular atrioventricular (AV) septum. Anterior to this muscular atrioventricular septum is a second atrioventricular septal structure where the right atrium is separated from the left ventricular outflow tract. This is the atrioventricular (AV) membranous septum.

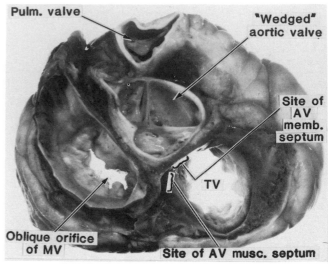

Figure 1. The dissected atrioventricular junction of the normal heart showing the clover leaf valve arrangement because of wedging of the aortic valve. Note the site and arrangement of the septal atrioventricular junction

1

2a & b

The position of these structures in the normal heart can best be appreciated by viewing a transilluminated specimen (*Figure 2a*). Examination of a so-called 'ostium primum defect' (*Figure 2b*) then shows that this and all other anomalies in this group exist because they have a defect (so-called 'endocardial cushion defect') at the site of the atrioventricular septum.

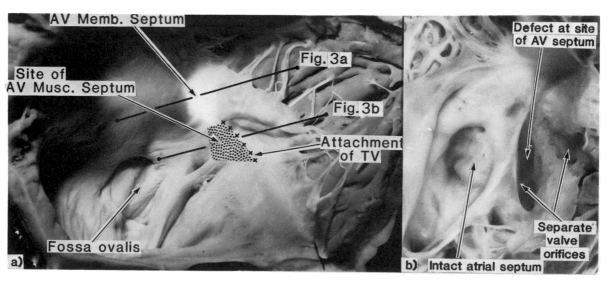

2a
2b

Figure 2. The basic lesion underscores a so-called 'endocardial cushion defect', a defect at the site of the atrioventricular septum. This is shown by comparing an 'ostium primum atrial septal defect' (Figure 2b) with a transilluminated normal heart (Figure 2a) (photographs by courtesy of Professor A. E. Becker, University of Amsterdam)

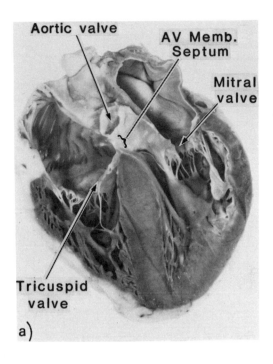

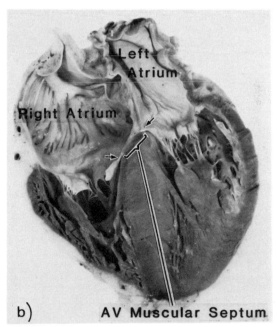

3a & b

The precise site of this atrioventricular septum, which has membranous and muscular components, is best appreciated by study of long-axis sections (*Figure 3*) taken in the planes shown in Figure 2.

Figure 3. Long axis sections through the normal heart at right angles to the inlet septum in the planes illustrated in Figure 2 show (a) the membranous septum and (b) the muscular components of the atrioventricular septum

4

Examination of the dissected atrioventricular junction in hearts with atrioventricular septal defects then shows that, because of the lack of wedging and absence of the septal atrioventricular junction, there is a common oval junction with the aortic valve positioned anteriorly in 'snowman' or 'cottage loaf' fashion (*Figure 4*). This altered anatomy affects mainly the left atrioventricular valve and the left ventricular outflow tract.

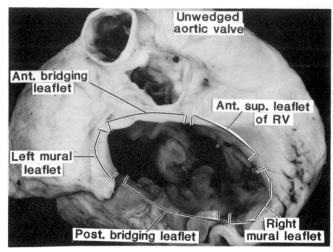

Figure 4. The dissected atrioventricular junction in an atrioventricular septal defect showing its sprung appearance because of the lack of wedging and the absence of any septal atrioventricular junction (photograph by courtesy of Professor A. E. Becker, University of Amsterdam)

4

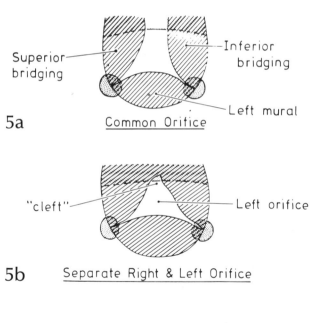

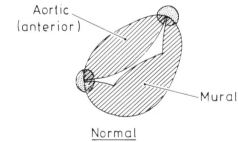

Figure 5. A comparison between the leaflet arrangement of the normal mitral valve (middle) or a common orifice (upper). All are orientated as they might be seen by the surgeon at operation

5a, b & c

Because of the 'wedged' position of the aortic valve in the normal heart (*Figure 1*) the orifice of the normal mitral valve is obliquely orientated between the anterolateral and posteromedial commissures, each supported by one of the paired left ventricular papillary muscles. The leaflets of the valve are eccentric, with a square anterior or aortic leaflet and a much longer mural leaflet, the latter usually having several scallops (*Figure 5c*). Because of the anterior position of the aorta in an atrioventricular septal defect and the absence of any septal atrioventricular junction the left atrioventricular valve is a half-oval structure with commissures in directly anterior and posterior position (*Figure 5a* and *b*). Because two of the leaflets guarding the common atrioventricular junction have both left and right ventricular papillary muscle attachments they are bridging leaflets. All of this means that the left valve in an atrioventricular septal defect is a trileaflet valve[2] and that the so-called 'mitral cleft' is the space between the facing edges of the left ventricular components of the bridging leaflets (*Figure 5b*).

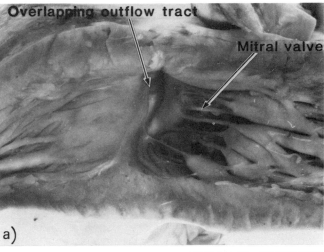

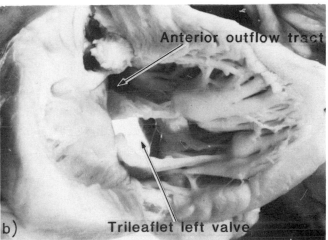

6a & b

In the normal heart, again because of the 'wedged' position of the aortic valve, the left ventricular outflow tract has an extensive posterior diverticulum and is overlapped by the aortic leaflet of the mitral valve (*Figure 6a*). In atrioventricular septal defects this does not occur (*Figure 6b*).

Figure 6. A comparison between the architecture of the normal left ventricular outflow tract (Figure 6a) and that found in atrioventricular septal defects (Figure 6b). Both are orientated in anatomic fashion having opened the left ventricle like a clam (reproduced from Anderson et al., Morphology of Congenital Heart Disease, by kind permission of Castle House Publications Ltd., Tunbridge Wells, UK)

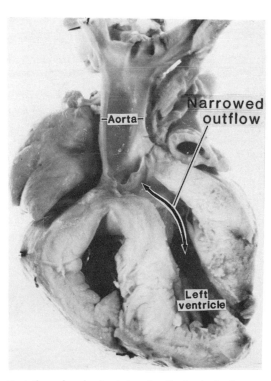

7

Figure 7. A 'four chamber' cut showing the intrinsically narrowed left ventricular outflow tract of an atrioventricular septal defect (reproduced from Anderson et al., Morphology of Congenital Heart Disease, by kind permission of Castle House Publications Ltd., Tunbridge Wells, UK)

7

Compared with the normal heart the left ventricular outflow tract, shown here in a 'four-chamber cut', is intrinsically narrowed (*Figure 7*), although the narrowing rarely produces a gradient between left ventricle and aorta. However, any lesion which further compromises the outflow tract does produce organic stenosis[3].

Overall, therefore, atrioventricular septal defects are characterized by the possession of a common atrioventricular junction guarded by a five-leaflet atrioventricular valve (*Figure 4*). One of these leaflets is confined to the left ventricle and is relatively insignificant, the left mural leaflet. The right anterosuperior and mural leaflets are confined to the right ventricle. The remaining two leaflets are tethered in both right and left ventricles and are the superior (anterior) and inferior (posterior) bridging leaflets[1].

Subcategorization of atrioventricular septal defects

There are several ways in which these lesions differ from one another. Most relate to the morphology of the atrioventricular valve leaflets. These vary first in terms of whether the bridging leaflets are separate and discrete structures (*Figure 5a*) or whether they are connected to each other by a connecting tongue of leaflet tissue running in the plane of the ventricular septum (*Figure 5b*).

When the bridging leaflets are separate structures, then there is a common atrioventricular orifice. When they are joined by the tongue, then there are separate right and left atrioventricular orifices.

8a–d

The second variation depends on the relationship of the valve leaflets to the facing edges of the ventricular and atrial septa (*Figure 8*). When the leaflets are attached completely to the ventricular septum there is only interatrial shunting through the septal defect. When the leaflets are attached to the underside of the atrial septum there is only the possibility for interventricular shunting. When attached to neither septum, then both interatrial and interventricular shunting can occur above and below the leaflets. The degree of shunting permitted depends on the extent to which the leaflets and the connecting tongue (if present) are attached to the septal structures. The combined variability in these two features – namely, the connection of the two bridging leaflets to each other and to the septal structures – accounts for all the different types of lesion which previous investigators have categorized as the complete, intermediate and partial forms of the malformation[4–7].

9a–e

The third variation is the way in which the atrioventricular junction is related to, on the one hand, the ventricular chamber and, on the other hand, the atrial chambers. Usually the junction is equally shared between the atria and the ventricles, producing the typical balanced atrioventricular septal defect (*Figure 9c*, centre). Sometimes the junction is connected eccentrically to the ventricles so that it connects predominantly to either the right ventricle or the left ventricle, the complementary ventricle being hypoplastic. This produces so-called right ventricular or left ventricular dominance[8] (*Figure 9d* and *9e*). Much more rarely the junction may be eccentrically connected to the atria so that one atrium connects to both ventricles. Although termed 'double outlet atrium'[9] it is reasonable to consider these malformations as the right or left atrial dominant variants of atrioventricular septal defect (*Figure 9a* and *b*).

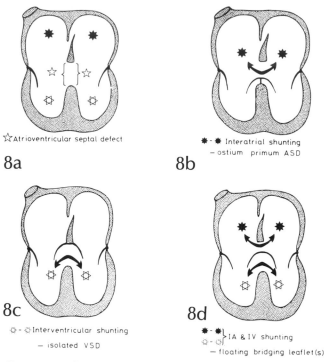

☆ Atrioventricular septal defect

✸ - ✸ Interatrial shunting
– ostium primum ASD

✧ - ✧ Interventricular shunting
– isolated VSD

✸ - ✸ ⎫ IA & IV shunting
✧ - ✧ ⎭
– floating bridging leaflet(s)

Figure 8. An illustration of how the attachments of the bridging leaflets determine the direction of shunting in an atrioventricular septal defect. The orientation is in the so-called 'four chamber plane' (reproduced with kind permission from the same source as Figures 6 and 7)

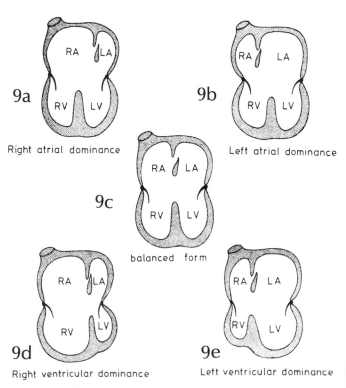

Right atrial dominance

Left atrial dominance

balanced form

Right ventricular dominance

Left ventricular dominance

Figure 9. A diagram, also in 'four chamber plane', showing the concept of atrial (a and b) and ventricular (d and e) dominance as opposed to the usual balanced form of atrioventricular septal defect

10

The final variation in leaflet anatomy concerns the way in which the bridging leaflets are shared between the two ventricles. Almost always when there are separate right and left valve orifices the superior bridging leaflet is placed mostly in the left ventricle and barely stretches over the septal crest, its right margin usually being turned in and attached along its length to the septum. This is also the pattern seen in the most frequently encountered variant with common orifice. There is minimal bridging of the superior leaflet and it is attached within the right ventricle to the medial papillary muscle, having multiple additional chordal attachments as it crosses the septum. This is the so-called Rastelli Type A variant[10]. The other variants described by Rastelli and his colleagues[10], as shown in this illustration, simply reflect increased bridging of the superior leaflet with concomitant decrease in size of the right anterosuperior leaflet (*Figure 10*). In the so-called Type B the commissure between the superior bridging and anterosuperior leaflets is attached to an anomalous apical papillary muscle and the medial papillary muscle is absent. In the Type C lesion there is extreme bridging of the superior leaflet and its right ventricular commissure attaches, along with the superomural commissure, to the anterior papillary muscle, which is often bifid[11]. There is further variability in the morphology of the inferior bridging leaflet. This is found not so much in the degree of bridging as in the shape of the leaflet. Sometimes it is a confluent structure extending over the septum but at other times it is almost completely divided by a well formed septal raphe.

All of this variable morphology is pertinent to surgical repair. It is clear that the atrioventricular junction in an atrioventricular septal defect bears no resemblance to the normal heart. There is therefore no justification for the surgeon to attempt to reconstruct the heart in the image of the normal. The five-leaflet valve can be a complete structure in its own right, and therefore reconstruction should be designed according to this five-leaflet template[2]. There is no anatomical evidence to support the concepts either of closure of the so-called 'mitral cleft' or of suspension of the valve leaflets higher in the junction than their naturally occurring position. Each lesion should be repaired on its own merits. The intrinsically narrow nature of the left ventricular outflow tract also influences surgical repair. Should left atrioventricular valve replacement be necessary it is wise to use a model with very low profile or else attach the valve within the left atrium lest the prosthesis obstruct the already narrowed outflow tract.

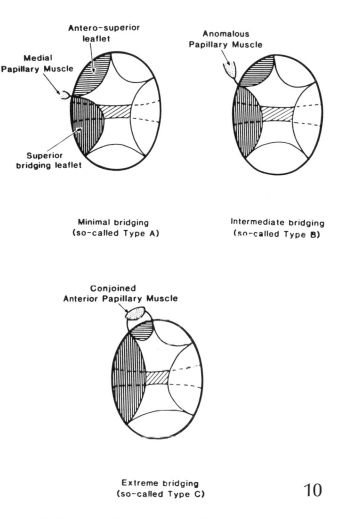

Figure 10. The variability in the degree of bridging of the superior leaflet which determines the Rastelli classification of atrioventricular septal defect with common orifice. Note that the size of the anterosuperior leaflet decreases concomitantly with the increasing bridging of the superior leaflet

The atrioventricular conduction tissues

11

The absence of any atrioventricular septal structures produces a marked deviation from normal in the course of the atrioventricular conduction tissue axis. The triangle of Koch is in its expected position but has no ventricular septum beneath it. Because of this the site of the atrioventricular node is deviated posteriorly. Here its position is indicated by the apex of a nodal triangle formed by the edge of the atrial septum and the attachment of the inferior bridging leaflet to the atrioventricular junction (*Figure 11*). The penetrating bundle is found at the apex of this nodal triangle. There is then a long non-branching bundle found beneath the inferior bridging leaflet, usually on the septal crest. The bundle branches beneath the connecting tongue when this is present but is exposed on the septal surface where there is a common orifice. The axis is therefore at risk when sutures are placed along the ventricular edge of the defect and when they are carried around its posteroinferior margin[12].

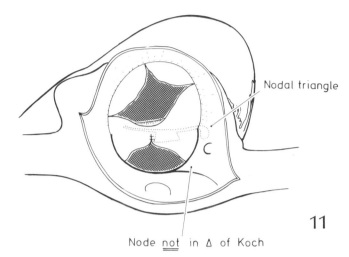

Figure 11. The arrangement of the conduction tissues in an atrioventricular septal defect with separate valve orifices as would be viewed by the surgeon

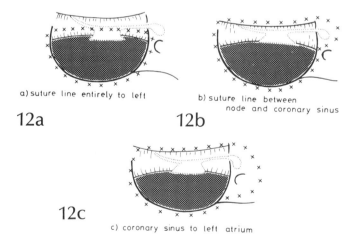

Figure 12. The options for securing the patch to close an 'ostium primum' defect so as to avoid the conduction tissues

12a, b, & c

The safest way to avoid the conduction system in the posteroinferior margin is to place the atrial components of the patch so that the coronary sinus drains to its left atrial side (*Figure 12c*). The ventricular sutures are then placed some distance away from the septal crest. However, an equally safe option when there are separate right and left orifices is to keep all sutures on the left ventricular aspect of the defect. This then obviates the need to cross the conduction axis (*Figure 12*).

Associated malformations

An atrioventricular septal defect results from a malformation of only a small part of the heart. Associated lesions in other parts of the heart which can seriously compromise the success of surgery should be anticipated. Additional defects of the atrial septum are frequent, producing a common atrium in their extreme form. An atrioventricular septal defect is particularly frequent in the presence of atrial isomerism ('splenic syndromes')[13]. When these are present a careful search should be made for venous malformations, anomalous pulmonary connection being the rule with right isomerism and azygos return of the inferior caval vein with left isomerism. Abnormal ventriculoarterial connections are also found with isomerism but can also occur in patients with usually arranged atrial chambers, as can tetralogy of Fallot. In these latter circumstances there is almost always a common valve orifice with extreme bridging of the superior leaflet ('Type C malformation')[14]. Finally, the surgeon should be aware that a common valve orifice can exist in the setting of a univentricular atrioventricular connection. In this circumstance, because a second ventricle if present will be rudimentary, the chances of direct surgical repair are almost non-existent. The operation should then be directed towards a Fontan procedure or similar options.

References

1. Becker, A. E., Anderson, R. H. Atrioventricular septal defects: what's in a name? Journal of Thoracic and Cardiovascular Surgery 1982; 83: 461–469

2. Carpentier, A. Surgical anatomy and management of the mitral component of atrioventricular canal defects. In: Anderson, R. H., Shinebourne, E. A., eds. Paediatric Cardiology. Vol. 1. Edinburgh: Churchill Livingstone, 1978: 477–486

3. Piccoli, G. P., Ho, S. Y., Wilkinson, J. L., Macartney, F. J., Gerlis, L. M., Anderson, R. H. Left-sided obstructive lesions in atrioventricular septal defects. Journal of Thoracic and Cardiovascular Surgery 1982; 83: 453–460

4. Wakai, C. S., Edwards, J. E. Symposium on persistent common atrioventricular canal: developmental and pathologic considerations in persistent common atrioventricular canal. Proceedings of the Staff Meeting of the Mayo Clinic 1956; 31: 487–500

5. Bedford, D. E., Sellors, T. H., Somerville, W., Belcher, J. R., Besterman, E. M. M. Atrial septal defect and its surgical treatment. Lancet 1957; 1: 1255–1126

6. Brandt, P. W. T., Clarkson, P. M., Neutze, J. M., Barratt-Boyes, B. G. Left ventricular cineangio-cardiography in endocardial cushion defect (persistent common atrioventricular canal). Australasian Radiology 1972; 16: 367–376

7. Bharati, S., Lev, M., McAllister, H. A. Jr., Kirklin, J. W. Surgical anatomy of the atrioventricular valve in the intermediate type of common atrioventricular orifice. Journal of Thoracic and Cardiovascular Surgery 1980; 79: 884–889

8. Bharati, S., Lev, M. The spectrum of common atrioventricular orifice (canal). American Heart Journal 1973; 86: 553–561

9. Otero Coto, E. Doble salida de auricula. Revista latina de Cardiologia 1982; 3: 289–292

10. Rastelli, G. C., Kirklin, J. W., Titus, J. L. Anatomic observations on complete form of persistent common atrioventricular canal with special reference to atrioventricular valves. Mayo Clinic Proceedings 1966; 41: 296–308

11. Piccoli, G. P., Wilkinson, J. L., Macartney, F. J., Gerlis, L. M., Anderson, R. H. Morphology and classification of complete atrioventricular defects. British Heart Journal 1979; 42: 633–639

12. Thiene, G. et al. The surgical anatomy and pathology of the conduction tissues in atrioventricular defects. Journal of Thoracic and Cardiovascular Surgery 1981; 82: 928–937

13. De Tommasi, S. M., Daliento, L., Ho, S. Y., Macartney, F. J., Anderson, R. H. Analysis of atrioventricular junction, ventricular mass and ventricular junction, ventricular mass and ventriculoarterial junction in 43 specimens with atrial isomerism. British Heart Journal 1981; 45: 236–247

14. Thiene, G., Frescura, C., Di Donato, R., Galluci, V. Complete atrioventricular canal associated with conotruncal malformations: anatomical observations in 13 specimens. European Journal of Cardiology 1979; 9: 199–213

Atrioventricular septal defect

Alain Carpentier　MD, PhD
Professor of Cardiovascular Surgery, University of Paris;
Chief, Department of Cardiovascular Surgery, Hôpital Broussais, Paris, France

Introduction

Atrioventricular septal defect (AVSD) is a complex cardiac malformation resulting from the incomplete development of the lower part of the atrial septum (inconstant feature), the upper part of the ventricular septum (constant feature) and the atrioventricular valves (constant feature).

SEPTAL MORPHOLOGY

Depending on the structures involved, a distinction can be made between three types of AVSD.

1a

In the partial type, an atrial septal defect (ostium primum type) is present and the junction between the left and right atrioventricular (AV) valves is directly attached to the crest of the ventricular septum, which is displaced downwards. A shunt is found at the atrial level.

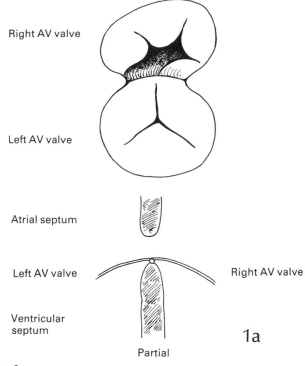

Partial   1a

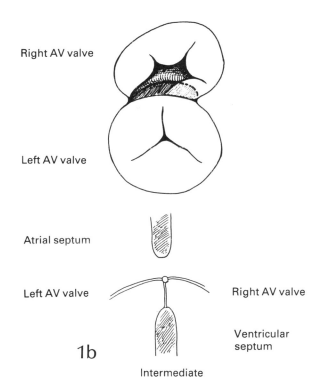

Intermediate   1b

1b

In the intermediate type, an ostium primum defect is present and the junction between the left and right AV valves is distant from the crest of the ventricular septum but attached to it by a thin ventricular membranous septum. A shunt is found at the atrial level. There is no shunt at the ventricular level, although the pellucid ventricular membranous septum may present with tiny holes.

1c

In the complete type, an ostium primum defect is generally present and a ventricular septal defect is constant. The right and left AV valves form a common AV valve with anterior and posterior bridging leaflets overriding the crest of the ventricular septum. A shunt is present at the ventricular level and in most cases also at the atrial level.

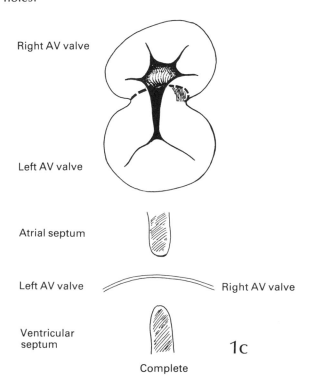

Complete   1c

VALVE MORPHOLOGY

The 'classical' interpretation of the valve morphology is that the left AV valve is a mitral valve with a cleft separating the anterior leaflet into two components, anterior and posterior. Accordingly, one major step of the 'classical' operation is to close the 'cleft' so as to restore the mitral valve configuration. In complete AV defect the anterior component is divided and attached to the septum (Rastelli Type I) or undivided and free-floating (Rastelli Type C).

Another interpretation (Carpentier) is that the left AV valve is not a normal mitral valve with a cleft anterior leaflet but a trileaflet valve with three components, anterior, posterior and lateral, separated by three commissures: septal (the so-called cleft), anterolateral and posterolateral. The malformation involves also the two papillary muscles, which are displaced laterally. Since the septal commissure is not a cleft it should be left intact when no leak is present (30 per cent of cases) and should be repaired (but not closed) when a leak is present. Variations of this trileaflet configuration exist in 15 per cent of cases and may present three aspects: (1) bicuspid valve resulting from a complete fusion between the lateral leaflet and the anterior or posterior leaflet; (2) double orifice valve resulting from a partial fusion between the lateral leaflet and the anterior or posterior leaflet; or (3) parachute valve resulting from the fusion of the two papillary muscles in a single papillary muscle attaching all the chordae.

The trileaflet concept with reconstruction of the septal commissure is of particular interest in these variations since the closure of the septal commissure would lead to a severe valve stenosis. The techniques described in this chapter are based on this concept and therefore differ significantly from the classical techniques.

Preoperative

Indications

The presence of an AVSD with significant AV valve regurgitation, no matter what its clinical manifestations, is an indication for surgical repair.

In complete AVSD the operation should be carried out between 6 and 18 months of age so as to prevent the development of pulmonary vascular disease secondary to the associated elevated pulmonary artery pressure. An operation may be mandatory before the age of 6 months in patients with pulmonary vascular resistance exceeding 8 units m^2 or severe valvular regurgitation.

In intermediate and partial forms of AVSD the operation should be performed between 2 and 4 years of age so as to prevent the development of 'secondary' valve lesions.

Contraindications

Fixed elevated pulmonary vascular resistance (>10 units/m^2) beyond the age of 2 years is a contraindication. Below 2 years of age a lung biopsy can be performed so as to evaluate the lesions of the distal pulmonary arteries. Down's syndrome (trisomy 21), which is present in 25 per cent of cases of complete AVSD, does not carry a higher operative risk and therefore is not a medical contraindication.

Diagnosis

The diagnosis is made by two-dimensional echocardiography, cardiac catheterization and angiocardiography. The anteroposterior view of the left ventriculogram shows the typical 'goose-neck' deformity resulting from the elongated outflow tract of the left ventricle and demonstrates left AV valve incompetence when present.

The operations

COMPLETE AVSD

A median sternotomy is used. When the pericardial sac is opened a piece of pericardium 5–7 cm long and 3 cm wide is excised and placed in a solution of 0.6 per cent glutaraldehyde. On exploring the heart increased pulmonary artery pressure and enlarged right atrium are common findings. The aortic cannula is placed in the ascending aorta. The vena cavae are cannulated through the right atrium as posteriorly as possible and then surrounded by tapes. Cardiopulmonary bypass is instituted and the patient is cooled to 24°C. A suction needle is placed in the aortic root. Once the heart fibrillates (around 28°C) the right atrium is opened with a horizontal anterior incision parallel to the right AV groove.

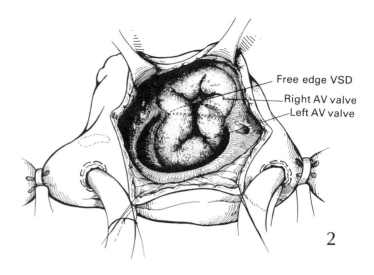

Free edge VSD
Right AV valve
Left AV valve

2

Analysis of lesions

2

The analysis of the lesions is carried out in two steps. With the aorta unclamped the septal configuration is analyzed with the valves in the open position. At the atrial level the ostium primum and an occasional ostium secundum defect are recognized. At the ventricular level the ventricular septal defect should be carefully identified and measured.

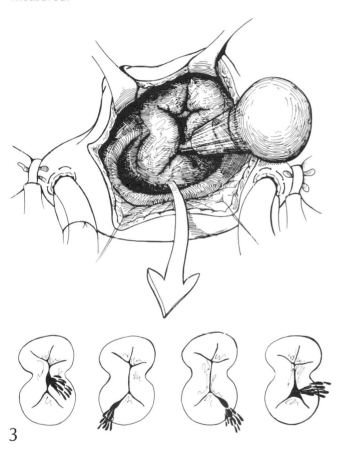

3

3

The aorta is then cross-clamped and cold saline is injected with a bulb syringe into the left ventricular cavity so as to assess the morphology of the valves in the closed position and to recognize the sites of leakage. Leaking of the left AV valve may be located at the septal, anterolateral and posterolateral commissures and/or at the centre of the orifice. Leakage of the right AV valve may be located at the septal commissure or at the centre of the orifice.

4

A stay suture is placed at the projected intercept of ventricular septum and valve leaflets, care being taken to approximate the anterior and posterior components and to restore their surfaces of coaptation. Another suture approximates the three leaflets in the centre. After suction has been established through the aortic needle the aorta is unclamped for 2 minutes so as to revascularize the heart. Then the aorta is cross-clamped once again and cardioplegia instituted through the aortic needle.

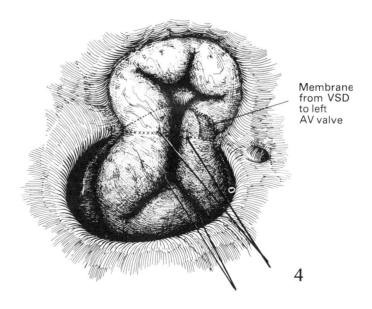

Membrane from VSD to left AV valve

4

5

Leaflet mobilization

The posterior component of the right AV valve is separated from the posterior component of the left AV valve and its membranous attachment to the septum. The incision is prolonged beyond the posteroseptal commissure. This extensive mobilization gives excellent exposure of the area of the conduction tissue and facilitates the proper placement of the ventricular patch away from this tissue.

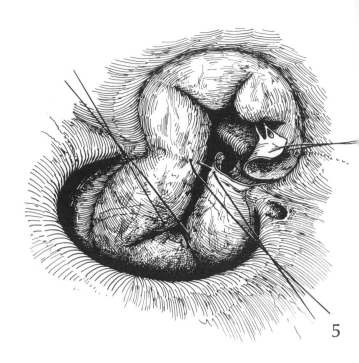

5

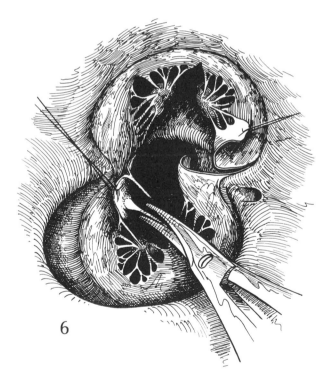

6

6

The anterior and posterior components of the left AV valve are mobilized by resection of the 'secondary' chordae attached to the ventricular aspect of the leaflet. The 'marginal' chordae attached to the free edge of the leaflets are carefully preserved so as to avoid leaflet prolapse.

7

Septal patch

The glutaraldehyde-treated autologous pericardium is rinsed for 5 minutes in saline and a semilunar patch tailored according to the measurement of the ventricular septal defect and the exposed area of the conduction tissue. The two upper angles of the ventricular patch are sutured to the annulus of the right AV valve at the appropriate points. A double-armed 4/0 monofilament suture secures the lower part of the patch to the right aspect of the ventricular septum 5 mm below the free edge of the ventricular septal defect. The two ends of this suture are used to secure the lower edge of the patch up to the two angles, care being taken that the posterior suture line remains away from the area of the conduction tissue. A 5 mm vertical incision is made in the free edge of the septal patch in front of the coapting surface of the anterior and posterior components. The free edge of these two components will be secured later within this incision.

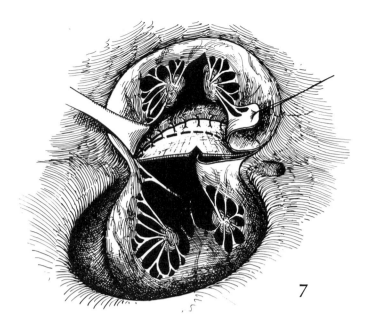

7

8

Atrial patch

From the glutaraldehyde-fixed autologous pericardium an atrial patch is tailored in a semilunar configuration, a little larger than the size of the ostium primum defect. Horizontal 5/0 mattress sutures are placed successively through the posterior component of the right AV valve, the septal patch, the posterior component of the left AV valve and then the atrial patch.

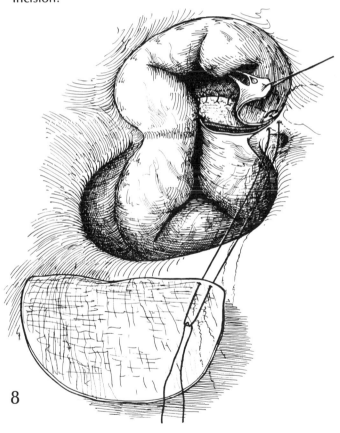

8

9

Then, if the anterior component is undivided (Type C), mattress sutures are placed successively through the crest of the septal patch, the superior component and the atrial patch.

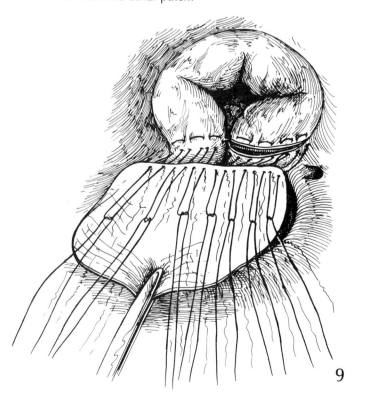

9

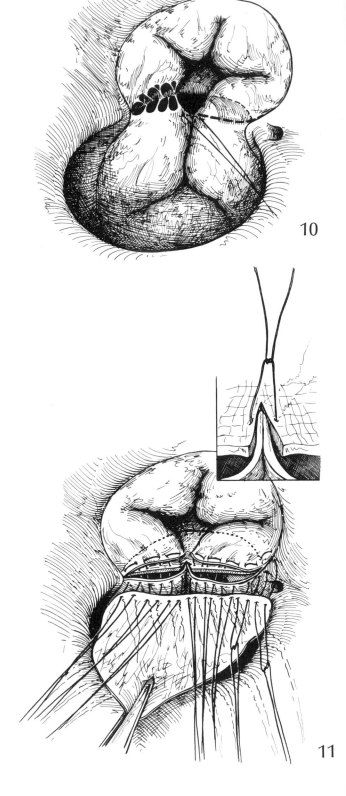

10 & 11

If the anterior component is divided (Type A) mattress sutures are passed successively through the anterior component of the right AV valve, the septal patch, the anterior component of the left AV valve and the atrial patch. The sutures are tied. The free edge of the anterior and posterior components of the left AV valve is sutured within the incision made in the free edge of the septal patch so as to restore the coaptation of these two components.

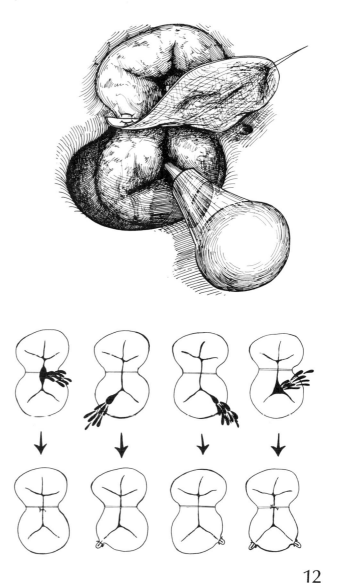

12

At this time the competence of the left AV valve is assessed by injecting saline into the ventricular cavity with a bulb syringe. A persistent leak at the septal commissure requires one or two sutures to improve approximation. A leak at the anterolateral or posterolateral commissure requires a commissuroplasty with a mattress suture, plicating the annulus. A central leak requires a triple commissuroplasty.

The right AV valve is also checked by injecting saline into the right ventricular cavity. An occasional central leak can be treated by an anteroposterior commissuroplasty with a mattress suture placed within the annulus at the junction between the anterior and posterior components of this valve.

A left ventricular vent is introduced through the left atrium at the origin of the right superior pulmonary vein and through the left AV valve.

12

13

Atrial patch

The circumference of the atrial patch is sutured to the free edge of the ostium primum defect, leaving the coronary sinus either on the left side if it is close to the edge of the ostium primum or on the right side if it is distant from it. An occasional ostium secundum defect is either sutured separately or 'patched' together with the ostium primum. The aorta is then unclamped after air has been evacuated from the left cavities. The patient is rewarmed and the heart defibrillated.

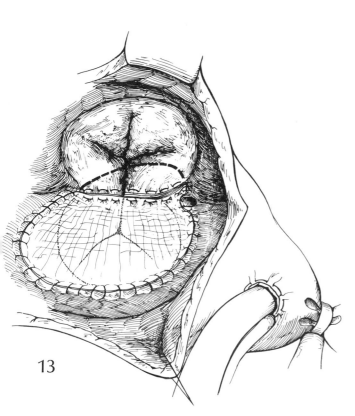

13

PARTIAL AVSD

14

A partial AVSD is recognized by the presence of an ostium primum defect, the absence of any ventricular septal defect and the adherence of the valve junction to the crest of the muscular ventricular septum. The right and left AV valves are abnormal. As in the other types of AVSD, the left AV valve is a trileaflet valve.

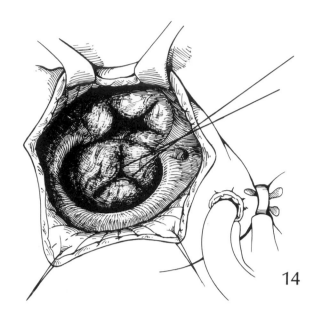

14

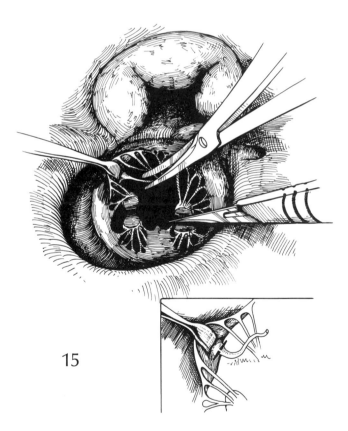

15

15

Leaflet mobilization

Leaflet mobilization is an important step to facilitate the approximation of the anterior and posterior components of the left AV valve. It is achieved by resection of secondary chordae attached to the ventricular surface of the anterior and posterior components. Fibrous bands connecting the base of the leaflets to the interventricular septum should also be resected, while the marginal chordae attached to the free edge of the anterior and posterior components are carefully preserved.

Leaflet mobilization is also obtained by splitting the papillary muscles so as to separate the portion of the papillary muscle supporting the main chordae of the anterior and posterior components from the portion giving rise to the insertion of the commissural chordae.

16

Valve reconstruction

Valve reconstruction in partial AVSD is often more difficult than in complete AVSD because secondary lesions such as thickening and rolling of the free edge of the leaflets are more frequent (inset a). A septal commissure regurgitation is ideally treated by restoring the apposition of the anterior and posterior components. This can be achieved only if the free edges of the leaflets are attached by marginal chordae and if there are minimal secondary lesions. Reapproximation of the leaflets is obtained by placing a 2/0 mattress suture within the crest of the septum at the origin of the commissure. If the tissue is fragile this suture should be pledgeted with two small squares of pericardium. A 5/0 suture is subsequently placed within the leaflet tissue at the base of the commissure to ensure excellent approximation of the leaflets.

Reconstruction of the septal commissure may be extremely difficult when important secondary lesions of the edges of the anterior and posterior leaflets are present, with a large gap between the two leaflets. In some cases it is possible to correct the lesions by removing the secondary chordae and resecting those fibrous bands attached to the ventricular surface of the leaflets responsible for leaflet rolling and retraction. The additional splitting of the papillary muscles restoring an appropriate orientation of the main chordae of the anterior and posterior components is a critical factor in the success of the repair. In many cases in which major secondary lesions are present it is necessary to close the septal commissure, at least partially (inset b). This is achieved by placing 5/0 sutures so as to restore a surface of apposition of the leaflets. The extent of closure of this commissure depends upon the possibility of restoring a surface of closure between the two leaflets.

An anterolateral or posterolateral commissure regurgitation is corrected by a commissuroplasty – that is, placement of a mattress suture within the annulus to achieve plication of the stretched commissure.

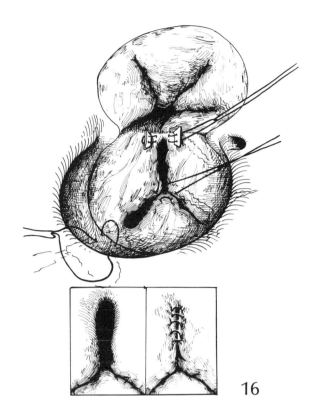

16

17

Ostium primum closure

The ostium primum defect is closed with an appropriately shaped and sized semilunar Dacron patch whose size should be a little larger than that of the defect. Fixation to the valvar-septal junction is achieved by placing mattress sutures through the base of the posterior component of the right AV valve and then through the base of the anterior component of the left AV valve.

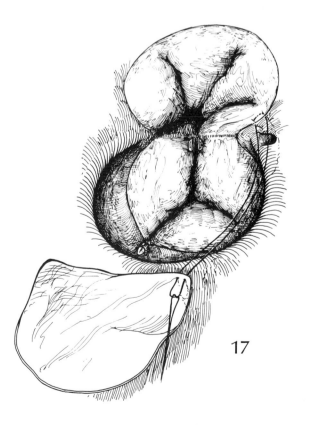

17

18

The remainder of the patch is sutured to the edge of the ostium primum with the exception of the area of the bundle of His, where the sutures are displaced towards the superior edge of the coronary sinus or even further away so as to leave the coronary sinus on the left side (inset).

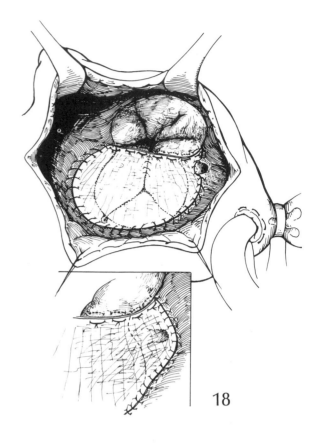

18

INTERMEDIATE AVSD

The intermediate type of AVSD looks very similar to the partial type. An ostium primum can be recognized and the junction between the right and left AV valves is clearly delineated. However, as opposed to partial AVSD this junction is not adherent to the muscular ventricular septum but connected to it by a membranous septum which may be in continuity with the anterior component of the left AV valve. The membranous septum is pellucid,

flaccid and sometimes perforated by tiny holes which must be recognized and sutured. This type may raise difficult problems of surgical correction because of the fragility of the valve junction and the membranous septum, which leads to frequent patch dehiscence. Except in cases of a strong membranous septum we think it preferable to reinforce the membranous septum by a single AV patch sutured to the ventricular septum.

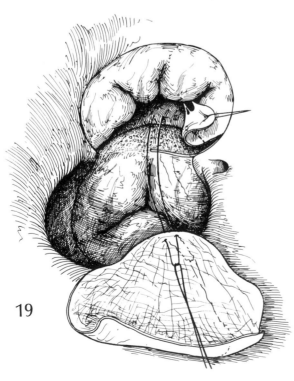

19

19

As in complete AVSD, the posterior component of the right AV valve is separated from the left AV valve so as to have a wide access to the area of the conduction tissue. Whenever a valvar leak is present the left AV valve is repaired according to the principles already indicated.

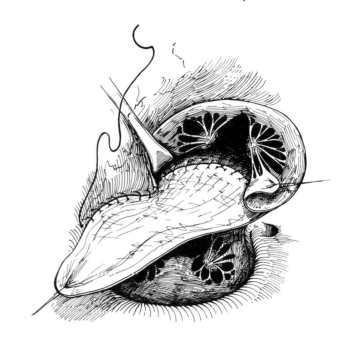

20

A large single patch is tailored so as to cover the interventricular membranous septum and the ostium primum. This patch is sutured to the right side of the muscular ventricular septum with a continuous 4/0 suture and then to the circumference of the ostium primum, leaving the coronary sinus either on the right or the left side.

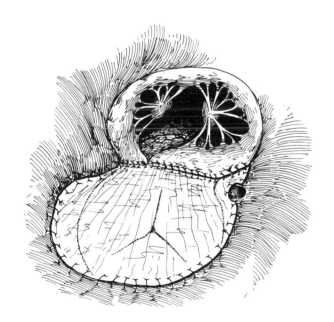

21

The posterior component of the right AV valve is then sutured to the patch so as to reconstruct this valve.

ANOMALIES

Single atrium, tetralogy of Fallot and absent coronary sinus are potential anomalies associated with AVSD. The most difficult problems are raised by valvar anomalies – in particular by three variations of the trileaflet configuration of the left AV valve, seen in 15 per cent of cases.

Bileaflet valve

A bileaflet valve results from the complete fusion of the lateral component to either the anterior or the posterior component of the left AV valve. There are only two commissures in this configuration and the closure of the septal commissure would lead to severe valvar stenosis. On the other hand restoring the trileaflet configuration by separating the lateral leaflet from the other leaflet may lead to severe regurgitation. The ideal operation in this case is to restore a surface of coaptation between the two leaflets by a double commissuroplasty.

Double orifice

A double orifice valve results from a partial fusion of the lateral leaflet to either the anterior or the posterior component. The remarks made about the bileaflet valve apply also to the double orifice valve. The double orifice should be left intact and the septal commissure should not be closed. Whenever a leak is present it should be treated by a double commissuroplasty.

Parachute valve

In this condition the chordae supporting the leaflets arise from a single papillary muscle. The interchordal spaces may be imperforate, resulting in some degree of valvar stenosis. The only commissure present is the septal commissure, which should be left intact so as to prevent severe stenosis. A septal commissuroplasty with papillary muscle splitting and interchordal space fenestration are mandatory (see chapter on 'Mitral valve reconstructive surgery', pp. 405–414).

Complications

Severe residual or recurrent valvar regurgitation requiring reoperation and valve replacement have been rare in our experience since we introduced the techniques described above. The incidence of AV block has been reduced by the introduction of mobilization of the inferior component of the right AV valve. It has not been completely eliminated, however, probably because of variations in the conduction tissue pathways, and has a current incidence of 4 per cent in our experience.

Double inlet ventricle

Robert H. Anderson BSc, MD, MRCPath
Joseph Levy Professor of Paediatric Cardiac Morphology, Cardiothoracic Institute, Brompton Hospital, London, UK

Introduction

The group of cardiac anomalies to be described in this chapter are often termed 'single ventricles'. Considerable confusion surrounds the use of this term since nearly all the hearts thus described possess two ventricular chambers, albeit that one is rudimentary to a greater or lesser degree. Some of the hearts have considerable affinities with the commonest examples of tricuspid atresia, yet conventional wisdom has decreed that the latter anomalies are not univentricular. Our attempts to show the similarity between 'single ventricle' and tricuspid atresia using the overall banner of univentricular heart have only added to the confusion[1-3]. It is pertinent to start this section, therefore, with a brief review of the background to these semantic problems.

Terminology

Hearts with both atria connected to the same ventricular chamber were initially described as 'cor triloculare biatriale'. Taussig[4] showed that most anomalous hearts of this type possessed a smaller ventricular chamber which usually supported the aorta, and she called this the 'rudimentary outlet chamber'. Subsequent to this it became conventional to distinguish these hearts with a rudimentary outlet chamber as having a 'single' ventricle, while hearts with a truly solitary ventricle were described as having a 'common' ventricle[5]. In a seminal paper Van Praagh, Ongley and Swan[6] then pointed to the semantic deficiencies in these usages and argued that the terms 'single' and 'common' should be used interchangeably to describe hearts unified by a double inlet atrioventricular connection. In doing so they arbitrarily excluded from their single ventricle group hearts with tricuspid and mitral atresia, despite the fact that Taussig had earlier described such hearts as having 'single' ventricles and despite the fact that Elliott, Anderson and Edwards[7] had illustrated the similarities between hearts with valve atresia and those now considered to be univentricular. Subsequently it became accepted teaching that double inlet connection should be the criterion for single ventricle[8-10]. It was then shown that the majority of hearts with double inlet to a right ventricle possessed a second chamber of unequivocally left ventricular morphology which was hypoplastic and rudimentary[11-13]. Van Praagh, who had proposed double inlet as the criterion of single ventricle, would not accept double inlet right ventricle in the presence of a rudimentary left ventricle as a univentricular heart[14]. Indeed, because of the existence of these lesions he proposed that double inlet should no longer be used as the criterion of 'single' ventricle[15].

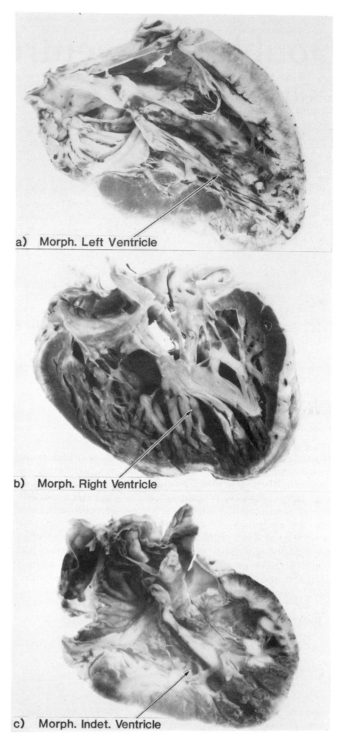

a) Morph. Left Ventricle

b) Morph. Right Ventricle

c) Morph. Indet. Ventricle

1a, b & c

The resolution of these semantic arguments is very simple. If the anomalies under discussion are grouped together because of their double inlet atrioventricular connection, then why not describe them for what they are – namely, double inlet ventricles? There is then no need to use the vexatious term 'single' ventricle. This has additional advantages. It then permits the similarities which exist between double inlet left ventricle and the commonest example of tricuspid atresia to be discussed without confusing the issue with the controversial use of the term 'univentricular heart'. Thus the hearts to be considered in this chapter all have both atrial chambers connected to the same ventricle[16]. Most usually they are connected to a left ventricle (a) and then almost always there is a rudimentary right ventricle found in antero-superior position. Less commonly the two atria are connected to the right ventricle (b) and then almost always there is a rudimentary left ventricle in posteroinferior position. Infrequently the atria may both be connected to a solitary indeterminate ventricle (c) and then there is never a second rudimentary ventricle.

Figure 1. Cross-sectional cuts in the four-chamber plane showing the different types of double inlet connection which in this section can be differentiated only by the trabecular pattern of the dominant ventricle. In the upper panel this is of left ventricular type; in the middle panel of right ventricular type and in the lower panel of indeterminate type. Sectioning in the long-axis at right angles to these sections would also differentiate the hearts, since an anterosuperior rudimentary right ventricle would then be demonstrated in (a), a posteroinferior rudimentary left ventricle in (b), and no other ventricle in (c)

2a & b

Hearts with double inlet ventricle, irrespective of the nature of the main ventricle, can be found with two valves (as seen in *Figure 1*), one of which may be imperforate or straddling, or with a common valve (as shown here). The presence of a common valve does not affect the presence of a double inlet connection with either left (*a*) or right (*b*) ventricle. A straddling valve can exist with double inlet as long as the degree of override of its annulus is such that it is connected mostly to the ventricle connected also to the other valve.

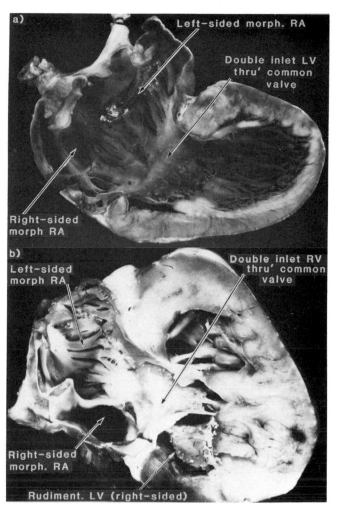

Figure 2. *Cross-sections in the four-chamber plane showing how double inlet can occur to a left ventricle (a) or a right ventricle (b) through a common valve as opposed to two separate valves as shown in Figure 1. In these examples both hearts have right atrial isomerism and a posteroinferior rudimentary left ventricle is seen in right-sided position in the heart with double inlet right ventricle (b)*

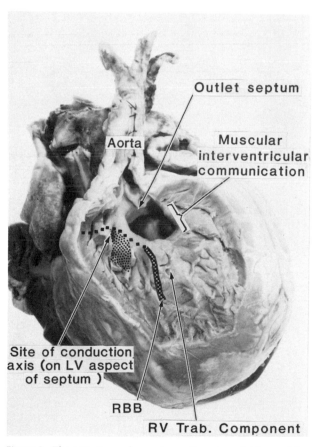

Figure 3. *The anterior and superior rudimentary right ventricle found in hearts with double inlet left ventricle. Note that the interventricular communication has completely muscular boundaries and that the rudimentary ventricle possesses outlet and trabecular components. The site of the conduction axis, carried on the left ventricular aspect of the trabecular septum, has been superimposed*

Double inlet left ventricle

3

This is the commonest type of double inlet. Both atrial chambers are connected to the main (left) ventricle through two valves or a common valve attached posterior to a septum which never extends to the crux. Of necessity in hearts with double inlet the inlet part of the ventricular septum is lacking and the anterior septum has only apical trabecular and outlet components. The interventricular communication is almost always placed between these septal components and has exclusively muscular margins (*Figure 3*).

4a & b

The rudimentary right ventricle, always located on the anterosuperior margin of the dominant left ventricle, possesses only apical trabecular and outlet components (*see* Illustration 3). Its precise morphology depends on the ventriculoarterial connection. Usually there is ventriculo-arterial discordance ('transposition'). In this case the apical trabecular component is hypoplastic and the outlet component very short. The rudimentary right ventricle with this combination may be either right-sided (a) or left-sided (b). Often, when left-sided, the apical trabecular component points backwards as a posterior 'tail'.

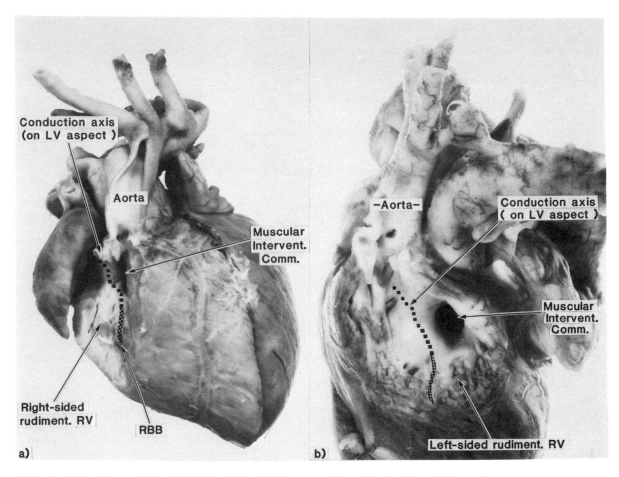

Figure 4. The typical positions of right-sided (a) and left-sided (b) rudimentary right ventricles in hearts with double inlet left ventricle. Both are carried basically in the anterosuperior position.

Note also that the sidedness of the rudimentary ventricle does not alter the basic position of the conduction tissue axis (superimposed)

5a & b

Less commonly there may be ventriculoarterial concordance. Here the great arteries are usually 'normally related' and the apical trabecular component is well formed and right-sided. There is an extensive outlet component which swings across the front of the heart to the left-sided pulmonary trunk (a). Sometimes, however, with ventriculoarterial concordance both apical trabecular component and outlet component, together with the pulmonary trunk, are left-sided (b). In these circumstances the rudimentary right ventricle can sometimes achieve considerable size[17].

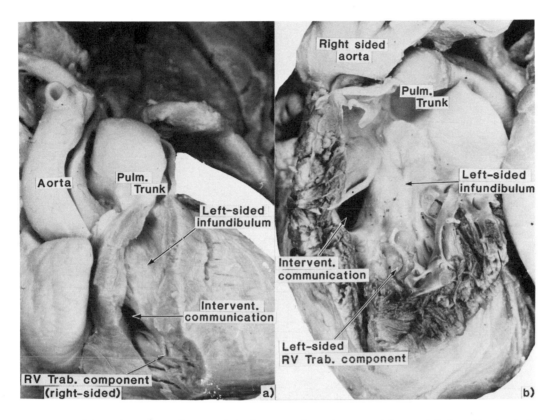

Figure 5. The morphology of the rudimentary right ventricle in the two variants found in double inlet left ventricle with ventriculoarterial concordance. The left-hand panel shows the more usual variant, typically called the 'Holmes Heart'. Note the similarity to the rudimentary right ventricle found in classical tricuspid atresia. The right-hand panel shows the rarer type where both pulmonary trunk and the trabecular component of the rudimentary ventricle are left-sided

6a & b

More rarely there may be double outlet from, as well as double inlet to, the dominant left ventricle (a) and then the rudimentary right ventricle is represented solely by its apical trabecular component (b), which is still in antero-superior position. Very rarely both great arteries may arise from the rudimentary right ventricle or else there may be a single outlet of the heart via a truncus. Pulmonary atresia is more frequent but usually in the setting of biventricular ventriculoarterial connection. Aortic atresia with double inlet left ventricle is exceedingly rare.

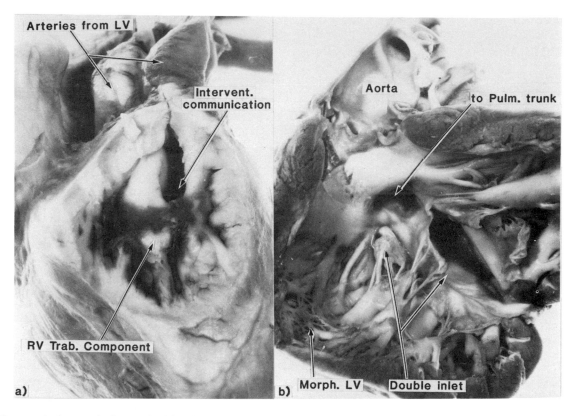

Figure 6. The ventricular morphology in double inlet left ventricle with double outlet also present from the dominant ventricle. The left-hand panel shows that the rudimentary right ventricle is represented only by the apical trabecular component which is still in anterosuperior position. The right-hand panel shows the dominant left ventricle

7

Malformations of the atrioventricular valves are frequent, particularly stenosis or atresia of one or other valve[18]. These severely compromise possibilities for surgical septation. In most examples of double inlet left ventricle surgical septation is favoured by the clear plane of cleavage which exists between the atrioventricular valves and their tension apparatus. Although cases will certainly be encountered in which there is crossing of the tension apparatus, this is the exception rather than the rule. Outflow tract stenosis is most usually encountered at the interventricular communication. Thus the outflow tract involved depends upon the ventriculoarterial connection. Most usually this is discordant and then the restrictive communication results in subaortic obstruction, usually with hypoplasia or coarctation of the aortic arch. When the ventriculoarterial connection is concordant, obstruction at the interventricular communication produces subpulmonary stenosis and in these cases there may be confusion with tetralogy of Fallot. Outflow tract stenosis of the arterial trunk arising from the dominant left ventricle is most frequently due to posterior deviation of the outlet septum. However, the obstruction may be due also to either anomalous insertion of papillary muscles across the outflow tract or to fibrous tissue tags.

Surgery of double inlet left ventricle can be either palliative or corrective[19]. The options for corrective surgery are either septation or a modified Fontan procedure. Both of these options are significantly influenced by the anatomy and in particular by the abnormal disposition of the atrioventricular conduction tissues. For septation to be successful it must be possible to place the septation patch between the atrioventricular valves so as to connect the left atrioventricular valve to the interventricular communication and thence to the aorta, presuming the presence of ventriculoarterial discordance. This is favoured by a left-sided position of the rudimentary right ventricle. Ideally, the patch should be placed so as to avoid the conductive system.

Because there is no inlet septum in hearts with double inlet ventricle the normal node lying in the triangle of Koch does not make contact with the ventricular conduction tissues in the anterior and malaligned apical trabecular septum. Instead, an anterior node assumes the role of effecting an atrioventricular conduction system[20]. This node is located in the anterior wall of the right atrioventricular orifice immediately beneath the ostium of

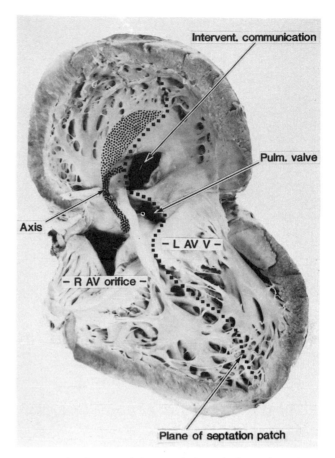

Figure 7. The dominant left ventricle from the heart shown in Figure 3 with double inlet left ventricle and ventriculoarterial discordance. Note the cleavage plane between the atrioventricular valves and the disposition of the conduction tissue axis. The plane of potential septation has been superimposed

the right atrial appendage. In hearts with a left-sided rudimentary right ventricle the penetrating bundle passes through the lateral margin of the fibrous continuity almost always present between the right atrioventricular and pulmonary valves. A long non-branching bundle then encircles the lateral aspect of the pulmonary valve attachment before descending on to the margin of the apical trabecular septum closest to the right valve.

8a & b

The perception of the relationship of bundle and interventricular communication varies according to whether the defect is viewed from the dominant left ventricle or from the rudimentary right ventricle.

When seen from the left ventricle, either via a ventriculotomy or an atriotomy the bundle runs round the lateral margin of the subpulmonary outflow tract and then passes anterocephalad to the interventricular communication before branching on the left ventricular aspect of the apical trabecular septum. The left bundle branch then streams down the smooth septal surface of the main left ventricle while the right bundle branch burrows intramyocardially to reach the apical trabecular component of the rudimentary right ventricle. However, when seen from the rudimentary right ventricle (*Figure 8*), then the conduction tissue axis is carried on the left ventricular aspect of the septum but is positioned posteroinferior to the interventricular communication, only the right bundle branch penetrating to become subendocardial within the rudimentary chamber.

In addition to the vulnerability of this axis during septation the conduction tissues are also at risk when it is necessary to enlarge the interventricular communication. This may be an initial palliative measure or may be needed to remove the hypertrophied muscle which is known to develop in this area after pulmonary artery banding[21, 22]. The rule for avoidance of the axis during this procedure is that it is carried on the left ventricular aspect of the apical trabecular septum, descending to this position from the anterior aspect of the right atrioventricular valve. The safe areas for resection are therefore the outlet septum and the margin of the defect towards the left atrioventricular valve (*see* shaded areas in Figure 8).

As indicated above, the septation procedure is most readily performed when there is ventriculoarterial discordance and the rudimentary right ventricle is left-sided. All the above discussion has presumed these features to be present. On occasion, however, it may be considered desirable to septate double inlet left ventricle when the rudimentary right ventricle is right-sided, combining this in the presence of ventriculoarterial discordance with either an atrial redirection procedure or an arterial switch. In either of these eventualities the conduction tissue disposition is as described above for left-sided right ventricle, except that when the rudimentary ventricle is right-sided the bundle descends directly on to the apical trabecular septum without encircling the pulmonary root[23]. The other condition in which septation might be considered is when there is double inlet left ventricle, rudimentary right ventricle and ventriculoarterial concordance with 'normally related' great arteries. Usually this combination is associated with a restrictive interventricular communication, but if it is possible to relieve the subpulmonary obstruction thus produced the morphology then favours septation by connecting the right atrioventricular valve to the rudimentary right ventricle. In the first case of this type that we studied histologically we found a grossly abnormal disposition of conduction tissue

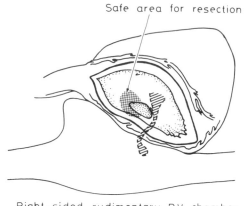

Safe area for resection

Right-sided rudimentary RV chamber

8a

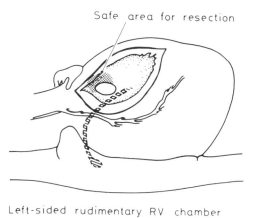

Safe area for resection

Left-sided rudimentary RV chamber

8b

Figure 8. Artist's impression showing the course of the conduction tissue axis as seen from the rudimentary right ventricle in hearts with double inlet left ventricle with a right-sided (a) and a left-sided (b) rudimentary right ventricle. The safe area for enlargement of the interventricular communication has been marked

in which the bundle encircled the right atrioventricular orifice completely, originating from a normal node. Since then we have studied several other similar hearts and the disposition was as described above for cases with ventriculoarterial discordance[24].

If the septation option is discarded, then all hearts with double inlet ventricle can be 'corrected' by the modified Fontan procedure. It should then be remembered that the conduit can be placed to the rudimentary right ventricle when there is ventriculoarterial concordance; otherwise, an atriopulmonary connection must be made. Conduction tissues are most at risk during closure of the right atrioventricular valve, and the connecting node will always be directly adjacent to the annular attachment of the right atrioventricular valve. It is therefore prudent to close this valve with a suture line placed approximately 1 cm from the atrioventricular junction.

Double inlet right ventricle

Although much rarer than double inlet left ventricle, this variant of double inlet is now being recognized with more frequency in both clinical and autopsy studies[12, 13]. Although it was initially described in the absence of a rudimentary left ventricle[6], most examples encountered since have possessed such a ventricle, which has always been located in posteroinferior position, usually to the left but occasionally to the right.

Double inlet right ventricle is found with some frequency in patients with right atrial isomerism and is almost always associated with a common valve, double outlet right ventricle and the venous anomalies which are part of the isomeric complex. Such patients are unlikely to be candidates for corrective surgery. Even when found in patients with lateralized atrial chambers a common atrioventricular valve is still frequent, and this would make corrective surgery exceedingly difficult.

9

Those patients with double outlet right ventricle most suitable for correction are those with two separate atrioventricular valves and the aorta in left-sided position. Indeed, one such patient with this morphology underwent successful septation at the Brompton Hospital. There was a straddling left atrioventricular valve with 90 per cent of its circumference connected to the right ventricle and the great arteries were positioned with the aorta anterior and to the left. It was possible to place the septation patch so as to connect the left atrioventricular valve to the aorta (*Figure 9*). Unfortunately the suture line traumatized the normal atrioventricular conduction axis, and although the patient was paced, he died suddenly 6 months later from pacemaker failure. However, this does suggest that patients with two atrioventricular valves and double outlet right ventricle are potential candidates for correction, although the rudimentary left ventricle will not be of much value in the circulation.

10

We have seen one heart with ventriculoarterial concordance and a common atrioventricular valve in which it might have been feasible to incorporate the rudimentary left ventricle in the circulation, but the left ventricle, which was in posteroinferior and left-sided position, was hypoplastic and the chances of success of such a procedure must be small (*Figure 10*). This leaves the modified Fontan procedure as the most likely option for these hearts. The rules for conduction tissue disposition are then that the conduction axis arises from a normal atrioventricular node whenever the rudimentary left ventricle is left-sided.

In the single case we have studied with a right-sided rudimentary left ventricle (left-hand pattern ventricular topology) there were both normal and anterior nodes with a conduction tissue sling between them. Placing a patch to close the right valve as suggested for double inlet left ventricle would avoid all the danger areas.

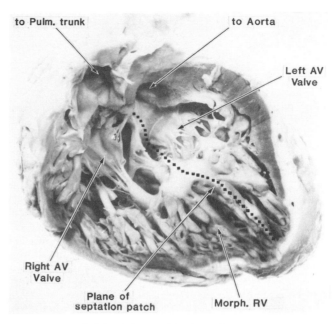

Figure 9. Double inlet right ventricle through two separate atrioventricular valves with double outlet from the dominant right ventricle and the aorta in left-sided position. The plane for potential septation of this ventricle is marked

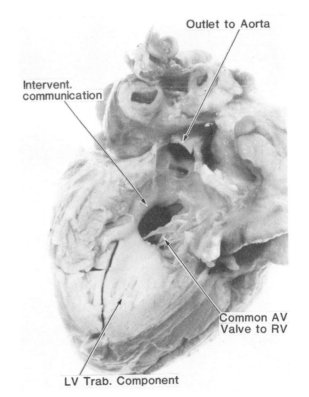

Figure 10. The rudimentary left ventricle which gives rise to the aorta in a heart with double inlet right ventricle and ventriculoarterial concordance. The double inlet was via a common atrioventricular valve. Note the posteroinferior and left-sided position of the rudimentary ventricle

Double inlet indeterminate ventricle

This is probably the rarest type of double inlet ventricle. Care must be taken to distinguish such hearts from those with huge ventricular septal defects. In the latter combination the apparently solitary ventricular mass has a right ventricular trabecular pattern to one side of its apex and a left ventricular pattern to the other (the Type C of Van Praagh, Ongley and Swan[6]). There is then almost always a rudiment of the ventricular septum between the apical trabecular components, and a posterior ridge carrying the conduction tissue axis runs down to join the septal rudiment[25]. In these hearts there is therefore a well demarcated plane of cleavage between the atrioventricular valves. Since the great arteries are often 'normally related' it is not unduly difficult to perform septation on these hearts.

11

When there is a truly solitary and indeterminate ventricle the difficulties are much greater. Often these hearts are found with a common atrioventricular valve in the presence of right atrial isomerism and then the combination is formidable, but sometimes they are found with two separate atrioventricular valves and with patent subarterial outflow tracts (*Figure 11*). Septation is possible in such hearts but is made difficult by two factors. The first is the nature of the apical trabecular component. This is criss-crossed by coarse trabeculae, often with crossing of the tension apparatus of the two valves. This arrangement gave considerable problems to Hamilton in his experience with this type of heart[26]. The second problem is the anomalous disposition of the conduction tissue. Since there are neither inlet nor apical trabecular septal structures in these hearts the disposition is truly bizarre. In our experience the conduction axis has usually originated from an anterolateral node and then descended either into the lateral wall of the chamber or else on to a free-standing trabecula[27]. However, in another heart in which a free-standing trabecula ran to the underside of the atrial septum the conduction bundle descended on to the trabecula from a normal node[28].

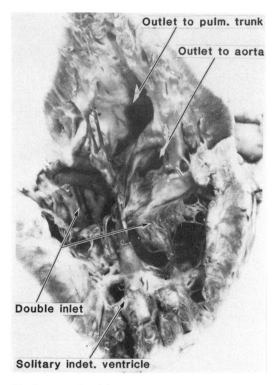

Figure 11. An example of the rare type of double inlet to a solitary indeterminate ventricle. There is also double outlet from the solitary chamber

References

1. Anderson, R. H., Becker, A. E., Macartney, F. J., Shinebourne, E. A., Wilkinson, J. L., Tynan, M. J. Is 'tricuspid atresia' a univentricular heart? Pediatric Cardiology 1979; 1: 51–56

2. Bharati, S., Lev, M. The concept of tricuspid atresia complex as distinct from that of the single ventricle complex. Pediatric Cardiology 1979; 1: 57–62

3. Rao, P. S. Terminology: tricuspid atresia or univentricular heart. In: Rao, P. S., ed. Tricuspid Atresia. New York: Futura Publishing Co, 1982: 3–6

4. Taussig, H. B. A single ventricle with a diminutive outlet chamber. Journal of Technical Methods 1939; 19: 120–128

5. Gasul, B. M., Arcilla, R. A., Lev, M. Persistent common atrioventricular canal (orifice). In: Gasul, B. M. et al. eds. Heart Disease in Children. Philadelphia: J. B. Lippincott Co, 1966: 404–423

6. Van Praagh, R., Ongley, P. A., Swan, H. J. C. Anatomic types of single or common ventricle in man: morphologic and geometric aspects of sixty necropsied cases. American Journal of Cardiology 1964; 13: 367–386

7. Elliott, L. P., Anderson, R. C., Edwards, J. E. The common cardiac ventricle with transposition of the great vessels. British Heart Journal 1964; 26: 289–301

8. Lev, M., Liberthson, R. R., Kirkpatrick, J. R., Eckner, F. A. O., Arcilla, R. A. Single (primitive) ventricle. Circulation 1969; 39: 577–591

9. Ellis, K. Angiography in complex congenital heart disease: single ventricle, double inlet, double outlet and transposition. In: Davila, J. C., ed. 2nd Henry Ford Hospital International Symposium on Cardiac Surgery. New York: Appleton-Century-Crofts, 1977: 222–224

10. Edwards, J. E. Discussion. In: Davila, J. C., ed. 2nd Henry Ford Hospital International Symposium on Cardiac Surgery. New York: Appleton-Century-Crofts, 1977: 242

11. Quero-Jimenez, M., Martinez, V. M. P., Azcarate, M. J. M., Batres, G. M., Granados, F. M. Exaggerated displacement of the atrioventricular canal towards the bulbus cordis (rightward displacement of the mitral valve). British Heart Journal 1973; 35: 65–74

12. Keeton, B. R., Macartney, F. J., Hunter, S. et al. Univentricular heart of right ventricular type with double or common inlet. Circulation 1979; 59: 403–411

13. Soto, B., Bertranou, E. G., Bream, P. R., Souza, A. Jr., Bargeron, L. M. Jr. Angiographic study of univentricular heart of right ventricular type. Circulation 1979; 60: 1325–1334

14. Van Praagh, R., Plett, J. A., Van Praagh, S. Single ventricle: pathology, embryology, terminology and classification. Herz 1979; 4: 113–150

15. Van Praagh, R., David, I., Van Praagh, S. What is a ventricle? The single ventricle trap. Pediatric Cardiology 1982; 2: 79–84

16. Anderson, R. H. Weasel words in paediatric cardiology: single ventricle. International Journal of Cardiology 1982; 2: 425–429

17. Freedom, R. M., Nanton, M., Dische, M. R. Isolated ventricular inversion with double inlet left ventricle. European Journal of Cardiology 1977; 5: 63–86

18. Quero-Jimenez, M., Cameron, A. H., Acerete, F., Quero-Jimenez, C. Univentricular hearts: pathology of the atrioventricular valves. Herz 1979; 4: 161–165

19. Pacifico, A. D., McKay, R., Kirklin, J. W., Kirklin, J. K. Surgical management of the univentricular heart. In: Anderson, R. H., Macartney, F. J., Shinebourne, E. A., Tynan, M., eds. Paediatric Cardiology Vol. 5. Edinburgh: Churchill Livingstone, 1983: 276–293

20. Anderson, R. H., Arnold, R., Thaper, M. K., Jones, R. S., Hamilton, D. I. Cardiac specialized tissues in hearts with an apparently single ventricular chamber (double inlet left ventricle). American Journal of Cardiology 1974; 33: 95–106

21. Somerville, J., Becu, L., Ross, D. Common ventricle with acquired subaortic obstruction. American Journal of Cardiology 1974; 34: 206–214

22. Freedom, R. M., Sondheimer, H., Dische, R., Rowe, R. D. Development of 'subaortic stenosis' after pulmonary arterial banding for common ventricle. American Journal of Cardiology 1977; 39: 78–83

23. Wenink, A. C. G. The conducting tissues in primitive ventricle with outlet chamber: two different possibilities. Journal of Thoracic and Cardiac Surgery 1978; 75: 747–753

24. Anderson, R. H., Lenox, C. C., Zuberbuhler, J. R., Ho, S. Y., Smith, A., Wilkinson, J. L. Double inlet left ventricle with rudimentary right ventricle and ventriculoarterial concordance. American Journal of Cardiology 1983; 52: 573–577

25. Edie, R. N., Ellis, K., Gersony, W. M., Krongrad, E., Bowman, F. O., Malm, J. R. Surgical repair of single ventricle. Journal of Thoracic and Cardiac Surgery 1973; 66: 350–360

26. Hamilton, D. A., Arnold, R., Wilkinson, J. L. Surgery of univentricular heart without outlet chamber. In: Anderson, R. H., Shinebourne, E. A., eds. Paediatric Cardiology. Vol. 1. Edinburgh: Churchill Livingstone, 1978: 388–395

27. Wilkinson, J. L., Anderson, R. H., Arnold, R., Hamilton, D. I., Smith, A. The conducting tissues in primitive ventricular hearts without an outlet chamber. Circulation 1976; 53: 930–938

28. Essed, C. E., Ho, S. Y., Hunter, S., Anderson, R. H. Atrioventricular conduction system in univentricular heart of right ventricular type with right-sided rudimentary chamber. Thorax 1980; 35: 123–127

Tricuspid atresia: surgical anatomy

Robert H. Anderson   BSc, MD, MRCPath
Joseph Levy Professor of Paediatric Cardiac Morphology, Cardiothoracic Institute, Brompton Hospital, London, UK

1

Introduction

Many and diverse cardiac anomalies have been described under the name 'tricuspid atresia'. Most have no communication between the systemic venous atrium and the ventricular mass. A few have been described as 'tricuspid atresia' when the pulmonary venous atrium has no communication with the ventricular mass[1]. Although most of the hearts in this group have a blind atrial chamber with a completely muscular floor, the term 'tricuspid valve atresia' usually conveys the concept that there is an imperforate membrane between the right atrium and the underlying right ventricle. This is rarely the case.

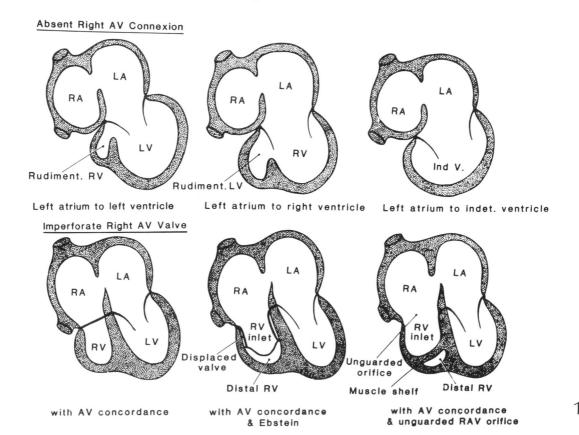

Figure 1. The basic type of right atrioventricular valve atresia which can exist in the settings of absent atrioventricular connection (upper panels) and atrioventricular concordance (lower panels). Imperforate right valves, as shown in the lower panels, can also be found with atrioventricular discordance, double inlet ventricle and ambiguous atrioventricular connection

1

Classical tricuspid atresia

2a & b

In the classical type of tricuspid atresia there is complete absence of the right atrioventricular connection, the left atrium being connected to the left ventricle in the presence of a rudimentary right ventricle[2]. The anatomy is best demonstrated by sections through the heart in 'four-chamber' plane[3]. Posterior sections (a) show that the floor of the right atrium is completely separated from the ventricular mass by the atrioventricular sulcus, with branches of the right coronary artery running through the sulcus. More anterior sections (b) show that the floor of the right atrial appendage may overlay the rudimentary right ventricle, but always the two are separated by the atrioventricular sulcus.

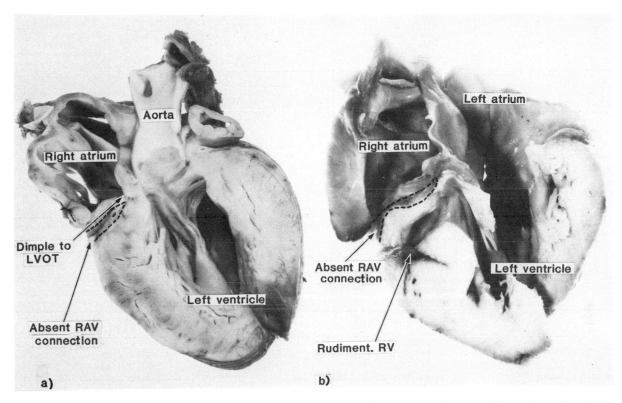

Figure 2. 'Four chamber' sections through hearts with classical tricuspid atresia (absent right atrioventricular connection, left atrium connected to left ventricle with rudimentary right ventricle). The left hand panel shows a posterior cut in which the floor of the right atrium is completely separated from the ventricular mass by sulcus tissue. The right hand panel shows a more anterior and oblique section in a different heart, showing how the atrial floor is related to the rudimentary right ventricle but separated from it by sulcus tissue

3

This anatomy can then be appreciated by examining the different cardiac chambers. The right atrium has a muscular floor and the commissure of the Eustachian and Thebesian valves runs forward through the sinus septum to be inserted into the central fibrous body at the site of the dimple. Almost without exception there is an interatrial communication within the oval fossa and the entire oval fossa is deviated posteriorly. There may be a defect of sinus venosus type; ostium primum defects may rarely be found. The atrioventricular (AV) node is a prominent structure and overlaps the dimple, lying at the apex of the triangle of Koch. The conduction axis penetrates the central fibrous body to reach the left ventricular outflow tract.

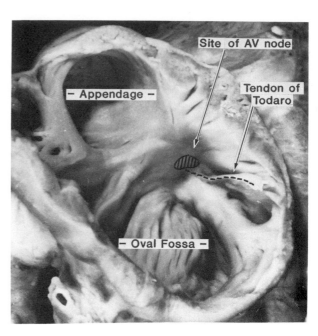

Figure 3. The muscular floor of the right atrium in typical tricuspid atresia showing the site of the atrioventricular node

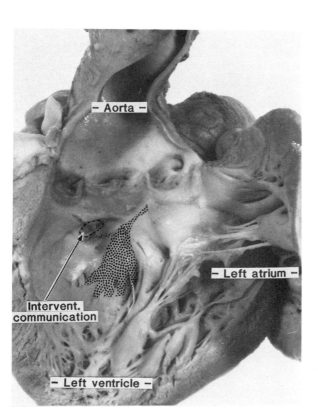

Figure 4. The left ventricle in classical tricuspid atresia with ventriculoarterial concordance showing the muscular interventricular communication and the site of the atrioventricular conduction tissue axis

4

The left atrium is an enlarged but otherwise anatomically normal chamber. It connects through a normally structured mitral valve with the left ventricle. The septum between the left ventricle and the rudimentary right ventricle does not reach to the crux, extending instead only to the acute margin of the ventricular mass.

The interventricular communication has completely muscular borders and is directly comparable to that found in double inlet left ventricle, as is the relationship of the atrioventricular conduction axis to the outflow tract and the interventricular defect. The non-branching bundle enters the left ventricle some distance behind the interventricular communication and branches on the smooth left ventricular aspect of the apical trabecular septum[4]. The right bundle branch then penetrates through the septum to ramify in the apical trabecular component of the rudimentary right ventricle.

5a & b

The rudimentary right ventricle itself is carried on the anterosuperior aspect of the main left ventricle. The precise morphology of the rudimentary right ventricle depends on the ventriculoarterial connection. Most usually this is concordant and then there is a well formed right-sided apical trabecular component which swings across into an extensive outlet component leading to the left-sided pulmonary trunk (a). Less frequently there is a discordant ventriculoarterial connection and then the apical trabecular component is more hypoplastic and is on the same side as the outlet component and the aorta (b).

More rarely there may be double outlet left ventricle and then the right ventricle is composed solely of its apical trabecular component, or else there may be ventriculoarterial concordance with 'anatomically corrected malposition' (anterior left-sided aorta arising from the left ventricle).

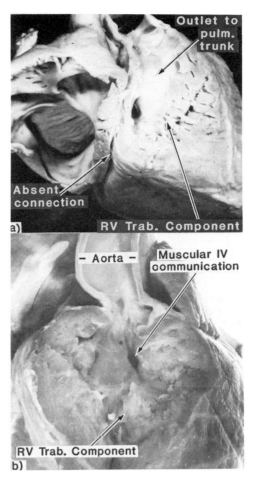

Figure 5. The rudimentary right ventricle in classical tricuspid atresia with (a) ventriculoarterial concordance and (b) ventriculoarterial discordance. Note the differing size of the trabecular and outlet components of the ventricles with the different ventriculoarterial connections

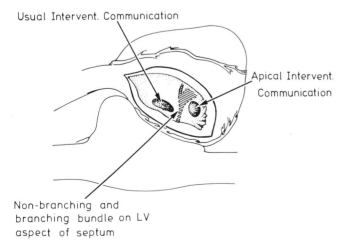

Figure 6. The course of the conduction axis in classical tricuspid atresia as would be seen from the rudimentary right ventricle. The axis is shown relative to the usual interventricular communication and also the much rarer, but highly significant, apical defect

6

As may be anticipated, the relationship of the conduction tissue axis to the interventricular communication when viewed from the rudimentary right ventricle in tricuspid atresia is directly comparable to that seen in double inlet left ventricle.

Variants of tricuspid atresia

7a & b

In our studies of autopsied hearts we have encountered several rare but significant lesions which result in absence of direct communication between the morphologically right atrium and the ventricular mass. The lesion in this group may indeed be due to an imperforate tricuspid valve. We have seen this once in the setting of atrioventricular concordance with a normally positioned tricuspid valve membrane (a) but more frequently in the setting of Ebstein's malformation (b). However, taken overall, imperforate right valve membranes are probably more frequent in the setting of double inlet left ventricle.

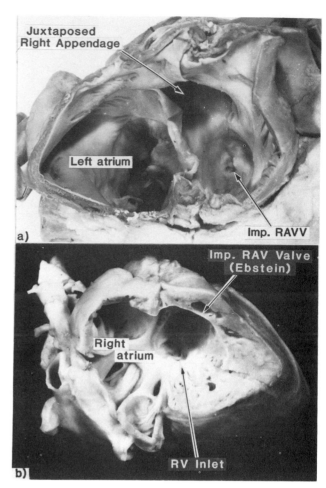

Figure 7. The variants of imperforate right atrioventricular valve with atrioventricular concordance shown (a) with the valve at its expected site and (b) with Ebstein's malformation. The lower heart is photographed with kind permission of Dr J. L. Wilkinson, University of Liverpool

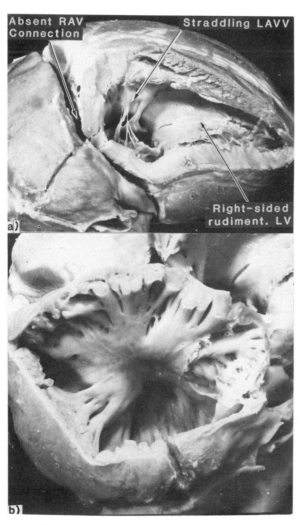

Figure 8. The variant of absent right atrioventricular connection seen when the left atrium connects to a right ventricle and the rudimentary left ventricle is posterior and to the right. There is straddling of the left atrioventricular valve (a). Note that the right atrial morphology is indistinguishable from that found in classical tricuspid atresia (compare (b) with Figure 2)

8a & b

Absence of the right atrioventricular connection has been found when the left atrium is connected to the morphologically right ventricle. In the hearts we have studied of this kind the rudimentary left ventricle was posterior and right-sided (left-hand pattern ventricular topology) (a) and the left valve was straddling[5]. Although it could be argued on embryological grounds that these anomalies represent mitral atresia, the right atrial chambers are indistinguishable from classical tricuspid atresia when viewed in isolation (b) – (compare with Illustration 3) and the basic haemodynamics are the same.

9

The final variant producing tricuspid atresia was found in the basic setting of atrioventricular concordance with Ebstein's malformation. The peculiar feature of this type, however, was that the right atrioventricular junction was completely unguarded, there being no evidence of tricuspid valve leaflet tissue. The right atrium communicated with the inlet portion of the right ventricle, which was blind-ending. A muscular partition interposed between the inlet of the right ventricle and the distal right ventricular chamber.

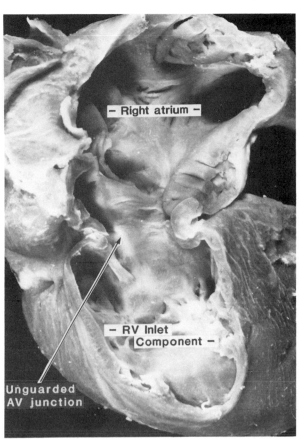

Figure 9. The variant of tricuspid atresia with atrioventricular concordance in which the right atrioventricular junction is unguarded. A muscular partition separates the right ventricular inlet from the distal components of the right ventricle (see Figure 10)

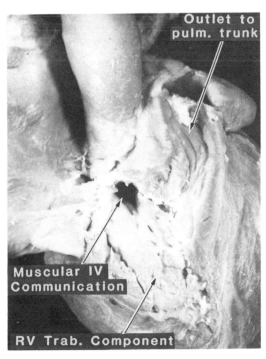

Figure 10. The distal right ventricle from the heart illustrated in Figure 9. Its morphology is directly comparable with that found in the rudimentary right ventricle in classical tricuspid atresia (compare with Figure 5a)

10

This distal chamber had apical trabecular and outlet components, communicated with the left ventricle through an interventricular communication with completely muscular margins and in all respects was indistinguishable from the typical rudimentary right ventricle found in classical tricuspid atresia (compare with illustration 5a).

Acknowledgement

The heart in illustration 7b is photographed with the kind permission of Dr J. L. Wilkinson, University of Liverpool.

References

1. Tandon, R., Edwards, J. E. Tricuspid atresia: a re-evaluation and classification. Journal of Thoracic and Cardiovascular Surgery 1974; 67: 530–542

2. Anderson, R. H., Wilkinson, J. L., Gerlis, L. M., Smith, A., Becker, A. E. Atresia of the right atrioventricular orifice. British Heart Journal 1977; 39: 414–428

3. Thiene, G., Anderson, R. H. The clinical morphology of tricuspid atresia: atresia of the right atrioventricular valve. Giornale Italiano di Cardiologia 1981; 11: 1845–1859

4. Dickinson, D. F., Wilkinson, J. L., Smith, A., Becker, A. E., Anderson, R. H. Atrioventricular conduction tissues in univentricular hearts of left ventricular type with absent right atrioventricular connection ('tricuspid atresia'). British Heart Journal 1979; 42: 1–8

5. Ho, S. Y., Anderson, R. H., Macartney, F. J. et al. Straddling atrioventricular valve with absent atrioventricular connection: report of 10 cases. British Heart Journal 1982; 47: 344–352

The Fontan operation

John C. Baldwin MD
Department of Cardiovascular Surgery, Stanford University School of Medicine, Stanford, California, USA

Francis Fontan MD
Hopital Cardiologique du Haut-Leveque, Universite de Bordeaux, Bordeaux (Pessac), France

Introduction

Palliative surgery may improve the clinical status of patients with tricuspid atresia and physiologically related disturbances, but it does not offer good long-term results. Corrective surgery, providing elimination of venoarterial mixing and definitive diversion of systemic venous return to the lungs without dependence on the normal right ventricle, has offered steadily improving results in tricuspid atresia and several other conditions[1].

History

There were unsuccessful early clinical attempts to bypass the right ventricle through connection of the right atrial appendage to the pulmonary artery in the mid and late 1950s, but in the late 1960s Fontan developed successful surgery involving the concept of right atrium-to-pulmonary artery bypass for physiological, but not anatomical, correction of tricuspid atresia[2-4]. Fontan's original report in 1971 described 3 patients, of whom 2 survived. These patients underwent surgery to 'ventriclize' the right atrium. This operation entailed a superior vena cava to right pulmonary artery anastomosis of the Glenn type, closure of the atrial septal defect and insertion of a homograft valve in the inferior vena caval orifice. In addition, a valved aortic homograft was placed between the right atrium and left pulmonary artery. These two valves were employed in the hope of avoiding difficulties with elevated systemic venous pressure, a complication which has persisted in the application of this technique. One patient had a direct right atrium-pulmonary artery anastomosis.

Kreutzer et al.[5] noted Fontan's approach to physiological correction and emphasized direct end-to-end anastomosis between the right atrial appendage and the pulmonary artery. They reported 2 cases of Type I tricuspid atresia in which they performed end-to-end right atrium-to-pulmonary artery anastomoses. In one case they used a pulmonary artery homograft and in another direct anastomosis of the right atrial appendage to the patient's own detached pulmonary valve annulus. Partial closure of the foramen ovale was accomplished through the opening in the right atrial appendage.

The physiological principle of the Fontan operation has received wide attention and has undergone various technical modifications over the ensuing years. Furthermore, applications have been extended into other areas, including the univentricular heart and pulmonary atresia with intact ventricular septum. However, in most centres the technique retains its principal usefulness in the treatment of tricuspid atresia. Relatively high mortality was experienced at first, but results have improved, as exemplified in Fontan's later report of 21 consecutive operations without a death[6, 7].

Indications

Successful application of this technique depends on careful patient selection, and similar principles apply for the various anomalies which may be treated with the operation. In the 'classic' instance of tricuspid atresia specific criteria have been laid down by Fontan and his colleagues[8]. Clinical criteria include age restrictions based on the finding that patients between the ages of 4 and 15 years are best suited for the technique. By the age of 4 and with a weight of approximately 13 kg most patients can accommodate a conduit 20 mm in diameter. Younger patients have generally been found to tolerate the operation less well, and Cleveland et al.[9] found that young age was a statistically significant ($P < 0.0003$) incremental risk factor for hospital mortality with the Fontan procedure. Others have suggested early intervention with the Fontan operation to improve the long-term outlook for left ventricular function, and the upper age limit of 15 years suggested by Fontan and his associates is based on the likelihood of diminution of ventricular function after that age[10]. There has been limited experience with the Fontan procedure in adults, but these patients must be carefully selected on a physiological basis[11]. Children should be selected for the operation on symptomatic grounds, usually exercise intolerance, anoxic spells and cyanosis.

Electrocardiographic criteria include the presence of sinus rhythm and the absence of recurrent or persistent supraventricular tachycardias. The presence of right atrial hypertrophy is a relatively auspicious finding.

Fontan and his associates have stressed the importance of normal vena caval drainage and normal right atrial volume as determined by angiography. Mean pulmonary artery pressure should be less than 15 mm Hg and pulmonary vascular resistance less than 4 units/m². The ratio of the diameter of the pulmonary artery to that of the aorta should be greater than 0.75 and there should be normal left ventricular function (ejection fraction >60 per cent). There should be no uncorrectable mitral regurgitation, and any possible deleterious effects of previous shunts (e.g., possible influences on pulmonary vascular resistance) should be taken into consideration.

Several conditions other than tricuspid atresia have been successfully treated with modifications of the Fontan operation. It should be noted, however, that Cleveland et al.[9] found a diagnosis other than tricuspid atresia to be a statistically significant ($P < 0.03$) incremental risk factor in hospital mortality after the Fontan procedure. Considerable attention has been focused upon application the Fontan operation to the condition of univentricular heart[12-14]. De la Riviere and Malm[15] have noted that hospital mortality for patients with univentricular heart treated with modifications of the Fontan operation is much less than that observed among patients treated with septation and that complete heart block is less frequent, though long-term follow-up is still lacking. They have suggested that application of the Fontan principle is the treatment of choice for univentricular heart when there is a single atrioventricular valve. McGoon et al.[16] have described their experience with the Fontan operation in univentricular heart and noted that, as in the case of tricuspid atresia, elevation of pulmonary vascular resistance was a significant risk factor; other risk factors in their experience included increasing heart size and ventricular failure as well as atrioventricular valve regurgitation.

The principle of the Fontan operation has been used successfully in the treatment of pulmonary atresia with intact ventricular septum; most surgeons currently employ early prostaglandin (PGE₁) infusion with transarterial valvotomy[17, 18]. Other applications of this same physiological surgical approach have been in Ebstein's anomaly, transposition of the great vessels, double outlet right ventricle with common atrioventricular canal, 'criss-cross' heart and hypoplastic right ventricle[19-22].

The operation

Anaesthesia

Standard cardiac surgical anaesthetic technique is employed with the Fontan operation except that the patient should be allowed to breathe spontaneously, if at all possible, at the conclusion of the operation so as to permit early extubation and avoidance of the need for positive-pressure ventilation[23]. The patient's clinical status is generally observed to be much improved as soon as he is breathing spontaneously, and significant diminution in the cardiac index has been demonstrated when positive end expiratory pressure (>6 cmH$_2$O) is applied[24].

Positioning

The patient lies supine with the shoulders slightly elevated, in the standard position for median sternotomy. Appropriate arterial and venous cannulae are placed for monitoring of blood pressure and administration of fluids and vasoactive agents.

TRICUSPID ATRESIA

As indicated above, the principal application for the Fontan operation has been in cases of tricuspid atresia. Depending on the type and specific anatomy, two basic techniques may be used for physiological correction. One involves right atrial-to-right ventricular anastomosis, and the other involves right atrial-to-pulmonary arterial connection.

Right atrial-to-right ventricular anastomosis

If there are normally related great arteries, with the pulmonary artery arising from the outlet chamber, a connection may be made between the right atrium and the outlet chamber of the right ventricle, preserving the patient's own pulmonary valve. In this instance it is essential to ascertain that there is no significant pulmonary stenosis, and if any such obstruction is encountered it should be relieved at the time of operation.

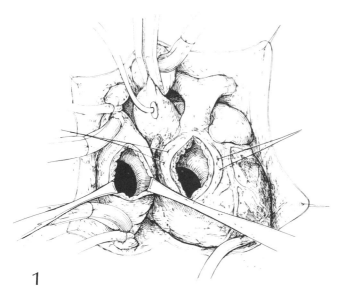

1

1

Median sternotomy is performed and extracorporeal circulation with systemic cooling is established. Cardioplegic solution is administered via the aortic root. Atriotomy is performed through the right atrial appendage and ventriculotomy in the outflow tract of the right ventricle. These incisions facilitate detailed inspection of the cardiac anatomy and, in particular, the exclusion of unexpected contraindications such as single atrium or small pulmonary valve ring.

Since right atrial function is of paramount importance it is important to cannulate the venae cavae directly, to preserve the Eustachian valve and to be meticulous in the performance of the atriotomy and conduit anastomosis from the right atrial appendage and not the atrium itself, thus preserving the atrial muscle and its arterial supply.

2a & b

Before operation the conduit is prepared. A variety of conduits have been used, including non-valved Dacron conduits, porcine and pericardial-valved Dacron conduits, autologous pericardial conduits and fresh aortic valve homograft conduits[25, 26]. Controversy exists regarding the need for a valve within the conduit, and the argument for the valve is most compelling and has most following in the case of the right ventricular anastomosis, where the possibility of subsequent right ventricular development and enlargement raises the possibility of development of significant regurgitation[1]. Various problems related to prosthetic conduits, and in particular the valved conduits, have been reported, including the development of valve conduit gradients, neointimal proliferation and obstruction, delayed valve closure and late deterioration. Consequently, autogenous or aortic valve homograft techniques (a) currently enjoy widest acceptance[27–30]. It should be noted that another alternative is the pericardial patch (b), which may be employed with or without malposition of the great arteries.

The right ventricular outlet chamber is approached through a high vertical ventriculotomy approximately 1 cm below the pulmonary valve ring, with careful avoidance of the coronary vessels. If the outlet chamber is small the pulmonary artery can be opened and a probe passed retrograde through the pulmonary valve to facilitate the correct siting of the ventriculotomy.

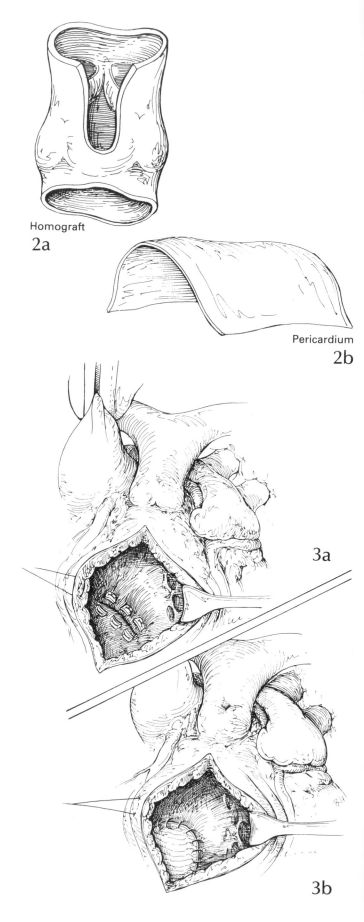

Homograft

2a

Pericardium

2b

3a

3a & b

The ventricular septal defect is closed with interrupted sutures buttressed by Teflon pledgets in the case of a small defect (a). Larger defects are closed with an elastic Dacron patch (b). Atrioventricular block is avoided by placement of the sutures on the right side of the septum in all cases, even if two defects are present.

3b

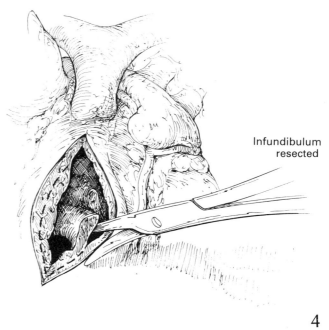

Infundibulum
resected

4

In order to ensure adequacy of right ventricular outflow when the right atrial-to-right ventricular technique is employed infundibular resection may occasionally be required. Fontan (unpublished observations) has noted that in certain instances of small outlet chamber it may be advantageous to leave the ventricular septal defect itself open and to effect patch closure at the level of the ostium infundibule.

4

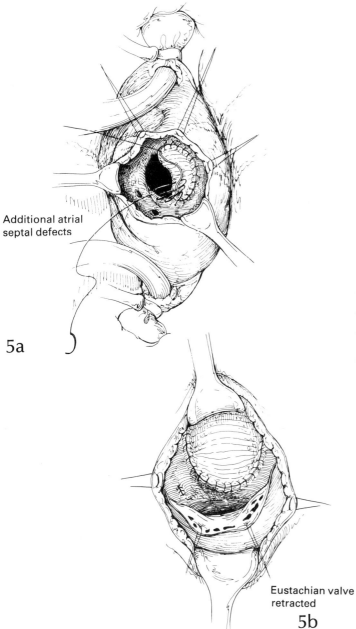

Additional atrial
septal defects

5a

5a & b

Through the incision in the right atrial appendage the atrial septal defect (ASD) is closed with a patch (a). It should be noted that additional defects may be present and these can frequently be closed primarily (b).

Eustachian valve
retracted

5b

6

The distal anastomosis is performed with the aortic valve homograft (or Dacron conduit if necessary), a continuous 5/0 polypropylene suture being used. With the heart beating, careful inspection of the atrial septum and the atrial septal defect patch is made to exclude the possibility of leaks around the suture line and other small defects in the atrial septum, particularly in its lower part. This can also be accomplished with the aortic cross-clamp in place, by discontinuation of left-sided venting or by instillation of saline on the right side.

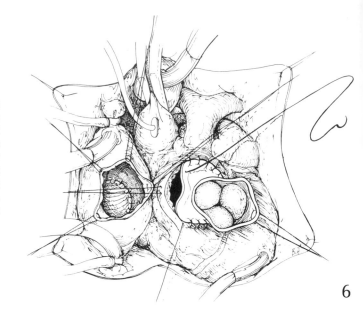

6

7

The proximal anastomosis between the homograft and the right atrial appendage is then carried out, again with a continuous 5/0 polypropylene suture. All suture lines are then carefully inspected for haemostasis, the patient is weaned from cardiopulmonary bypass and routine decannulation is carried out.

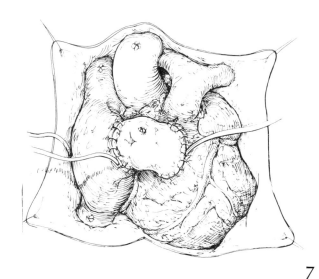

7

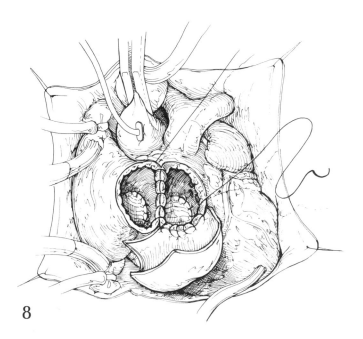

8

8

As noted previously, the pericardial patch procedure for direct right atrial-outlet chamber connection is frequently applicable (*see illustration 2b*). The relevant anastomotic technique, after septal defect closure, is shown here.

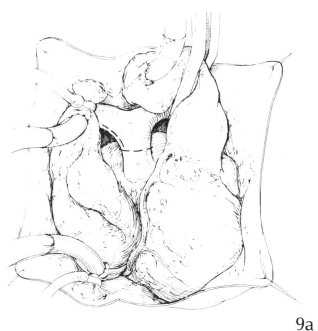

9a

Right atrial-to-pulmonary arterial anastomosis

If the right ventricular chamber is absent or too small and if there is ventriculoarterial discordance the right atrial-to-pulmonary arterial anastomosis is preferred. In this instance it is generally accepted that no valve is truly required in the circuit, although accumulating experience with aortic-valved homografts has been favourable. Several alternatives have been developed in this regard.

9a–c

Fontan[31] has previously described the use of the aortic valve homograft, with end-to-side anastomosis to the main pulmonary artery-right pulmonary artery junction or with end-to-end anastomosis to the transected main pulmonary artery. The currently preferred version of this technique is performed entirely on cardiopulmonary bypass. This technique involves initial transection of the main pulmonary artery (a) with oversewing of the proximal stump. This is accomplished with two rows of continuous sutures, one closing the pulmonary valve leaflets (b) and the second closing the end of the artery (c).

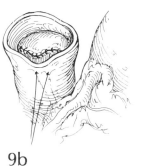

9b

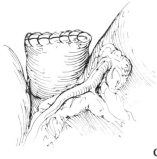

9c

10a–d

Performance of the distal homograft to pulmonary arterial anastomosis is then carried out with a continuous 5/0 polypropylene suture (a, b), and the distal suture line is inspected (c). Following this the atrial septal defect is closed as described previously (d).

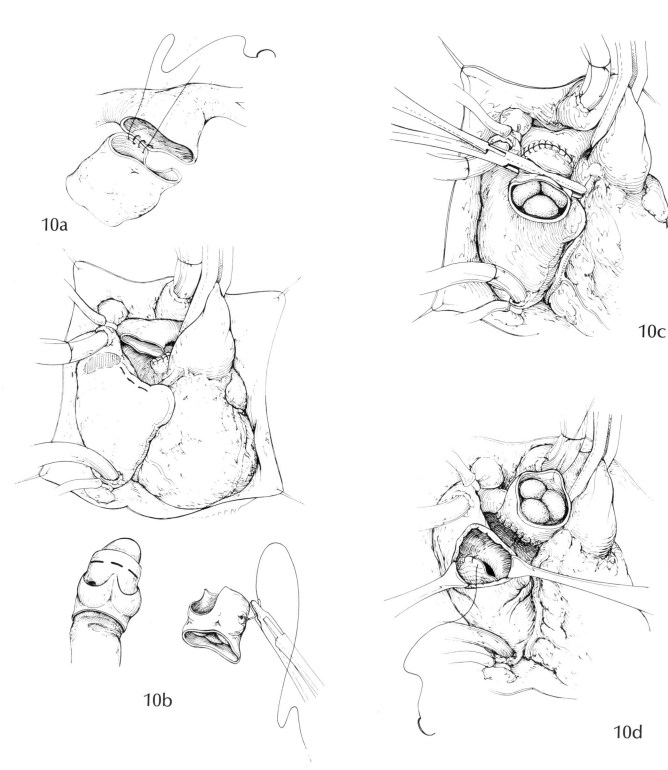

10a

10b

10c

10d

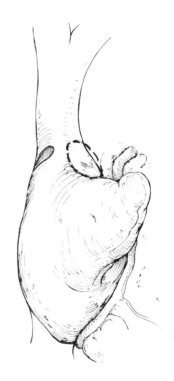

11

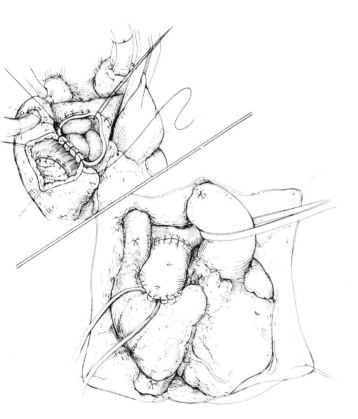

11

It should be noted that in this case and with similar homograft anastomoses in other conditions (e.g. univentricular heart) avoidance of kinking of the conduit is critical. This depends in part on correct siting of the atriotomy. An incision at the base of the right atrial appendage, extending towards the superior vena cava with avoidance of the sinus node and right atrial blood supply, may facilitate this effort.

11

12

The proximal anastomosis, between the right atrium and the homograft, is performed with continuous 5/0 polypropylene. In the performance of all anterior conduits it is important to check carefully when closing the sternum that there is no compression of the conduit. When this does occur it may be necessary to resect the posterior table of the sternum in the area of the anterior aspect of the conduit. The pericardium is left widely open.

12

13a & b & 14a & b

Some attention has been given to avoidance of compression of the anterior conduit through the use of posterior right atrial-to-pulmonary arterial connections[32]. When anatomically feasible this posterior technique may be performed either with transposed or non-transposed great vessels and with left juxtaposition of the atria.

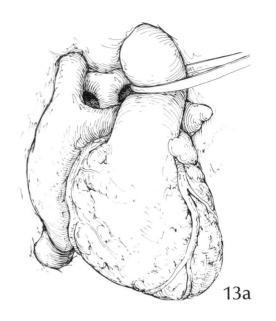

13a

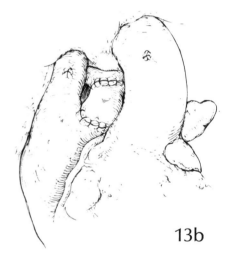

13b

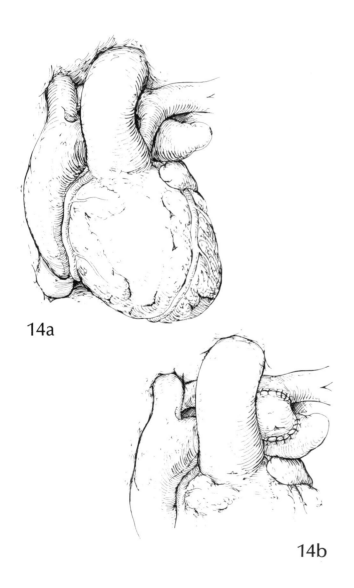

14a

14b

UNIVENTRICULAR HEART

15

The Fontan operation has been widely used in the treatment of univentricular heart because of generally poor results with septation. This technique involves patch closure of the right-sided atrioventricular orifice in combination with the Fontan physiological principle of redirection of systemic venous return into the pulmonary artery[16]. Here again emphasis is placed on limitation of the atriotomy to the right atrial appendage as far as possible. With this approach it is possible to close both the atrial septal defect and the right atrioventricular valve. The illustration shows the essential aspects of this technique, employing the homograft conduit.

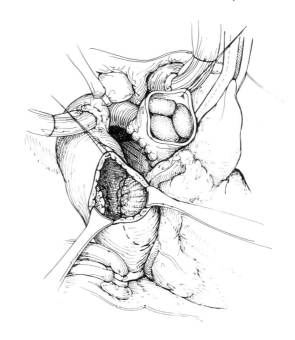

15

16

One of the principal problems which has been experienced in application of the Fontan operation to this anomaly has been the patch closure of the right atrioventricular valve[33, 34]. Difficulties with heart block have been widely encountered and efforts at pledgeted closure of the valve leaflets have been associated with dehiscence and failure of closure. One alternative is to place the patch, which can be fashioned from pericardium or Dacron, 1–2 cm above the valve annulus. As shown, this patch may be placed above the level of the coronary sinus. This specific technique has been widely employed and there appear to be no untoward effects as long as there is no significant atrioventricular (A-V) valve regurgitation. It has been suggested that placement of the patch above the coronary sinus may be preferable in these cases because of more effective coronary sinus drainage from the low-pressure chamber and because of avoidance of iatrogenic heart block (Fontan, unpublished observations). If there is A-V valve regurgitation and especially if the valve commissures do not extend all the way to the annulus placement of the patch at the annular level is preferable. One may also consider concomitant left translocation of the coronary sinus to achieve low-pressure chamber (left atrial) drainage.

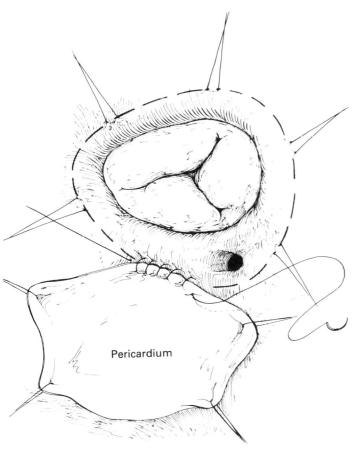

Pericardium

16

Postoperative care

The patient is placed in the head-up (45°) and feet-up (30°) position to facilitate systemic venous return and pulmonary artery perfusion. As indicated earlier, it is important to allow the patient to breathe spontaneously as early as possible and to achieve early extubation. Pharmacological support, including pressor agents as well as vasodilators for reduction of pulmonary vascular resistance, may be of considerable help in the early postoperative phase[35].

In connection with the general observance of the principle of preservation of right atrial systolic function emphasis has been placed on the importance of sinus rhythm after the Fontan operation. Most patients are observed to maintain sinus rhythm, and in those who develop supraventricular arrhythmias cardioversion is usually successful. Adequate pulsatile pulmonary arterial bloodflow does appear to depend on atrial systole[36]. Although not generally applied, a technique of external compression of the systemic venous circulation has been employed by some investigators with apparent improvement in systemic arterial pressure[37]. The Bordeaux group currently uses an external compressing device, timed with the ventilator to inflate with expiration, in selected postoperative patients with elevated right-sided pressure and low output (Fontan, unpublished observations).

Results

More than 16 years of follow-up has now been accumulated with the Fontan operation for physiological correction. After early reports of relatively high mortality there has been a steady decline in the operative death rate, mortality in a variety of conditions having been reduced to the 5–20 per cent range[38–40]. Indeed, some centres have reported impressive series of tricuspid atresia repairs without operative death[41]. Kirklin and his associates have reported 71 per cent actuarial survival at 5 years in patients with tricuspid artresia[9].

Catheterization follow-up has been performed and most studies have shown some depression of the cardiac index at rest and with exercise, although some have shown near-normal results[42–44]. However, nearly all patients experience prompt and dramatic symptomatic improvement. Ascites and other difficulties related to elevated right-sided pressures are generally temporary, resolving within a few weeks[45]. Laks et al.[46] found that 78 per cent of their patients achieved New York Heart Association Class I symptom status after the operation. De Brux et al.[47], reporting 24 Fontan operations for tricuspid atresia, noted that 88 per cent of their patients were leading a normal life and that two-thirds of these required no medical therapy.

References

1. Laks, H. Tricuspid atresia. Glenn W. W. L. ed. Thoracic and cardiovascular surgery, 4th ed. pp. 914–925. Norwalk: Appleton-Century-Crofts, 1983

2. Sade, R. M. Tricuspid atresia. In Sabiston, D., Spencer, F. eds. Gibbon's Surgery of the chest, 4th ed. pp. 1186–1203. Philadelphia: Saunders, 1983

3. Fontan, F., Baudet, E. Surgical repair of tricuspid atresia. Thorax 1971; 26: 240–248

4. Fontan, F., Mounicot, F. B., Baudet, E., Simonneau, J., Gordo, I., Gouffrant, J. M. Correction de la'atrésie tricuspideienne: rapport de deux cas corrigés par l'autilisation d'une technique chirurgicale nouvelle. Annales de Chirurgie Thoracique et Cardiovasculaire 1971; 10: 39–00

5. Kreutzer, G., Galindez, E., Bono, H., De Palma, C., Laura, J. P. An operation for the correction of tricuspid atresia. Journal of Thoracic and Cardiovascular Surgery 1973; 66: 613–621

6. Fontan, F., Choussat. A., Brom, A. G., Chauve, A., Deville, C., Castro-Cels, A. Repair of tricuspid atresia: surgical considerations and results. In: Anderson, R. H., Shinebourne, E. A., eds. Paediatric Cardiology, pp. 567–580 Edinburgh: Churchill-Livingstone, 1977

7. Fontan, F., et al. Repair of tricuspid atresia in 100 patients. Journal of Thoracic and Cardiovascular Surgery 1983; 85: 647–660

8. Choussat, A., Fontan, F., Besse, P., Vallot, F., Chauve, A., Bricaud, H. Selection criteria for Fontan's procedure. In: Anderson, R. H., Shinebourne, E. A. eds. Paediatric cardiology, pp. 559–566. Edinburgh: Churchill-Livingstone, 1977

9. Cleveland, D. C. et al. Surgical treatment of tricuspid atresia. Annals of Thoracic Surgery 1984; 38: 447–457

10. Hassoulas, J., Barnard, M. S., Sanchez, H., Barnard, C. N. Tricuspid atresia corrected by the Fontan method. South African Medical Journal 1982; 62: 356–358

11. Patterson, W., Baxley, W. A., Karp, R. B., Soto, B., Bargeron, L. L. Tricuspid atresia in adults. American Journal of Cardiology 1982; 49: 141–152

12. Corno, A. et al. Univentricular heart: can we alter the natural history? Annals of Thoracic Surgery 1982; 34: 716–727

13. Eijgelaar, A., Hess, J., Hardjowijono, R., Karliczek, G. F., Rating, W., Homan van der Heide, J. N. Experiences with the Fontan operation. Journal of Thoracic and Cardiovascular Surgery 1982; 30: 63–68

14. Moreno-Cabral, R. J., Miller, D. C., Oyer, P. E., Stinson, E. B., Reitz, B. A., Shumway, N. E. An approach for S,L,L single ventricle incorporating total right atrium-pulmonary artery diversion. Journal of Thoracic and Cardiovascular Surgery 1980; 79: 202–210

15. de la Riviere, A. B., Malm, J. R. Univentricular heart. In: Sabiston, D., Spencer, F. eds. Gibbon's Surgery of the chest, 4th ed. pp. 1177–1185. Philadelphia: Saunders, 1983

16. McGoon, D. C., Danielson, G. K., Puga, F. J. Univentricular heart. In: Glenn, W. W. L. ed. Thoracic and cardiovascular surgery, 4th edn, pp. 770–784. Norwalk: Appleton-Century-Crofts, 1983

17. de Leval, M., Bull, C., Stark, J., Anderson, R. H., Taylor, J. F., Macartney, F. J. Pulmonary atresia and intact ventricular septum: surgical management based on a revised classification. Circulation 1982; 66: 272–280

18. Moulton, A. L., Malm, J. R. Pulmonary stenosis, pulmonary atresia, single pulmonary artery, and aneurysm of the pulmonary artery. In: Glenn, W. W. L. ed. Thoracic and cardiovascular surgery, 4th edn, pp. 829–850. Norwalk: Appleton-Century-Crofts, 1984

19. Kreutzer, G. O. et al. Atrial pulmonary anastomosis. Journal of Thoracic and Cardiovascular Surgery 1982; 83: 427–436

20. Marcelletti, C., Diren, D. R., Schuilenburg, R. M., Becker, A. E. Fontan's operation for Ebstein's anomaly. Journal of Thoracic and Cardiovascular Surgery 1980; 79: 63–66

21. Marcelletti, C. et al. Fontan's operation: an expanded horizon. Journal of Thoracic and Cardiovascular Surgery 1980; 80: 764–769

22. De Vivie, E. R., Ruschewski, W., Koveker, G., Risch, D., Weber, H., Beuren, A. G. Fontan procedure: indication and clinical results. Thoracic and Cardiovascular Surgery 1981; 29: 348–354

23. Schuller, J. L., Sebel, P. S., Bovill, J. G., Marcelletti, C. Early extubation after Fontan operation: a clinical report. British Journal of Anaesthesia 1980; 52: 999–1004

24. Williams, D. B., Kiernan, P. D., Metke, M. P., Marsh, M. M., Danielson, G. K. Hemodynamic response to positive end-expiratory pressure following right atrium-pulmonary artery bypass (Fontan procedure). Journal of Thoracic and Cardiovascular Surgery 1984; 87: 856–861

25. Bowman, F. O., Malm, J. R., Hayes, C. J., Gersony, W. M. Physiologic approach to surgery for tricuspid atresia. Circulation 1978; 58 (Suppl. I): 83–86

26. Bjork, V. O., Olin, C. L., Bjarke, B. B., Thoren, C. A. Right atrial-right ventricular anastomoses for correction of tricuspid atresia. Journal of Thoracic and Cardiovascular Surgery 1979; 77: 452–458

27. DeLeon, S. Y., Idriss, F. S., Ilbawi, M. N., Rastegar, H., Muster, A. J., Paul, M. H. Neointimal obstruction of Carpentier-Edwards valved conduits in two patients with modified Fontan procedure. Annals of Thoracic Surgery 1982; 34: 586–589

28. Doty, D. B., Marvin, W. J., Jr, Lauer, R. M. Modified Fontan procedure: Methods to achieve direct anastomosis of right atrium to pulmonary artery. Journal of Thoracic and Cardiovascular Surgery 1981; 81: 470–475

29. Serratto, M., Miller, R. A., Tatooles, C., Ardekani, R. Hemodynamic evaluation of Fontan operations in tricuspid atresia. Circulation 1975; 51–52 (Suppl. II): 102

30. Mair, D. D., Fulton, R. E., Danielson, G. K. Thrombotic occlusion of Hancock conduit due to severe dehydration after Fontan operation. Mayo Clinic Proceedings 1978; 53: 397–402

31. Fontan, F. Tricuspid atresia. In: Jackson, J. W. ed. Rob and Smith's Operative surgery: Cardiothoracic Surgery, 3rd ed. pp. 152–157. London: Butterworths, 1978

32. Molina, J. E., Wang, Y., Lucas, R., Molar, J. The technique of the Fontan procedure with posterior right atrium-pulmonary artery connection. Annals of Thoracic Surgery 1985; 39: 371–375

33. Didonato, R. et al. Ventricular exclusion during Fontan operation: an evolving technique. Annals of Thoracic Surgery 1985; 39: 283–285

34. Nunez, L., Aguado, M. G., Celemin, D., Larrea, J. L. Closure of the right atrio-ventricular valve in the modified Fontan operation for univentricular heart. Annals of Thoracic Surgery 1982; 34: 714–715

35. Williams, D. B., Kiernan, P. D., Schaff, H. V., Marsh, H. M., Danielson, G. K. The hemodynamic response to dopamine and nitroprusside following right atrium-pulmonary artery bypass (Fontan procedure) Annals of Thoracic Surgery 1982; 34: 51–57

36. Sharratt, G. P., Johnson, A. M., Monro, J. L. Persistence and effects of sinus rhythm after Fontan procedure for tricuspid atresia. British Heart Journal 1979; 42: 74–80

37. Heck, H. A., Doty, D. B. Assisted circulation by phasic external lower body compression. Circulation 1981; 64 (Suppl. II): 118–122

38. Tatooles, C. J., Ardekani, R. G., Miller, R. A., Serratto, M. Operative repair for tricuspid atresia. Annals of Thoracic Surgery 1986; 21: 499–503

39. Gale, A. W., Danielson, G. K., McGoon, D. C., Wallace, R. B., Mair, D. D. Fontan procedure for tricuspid atresia. Circulation 1980; 62: 91–96

40. Laks, H. et al. Results of right atrial to right ventricular, and right atrial to pulmonary artery conduits for complex congenital heart disease. Annals of Surgery 1980; 192: 382–389

41. Ottenkamp, J., Rohmer, J., Quagebeur, J. M., Brom, A. G., Fontan, F. Nine years experience of physiologic correction of tricuspid atresia: long-term results and current surgical approach. Thorax 1982; 37: 718–726

42. Shachar, G. B., Fuhrman, B. P., Wang, Y., Lucas, R. V., Lock, J. E. Rest and exercise hemodynamics after the Fontan procedure. Circulation 1982; 65: 1043–1048

43. Laks, H., Hellenbrand, W. E., Kleinman, C. S., Stansel, H. C., Talner, N. S. Patch reconstruction of the right ventricular outflow tract with pulmonary valve insertion. Circulation 1981; 64 (Suppl. II): 154–161

44. Peterson, R. J., Franch, R. H., Fajman, W. A., Jennings, J. G., Jones, R. H. Non-invasive determination of exercise cardiac function following Fontan operation. Journal of Thoracic and Cardiovascular Surgery 1984; 88: 263–272

45. Behrendt, D. M., Rosenthal, A. Cardiovascular status after repair by Fontan procedure. Annals of Thoracic Surgery 1980; 29: 322–330

46. Laks, H. et al. Experience with the Fontan procedure. Journal of Thoracic and Cardiovascular Surgery 1984; 88: 939–951

47. de Brux, J. L. et al. Tricuspid atresia: results of treatment in 115 children. Journal of Thoracic and Cardiovascular Surgery 1983; 85: 440–446

Ebstein's anomaly: surgical anatomy

Robert H. Anderson BSc, MD, MRCPath
Joseph Levy Professor of Paediatric Cardiac Morphology, Cardiothoracic Institute, Brompton Hospital, London, UK

Introduction

The lesion which is nowadays described under the eponym of Wilhelm Ebstein[1] has two major features: (1) some part of the tricuspid valve leaflets have their proximal attachment to the ventricular walls placed more distally than in the normal heart and (2) the leaflets themselves are dysplastic, thickened and malformed.

There is argument about whether Ebstein himself described more than valve dysplasia, but nowadays it is the downward displacement of the proximal attachment of the valve leaflets which is the hallmark of the anomaly[2]. The degree of abnormality varies considerably from heart to heart and in some cases presenting at autopsy only mild abnormal downward displacement of the septal leaflet is found. But in patients who require surgical treatment the lesion will almost always be encountered in its 'fullblown' form with downward displacement of the mural and septal leaflets, which are often adherent to the wall of the right ventricle.

Rarely an Ebstein-like lesion can affect the mitral valve[3]. Usually, however, when Ebstein's malformation affects the left-sided atrioventricular valve it does so in the setting of congenitally corrected transposition, and then the valve is of tricuspid morphology[4, 5].

When Ebstein's disease affects the tricuspid valve it afflicts the different valve leaflets in different fashions[6, 7]. It is the septal and mural (inferior) leaflets which become downwardly displaced (see Figure 1). These are the leaflets of the tricuspid valve which, during diastole, fall back against the septum and inferior wall of the inlet portion of the right ventricle. In severe cases these leaflets may cease to exist or become adherent to the right ventricular wall.

The parietal wall of the ventricular inlet portion undergoes thinning to varying degrees, a process often termed 'atrialization'. Irrespective of the thinning of the wall the inlet portion always becomes an effective part of the right atrium and gives atrial pressure tracings. This is because the remaining leaflet of the tricuspid valve, the anterosuperior leaflet, retains its usual proximal attachment to the inner heart curvature.

The attachments of the distal edge of the anterosuperior leaflet determine the vital surgical anatomy of the valve (see Figures 1 and 2). In some hearts with 'fullblown' displacement of the septal and mural leaflets the anterosuperior leaflet retains its usual chordal attachments to the medial and anterior papillary muscles and has its anticipated normal appearance when seen from the right ventricular outlet (compare Figures 1 and 3).

In other hearts with similar downward displacement of the septal and mural leaflets the anterosuperior leaflet has completely abnormal morphology. Instead of having a free leading edge as seen in the normal heart the leaflet is enlarged to form a square sail-like structure (see Figure 3). The bottom edge of this 'sail' is attached to a prominent muscular shelf between the inlet and apical trabecular components of the ventricle (see Figure 2a). The blood is therefore unable to pass through the ventricle in usual fashion. Instead it must pass through the sites of the anticipated commissures (see Figure 2b), but since the other leaflets of the valve are abnormal, so are the commissural areas. When these areas are examined in autopsy specimens the impression is gained of an attempt to produce a competent valve at the inlet-trabecular junction (see Figure 4).

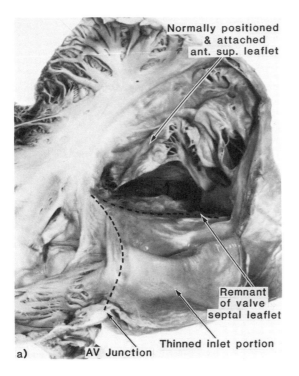

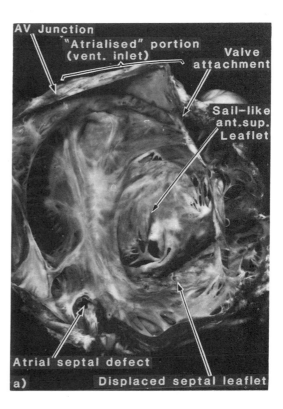

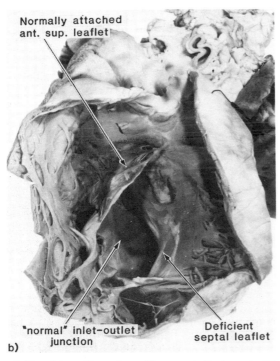

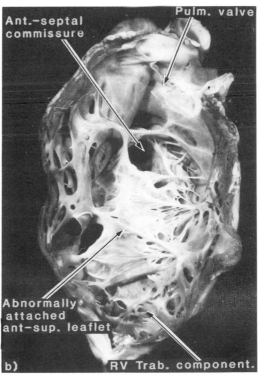

Figure 1. Ebstein's malformation with normal attachment of the distal edge of the anterosuperior leaflet (compare with Figure 3) but virtual absence of the septal and mural leaflets; (a) shows the inlet and (b) the outlet aspects. Specimen provided by Dr Luis Becu, Buenos Aires, and photographed with his kind permission together with that of Drs Jane Somerville and Patrizia Presbitero

Figure 2. Ebstein's malformation with grossly abnormal morphology and attachments of the anterosuperior leaflet (compare with Figures 1 and 3); (a) shows the inlet and (b) the outlet aspects. Specimen provided and photographed by kind permission of Dr Nuala Fagg, Guy's Hospital, London

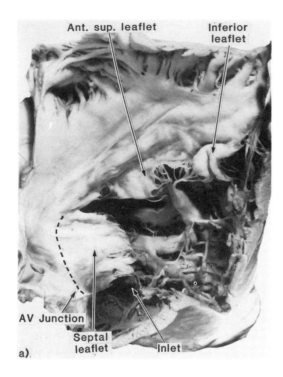

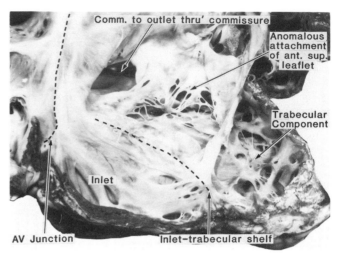

Figure 4. A close-up of the inlet-trabecular junction of the heart shown in Figure 2. Note the abnormal attachments to the shelf between inlet and trabecular components

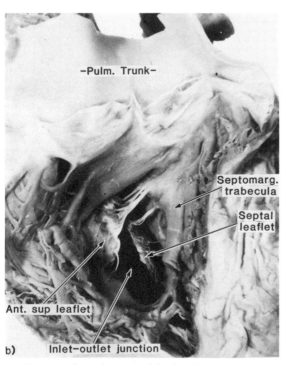

Figure 3. The normal attachments of the distal edge of the anterosuperior leaflet of the tricuspid valve (compare with Figures 1 and 2)

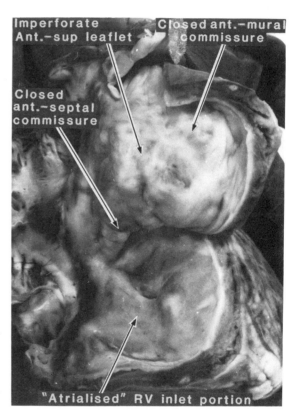

Figure 5. Ebstein's malformation with abnormal attachment of the anterosuperior leaflet as shown in Figure 2 but with additional obliteration of the commissures resulting in tricuspid atresia

Sometimes the sail-like leaflet is additionally attached to the ventricular wall along its side edges and this then results in an imperforate Ebstein lesion, giving tricuspid atresia (see Figure 5). Alternatively the leaflet may be fenestrated. Very rarely the anterosuperior leaflet may also be displaced distally along a shelf of the ventriculoinfundibular fold[7].

The morphology of the valve leaflet and its precise attachments are crucial in determining the feasibility of valve replacement or reconstruction as the optimal surgical option[8-11]. Each case must be treated on its merits, but it would seem from the anatomy that only patients with normal distal attachment of the anterosuperior leaflet would be suitable for reconstructive surgery. Whether reconstruction or valve replacement is attempted it is likely that obliteration of the atrialized segment will be necessary when the wall of the inlet is excessively thin. In severe cases coming to autopsy the trabecular and outlet components of the right ventricle are also dilated and thinned. Anatomical observations would suggest a poor prognosis for these patients. It should also be noted that the left ventricle is not normal in these hearts[12]. Particularly noticeable is the bulging of the inlet septum towards the left.

Ebstein's malformation may coexist with other lesions. An atrial septal defect within the oval fossa is particularly frequent but ventricular septal defects may be found, communicating with either the distal or proximal components of the right ventricle. When the displaced valve is imperforate the defect represents the only route to the distal right ventricle. Ebstein's malformation may also be found in the setting of an atrioventricular septal defect with either separate valve orifices[13] or a common valve[7]. The fact that Ebstein's malformation may affect the left-sided valve in corrected transposition has been mentioned above. It is a particularly common finding in this segmental combination[4, 5]. Whenever Ebstein's anomaly affects the morphologically tricuspid valve accessory atrioventricular connections and the Wolff-Parkinson-White syndrome are to be anticipated. These produce right-sided pre-excitation in the normal heart but left-sided pre-excitation with discordant atrioventricular connection.

References

1. Ebstein, W. Ueber einen sehr seltenen Fall von Insufficienz der Valvula triscuspidalis, bedingt eine angeborene hochgradige Missbildung derselben. Archiv für Anatomie, Physiologie und Wissenschaftliche Medicin (Müller's Archiv). 1866: 238–254

2. Becker, A. E., Becker, M. J., Edwards, J. E. Pathologic spectrum of dysplasia of the tricuspid valve: features in common with Ebstein's malformation. Archives of Pathology 1971; 91: 167–178

3. Ruschhaupt, D. G., Bharati, S., Lev, M. Mitral valve malformation of Ebstein type in absence of corrected transposition. American Journal of Cardiology 1976; 38: 109–112

4. Anderson, K. R., Danielson, G. K., McGoon, D. C., Lie, J. T. Ebstein's anomaly of the left-sided tricuspid valve; pathological anatomy of the valvular malformation. Circulation 1978; 57: Supp. I: 187–191

5. Anderson, K. R., Zuberbuhler, J. R., Anderson, R. H., Becker, A. E., Lie, J. T. Morphologic spectrum of Ebstein's anomaly of the heart: a review. Mayo Clinic Proceedings 1979; 54: 174–180

6. Zuberbuhler, J. R., Allwork, S. P., Anderson, R. H. The spectrum of Ebstein's anomaly of the tricuspid valve. Journal of Thoracic and Cardiovascular Surgery 1979; 77: 202–211

7. Zuberbuhler, J. R., Becker, A. E., Anderson, R. H., Lennox, C. C. Further observations on Ebstein's malformation pertinent to the embryological development of the tricuspid valve, with a note on the nature of 'clefts' in the atrioventricular valves. Pediatric Cardiology

8. Danielson, G. K., Maloney, J. D., Devloo, R. A. E. Surgical repair of Ebstein's anomaly. Mayo Clinic Proceedings 1979; 54: 185–192

9. Schmidt-Hablemann, P., Meisner, H., Struck, E., Sebening, F. Results of valvuloplasty for Ebstein's anomaly. The Thoracic and Cardiovascular Surgeon 1981; 29: 155–157

10. Barbero-Marcial, M., Verginelli, G., Awad, M., Ferreira, S., Ebaid, M., Zerbini, E. J. Surgical treatment of Ebstein's anomaly: early and late results in 20 patients subjected to valve replacement. Journal of Thoracic and Cardiovascular Surgery 1979; 78: 416–422

11. Westaby, S., Karp, R. B., Kirklin, J. W., Waldo, A. L., Blackstone, E. H. Surgical treatment in Ebstein's malformation. Annals of Thoracic Surgery 1982; 34: 388–395

12. Castaneda-Zuniga, W., Nath, H. P., Moller, J. H., Edwards, J. E. Left-sided anomalies in Ebstein's malformation of the tricuspid valve. Pediatric Cardiology 1982; 3: 181–185

13. Caruso, G., Losekoot, T. G., Becker, A. E. Ebstein's anomaly in persistent common atrioventricular canal. British Heart Journal 1978; 40: 1275–1279

Ebstein's anomaly: surgical treatment

Gordon K. Danielson MD

Professor or Surgery, Mayo Medical School;
Consultant in Thoracic and Cardiothoracic Surgery, Mayo Clinic, Rochester, Minnesota, USA

Introduction

1

The typical appearance of the anomalous development of the tricuspid valve described by Ebstein, characterized by a deformity of the valve with downward displacement of the posterior and septal leaflets in a spiral fashion below the true annulus, is illustrated. The displaced leaflets leave a portion of the ventricle above the valve as an integral part of the right atrium – the 'atrialized ventricle'. The larger than normal anterior leaflet of the tricuspid valve is shown.

The chordae tendineae and papillary muscles of the tricuspid valve are anomalous and abnormally positioned. The atrioventricular node is located at the apex of the triangle of Koch, and the conduction system is normally situated. The common atrial septal defect is shown.

The diagnosis can be made by cardiac catheterization and angiocardiography. More recently the two-dimensional echocardiogram has been of great assistance in the diagnosis and assessment of Ebstein's anomaly; indeed, in most cases it has made cardiac catheterization unnecessary. Two-dimensional echocardiography allows precise anatomical assessment and can define with high probability the subgroup of patients who may require tricuspid valve replacement at operation[1].

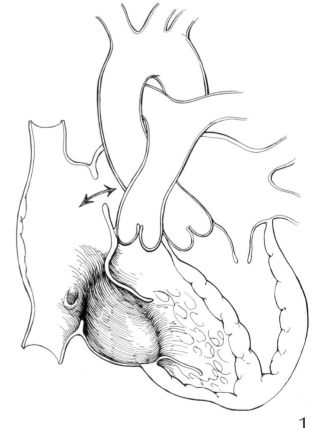

1

The operation

Surgical treatment for Ebstein's anomaly has followed two parallel paths: tricuspid valve replacement and various types of plastic reconstruction. Because of the relatively limited surgical experience reported at the present time and the variable natural history of Ebstein's anomaly there is controversy over indications for operation. Important considerations include the risk of operation, the expected benefits and late complications. The currently low mortality for repair, the fact that the majority of patients can be repaired with a plastic procedure, and the long-term results all make operation advisable for patients who have deteriorated into Class III or IV, along with those who are less symptomatic but have moderate to severe cyanosis, paradoxical emboli, or a progressive increase in cardiac size. There is a natural reluctance to advise operation if tricuspid valve replacement is required since this introduces new potential problems of thromboembolism, anticoagulation-related complications and prosthetic valve dysfunction. It is clear, however, that tricuspid valve replacement with a prosthesis can offer substantial long-term improvement for some symptomatic patients. Most of the valve replacement series are composed of older children and adults; few successful results in infants have been reported[2].

Although some patients do well for many years with a mechanical tricuspid prosthesis, tricuspid valve replacement generally has a higher incidence of complications and a lower standard of long-term record than does replacement of the mitral or aortic valve. The introduction of the bioprosthesis has not completely solved the problem of tricuspid valve replacement as this valve is subject to accelerated deterioration in infants, children and young adults. In our experience the failure-free rate of porcine heterograft valves in children is only 58.5 per cent at 5 years[3]. In addition, for all types of prosthetic valve there is the problem of the need for valve replacement because of growth of the patient. For these reasons it seems preferable to perform a plastic repair for Ebstein's anomaly whenever feasible.

Since 1972 we have used a repair technique that consists of plication of the free wall of the atrialized portion of the right ventricle, posterior tricuspid annuloplasty and right atrial reduction[4, 5]. The operation is based on the construction of a monocusp valve using the anterior leaflet of the tricuspid valve. Because this repair depends on the presence of a normal or enlarged anterior leaflet major abnormalities of the leaflet may compromise the result. For most patients with fenestrations or perforations of the anterior leaflet the defects can be satisfactorily repaired with a fine continuous suture. If greater abnormalities are present, such as attachment of the free edge of the leaflet to the ventricular wall or complete failure of delamination of the tricuspid valve so that there are no chordae or papillary muscles, this plastic repair will not be applicable and prosthetic valve replacement will be required.

Our operative management of patients with Ebstein's malformation consists of: (1) electrophysiological mapping for localization of the accessory conduction pathways in those patients with ventricular pre-excitation; (2) patch closure of the atrial septal defect or patent foramen ovale; (3) plication of the atrialized portion of the right ventricle; (4) plastic repair of the tricuspid valve, when feasible, or valve replacement; (5) correction of associated anomalies such as relief of pulmonary stenosis or division of accessory conduction pathways; and (6) excision of redundant right atrial wall.

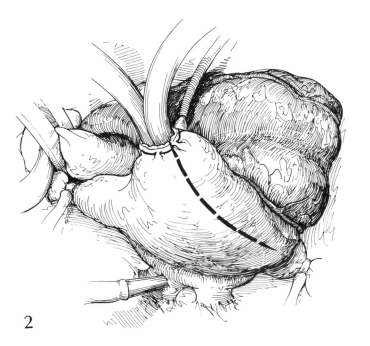

2

Electrophysiological mapping and cannulation

After a median sternotomy adhesions are freed and the external cardiac anatomy is confirmed. Electrophysiological mapping is performed if the Wolff-Parkinson-White syndrome is diagnosed or suspected[6].

2

Cannulation is accomplished by using the ascending aorta for arterial inflow and inserting separate caval cannulae through the right atrial appendage for venous outflow to the pump. A vent is required. The right atrium is opened widely with an incision made from the appendage towards the inferior vena cava and the caval cannulae are retracted to provide maximum exposure.

3

Closure of defects

The repair is begun by closing the atrial septal defect. We prefer to patch all atrial septal defects in patients with Ebstein's anomaly because of our experience and that of others in which sutured atrial septal defects in patients with a high-pressure right atrium may reopen either early or late as a result of sutures pulling through the septal tissue.

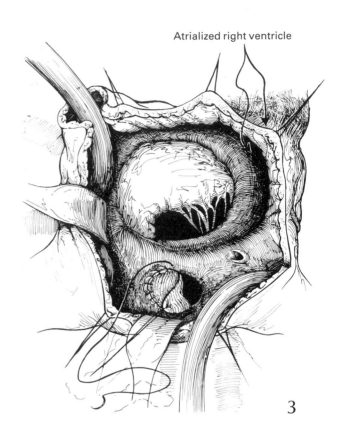

Atrialized right ventricle

3

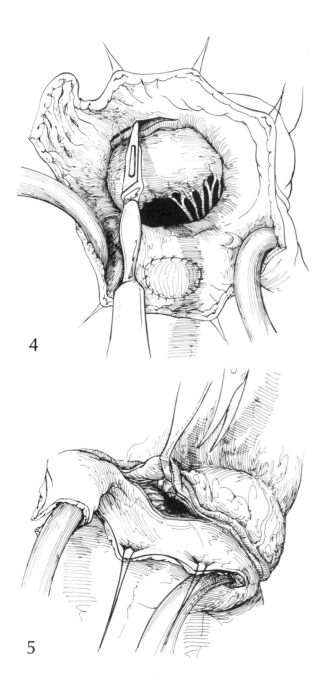

4

5

4 & 5

In symptomatic patients with accessory conduction pathways in the right free wall surgical interruption of the pathway is performed next[6]. The right atrium is incised just proximal to the tricuspid annulus opposite the point of earliest epicardial activation. Dissection is carried down the right ventricular wall for 1 cm and is extended along the annulus medially and laterally for a least 2 cm. A second incision is made in the epicardium cephalad to the right artery, joining the endocardial incision.

6

The edges of the incision and exposed right ventricle are electrocoagulated and the endocardial incision is closed with a double suture line. The epicardial incision is closed as a separate layer in a similar manner.

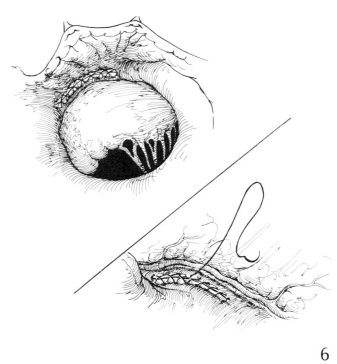

6

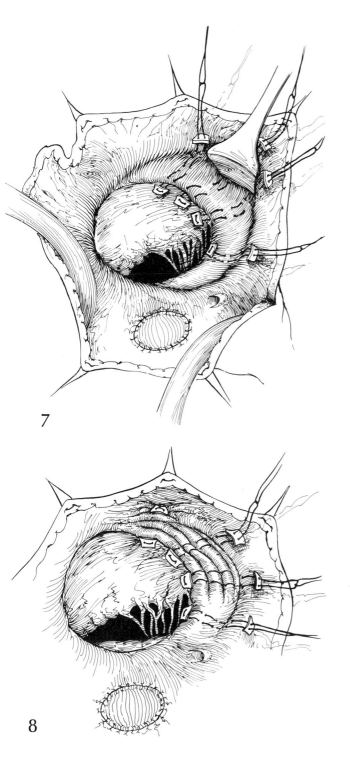

7

8

7 & 8

Plication of atrialized right ventricle

Mattress sutures passed through pledgets of Teflon felt are used to pull the tricuspid annulus down to the insertion of the tricuspid valve in the wall of the right ventricle. Sutures are placed in the atrialized portion of the right ventricle (*see* Illustration 4) so that when they are subsequently tied the atrialized ventricle is plicated and no aneurysmal cavity is formed. The plication sutures are placed so as to avoid the posterior descending coronary artery and obvious large branches of the right coronary artery.

In those instances in which the tricuspid valve is only moderately displaced from the annulus but in which the leaflets are adherent to the ventricular endocardium the plicating sutures are extended across the leaflet down towards the apex of the right ventricle to the same level that would be appropriate if the leaflets had been displaced to the level of their adherence to the ventricular wall. This modification has given results as good as for those cases in which there is no adherence of the displaced leaflet to the right ventricle.

The sutures are tied down sequentially to obliterate the atrialized ventricle. The anterior and posterior aspects of the right ventricle are inspected to be certain that no injury has occurred to the major coronary arteries.

9 & 10

Posterior tricuspid annuloplasty

A posterior annuloplasty is performed to narrow the diameter of the tricuspid annulus. The coronary sinus marks the posterior and leftward extent of the annuloplasty, which is terminated there to avoid injury to the conduction bundle. Occasionally one or two additional mattress sutures are required to obliterate the posterior aspect of the annuloplasty repair in order to render the valve totally competent.

The completed repair allows the anterior tricuspid leaflet to function as a monocusp valve. The competence of the valve is tested by injecting saline under pressure into the right ventricle with a bulb syringe and large catheter.

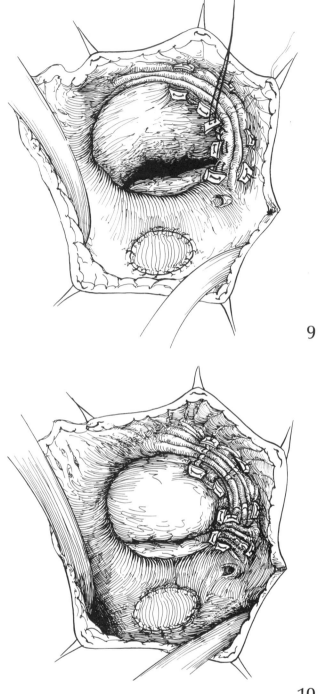

9

10

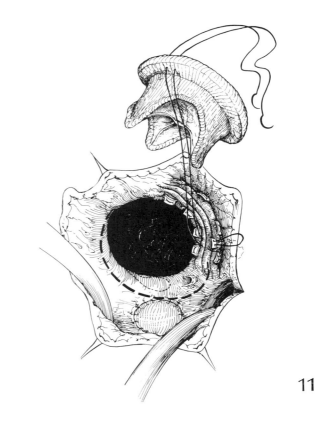

11

11 & 12

Tricuspid valve replacement

When valve replacement is required in Ebstein's anomaly because of significant abnormalities of the anterior leaflet suture of the prosthesis in the anatomical position at the level of the annulus is associated with a high incidence of complete heart block. The accepted technique today is to carry the suture line cephalad to the coronary sinus and atrioventricular node. This has reduced, but not completely eliminated, the occurrence of permanent complete heart block. We prefer to place interrupted felt-buttressed sutures through the tissues from the atrial to the ventricular side and then through the sewing ring of the prosthesis. The struts of the prosthesis are positioned so that they will not impinge on the bundle of His.

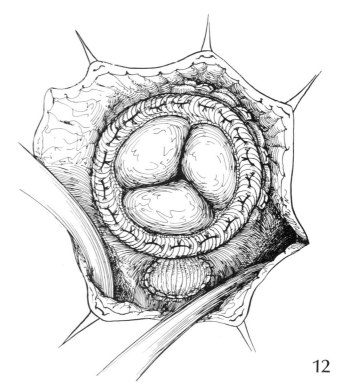

12

13

Closure of atriotomy and decannulation

The redundant portion of the right atrium is excised so that the final size of the right atrium is normal and the atriotomy is closed up to the appendage, leaving room for the caval cannulae, with a running mattress suture followed by an over-and-over suture. The cannulae are controlled with a tourniquet. After venous decannulation an exploring finger is introduced into the right atrium for direct palpation of the tricuspid valve in the beating heart. This allows a final assessment of tricuspid valve competence. Temporary pacemaker wires are attached to the right atrium and the right ventricle for postoperative monitoring of rhythm and for pacing in selected cases.

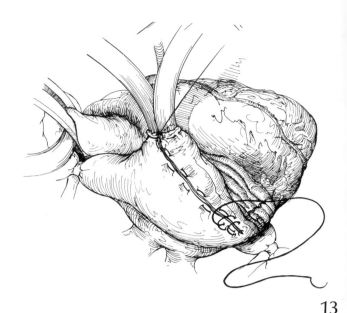

13

Postoperative

There is a known high incidence of atrial and ventricular arrhythmias in Ebstein's anomaly both before and after operation. Postoperative ventricular arrhythmias appear to be particularly lethal in patients who have massive cardiomegaly. We advise the administration of intravenous lidocaine prophylactically for the first 48 hours and then change to procainamide when oral intake is begun. We are uncertain how long the procainamide should be continued but currently advise its use for 3 months.

References

1. Shiina, A., Seward, J. B., Tajik, A. J., Hagler, D. J., Danielson, G. K. Two-dimensional echocardiographic-surgical correlation in Ebstein's anomaly: preoperative determination of patients requiring tricuspid valve plication vs replacement. Circulation 1983; 68: 534–544

2. Danielson, G. K. Ebstein's anomaly: editorial comments and personal observations. Annals of Thoracic Surgery 1982; 34: 396–400

3. Williams, D. B., Danielson, G. K., McGoon, D. C., Puga, F. J., Mair, D. D., Edwards, W. D. Porcine heterograft valve replacement in children. Journal of Thoracic and Cardiovascular Surgery 1982; 84: 446–450

4. Danielson, G. K., Maloney, J. D., Devloo, R. A. E. Surgical repair of Ebstein's anomaly. Mayo Clinic Proceedings 1979; 54: 185–192

5. Danielson, G. K., Fuster, V. Surgical repair of Ebstein's anomaly. Annals of Surgery 1982; 196: 499–504

6. Holmes, D. R., Jr, Osborn, M. J., Gersh, B., Maloney, J. D., Danielson, G. K. The Wolff-Parkinson-White syndrome. Mayo Clinic Proceedings 1982; 57: 345–350

Ventricular septal defect: surgical anatomy

Robert H. Anderson BSc, MD, MRCPath
Joseph Levy Professor of Paediatric Cardiac Morphology, Cardiothoracic Institute, Brompton Hospital, London, UK

Introduction

When repairing a ventricular septal defect the surgeon will, by examining its margins, take care not to damage unduly any valve leaflets which may form part of the borders. This danger can readily be assessed by simple inspection of the defect. However, when making the repair the surgeon will be equally concerned to avoid damage to the atrioventricular conduction tissue axis. In this respect direct observation is of less immediate value since the conduction tissue axis cannot be identified by gross inspection with complete confidence. In any event it is usually carried on the left ventricular aspect of the septum – that is, on the other side from the usual surgical approach. Furthermore, histological and anatomical studies[1-4] have shown that the conduction axis bears a different relationship to different types of ventricular septal defect. It is therefore of great help to the surgeon to categorize ventricular septal defects in such a way that the system employed conveys the vital information concerning the likely disposition of the conductive tissue axis. The system we advocate[5,6] provides this information. Before describing categorization of defects we shall briefly review the usual disposition of the atrioventricular conduction axis.

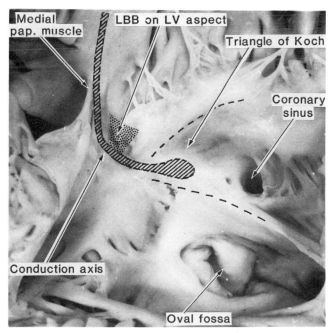

Figure 1. The course of the atrioventricular conduction tissue axis has been superimposed on a photograph of the normal heart taken as might be viewed by the surgeon via the right atrium. The major landmark to the most vulnerable segments is a line joining the medial papillary muscle and the apex of the triangle of Koch

1

Atrioventricular conduction axis

The atrial components of the axis, the compact atrioventricular node and its transitional cell zones, are contained exclusively within the triangle of Koch. The borders of this triangle are, on the atrial side, the passage of the commissure of the valves of the inferior vena cava and coronary sinus (tendon of Todaro) through the sinus septum to the central fibrous body (tricuspid-aortic-mitral continuity) and, on the ventricular side, the annular attachment of the septal leaflet of the tricuspid valve. The axis penetrates into the atrioventricular membranous septal component at the apex of the triangle and surfaces in the left ventricular outflow tract. Here it is usually sandwiched between the interventricular component of the membranous septum and the crest of the muscular septum. After a short non-branching segment it branches beneath the non-coronary–right-coronary commissure of the aortic valve. The fan-like left bundle branch (LBB) spreads out subendocardially on the septal surface while the cord-like right bundle branch burrows through the septum and surfaces beneath the medial papillary muscle on the right ventricular aspect of the septum.

Categorization of ventricular septal defects

There are basically three discrete types of ventricular septal defect[5]. Identifying the type of defect and knowing the disposition of the conduction tissue axis as described above enables the danger area of each defect to be predicted with a high degree of accuracy.

PERIMEMBRANOUS VENTRICULAR SEPTAL DEFECTS

2a & b

The commonest type of ventricular septal defect is found in the environs of the central fibrous body. Although usually called 'membranous' defects they do not exist because of absence of the membranous component of the ventricular septum. The atrioventricular component of the septum is always present in these defects and forms the direct posteroinferior margin of their edge. In this area the tricuspid valve is always in fibrous continuity with the aortic valve, usually also with the mitral valve. This can be seen best from the left ventricle (Figure 2a) but is also demonstrated by retraction of the septal leaflet of the tricuspid valve (Figure 2b). If the tricuspid valve is not in fibrous continuity with the aortic valve, then the defect cannot be perimembranous. In many cases, in addition to the atrioventricular component of the membranous septum forming the posterior margin of the defect, a remnant of the interventricular part of the membranous septum is also found hanging down like a fold from the central fibrous body. The defect is perimembranous, therefore, because it surrounds these persisting membranous septal structures as a consequence of deficiency of the muscular septum.

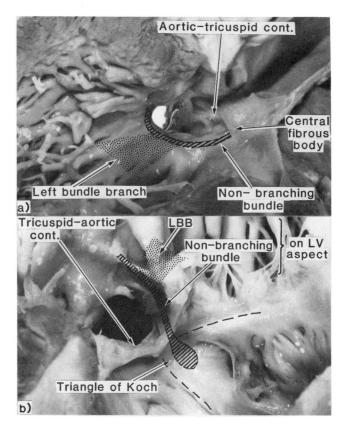

Figure 2. A perimembranous ventricular septal defect is defined as one in which the central fibrous body (tricuspid-aortic-mitral continuity) forms a direct border. This is best seen from the left ventricle (Figure 2a). This photograph is taken in anatomical orientation. It can also be seen (demonstrated in a different heart, as might be viewed by the surgeon via the right atrium) when the septal leaflet of the tricuspid valve is retracted (Figure 2b). The course of the conduction tissue axis is superimposed on the figures

3a–d

The precise morphology and extent of a perimembranous ventricular septal defect can then vary depending on which part of the muscular septum is deficient. This in turn affects the proximity of the conduction axis to the edge of the defect. As expected, since the atrioventricular component of the membranous septum forms the posteroinferior corner of the defect and the axis penetrates through this part of the septum, this is the most vulnerable area. When viewed by the surgeon through the tricuspid valve this area is to his right hand.

The initial ventricular segment of the axis (the nonbranching bundle) is closest to the rim of the defect when it extends predominantly into the inlet part of the septum. The defect is then shielded by the tricuspid valve septal leaflet and is caudal to the medial papillary muscle (*Figure 3a*). However, the important anatomical feature which proclaims the perimembranous nature of the defect is that its roof is formed by an area of aortic-mitral-tricuspid valve continuity. When the defect extends mostly into the trabecular septum it points towards the ventricular apex. The medial papillary muscle is then more towards the apex of the defect and the conduction axis tends to be away from the posterior rim of the defect, being carried on the left ventricular aspect (*Figure 3b*).

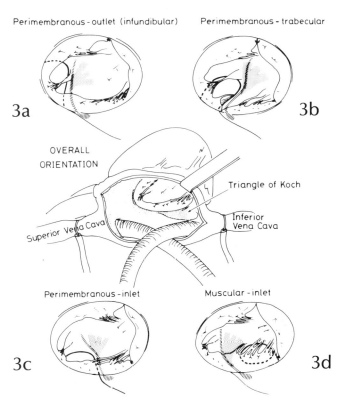

Figure 3. *An artist's impression of the likely disposition of the conduction tissue axis as would be viewed by the surgeon in perimembranous ventricular septal defects extending (a) into the inlet, (b) into the trabecular and (c) into the outlet parts of the septum. The disposition is significantly different when there is a muscular inlet defect (d).*

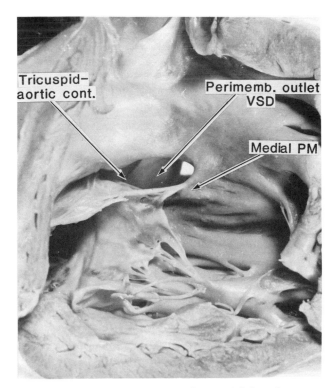

Figure 4. *A perimembranous ventricular septal defect photographed from the apex of the right ventricle and showing anatomical orientation*

4

The other variant in this type of defect is when the outlet septum is either deficient or malaligned. Then it is cephalad to the medial papillary muscle (PM) and the aortic-tricuspid continuity is much more obvious (*Figure 4*).

Often, particularly when the outlet septum is malaligned, the aortic valve overrides the septum. In this outlet type of perimembranous ventricular septal defect the conduction axis is usually carried well away from the septal crest, branching on the left ventricular aspect of the septum (*Figure 3c*).

In all these variants of perimembranous ventricular septal defect the major danger area is that part of the central fibrous body formed by the atrioventricular component of the membranous septum, since this is the site of penetration of the conduction tissue axis. When a remnant of the interventricular component of the membranous septum is present it usually overlies the nonbranching bundle. Although an obvious site for sutures, care must be taken if it is used for this purpose because of its close relation to the conduction axis. It is much safer to place sutures in this area in the tricuspid leaflet tissue since this never harbours the conduction tissue axis.

MUSCULAR VENTRICULAR SEPTAL DEFECTS

5a & b

Muscular ventricular septal defects differ from the perimembranous type in that their edges are exclusively formed by the muscular tissue of the septum and, unless there is a coexisting perimembranous ventricular septal defect, the membranous part of the septum is intact. The relation of muscular ventricular septal defects to the conduction axis depends upon their position within the septum (*Figure 5*).

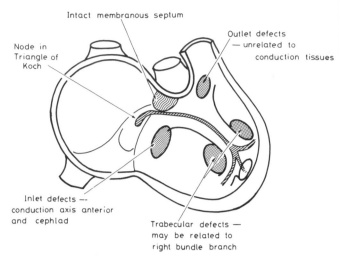

Figure 5. A diagram drawn in anatomical orientation showing how muscular ventricular septal defects in different parts of the septum have differing relationships to the conduction axis

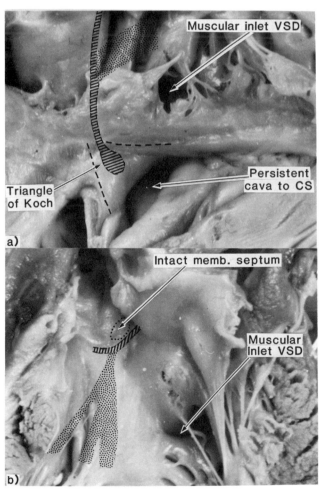

Figure 6. The salient features of a muscular inlet ventricular septal defect. Figure 6a shows how, as might be viewed by the surgeon from the right atrium, the defect is shielded by the tricuspid valve. The left ventricular aspect, seen in anatomical orientation, shows the site of the defect and its relationship to the conduction tissue axis (Figure 6b). The differentiation from a perimembranous ventricular septal defect is much harder when the muscular defect extends closer towards the central fibrous body

6a & b

The most significant type of defect is that within the inlet septum. When seen from the right atrium (a) the defect is shielded by the tricuspid valve septal leaflet (*Figure 6a*). When this leaflet is retracted it will be found that a muscular rim separates the defect from the annular attachment of the valve. Because of this the conduction axis passes superior and cephalad to the defect (*Figure 6b*). When viewed from the right atrium this is to the surgeon's left hand, exactly the opposite to that found with a perimembranous ventricular septal defect (*Figure 3a*).

Muscular ventricular septal defects in the apical part of the trabecular septum can either be large and single or small and multiple. The latter are often collectively called the 'Swiss cheese' type of defect. These defects are not immediately related to the proximal segments of the conduction axis but may have the bundle branches ramifying over their inferior margins[4].

7

The final type of muscular ventricular septal defect is that located within the outlet part of the septum. Its cardinal feature is fusion of the posterior limb of the septomarginal trabecula (TSM) with the ventriculoinfundibular fold (*Figure 7*). This produces the muscular posteroinferior margin of the defect behind which the membranous septum is intact. This muscular rim distances the conduction tissue axis from the septal crest. In these defects, therefore, it is safe to place sutures all round the muscular margins. The roof of these defects is the muscular outlet septum separating the aortic and pulmonary valves.

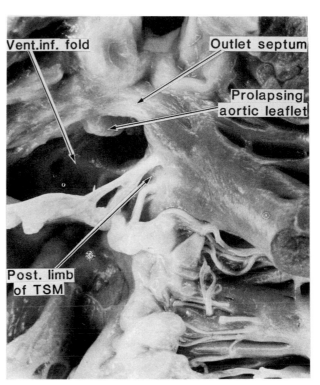

Figure 7. A muscular outlet ventricular septal defect seen from the apex of the right ventricle in anatomical orientation. Note the fusion of the posterior limb of the septomarginal trabecula with the ventriculoinfundibular fold. This produces the muscular posteroinferior rim (arrowed) which protects the conduction tissue axis. (Reproduced by kind permission of Dr J. R. Zuberbuhler, Children's Hospital of Pittsburgh, USA)

DOUBLY COMMITTED SUBARTERIAL VENTRICULAR SEPTAL DEFECTS

8a & b

These defects, often called supracristal defects, are closely related to the muscular outlet ventricular septal defect. Their characteristic feature, however, is complete absence of the muscular outlet septum. Because of this the aortic valve is in fibrous continuity with the pulmonary valve in their roof. The postero-inferior margin can vary in its morphology. When the septomarginal trabecular fuses with the ventriculo-infundibular fold then there is a safe muscular rim as in muscular outlet ventricular septal defects (*Figure 8a*). But when these muscular structures do not fuse there is aortic-tricuspid valvar continuity and then the defect is perimembranous (*Figure 8b*). The conduction axis is much more at risk in this latter variant. Because the outlet septum is lacking. The aortic valve leaflets show a tendency to prolapse, a feature shared with perimembranous outlet ventricular septal defects[7, 8].

'ATRIOVENTRICULAR CANAL' VENTRICULAR SEPTAL DEFECTS

Considerable confusion surrounds the so-called 'isolated ventricular septal defect of atrioventricular canal type'. There is no doubt that hearts with all the stigmata of an atrioventricular septal defect (*see* chapter on 'Atrioventricular septal defect', pp. 151–159) can have the valve leaflets attached to the atrial septum so that there is only the potential for interventricular shunting of blood. But then the valve is a typical five-leaflet common valve which guards a common atrioventricular junction, although the bridging leaflets may be connected so as to give separate right and left valve orifices. The defects more usually termed 'atrioventricular canal defects'[9, 10] are simply perimembranous defects with extensive deficiency of the inlet septum.

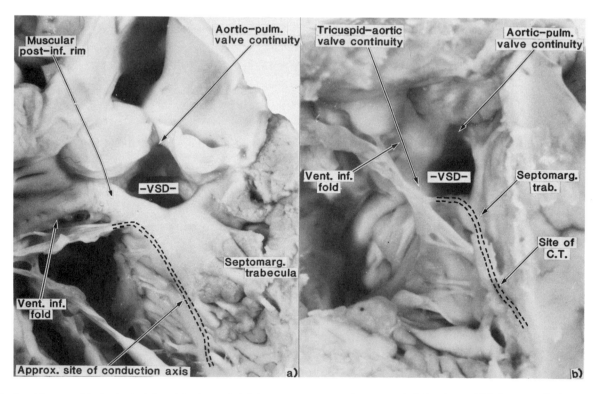

Figure 8. Doubly committed subarterial ventricular septal defects seen in anatomical orientation showing (a) the variant with a muscular posteroinferior rim and (b) the type which extends to become perimembranous

9

Alternatively these are defects associated with straddling of the tricuspid valve (TV). This variant (*Figure 9*) is not an atrioventricular septal defect but is of major surgical significance. This is because of the most unusual conduction tissue disposition[11]. The hallmark of the anomaly is the malalignment of the atrial and ventricular septa. The ventricular septum does not extend to the crux but is inserted into the posterior parietal margin of the atrioventricular junction. The 'regular' node in the triangle of Koch is then unable to make contact with the ventricular conduction axis carried on the ventricular septal crest. Instead an anomalous node is formed at the point where the malaligned septum reaches the posterior atrial wall[11].

MALALIGNMENT DEFECTS

The type of defect described above with straddling tricuspid valve can be regarded as an inlet malalignment ventricular septal defect. More usually it is the outlet septum which is malaligned. This occurs most frequently with deviation into the right ventricular outlet as seen in tetralogy of Fallot (see chapter on 'Tetralogy of Fallot', pp. 233–238). Equally significant is deviation into the left ventricular outlet portion because this finding is almost always a harbinger of either severe coarctation or interruption of the aortic arch[12, 13].

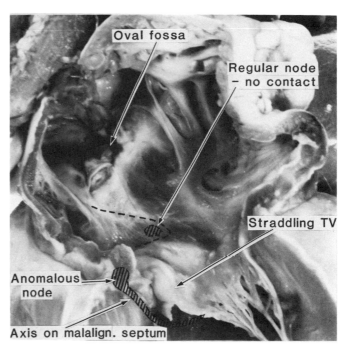

Figure 9. A heart with straddling tricuspid valve opened through the posterior aspect of the right atrioventricular junction and photographed in anatomical orientation. Note the malalignment between atrial and ventricular septum, the 'marooning' of the regular atrioventricular node and the anomalous position of the atrioventricular conduction axis

References

1. Truex, R. C., Bishof, J. K. Conduction system in human hearts with interventricular septal defects. Journal of Thoracic Surgery 1958; 35: 421–439

2. Lev, M. The architecture of the conduction system in congenital heart disease III. Ventricualar septal defect. Archives of Pathology 1960; 70: 529–549

3. Titus, J. L., Daugherty, G. W., Edwards, J. E. Anatomy of the atrioventricular conduction system in ventricular septal defect. Circulation 1963; 28: 72–81

4. Latham, R. A., Anderson, R. H. Anatomical variations in atrioventricular conduction system with reference to ventricular septal defects. British Heart Journal 1972; 34: 185–190

5. Soto, B., Becker, A. E., Moulaert, A. J., Lie, J. T., Anderson, R. H. Classification of ventricular septal defects. British Heart Journal 1980; 43: 332–343

6. Milo, S., Ho, S. Y., Wilkinson, J. L., Anderson, R. H. Surgical anatomy and atrioventricular conduction tissues of hearts with isolated ventricular septal defects. Journal of Thoracic and Cardiovascular Surgery 1980; 79: 244–255

7. Tatsuno, K., Konno, S., Sakakibara, S. Ventricular septal defect with aortic insufficiency: angiocardiographic aspects and a new classification. American Heart Journal 1973; 85: 13–21

8. Van Praagh, R., McNamara, J. J. Anatomic types of ventricular septal defect with aortic insufficiency. American Heart Journal 1968; 75: 604–619

9. Neufeld, H. N., Titus, J. L., Dushane, J. W., Burchell, H. B., Edwards, J. E. Isolated ventricular septal defect of the persistent common atrioventricular canal type. Circulation 1961; 23: 685–696

10. Titus, J. L., Rastelli, G. C. Anatomic features of persistent common atrioventricular canal. In: Feldt, R. H., ed. Atrioventricular Canal Defects. Philadelphia: W. B. Saunders, 1976: 1–35

11. Milo, S., et al. Straddling and overriding atrioventricular valves: morphology and classification. American Journal of Cardiology 1979; 44: 1122–1134

12. Van Praagh, R., Bernhard, W. F., Rosenthal, A., Parisi, L. F., Fyler, D. C. Interrupted aortic arch: surgical treatment. American Journal of Cardiology 1971; 27: 200–211

13. Freedom, R. M., Bain, H. H., Esplugas, E., Dische, R., Rowe, R. D. Ventricular septal defect in interruption of aortic arch. American Journal of Cardiology 1977; 39: 572–582

Ventricular septal defect

Bruce A. Reitz MD
Professor of Surgery, Cardiac Surgeon-in-Chief, The Johns Hopkins University School of Medicine, Baltimore, Maryland, USA

Introduction

Ventricular septal defect is the most common congenital cardiac anomaly. During surgical repair, either of a primary defect or one associated with other complex congenital abnormalities, precise placement of sutures is essential to avoid recurrence of the defect, development of conduction abnormalities or injury to adjacent valvular structures. Because of the depth and poor exposure of these defects usually only the surgeon and first assistant can see exactly where sutures should be placed. In addition to a brief review of the physiology of left-to-right shunts and the timing of operative closure this chapter reviews the pertinent anatomy and techniques which have been successfully employed for the repair of ventricular septal defects. These are most commonly of the membranous type, defects in the muscular and outlet septum being found much less frequently.

Anatomy and physiology

1

ANATOMICAL CLASSIFICATION

The various portions of the ventricular septum are illustrated here, defects being shown in the membranous area, the muscular trabecular septum and the outlet portion in the infundibulum. Not illustrated here or discussed in this chapter are the ventricular septal defects in the inlet portion of the septum associated with the tricuspid valve. These defects come within the broad category of atrioventricular canal defects and are dealt with separately elsewhere (see chapter on 'Atrioventricular septal defect', pp. 151–159).

FUNCTIONAL CLASSIFICATION

The haemodynamic consequences of defects in the ventricular septum can be quantified by means of cardiac catheterization. The size of the ventricular septal defect and the resulting left-to-right shunt, its effect on right ventricular and pulmonary artery pressures and, ultimately, its effect on pulmonary vascular resistance are important considerations for the timing of operative closure.

Functionally small defects produce left-to-right shunts of less than 1.5 to 1. Right ventricular and pulmonary artery pressures are normal and pulmonary vascular resistance is low. Moderate sized left-to-right shunts are in the range of 1.5–2 to 1, with right ventricular and pulmonary artery pressures between 0.25 and 0.5 of the left ventricular pressure. A moderate sized defect will have slightly increased pulmonary vascular resistance, but generally less than 5 units/m². Functionally large ventricular septal defects have left-to-right shunts of more than 2 to 1 and right ventricular pressure may be equal to left ventricular pressure. These defects usually result in increased pulmonary vascular resistance – for example 5–7 units/m² – or progressively increasing resistance to more than 7 units/m².

INDICATIONS FOR CLOSURE

Closure of the ventricular defect is recommended at any age if it is large and medical treatment is unable to control symptoms of congestive heart failure. Failure of medical therapy may also be manifested by poor growth and development. Even with successful medical treatment unrestrictive large ventricular septal defects should be

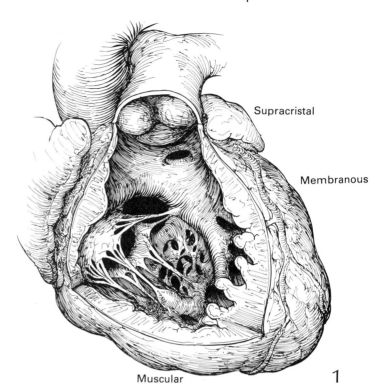

Supracristal

Membranous

Muscular   1

closed by 6–12 months of age to prevent development of pulmonary vascular disease. If the ventricular septal defect is restrictive or there is some element of pulmonary stenosis the timing can be variable and may be elective. In these instances one should take into account the actual degree of pulmonary vascular resistance, symptoms of cardiac failure, the growth and size of the patient, the position of the ventricular septal defect and the presence of associated lesions.

For ventricular septal defects of moderate size and haemodynamic significance, observation for several years is reasonable to see whether spontaneous closure will occur. Perhaps as many as 50 per cent of patients with this type of defect will show spontaneous closure by 2 or 3 years of age, after which closure is unlikely and surgery should be considered.

For small ventricular septal defects of negligible haemodynamic significance closure is not generally recommended except for potential prophylaxis against bacterial endocarditis. For patients with a large ventricular septal defect who have established elevated pulmonary vascular resistance of more than 10 units/m² and if the shunt is less than 1.5 to 1, surgical closure is not recommended. These patients should undergo catheterization with the administration of 100 per cent oxygen or tolazoline in order to see whether a larger shunt will develop in association with a measurable fall in pulmonary vascular resistance. If there is a large dynamic component the defect should be closed.

The operations

The operation for closure of ventricular septal defect is performed through a standard median sternotomy incision with cardiopulmonary bypass and moderate hypothermia. In the case of children less than 4 kg in weight cardiopulmonary bypass is combined with hypothermia and circulatory arrest for improved operative exposure.

Cardiopulmonary bypass is instituted with central cannulation, an arterial return catheter being inserted in the high ascending aorta and two caval catheters in the right atrium to both venae cavae. A vent is placed through the left atrial appendage in order to remove return resulting from the bronchial circulation.

The defects themselves can be approached through an incision in the right atrium or in the infundibulum of the right ventricle. The principles of closure of the defects are the same regardless of the approach and the anatomical landmarks are similar. Most defects are viewed first through a small incision in the right atrium to assess exposure from this approach. This also allows examination of the interatrial septum for the presence of a patent foramen ovale.

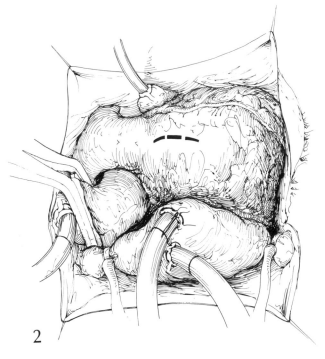

2

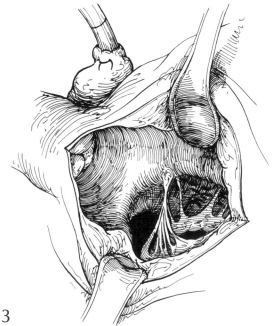

3

DEFECTS OF THE MEMBRANOUS SEPTUM

Location of the defect: right ventricular approach

2 & 3

When the right ventricle is opened with a vertical incision in the infundibulum the defect is located posterior to the crista of the right ventricle and beneath the attachments of the septal leaflet of the tricuspid valve to the right side of the ventricular septum.

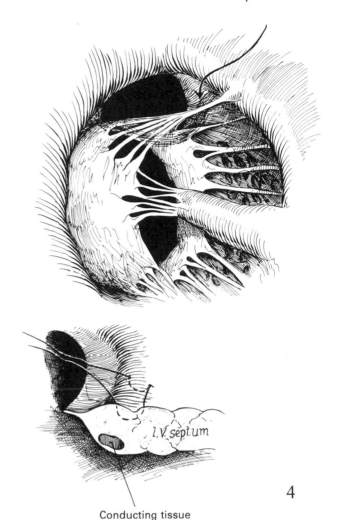

4

Conducting tissue

4

Of crucial importance to avoiding interference with the conduction mechanism is an understanding of the position of the bundle of His and its branches. The bundle arises from the atrioventricular node, penetrates the central fibrous body near the posteroinferior rim of the ventricular septal defect and courses on the left ventricular aspect of the rim of the defect. The bundle branches have usually spread on to the ventricular septum posterior to the base of the papillary muscle of the conus. The bundle lies towards the left ventricular aspect of the rim of the septum so that suture placement should be confined to the right ventricular side of the septum and several millimetres from the actual rim of the defect.

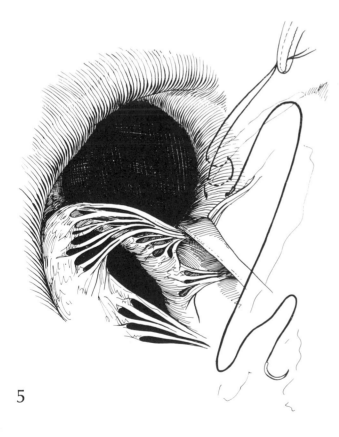

5

Placement of sutures

5

Suture placement begins with interrupted mattress sutures. These sutures may either be bolstered with Teflon felt pledgets or used by themselves, as illustrated. A braided Teflon-Dacron material of 4/0 size is preferred, with a small half-circle needle. The sutures are begun at the area of insertion of the papillary muscle to the septal leaflet and are continued in a clockwise fashion.

6

As the sutures are brought towards the area of transition between the ventricular septum and the annulus of the tricuspid valve particular care must be taken. This is the most difficult area of closure of the ventricular septal defect because of the complex relationship of the tricuspid valve and the septum. Usually, at the transition between the muscle of the septum and the valve annulus, sutures are brought from within the right atrium through the fibrous portion of the tricuspid valve and into the interior of the ventricle in order to buttress them with the fibrous annular tissue. Approximately three sutures can be placed in this fashion at that part of the circumference of the defect where the tricuspid valve annulus is in continuity. One should be extremely careful that these sutures are in the annular fibrous tissue and not in the thinner tissue of the septal leaflet, through which they may be pulled to leave a potential shunt from left ventricle to right atrium.

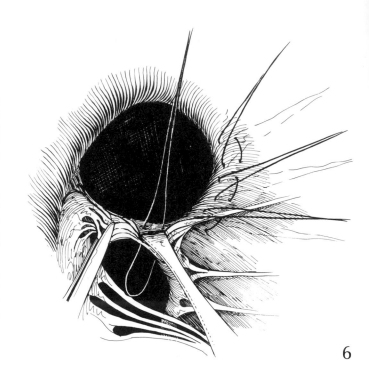

6

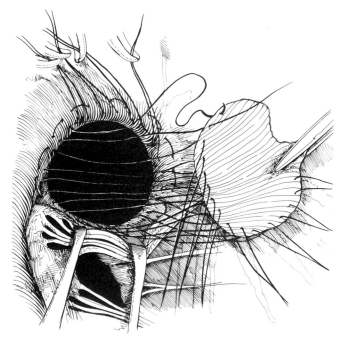

7

7

After the region of the tricuspid valve annulus has been traversed, sutures are once again placed from within the ventricle as the margin of the defect is formed by the muscle band of the crista supraventricularis. The non-coronary cusp of the aortic valve may be damaged if sutures are placed too deeply along the right lateral side of the crista.

The usual perimembranous defect may require from 10 to 14 interrupted mattress sutures in order to rim its margin effectively. These defects are closed with an approximately sized patch giving several millimetres of margin for placement of the suture material. We favour a loosely woven Dacron material for the patch since it can be rapidly endothelialized and incorporated with the host endothelium.

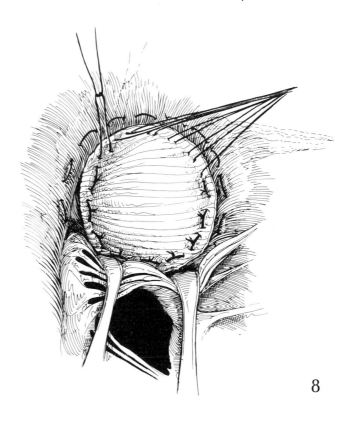

8

8

The mattress sutures are placed through the patch material, which is lowered into place and the sutures tied and cut.

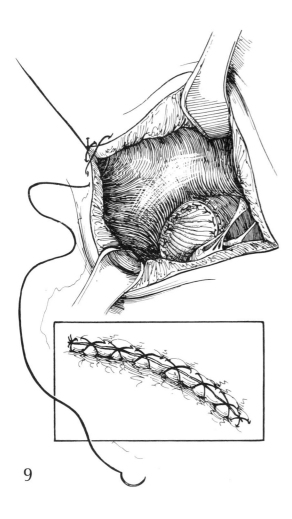

9

The ventriculotomy is then closed with monofilament polypropylene material in two running layers.

9

Right atrial approach

10

When the defect is approached through the right atrium and the exposure is satisfactory the defect may be closed without the need for a right ventriculotomy. Significant hypertrophy of the parietal extension of the crista supraventricularis may seriously compromise the exposure of the superior margin of the defect, making this approach too difficult.

Cannulation for cardiopulmonary bypass is facilitated by cannulation of the vena cava nearer the caval orifices, as shown, a vent again being placed in the left atrial appendage. An oblique incision is made in the right atrium and the tricuspid valve exposed.

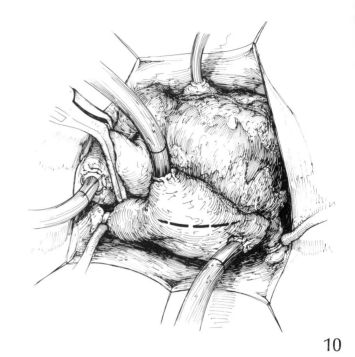

10

11

The interatrial septum is examined for the presence of a patent foramen ovale. A retractor is placed through the tricuspid valve annulus to expose perimembranous defects behind the septal leaflet of the tricuspid valve. In order to improve exposure of the defect further the attachment of the septal leaflet is occasionally incised several millimetres from the tricuspid valve annulus. This improves exposure, particularly along the margin of the defect formed by the crista supraventricularis.

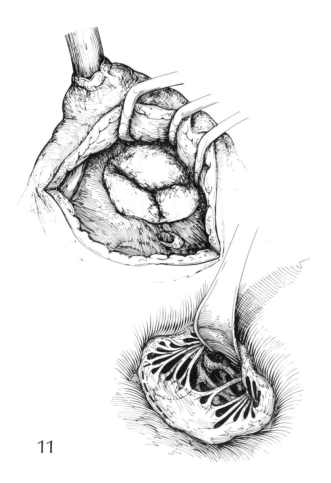

11

12, 13 & 14

Interrupted mattress sutures of 4/0 braided material are begun along the inferior margin of the defect in the same manner as are sutures placed through a right ventriculotomy. Along the rim of the defect in juxtaposition to the tricuspid valve ring sutures can again be placed from the right atrial side through to the ventricular side of the defect. After placement of all sutures around the rim of the defect they are passed through an appropriately sized patch, which is lowered into place and the sutures tied and cut. Finally any incision in the septal leaflet is repaired with 5/0 polypropylene material in two running layers.

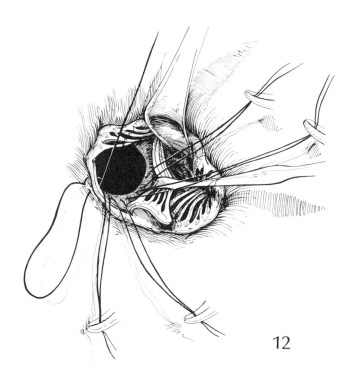

12

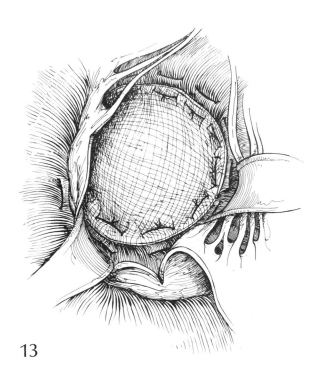

13

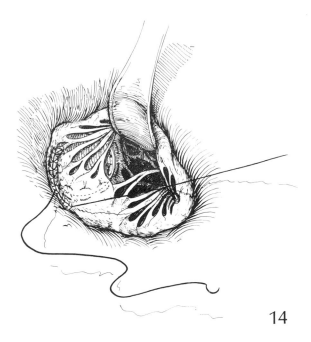

14

DEFECTS OF THE MUSCULAR SEPTUM

Although rare, haemodynamically important defects in the muscular or trabecular portions of the ventricular septum are among the most challenging defects to close. Each patient is individually assessed, depending upon the angiographic findings. The major problem is the trabecular nature of the right ventricular side of the septum which may obscure the primary or principal component of the defect. This type of pattern may lead one to close off several exit points of the defect within the right ventricle but to leave residual defects around other trabecular portions of the septum.

Exposure of the defect

Exposure may be through the right atrium, through a ventriculotomy in the body of the right ventricle or through a fish-mouth incision parallel to the distal portion of the left anterior descending coronary branch in the body of the left ventricle. This last incision may be required in unusual cases, giving a better view of the defect on the left ventricular side of the septum, where it is smoother and without the trabeculae of the right side.

15

In the patient illustrated here standard cannulation for cardiopulmonary bypass has been employed. A left atrial vent is used to instil blood into the left ventricle to look for the point of egress across the ventricular septum.

16 & 17

In order to delineate the defect further, muscle bands overlying the trabecular septum are excised in order to make the defect a larger and more single opening which can be more accurately closed.

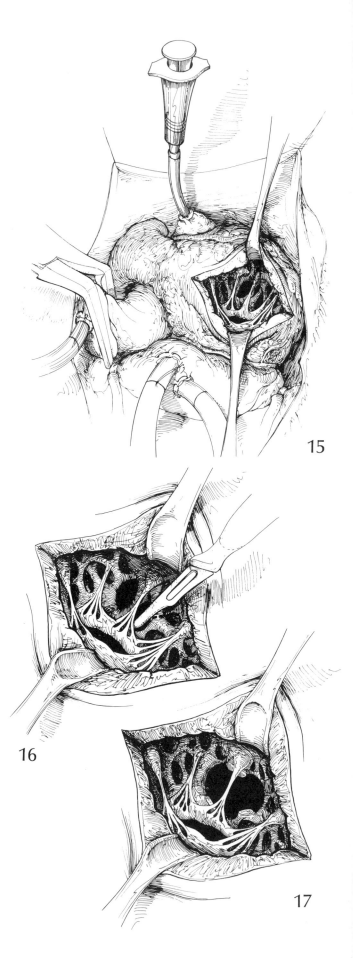

15

16

17

18, 19 & 20

Closure of the defect

Once the margins of the defect have been delineated interrupted mattress sutures with Teflon felt bolsters can be placed around the rim of the defect. Between eight and 12 sutures are generally required and these are passed through an appropriately sized Dacron patch which is lowered into place and the sutures tied and cut.

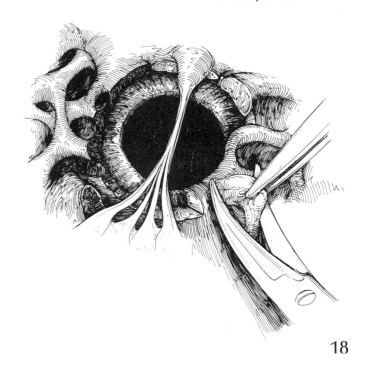

18

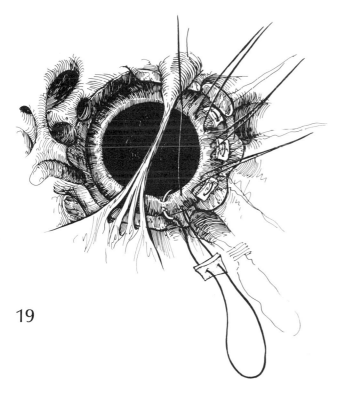

19

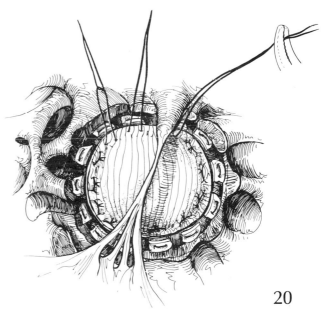

20

SUPRACRISTAL VENTRICULAR SEPTAL DEFECTS

21

Frequently defects below the pulmonary valve in the supracristal portion of the outlet septum can be approached through a vertical incision in the pulmonary artery. Because of the left-to-right shunt just below the pulmonary valve the pulmonary artery itself is enlarged and exposure is generally quite adequate. These defects frequently have a fibrous border from the turbulence of high flow.

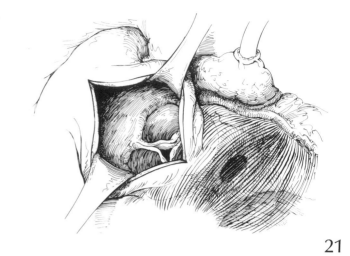

21

22

The defect exposed through the valve annulus is rimmed with interrupted mattress sutures of braided material and an appropriately sized patch inserted. The opening in the pulmonary artery is closed with 4/0 or 5/0 monofilament polypropylene material in two layers. If the incision in the pulmonary artery is inadequate for exposure a small vertical incision in the infundibulum of the right ventricle can be employed as previously described for membranous ventricular septal defects.

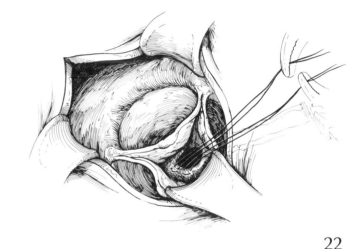

22

Results

Operative repair of ventricular septal defects is generally quite satisfying. Operative mortality is low for patients with typical defects and related to the age of the patient, the presence of associated defects and the degree of pulmonary vascular disease. Mortality is higher for patients under 1 year of age and for those with elevated pulmonary vascular resistance. In these patients mortality may range from 5 to 10 per cent.

For patients over 1 year of age and with normal pulmonary vascular resistance operative mortality is usually no higher than 1 per cent. Similarly the incidence of permanent complete heart block should be less than 1 per cent, and when this occurs it should be treated by insertion of a permanent pacemaker. Recurrent ventricu-

lar septal defect may be seen in up to 10 per cent of patients. This is particularly true in patients with defects of the muscular septum. In most instances the degree of residual shunt is low and generally less than 1.5 to 1. This degree of residual shunting does not require reoperation, but the patient must continue to take prophylactic antibiotics when indicated.

Patients with successful closure of ventricular septal defects in childhood show long-term actuarial survival near normal, the late results depending upon the degree of right ventricular dysfunction induced by the presence of the defect, the ventriculotomy or tricuspid valve deformity induced by repair.

Tetralogy of Fallot: surgical anatomy

Robert H. Anderson   BSc, MD, MRCPath
Joseph Levy Professor of Paediatric Cardiac Morphology, Cardiothoracic Institute, Brompton Hospital, London, UK

Introduction

It is well recognized that the four morphological features of tetralogy of Fallot are subpulmonary outlet obstruction, a ventricular septal defect, overriding of the aorta and right ventricular hypertrophy. It is also well known that the hypertrophy is a haemodynamic consequence of the three anatomical lesions and that the common feature underscoring the other three is anterior and cephalad deviation of the outlet (or infundibular) septum[1]. However, although nearly all examples of tetralogy have this anterior deviation (the exception being the rare variant with absence of the outlet septum), there is considerable variability within the overall group such that Baffes et al.[2] and Lev and Eckner[3] commented that no two hearts were ever exactly the same. While this is certainly true, it is possible to describe the variability in terms of variations in the morphology of the ventricular septal defect, variation in the degree of overriding of the aorta, different patterns of subpulmonary outflow tract obstruction and the presence or absence of associated lesions[4].

Ventricular septal defect

Since the essence of tetralogy is anterior deviation of the outlet septum the ventricular septal defect (VSD) is basically a malalignment defect between the outlet and trabecular parts of the septum, the latter being reinforced by the septomarginal trabecula. In the normal heart the outlet septum is inserted between the limbs of the septomarginal trabecula, the junction being overlaid laterally by the prominent ventriculoinfundibular fold interposed between the pulmonary and tricuspid valves (*Figure 1a*).

In tetralogy these three building-blocks of the subpulmonary outflow tract are sprung apart (*Figure 1b*) and the variability encountered in septal defect morphology depends upon their interrelationships. Most frequently

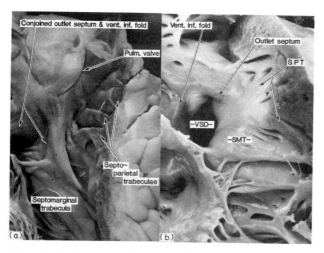

Figure 1 (a). The outlet of the normal right ventricle showing how the 'crista', composed of the conjoined outlet septum and ventriculoinfundibular fold is inserted between the limbs of the septomarginal trabecula (SMT). Note the series of septoparietal trabeculae (SPT) in anterior position. (b). In tetralogy the outlet septum is deviated anteriorly so as to be attached cephalad to the septomarginal trabecula (Anatomical orientation.). (a is reproduced by courtesy of Professor A. E. Becker and b by courtesy of Dr J. R. Zuberbuhler)

(in about four-fifths of cases) the defect is perimembranous, having the area of tricuspid-aortic-mitral continuity as part of its border (*Figure 2*). The defect extends to become perimembranous because there is discontinuity between the ventriculoinfundibular fold, separating tricuspid and aortic valves, and the posterior limb of the septomarginal trabecula.

The fibrous area between these two muscular structures is the major danger area for damage to the conduction tissue axis. This is because the axis penetrates through the area of aortic-tricuspid continuity to reach the subaortic outflow tract. Here it is usually carried on the left ventricular aspect of the septum some distance below the septal crest, and only the right bundle branch penetrates through the septum to become subendocardial in relation to the medial papillary muscle. Rarely, however, the branching bundle may be located directly astride the septum (*Figure 3*). It is then at risk from sutures placed directly in the muscular margin of the defect[5-7].

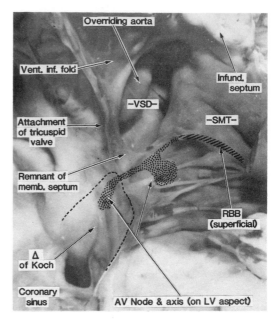

Figure 2. A dissection removing the septal leaflet of the tricuspid valve to demonstrate the nature of a perimembranous defect (VSD) and the usual course of the conduction tissue axis (Anatomical orientation.). RBB = right bundle branch

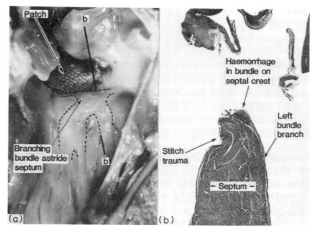

Figure 3. A rare variant of tetralogy with a perimembranous defect in which the conduction axis was astride the septal crest. A stitch through the crest, seen from the left ventricular aspect in (a) produced complete heart block with haemorrhage in the conduction axis (b). The plane of the section is indicated in (a) (Anatomical orientation.)

Apart from this posteroinferior margin of the defect up to the medial papillary muscle the remainder of the defect margins are free from conduction tissue. However, it should be remembered that deep stitches placed through the ventriculoinfundibular fold may damage the branches of the right coronary artery running through the inner heart curvature.

The most significant variation in morphology of the septal defect is found when the posterior limb of the septomarginal trabecula fuses with the ventriculoinfundibular fold (*Figure 4*). This produces a completely muscular rim to the defect and protects the conduction tissue axis. With this variant it is safe to place stitches along the muscular margin all round the defect, provided of course that the stitches are relatively superficial. This defect, with a muscular posteroinferior rim, is found in about one-fifth of cases.

The rarest type of defect among Caucasian populations, although much more frequent in the Far East[8] and in

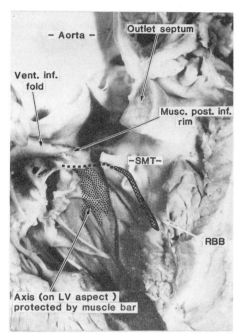

Figure 4. A defect in tetralogy which has a muscular posteroinferior rim produced by fusion of the posterior limb of the septomarginal trabecula with the ventriculoinfundibular fold. Note how the muscle bar protects the conduction axis (Anatomical orientation.)

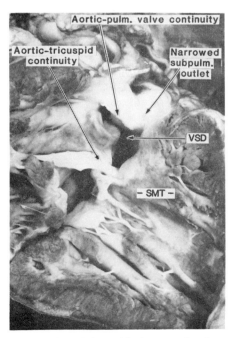

Figure 5. Rare defect with absence of outlet septum (VSD) roofed by conjoined rings of aortic and pulmonary valves (aortic-pulm. valve continuty)

Argentina[9], is that with absence of the outlet septum. The defect is therefore doubly committed and subarterial, being roofed by the conjoined rings of the aortic and pulmonary valves (Figure 5). Such defects may have a muscular posteroinferior rim which will protect the conduction axis or else may extend to become perimembranous, when the axis will be at risk in the posteroinferior corner of the defect.

Overriding of the aorta

There is a complete spectrum to be found in tetralogy between the aorta being almost exclusively connected to the left ventricle (ventriculoarterial concordance) and it being almost completely connected to the right ventricle (double-outlet right ventricle). There is some confusion as to whether double-outlet right ventricle can coexist with tetralogy of Fallot. Stances adopted in this respect devolve entirely upon the definition used for double-outlet right ventricle. If a bilateral infundibulum is considered the *sine qua non* of double outlet[10], then only very rarely will cases be seen with both double outlet and tetralogy[7]. However, if double outlet is defined in terms of a ventriculoarterial connection, i.e. more than half of both great arterial valves connected to the same ventricle, then the combination of tetralogy and double outlet will be found with considerably greater frequency[4]. The important point when using this latter definition is to know that tetralogy and double outlet coexist. It is not to be used as an excuse to weed out from surgical series those cases which may have poor outcome and group them along with double outlets. All tetralogies should be analysed together, taking cognizance of the ventriculoarterial connection if considered appropriate. Tetralogy with double outlet is a different lesion from the common variant of double outlet without subpulmonary stenosis but with subaortic ventricular septal defect.

Subpulmonary stenosis

The basis of subpulmonary stenosis is the anterior and cephalad deviation of the outlet septum. Added to this obstruction may be several other structures which compromise the subpulmonary outflow tract. In order to describe adequately these lesions, particularly with regard to their surgical resection, it is vital to have clear descriptive terms.

Description has been confused previously by indiscriminate use of the terms 'crista', 'septal band' and 'parietal band'. In the setting of tetralogy the term 'crista' was used by Kjellberg and his colleagues[11] to describe the body of the outlet septum. They then described the angiocardiographic appearances of the septal and parietal attachments of their crista (i.e. the septal and parietal attachments of the outlet septum). They termed these attachments the septal and parietal bands. However, earlier anatomists, starting with Keith in 1909[12], had described parietal and septal extensions of the crista of the normal heart, the septal band of Keith then being the extensive septal trabeculation which continued as the moderator band.

Tandler, in 1913[13], had called this the septomarginal trabecula. When Van Praagh[14] adopted the concept of Keith[12] for congenitally malformed hearts he used the term 'parietal band' to describe the entire outlet septum and its attachments, while the septomarginal trabecula of Tandler was called the 'septal band'. However, when surgeons refer to excision of the 'septal band', they refer in most cases to 'septal band' as defined by Kjellberg *el al*[11]. This is quite different from the 'septal band' of Keith and Van Praagh. This already complex situation has been further complicated by description of the muscle bundle between the aortic and tricuspid valves in hearts with tetralogy and muscular ventricular septal defect as 'parietal band 2'[15]. Because of all these various and different uses of the bands of the 'crista', we prefer to account for the subpulmonary outflow tract in tetralogy by using simple descriptive terms. Thus we describe the outlet septum and its parietal and septal attachments.

The parietal attachment is often an extensive structure which fuses with the ventriculoinfundibular fold, the latter structure being defined as the muscle bar separating the aortic and tricuspid valves. The extensive septal trabeculation which bifurcates at the base into limbs which clasp the septal defect and which extends towards the apex, where it gives rise to the moderator band and the anterior papillary muscle, is called the septomarginal trabecula.

Finally, cognizance is taken of the series of muscle bundles which, in the normal heart, spring from the anterior margin of the septomarginal trabecula and fan out into the parietal wall of the ventricle (*see Figure 1a*). These are termed the septoparietal trabeculae[16].

When these terms are used it is then an easy matter to describe the different types of subpulmonary obstruction found in tetralogy. Almost without exception the septal attachment of the outlet septum is either fused with or attached cephalad to the anterior limb of the septomarginal trabecula (*Figure 6*). This produces the major obstruction, often exacerbated by hypertrophy of the septum. Usually the outlet septum itself is of good size, although it may be hypoplastic or even absent, as in cases with doubly committed subarterial defects (*Figure 6*). It is incorrect to say that in tetralogy the subpulmonary infundibulum is too narrow, too short and too shallow[17]. It is certainly too narrow, but measurements and comparison with the normal heart show that in general the length of the outlet septum is greater than normal[1]. Hypertrophy of the parietal extension of the outlet septum is almost always present. This is the structure usually resected by the surgeon. On the septal side the septal attachment may be enlarged, but usually the obstruction here is produced by hypertrophied septoparietal trabeculae, and these can be completely removed at surgery. It is hypertrophy of these septoparietal trabeculae, particularly if one prominent bundle is enlarged, that is spoken of as a 'high take-off' of the moderator band and regarded as one form of double-chamber right ventricle. In fact, anatomical and electrophysiological studies[18, 19] have shown that the band is not a displaced moderator band but is one of the series of septoparietal trabeculae.

The other type of double-chamber right ventricle can also coexist with tetralogy and contribute to subpulmonary obstruction – namely the formation of an apical shelf from the septomarginal trabecula. Only in this circumstance, and in those rare instances when the body of the septomarginal trabecula is particularly hypertrophied, is it

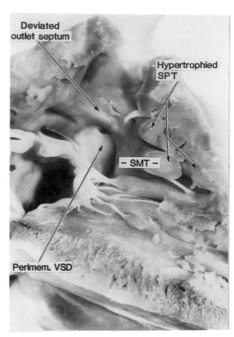

Figure 6. The opened sub-pulmonary outflow tract showing the cephalad deviation of the outlet septum and hypertrophied septoparietal trabeculae (Anatomical orientation.)

necessary to resect this structure. All the obstructive lesions described thus far have been located at subpulmonary level. Usually in tetralogy there is further obstruction at valve level, often in the setting of a bileaflet pulmonary valve. In those cases with doubly committed subarterial defects the major obstruction is at the level of the hypoplastic pulmonary valve ring. Although rare, it should also be remembered that subaortic obstruction can be found with tetralogy, usually due to a subvalvar fibrous shelf. Frequently this will not become manifest before closure of the ventricular septal defect.

Associated malformations

Any lesion which is morphologically possible must be anticipated to coexist with tetralogy. Some are sufficiently frequent to warrant special mention. The commonest variant of pulmonary atresia with ventricular septal defect is simply tetralogy of Fallot with muscular subpulmonary atresia. The major variation in this lesion then depends upon the source and pattern of pulmonary arterial supply[20].

In all types of tetralogy the presence of a second muscular inlet ventricular septal defect is highly significant. This is because the combination of perimembranous and muscular inlet defects leaves only a small muscle bundle through which the conduction axis must run (*Figure 7*). It may be difficult to repair these defects using separate patches without damage to the axis, particularly in infancy. The better option may be to repair the defects with a single all-embracing patch[21]. The combination of tetralogy with atrioventricular septal defect or with straddling tricuspid valve is also formidable for the surgeon.

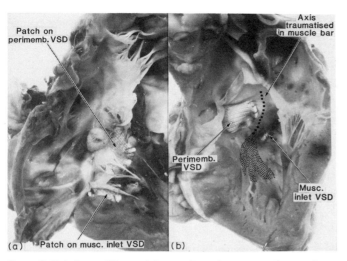

Patch on perimemb. VSD

Axis traumatised in muscle bar

Perimemb. VSD

Musc. inlet VSD

(a) Patch on musc. inlet VSD (b)

Figure 7. Tetralogy with coexisting perimembranous and muscular inlet defects viewed (a) from the right ventricular inlet and (b) from the left ventricle. The conduction axis runs through the narrow muscle bar between the defects and was traumatized during the placement of two separate patches (Anatomical orientation.)

Spontaneous closure of the ventricular septal defect occurs on occasion in tetralogy and is usually due to reduplication of tissue from the anteroseptal commissure of the tricuspid valve. This may present either as tissue tags or as a discrete hammock-like leaflet[22]. So-called 'absence' of the pulmonary valve with dilatation of the proximal pulmonary arteries is a bad complication. Found with absence of the duct, a recent study[23] showed that the abnormality in severe cases extended into the lung, with grossly abnormal branching patterns of the segmental pulmonary arteries. Also found in combination with tetralogy is so-called 'absence' of one pulmonary artery. As with the 'absent' valve (which is usually grossly hypoplastic rather than absent), in most cases the artery is not absent. It is discontinuous from the pulmonary trunk and supplied by a duct which may have closed. The whole arrangement of the pulmonary arterial pathways is of major significance in the surgical treatment of tetralogy. The elegant studies of the University of Alabama group have shown how all the necessary information concerning these pathways may best be assembled and utilized[24–26].

References

1. Becker, A. E., Connor, M., Anderson, R. H. Tetralogy of Fallot; a morphometric and geometric study. American Journal of Cardiology 1975; 35: 402–412

2. Baffes, T. G. Johnson, F. R., Potts, W. J., Gibson, S. Anatomic variations in the tetralogy of Fallot. American Heart Journal 1953; 46: 657–669

3. Lev, M., Eckner, F. A. O. The pathologic anatomy of tetralogy of Fallot and its variants. Diseases of the Chest 1964; 45: 251–261

4. Anderson, R. H., Allwork, S. P., Ho, S. Y., Lenox, C. C., Zuberbuhler, J. R. Surgical anatomy of tetralogy of Fallot. Journal of Thoracic and Cardiac Surgery 1981; 81: 887–896

5. Titus, J. L., Daugherty, G. W., Edwards, J. E. Anatomy of the atrioventricular conduction system in ventricular septal defect. Circulation 1963; 28: 72–81

6. Anderson, R. H., Monro, J. L., Ho, S. Y., Smith, A., Deverall, P. B. Les voies de conduction auriculo-ventriculaires dans le tetralogie de Fallot. Coeur 1977; 8: 793–807

7. Dickinson, D. F., Wilkinson, J. L., Smith, A., Hamilton, D. I., Anderson, R. H. Variations in the morphology of the ventricular septal defect and disposition of the atrioventricular conduction tissues in tetralogy of Fallot. The Thoracic and Cardiovascular Surgeon 1982; 5: 243–249

8. Ando, M. Subpulmonary ventricular septal defect with pulmonary stenosis. Circulation 1974; 50: 412

9. Neirotti, R., Galindez, E., Kreutzer, G., Coronel, A. R., Pedrini, M., Becu, L. Tetralogy of Fallot with sub-pulmonary ventricular septal defect. Annals of Thoracic Surgery 1978; 25: 51–56

10. Baron, M. G. Radiologic notes in cardiology: angiographic differentiation between tetralogy of Fallot and double outlet right ventricle: relationship of the mitral and aortic valves. Circulation 1971; 43: 451–455

11. Kjellberg, S. R., Mannheimer, E., Rudhe, U., Jonsson, B. Diagnosis of Congenital Heart Disease. 2nd ed. Chicago: Year Book Medical Publishers, 1959

12. Keith, A. Malformations of the heart. Lancet 1909; 2: 433–435

13. Tandler, J. Anatomie des Herzens. Jena: G. Fischer, 1913.

14. Van Praagh, R. What is the Taussig-Bing malformation? Circulation 1968; 38: 445–449

15. Rosenquist, G. C., Sweeney, L. J., Stemple, D. R., Christianson, S. D., Rowe, R. D. Ventricular septal defect in tetralogy of Fallot. American Journal of Cardiology 1973; 31: 749–754

16. Goor, D. A., Lillihei, C. W. Congenital malformations of the heart. New York: Grune and Stratton, 1975: 1–37

17. Van Praagh, R., Van Praagh, S., Nebesar, R. A., Muster, A. J., Sinha, S. N., Paul, M. H. Tetralogy of Fallot: underdevelopment of the pulmonary infundibulum and its sequelae. American Journal of Cardiology 1970; 26: 25–33

18. Gallucci, V., Scalia, D., Thiene, K. G., Mazzucco, A., Valfre, C. Double-chambered right ventricle: surgical experience and anatomical considerations. Journal of Thoracic and Cardiovascular Surgeon 1980; 28: 13–17

19. Byrum, C. J., Dick II, M., Behrendt, D. M., Hees, P. Rosenthal, A. Excitation of the double chamber right ventricle: electrophysiologic and anatomic correlation. American Journal of Cardiology 1982; 49: 1254–1258

20. Thiene, G., Anderson, R. H. Pulmonary atresia with ventricular septal defect: anatomy. In: Anderson, R. H. Macartney, F. J., Shinebourne, E. A., Tynan, M., eds. Paediatric Cardiology, Vol 5. Edinburgh: Churchill Livingstone, 1983: 80–101

21. Bharati, S., Lev, M., Kirklin, J. W. Cardiac Surgery and the Conduction System. New York. Wiley, 1983: 28–29

22. Faggian, G., Frescura, C., Thiene G., Bortolotti, U., Mazzucco, A., Anderson, R. H. Accessory tricuspid valve tissue causing obstruction of the ventricular septal defect in tetralogy of Fallot. British Heart Journal 1983; 49: 324–327

23. Rabinovitch, M., Grady, S., David, I. *et al.*, Compression of intrapulmonary bronchi by abnormally branching pulmonary arteries associated with absent pulmonary valves. American Journal of Cardiology 1982; 50: 804–813

24. Blackstone, E. H., Kirklin, J. W., Bertranou, E. G., Labrosse, C. J., Soto, B., Bargeron L. M., Jr. Preoperative prediction from cineagiograms of post-repair right ventricular pressure in tetralogy of Fallot. Journal of Thoracic and Cardiovascular Surgery 1979; 78: 542–552

25. Blackstone, E. H., Kirklin, J. W. Pacifico, A. D. Decision-making in repair of tetralogy of Fallot based on intraoperative measurements of pulmonary arterial outflow tract. Journal of Thoracic and Cardiovascular Surgery 1979; 77: 526–532

26. Kirklin, J. W., Blackstone, E. H., Pacifico, A. D., Brown, R. N., Bargeron, L. M., Jr. Routine primary repair vs two stage repair of tetralogy of Fallot. Circulation 1979; 60: 373–386

Tetralogy of Fallot: surgical treatment

Christopher Lincoln FRCS
Consultant Cardiothoracic Surgeon, Brompton Hospital, London;
Senior Lecturer in Paediatric Surgery, London University, London, UK

Introduction

Complete intracardiac repair would appear to be the operation of choice for patients with Fallot's tetralogy. However, although almost three decades have passed since this complex cardiac anomaly was first corrected the criteria for performing a preliminary palliative systemic artery–pulmonary artery shunt operation remain controversial. This procedure may be more suitable when the anatomy is unfavourable to corrective operation in patients below the age of one year and even in some above this age. Experience with complete correction at all ages suggests that an operative mortality of between 5 and 15 per cent can be achieved. The debate of two-stages versus one-stage corrective surgery for Fallot's tetralogy continues.

Preoperative

Preoperative investigation

Patients require investigation by cross-sectional echocardiography followed by cardiac catheterization and angiography. This should demonstrate:

1. Concordant atrioventricular relationships;
2. Right ventricular infundibular stenosis, pulmonary valve stenosis and/or pulmonary artery hypoplasia;

3. A single high ventricular septal defect or multiple ventricular septal defects;
4. The aorta overriding the right ventricle but placed above both ventricles.
5. The presence or absence of a persistent ductus arteriosus; and
6. A functioning systemic-pulmonary artery shunt (when previously palliated).

Previous cardiac surgery

A patient with tetralogy of Fallot presenting for correction may have undergone a previous palliative systemic artery–pulmonary artery shunt that must first be closed. This shunt may have been:

1. Right or left Blalock-Taussig subclavian artery–pulmonary artery anastomosis;
2. Waterston ascending aorta–right pulmonary artery anastomosis;
3. Pott's left pulmonary artery–descending aorta anastomosis;
4. Modified Blalock-Taussig polytetrafluroethylene (PTFE) prosthetic shunt.

The technique of closing the shunt differs in each case; it may be difficult and influence the subsequent corrective operation.

Anatomy

Summary of cardiac morphology

The aortic valve is dextroposed in relation to the origin of the tricuspid and mitral valves. The mitral valve is in fibrous continuity with the aortic valve.

The pulmonary valve is abnormally posterior, inferior and leftwards in its position. The valve commissures may or may not be fused and the pulmonary valve annulus is usually hypoplastic.

The infundibular septum is rotated and anteriorly deviated, forming a prominent supraventricular muscle mass. The septal and parietal insertions of the infundibular septum form two prominent muscle bundles on either side of the ventricular septal defect. The medial papillary muscle is a key structure in identifying the right lateral and inferior border of the ventricular septal defect.

The atrioventricular bundle of His and Kent lies in the inferior posterior wall of the ventricular septal defect on the left side beneath the crest of the ventricular septum. The left bundle branch (LBB) runs an endocardial course on the left side of the septum. The right bundle branch (RBB) passes through the inferior aspect of the defect and proceeds on the trabecula septomarginalis.

Surgical anatomy

1

Hypertrophied septal and parietal insertions of the infundibular septum encroach upon the outflow tract of the right ventricle and, in addition, the infundibular septum projects anterosuperiorly, thus raising the floor of the cavity of the right ventricular infundibulum and causing further obstruction to the outflow of blood. Therefore varying degrees of hypertrophy of these muscle bars will cause differences in the severity of the condition. Pulmonary valve stenosis may or may not be added to the above morphological abnormalities.

Damage to the LBB of the conducting tissue can be avoided by placing sutures to the right side of the interventricular septum 2–4 mm back from the crest of the interventricular septum and the rim of the ventricular septal defect. These sutures, however, invariably cause RBB block since it is difficult to avoid damage to this structure.

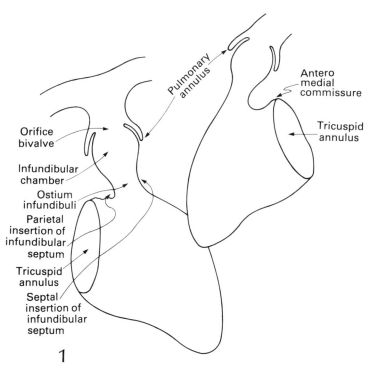

1

The operations

Extracorporeal circulation

The technique of extracorporeal circulation varies according to the surgeon's choice. Conventional cardiopulmonary bypass with moderate hypothermia and cold cardioplegia for myocardial preservation is preferred in children and adults. Below the weight of 8 kg surface cooling to 26°C is carried out, after which the heart and body are further cooled on bypass to 15°C when the circulation is stopped. After the correction cardiopulmonary bypass is reinstituted and, with a further limited period of extracorporeal circulation, the patient is rewarmed.

2

The incision

A median sternotomy incision offers good exposure for intracardiac repair as well as for closure of previously constructed shunts. The thymus, if large, is subtotally excised.

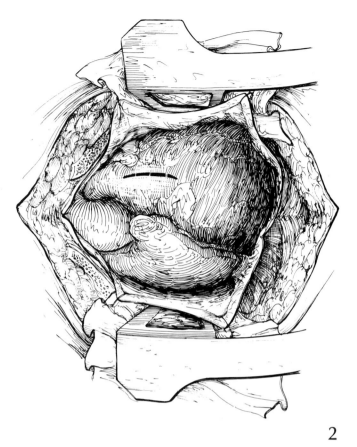

2

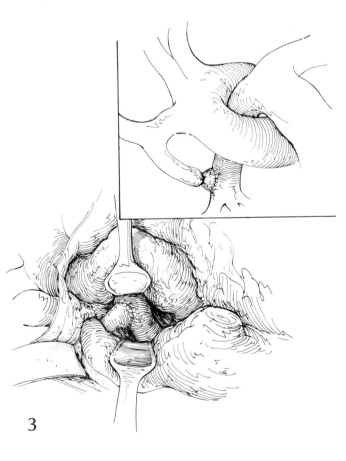

3

CLOSURE OF PREVIOUSLY CONSTRUCTED SHUNTS

Right Blalock-Taussig anastomosis (left aortic arch)

3

The subclavian artery is dissected out just proximal to its anastomosis to the right pulmonary artery and is located by retracting the superior vena cava laterally and to the right.

4

This shunt is easily closed by means of large tantalum clips. The use of these clips obviates the need to dissect round the posterior aspect of the subclavian artery, which on occasion can be difficult.

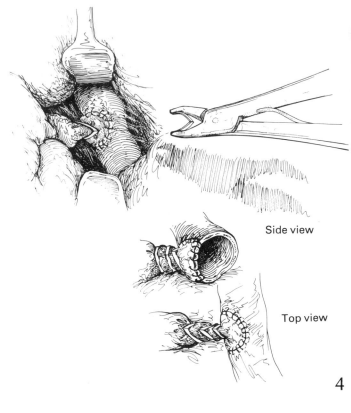

Side view

Top view

4

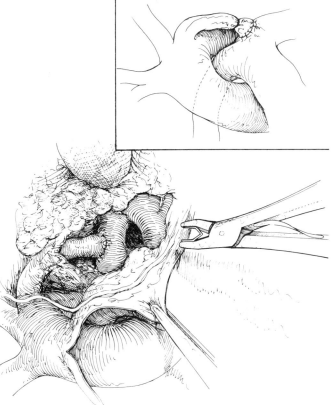

5

5

Left Blalock-Taussig anastomosis (left aortic arch)

Closure of this shunt in patients with a left aortic arch may be more difficult. The region of the anastomosis is exposed by careful extrapleural dissection and retraction of the cut edge of the pericardium to the right. This has the effect of retracting the hilum into the field of vision. The phrenic nerve must be identified to avoid injury. Final exposure of the subclavian artery before its anastomosis to the left pulmonary artery is carried out in a dissection which can be very posterior. As previously, the use of two metal clips is preferred to the classical ligature to close off the anastomosis.

6a & b

Waterston anastomosis

This can cause distortion of the right pulmonary artery. It is therefore necessary to detach completely the right pulmonary artery from the aorta and it is frequently necessary to enlarge the pulmonary artery at the site of the previous stoma. Closure of this anastomosis is carried out by first clamping the aorta proximal to the aortic perfusion cannula and cephalad to the Waterston anastomosis immediately on establishing cardiopulmonary bypass; failure to do this will result in overperfusion of the lungs. (Note that for clarity the aortic cross-clamp has been omitted from *Illustration 6a*). Further exposure can be obtained by rotating the ascending aorta by attaching haemostat forceps to its adventitia. The right pulmonary artery is completely detached from the back of the ascending aorta and the defect in the ascending aorta is then repaired by horizontal mattress sutures followed by a running suture (*b*). The aortic cross-clamp can now be removed. The right pulmonary artery is carefully inspected for any narrowing at the site of the previous stoma. It is almost always necessary to enlarge the right pulmonary artery in this area by means of a patch of pericardium or prosthetic material.

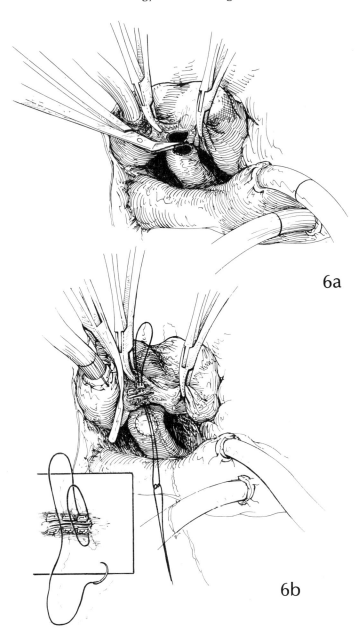

6a

6b

Pott's anastomosis

The ascending aorta, the right femoral artery and the venae cavae are prepared for cannulation before dissection of the left pulmonary artery. The left upper pulmonary artery is dissected as far as possible into the hilum up to and beyond the entry of the shunt, which is located by palpation of the thrill. The left pulmonary vein will be seen crossing the pulmonary artery in the area of the previously constructed shunt. It is important that dissection of the left pulmonary artery should allow obliteration of the shunt by the finger as this will be needed on institution of cardiopulmonary bypass to control the run-off.

Cardiopulmonary bypass is then instituted by means of femoral artery cannulation and superior and inferior caval cannulation, sequentially obliterating the shunt by finger pressure. Whole-body hypothermia is then achieved to 20°C. Perfusion is reduced to a 'trickle' such that there is a positive but minimal pressure of blood into the aorta. The left pulmonary artery is then opened in its long axis and the shunt stoma identified, This is not always easily apparent but can be positively identified by momentarily stopping the bypass and then reinstituting it, when blood will be seen flowing through the stoma. Excessive blood flow through the stoma can be occluded by means of a Foley or Fogarty catheter passed prograde through the

shunt into the aorta. The sutures for closure can then be placed more easily. During this procedure a head-down posture is adopted to guard against the possibility of air embolism to the cerebral vessels.

Modified Blalock-Taussig PTFE prosthetic shunt

The exposure of this shunt is similar to that used for the classical Blalock shunt but the dissection is easier since the position of the anastomosis is easily palpated and the prosthetic tube is surrounded by a pseudoadventitia with a grey coloration. Closure is effected by means either of a circumferential ligature or of the tantalum liga clip.

INTRACARDIAC REPAIR

Successful intracardiac repair of tetralogy of Fallot must fulfil the following criteria:

1. The ventricular septal defect or defects must be securely closed.
2. Right ventricular outflow tract obstruction must be relieved at ventricular, pulmonary valve and pulmonary artery levels.
3. The myocardium must be preserved from prolonged ischaemia and damage to coronary arteries must be avoided.

TRANSVENTRICULAR REPAIR

7

The intracardiac repair is performed through a vertical right ventriculotomy, avoiding branches of the coronary arteries.

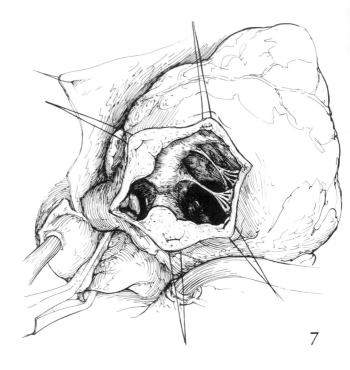

7

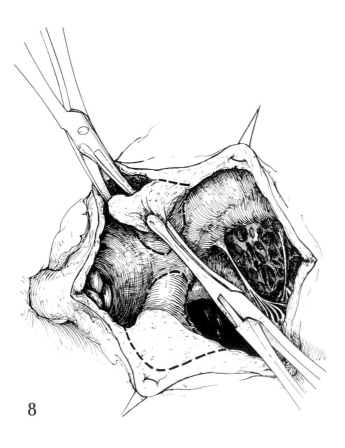

8

8

The region of infundibular stenosis is treated by excision of the hypertrophied parietal and septal insertions of the infundibular septum and mobilization of the free wall of the right ventricle. Between 40 and 60 per cent of patients will require outflow tract reconstruction to enlarge this channel.

Closure of ventricular septal defect

9

The ventricular septal defect is closed with a Teflon patch sutured in place with interrupted or continuous monofilament sutures. This is facilitated by a dry field in a non-beating heart and by knowledge of the pathways of the conducting bundle. The initial suture is placed at the base of the medial papillary muscle. Gentle traction on this suture delivers the base of the septal leaflet of the tricuspid valve into the operative field, where further sutures are placed.

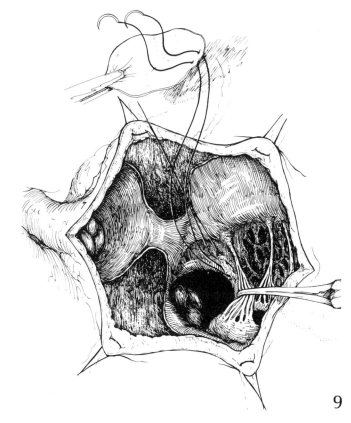

9

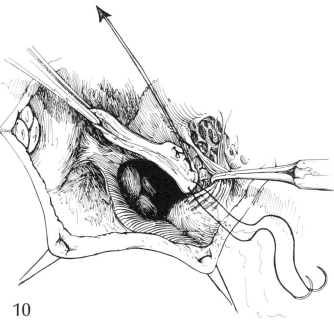

10

10

Continuing traction on the sutures as placed *pari passu* delivers the periphery of the ventricular septal defect into the field of vision, thus facilitating placement of the sutures throughout its circumference.

11

In the region of the muscular septum the sutures are placed well back from the margin of the defect until the region of the septal leaflet of the tricuspid valve is reached. (The medial papillary muscle is shown detached for illustrative purposes.) A metal probe is used to detect any small defects between sutures and if present they are closed with additional sutures. Sutures are placed around the superior edge of the defect, avoiding distortion of the aortic valve cusps.

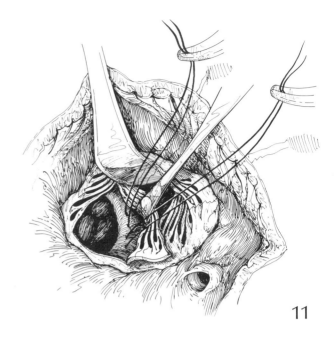

11

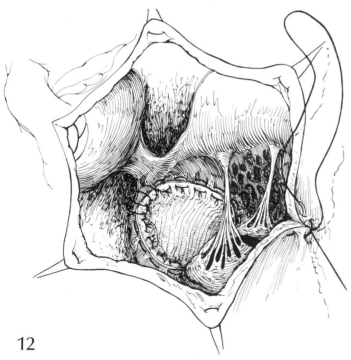

12

12

The ventriculotomy incision is closed with continuous 4/0 sutures. The left atrium, which has been vented either through the patent foramen if present or an incision made in the fossa ovalis, is then closed.

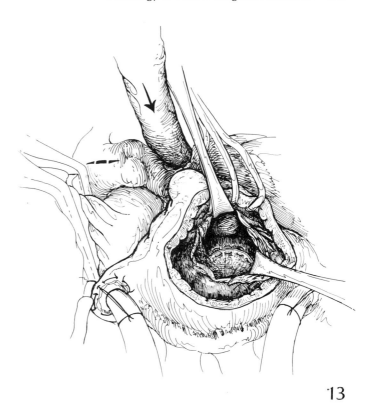

TRANSATRIAL—PULMONARY ARTERY CORRECTION

Closure of ventricular septal defect

Transatrial, transtricuspid valve closure of the ventricular septal defect in tetralogy of Fallot is technically similar to that of closure of an isolated perimembranous or subaortic ventricular septal defect. Careful traction on the inferior aspect of the ventricular septal defect and retraction of the septal leaflet of the tricuspid valve give excellent exposure for securing the patch for closure. Since the superior part of the circumference of the patch is attached to the anterior third of the aortic annulus the patch is considerably smaller than that placed through the transventricular route.

`13`

Resection of infundibular muscle

13 & 14

With the index finger it is possible to invaginate the free wall of the infundibulum of the right ventricle, bringing into view obstructing muscle bundles in the right ventricular outflow tract. These are identified and excised.

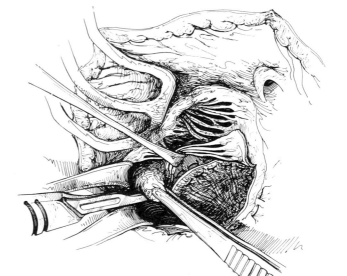

14

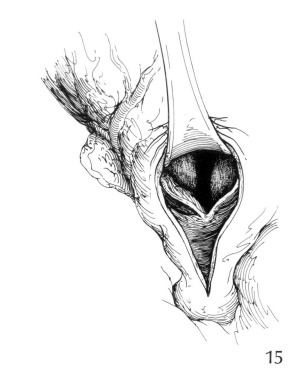

15 & 16

Two stay sutures are then placed on the infundibulum of the right ventricle and gentle retraction caudad exposes the area of the infundibulum and pulmonary artery in the field of surgery. A vertical incision is then made in the long axis of the pulmonary valve annulus and a pulmonary valvotomy performed. Exposure of the infundibulum through the pulmonary valve annulus is effected with appropriate retractors, and if the surgeon stands directly at the head of the patient (where the anaesthetist usually stands), having appropriately towelled up the area, a direct view is obtained of the infundibulum, when the septal and parietal insertions of the infundibular septum can be located and excised together with the anterior free wall of the right ventricle.

The incision in the pulmonary artery is closed and the operation continues as with the transventricular approach.

When correction has been completed care is taken to remove air from the left atrium, left ventricle and right ventricle. The heart is then allowed to beat and eject blood. Extracorporeal circulation is then gradually discontinued. After discontinuation of cardiopulmonary bypass the heart is allowed to support the circulation for approximately 5 minutes, when peak pressures in the left and right ventricles are measured. If the right ventricular peak pressure is 75 per cent of the left ventricular pressure or less relief of the right ventricular tract obstruction is considered adequate.

15

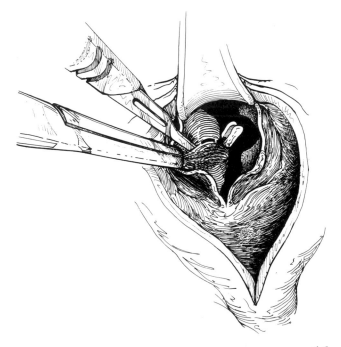

16

RIGHT VENTRICULAR OUTFLOW TRACT OBSTRUCTION

In approximately 40–60 per cent of patients it will be necessary to widen the right ventricular outflow tract. This may be due to: (a) extreme anterior position of the infundibular septum, (b) a small pulmonary valve annulus or (c) stenosis or hypoplasia of the main pulmonary artery and/or the right and left pulmonary arteries. In such cases, the initial longitudinal incision in the infundibulum of the right ventricle can now be extended as necessary.

17

Even when the infundibular septum and the septal and parietal insertions have been reduced in size by excision, when the heart is tonic the infundibular septum sometimes protrudes into the outflow part of the right ventricular infundibulum. If the pulmonary valve annulus and the main pulmonary artery are of satisfactory size a gusset of pericardium is inlaid in the ventriculotomy site, thus increasing the volume of the right ventricular infundibulum. The gusset does not cross the pulmonary valve annulus.

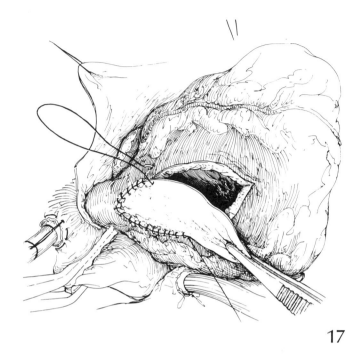

17

18 & 19

When extreme anterior position of the infundibular septum coexists with hypoplasia of the pulmonary valve annulus and main pulmonary artery however, the whole of the right ventricular outflow tract must be enlarged by a gusset of pericardium.

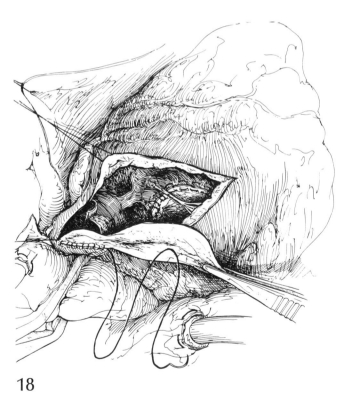

18

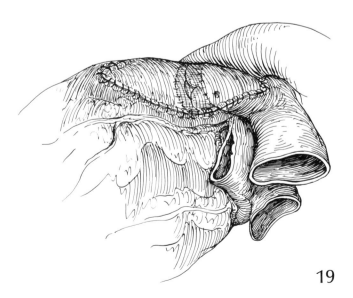

19

20

Alternatively, a section of an aortic valve homograft tailored into a monocusp can be used, thus preserving a competent pulmonary valve mechanism. Evidence to suggest that pulmonary valve regurgitation has a deleterious effect on right ventricular function is emerging in the long-term follow-up of these patients.

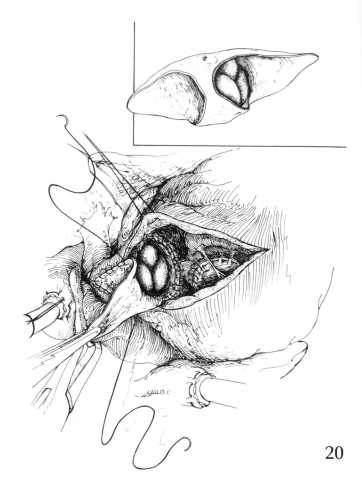

20

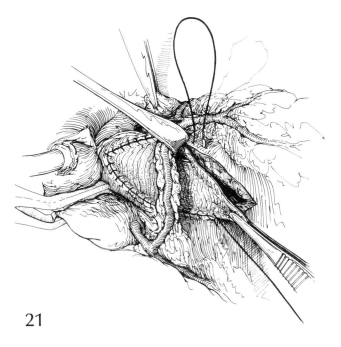

21

CORONARY ARTERY ANOMALIES IN TETRALOGY OF FALLOT

In 2 per cent of patients the left anterior descending coronary artery may either arise from or receive a major contribution from the right coronary artery. In such cases the anomalous coronary artery crosses the right ventricular outflow tract, obstruction of which cannot be relieved by extending the longitudinal incision in the right ventricular infundibulum because of the danger of damaging this critical coronary artery.

21

One method of overcoming this difficulty is to dissect the coronary artery free of the myocardium and to place a gusset behind the vessel.

22

An alternative method is to bypass the anomalous coronary artery by the insertion of a right ventricular-pulmonary artery external tube conduit containing a valve.

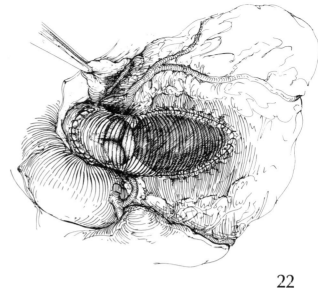

22

Further reading

Anderson, R. H., Wilkinson, J. L., Arnold, R., Becker, A. E., Lubkiewicz, K. Morphogenesis of bulboventricular malformations. II: Observations on malformed hearts. British Heart Journal 1974; 36: 948–970

Edmonds, L. H., Saxena, N. C., Friedman, S., Rashkind, W. J., Dodd, P. F. Transatrial resection of the obstructed right ventricular infundibulum. Circulation 1976; 54: 117–122

Kirklin, J. W., Karp, R. The tetralogy of Fallot from a surgical viewpoint. Philadelphia: Saunders, 1970

Pulmonary atresia: surgical anatomy

Robert H. Anderson BSc, MD, MRCPath
Joseph Levy Professor of Paediatric Cardiac Morphology, Cardiothoracic Institute, Brompton Hospital, London, UK

Introduction

1a, b & c & 2a & b

Pulmonary atresia is a congenital aberration in which there is complete blockage of the pathway from the pulmonary trunk to the ventricular mass. The atresia can take one of three forms, valvar or 'membranous' atresia, muscular atresia, and solitary arterial trunk, the differences being of considerable surgical significance.

The first variety (1a) exists when the cavity of the trunk is in potential communication with a ventricular cavity but the two are separated by an imperforate valve membrane (2a). The imperforate valve can be found in the setting of a bileaflet or trileaflet valve (rarely a quadrileaflet valve).

The second type is found when the base of the pulmonary trunk is itself connected to the ventricular mass (1b) but the cavity of the trunk is separated from the ventricular cavity by the musculature of the heart wall because of obliteration of the cavity of the ventricular outlet component. When this type is examined from the ventricular side there is usually evidence of the outlet component, but the roof is made of muscle tissue with no evidence of valve leaflet formation. When examined from the arterial aspect the absence of valve tissue is confirmed. Instead, the pulmonary sinuses radiate in triplicate fashion from a central fusion point (2b).

These two more common forms must be distinguished from the more rare third type, in which the pulmonary trunk itself is totally lacking, not even being represented by a fibrous cord (1c). This third type, which is found only in the presence of a ventricular septal defect, is usually described as solitary aortic trunk with pulmonary atresia. However, sometimes the entire intrapericardial pulmonary arteries may be lacking and the pulmonary blood supply is via systemic-pulmonary collateral arteries. In either circumstance there is no anatomical means of determining whether the arterial trunk leaving the base of the heart is a truncus arteriosus ('Truncus Type IV') or a solitary aorta. A strong case can therefore be made for describing this third arrangement simply as a solitary arterial trunk[1, 2] and then describing the pattern of pulmonary blood supply.

Indeed, in all hearts with pulmonary atresia, while the nature of the atresia itself is of significance, it is the arrangement of the rest of the heart which is paramount,

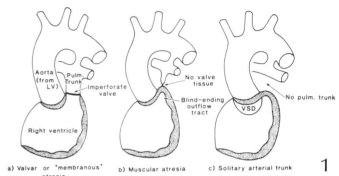

Figure 1. The different types of pulmonary atresia. The valvar and muscular types can be found with or without a ventricular septal defect. Solitary arterial trunk is found only in the presence of a ventricular septal defect

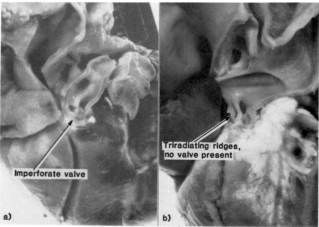

Figure 2. Illustrations of (a) valvar and (b) muscular pulmonary atresia as seen from the atretic trunk. Both are illustrated in the setting of an intact septum, but can exist with a ventricular septal defect. it is rare, however, to see triradiating sinuses (compare 2b with Figure 5) (reproduced from Anderson et al; Paediatric Cardiology Volume 5; p. 240; 1983; by kind permission of Churchill Livingstone, Edinburgh)

notably the chamber connections, the integrity of the ventricular septum and the pattern of the pulmonary arterial supply. Of these it is septal integrity which most clearly divides pulmonary atresia into clinical entities, although rarely there may be overlap between the two when a defect is closed by fibrous tissue tags[1, 3].

Pulmonary atresia with intact ventricular septum

To all intents and purposes this combination can be regarded as hypoplasia of the right heart. Almost always it exists with atrioventricular and ventriculoarterial concordance. Rarely it is found with atrioventricular and ventriculoarterial discordance ('corrected transposition'). In these latter settings it is the left ventricle which is hypoplastic[4, 5].

In the usual form it is the morphology of the right ventricle and its valves which determines the surgical options. Throughout the group the atrial septum is widely patent and the pulmonary arteries are usually confluent, of good dimensions and fed via a duct[6]. Rarely cases may be encountered with systemic-pulmonary collateral arteries. The options for surgical management are determined by the size and architecture of the right ventricle[7].

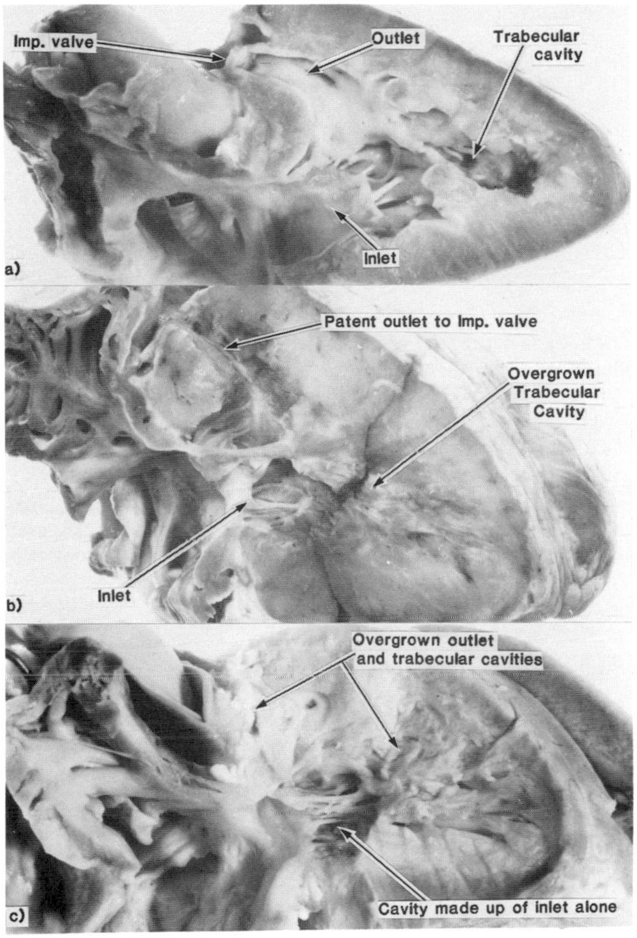

Figure 3. The different degrees of hypertrophy of the ventricular wall which produce corresponding hypoplasia of the ventricular cavity in pulmonary atresia with intact ventricular septum. (a) shows minimal hypoplasia of all components of the ventricular cavity with valvar atresia; (b) shows obliteration of the outlet with hypertrophy of the wall of the trabecular component, while the gross hypertrophy shown in (c) obliterates virtually all the cavity except for the inlet component (reproduced from Anderson et al: Paediatric Cardiology Volume 5; p. 237; 1983; by kind permission of Churchill Livingstone, Edinburgh)

3a, b & c

The most favourable cases have minimal hypoplasia of all ventricular components but with representation of all parts of the ventricular cavity. Thus the outlet portion is patent, but egress to the pulmonary trunk is blocked by an imperforate valve membrane (a). The trabecular component is well formed and sometimes may achieve normal dimensions. The tricuspid valve is usually dysplastic and often shows minimal features of Ebstein's malformation[6, 8] but is of good dimensions. These hearts are ideal for immediate valvotomy and direct restoration of ventriculoarterial continuity.

In an intermediate group of hearts (b) the outlet portion is present but has a muscular roof – i.e., there is no pulmonary valve tissue and the pulmonary trunk commences above the triradiating sinuses. The trabecular component is much less well formed, being obliterated by hypertrophy of its walls. The tricuspid valve is smaller in this group and it is questionable whether ventriculoarterial continuity can be adequately achieved at operation.

In the third and worst group (c) there is obliteration of the outlet component and overgrowth of the cavity of the trabecular component by gross muscular hypertrophy. The ventricular cavity is represented only by the tiny inlet component containing a small dysplastic tricuspid valve. It is hard to see how such a hypertrophied ventricle with such a hypoplastic cavity could ever be incorporated into the circulation.

4

A fourth discrete variant has an equally dismal surgical prognosis. In this type the atresia is usually of membranous type but in combination with severe Ebstein's malformation. The tricuspid orifice is hugely dilated along with the cavity of the right ventricle (RV), and the wall of the ventricle is paper-thin. These cases should not be confused with Uhl's anomaly, in which the pulmonary valve is normal. They present with 'wall-to-wall' heart in the neonatal period. As with the 'olive stone' variant, it is difficult to imagine how the right ventricle could ever serve a useful haemodynamic purpose.

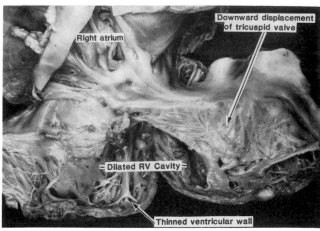

Figure 4. The discrete type of pulmonary atresia with intact ventricular septum associated with severe Ebstein's malformation and gross thinning and dilation of the wall of the entire right ventricle (Reproduced from Anderson et al: Paediatric Cardiology Volume 5; p. 235; 1983; by kind permission of Churchill Livingstone, Edinburgh)

Pulmonary atresia with ventricular septal defect

In pulmonary atresia with intact ventricular septum the feature of most surgical significance is the ventricular morphology, the pulmonary anatomy being relatively constant. In contrast, when there is a ventricular septal defect it is primarily the arrangement of the arterial tree which determines the feasibility of and options for surgery. Also of significance is the segmental arrangement of the heart itself. Thus in the presence of atrial isomerism or univentricular atrioventricular connection the problems created by the atresia are likely to be minor in comparison to those created by the other complex lesions present.

The problems of the associated lesions are less when pulmonary atresia with ventricular septal defect exists in the setting of complete or corrected transposition, since most usually in these cases the pulmonary arteries are confluent and fed by a duct. However, most surgical experience with this type of pulmonary atresia has been in cases with atrioventricular concordance and a 'normally related' atretic pulmonary trunk. It is the anatomical variablity of this type which will be discussed.

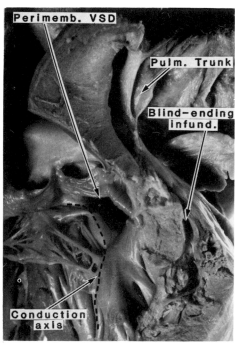

Figure 5. The typical ventricular morphology in pulmonary atresia and ventricular septal defect found in the setting of tetralogy of Fallot. Note the perimembranous nature of the ventricular septal defect and the site of the conduction tissue axis

5

The ventricular anatomy is relatively constant, being in essence tetralogy of Fallot with pulmonary atresia. Sometimes an imperforate valve is found, but usually the outlet septum is deviated so far in an anterocephalad direction that it totally blocks the subpulmonary outlet, producing muscular atresia. The pulmonary trunk is usually present and can be traced back as a fibrous cord to the roof of the atretic outflow tract, but it is rarely as well formed as when the ventricular septum is intact (compare illustrations 2 and 5). The ventricular septal defect is almost always of perimembranous type with aortic-tricuspid continuity so that the conduction tissue axis is at risk in the posteroinferior quadrant.

6a–e

As with tetralogy, cases may rarely be found with additional muscular inlet defects or with atrioventricular septal defects, and the defect may occasionally reduce its size spontaneously because of accessory tricuspid valve tissue tags[8]. The major variability of surgical significance is in the pulmonary pathways and the source of arterial supply[9–12].

In terms of the pulmonary arteries (PAs), the final common pathway is via the intraparenchymal pulmonary arteries (a). These are always present but are not always linked together. Usually they are, not only within each lung but across the midline via a pulmonary arterial confluence (b). However, sometimes the intraparenchymal arteries in each lung may be linked to the pulmonary artery of that side in the absence of a confluence (c), part of one lung may be connected via its pulmonary artery to a confluence and thence to the other lung (d) or there may be no intrapericardial pulmonary arteries whatsoever, the different parts of each lung being separately supplied in various patterns (e).

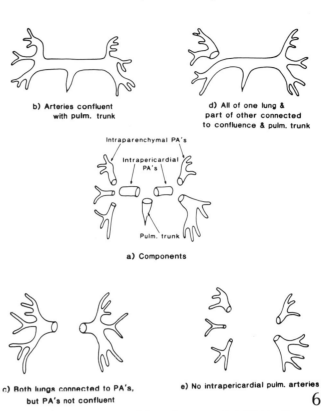

Figure 6. The components of the pulmonary arterial (PA) pathways (a) and the different ways they can be interconnected in presence of pulmonary atresia with ventricular septal defect

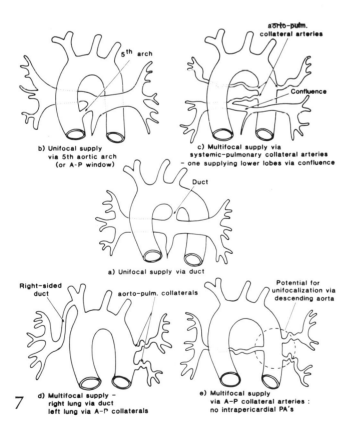

Figure 7. The different sources of blood supply to the intraparenchymal pulmonary arteries (PAs) in pulmonary atresia with ventricular septal defect (A-P; aortopulmonary)

7a–e

Equally significant, therefore, is the source of arterial supply to the intraparenchymal pulmonary arteries. The most favourable situation is when the pulmonary arteries are confluent and the confluence is supplied by a single source, an arrangement termed a unifocal supply[10]. The unifocal supply is most usually through a duct (a) but may occasionally be through a solitary major aortopulmonary (A-P) collateral artery or through a more esoteric conduit such as a persistent fifth aortic arch or an aortopulmonary window (b). It is significant to note that the presence of major aortopulmonary collateral arteries does not rule out the presence of a confluence (c).

8

Indeed, confluent pulmonary arteries are found in most cases in which the pulmonary supply is exclusively through aortopulmonary collateral arteries, although the confluence is usually small. In such circumstances it is important to establish how much of the pulmonary arterial supply is connected to the confluence. It is unusual to find a unifocal supply. Usually the supply is multifocal through between two and six major collateral arteries.

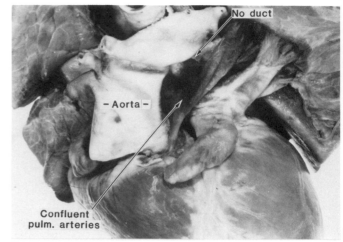

Figure 8. Hypoplastic but confluent pulmonary arteries in a case of pulmonary atresia with ventricular septal defect in which the pulmonary arterial supply was exclusively through aortopulmonary collateral arteries

9

These collateral arteries are *not* bronchial arteries[13] and it is a mistake to refer to them in that fashion. Collateral supply can be present via the bronchial and intercostal arteries, but then the collaterals are small and multiple, being acquired during life and of no value to the surgeon. The major aortopulmonary collateral arteries are present *ab initio* and usually arise directly from the descending aorta. More rarely they can arise from head and arm or even coronary arteries. If the supply is not unifocal through such arteries it is important to establish how much of the lung parenchyma is supplied through each collateral and how much is connected to a confluence or to intrapericardial pulmonary arteries if present.

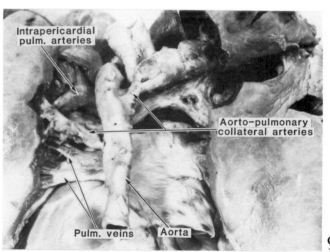

Figure 9. The origin of major aortopulmonary collateral arteries from the descending aorta in pulmonary atresia with ventricular septal defect

Intrapericardial arteries can be present for each lung in the absence of a confluence, and these may be supplied via bilateral ducts or by a duct on one side and aortopulmonary collaterals on the other (*see* Illustration 7d). Very rarely cases may be found in which a duct and aortopulmonary collateral arteries supply the same lung[14], but usually these two supplies (duct and collateral arteries) are mutually exclusive[15].

The least favourable type of arterial supply so far as the surgeon is concerned is when the intrapericardial arteries are totally lacking and the pulmonary arterial supply is provided exclusively by aortopulmonary collateral arteries (solitary arterial trunk or so-called 'truncus Type IV'[1, 2]. These are the hearts in which surgical unifocalization[16] is most difficult to achieve. It can be achieved when the

collaterals arise closely together from a segment of descending aorta (*see* Illustration 7e). It is possible to isolate this segment and connect it to the right ventricle, thus 'correcting' the circulatory pattern[17]. Whether this can be done together with closure of the ventricular septal defect to produce total 'correction' will depend on other factors such as the size of the pulmonary arteries and the pressure within them after isolation[18]. The existence of stenoses between the aortopulmonary collateral arteries, the true pulmonary arteries and the intraparenchymal arteries is highly significant in this respect.

It is clear that the options for pulmonary supply are many and varied. Highly skilled angiography is needed to determine the precise arrangement in each patient for the provision of optimal surgical treatment[14, 16, 18].

References

1. Thiene, G., Anderson, R. H. Pulmonary atresia with ventricular septal defect: anatomy. In: Anderson, R. H., Macartney, F. J., Shinebourne, E. A., Tynan, M. eds. Paediatric cardiology, vol. 5, pp. 80–101, Edinburgh: Churchill Livingstone, 1983

2. Anderson, R. H. Truncus Type IV: does it exist? Invited introduction. In: Moulton A. M., ed. Current controversies in techniques in congenital heart disease, pp. 101–105. New York: W. Saunders, 1984

3. Fisher, E. A., Tanopoulos, B. D., Eckner, F. A. O., Hastreiter, A. R., DuBrow, I. W. Pulmonary atresia with obstructed ventricular septal defect. Pediatric Cardiology 1980; 1: 209–217

4. Steeg, C. N., Ellis, K., Bransilver, B., Gersony, W. M. Pulmonary atresia and ventricular intact septum complicating corrected transposition of the great vessels. American Heart Journal 1971; 82: 382–386

5. Van Praagh, R. et al. Pulmonary atresia: anatomic considerations. In: Kidd, B. S., Rowe, R. D. eds. The child with congenital heart disease after surgery, pp. 103–134. New York: Futura Publishing Company, 1976

6. Zuberbuhler, J. R., Anderson, R. H. Morphological variations in pulmonary atresia with intact ventricular septum. British Heart Journal 1979; 41: 281–288

7. De Leval, M., Bull, C., Stark, J., Anderson, R. H., Taylor, J. F. N., Macartney, F. J. Pulmonary atresia and intact ventricular septum: surgical management based on a revised classification. Circulation 1982; 66: 272–280

8. Faggian, G., Frescura, C., Thiene, G., Bortolotti, U., Mazzucco, A., Anderson, R. H. Accessory tricuspid valve tissue causing obstruction of the ventricular septal defect in tetralogy of Fallot. British Heart Journal 1983; 49: 324–327

9. Somerville, J. Management of pulmonary atresia. British Heart Journal 1970; 32: 641–651

10. Macartney, F. J., Scott, O., Deverall, P. B. Haemodynamic and anatomical characteristics of pulmonary blood supply in pulmonary atresia with ventricular septal defect – including a case of persistent fifth aortic arch. British Heart Journal 1974; 36: 1049–1060

11. Haworth, S. G., Macartney, F. J. The pulmonary blood supply. In: Anderson, R. H., Macartney, F. J., Shinebourne, E. A., Tynan, M. eds. Paediatric cardiology, vol. 5, pp. 102–110. Edinburgh: Churchill Livingstone, 1983

12. Thiene, G., Bortolotti, U., Gallucci, V., Valente, M. D., Volta, S. D. Pulmonary atresia with ventricular septal defect. British Heart Journal 1977; 39: 1223–1233

13. Thiene, G., Frescura, C., Bini, R. M., Valente, M. L., Gallucci, V. Histology of pulmonary arterial supply in pulmonary atresia with ventricular septal defect. Circulation 1979; 60: 1066–1074

14. Macartney, F. J., Haworth, S. G. Investigation of pulmonary atresia with ventricular septal defect. In: Anderson, R. H., Macartney, F. J., Shinebourne, E. A., Tynan, M. eds. Paediatric cardiology vol. 5, pp. 111–125. Edinburgh: Churchill Livingstone, 1983

15. Thiene, G., Frescura, C., Bortolotti, U., Del Maschio, A., Valente, M. L. The systemic pulmonary circulation in pulmonary atresia with ventricular septal defect: concept of reciprocal development of the fourth and sixth aortic arches. American Heart Journal 1981; 101: 339–344

16. Stark, J., Huhta, J. C., Macartney, F. J. Palliative surgery for pulmonary atresia with ventricular septal defect. In: Anderson, R. H., Macartney, F. J., Shinebourne, E. A., Tynan, M. eds. Paediatric cardiology vol. 5, pp. 126–136. Edinburgh: Churchill Livingstone, 1983

17. Bowman, F. O. Jr. Operative approach to truncus arteriosus 'Type IV'. In: Moulton, A. L., ed. Current controversies in techniques in congenital heart disease, pp. 105–114. New York: W. Saunders, 1984

18. Alfieri. O., Blackstone, E. H., Kirklin, J. W., Pacifico, A. D., Bargeron, L. M. Jr. Surgical treatment of tetralogy of Fallot with pulmonary atresia. Journal of Thoracic and Cardiovascular Surgery 1978; 76: 321–335

Pulmonary atresia with ventricular septal defect

Marc de Leval MD
Consultant Cardiothoracic Surgeon, The Hospital for Sick Children, Great Ormond Street, London, UK

Introduction

The intracardiac anatomy of pulmonary atresia with ventricular septal defect is basically similar to the anatomy of tetralogy of Fallot. Its unique feature is the anatomy of the pulmonary circulation and the source of the pulmonary blood flow.

During normal early fetal development the vascular plexus forming in the lung buds is connected to segmental arteries arising from the dorsal aortae. The intrapulmonary vascular plexus has differentiated into definitive segmental arteries by the 40th day, at which time the lung is perfused both by the sixth aortic arch (central pulmonary arteries) and the segmental arteries. These normally disappear by the 50th day[1]; the lungs are then entirely and exclusively supplied by central pulmonary arteries derived from the sixth arch. In pulmonary atresia with ventricular septal defect it appears that the normal maturation process may be arrested, with resulting coexistence of some bronchopulmonary segments or lobules connected to the central pulmonary arteries and/or to segmental arteries. The latter must be differentiated from bronchial arteries, which develop late in fetal life and remain smaller. The bronchial arteries can be traced to the vascular plexus around the carina and the lower end of the trachea. The terms large systemic pulmonary collateral arteries and major aortopulmonary collateral arteries have both been used to describe these arteries[2].

Preoperative

Diagnosis

The majority of patients with pulmonary atresia with ventricular septal defect present with some degree of cyanosis. Sometimes, however, they present in congestive heart failure due to an excessive pulmonary blood flow through major aortopulmonary collateral arteries or they may be completely asymptomatic.

Detailed anatomical and haemodynamic studies of patients with this condition must be undertaken early in life, even if cyanosis is mild, in order to plan a repair which, ideally, should consist of connecting the right ventricle with a unifocal pulmonary circulation[3].

Preoperative investigations include an assessment of the intracardiac circulation. This consists of a detailed angiographic study of the central pulmonary arteries, their connection with the right ventricle, their sources of blood supply and their destination in the lung. Similarly the origin, course and destination of all major aortopulmonary collateral arteries must be demonstrated. Central pulmonary arteries are visualized best by aortography or selective injections into their source of blood supply (aortopulmonary collateral arteries, persistent ductus arteriosus and/or surgically created systemic-to-pulmonary shunts). When confluent, the pulmonary arteries produce a characteristic Y-shaped vessel running across the mediastinum immediately anterior to the trachea (seagull picture). Pulmonary vein wedge angiography is sometimes useful in visualizing central pulmonary arteries[4].

1 & 2

In most cases the right and left pulmonary arteries are confluent and it is either the right ventricular outflow tract, the pulmonary valve, the main pulmonary artery or all of the above which are atretic. If the right and left pulmonary arteries are not confluent either or both intrapericardial pulmonary arteries may be absent. Even so, a confluence of the intrapulmonary arteries of a given lung is usually present at the hilum.

The size, distribution and growth potential of the pulmonary arteries vary from patient to patient. Hypoplasia of the pulmonary arteries is not uncommonly associated with major aortopulmonary collateral arteries. With regard to their distribution there may be an arborization abnormality in that not all the intrapulmonary arteries in a given lung are connected to the central pulmonary arteries. This failure of connection was present in about half the segments in Haworth and Macartney's study[5].

Selective injection into each of the large collateral arteries is necessary to plan the surgical management of these patients. Most of these arteries arise from the descending aorta and run posterior to the bronchi. They may anastomose with either a central pulmonary artery or a normally connected lobar artery or else enter the lung parenchyma to branch within it without connecting with the central pulmonary arteries. In this situation two types of perfusion are encountered. Some segments are only connected to collateral arteries where the right upper lobe is so connected and the rest of the lung to the pulmonary artery. Sometimes lung segments are connected both to collateral and central pulmonary arteries. Localized stenosis may occur at the origin of collateral arteries, along their course or where they anastomose with a pulmonary artery. Approximately 50 per cent of major aortopulmonary collateral arteries are stenosed at some point. In the lung parenchyma the size and structure of the intrapulmonary arteries depend on the size of the perfusing vessel.

Indications for surgery

The aims of the surgical repair of these anomalies are: (1) eventually to connect the right ventricle with as many bronchopulmonary segments as possible; (2) to avoid excessive residual right ventricle hypertension, which has been shown to be an important determinant of hospital mortality[6]; and (3) to close those major aortopulmonary collateral arteries not connected to the right ventricle to prevent postoperative pulmonary overcirculation.

For those cases in which pulmonary arteries are confluent and perfuse the majority of all the bronchopulmonary segments operability can be assessed before operation by comparing the size of the right and left pulmonary arteries with that of the aorta at the diaphragm[7]. If the right and left pulmonary arteries have a total combined cross-sectional area greater than about one-half the cross-sectional area of the aorta just above the diaphragm they are probably adequate to receive the cardiac output after repair without excessive right ventricular hypertension. A refinement of this approach by developing quantitative interrelations between these and other variables such as peripheral stenosis and arborization anomalies increases the accuracy of prediction of right-to-left ventricular pressure ratio after repair[6].

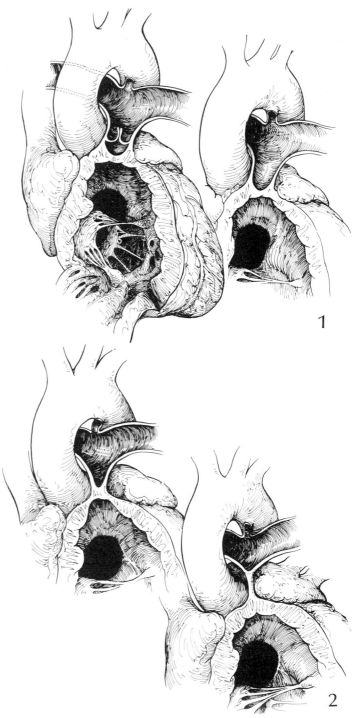

Because complete repair often includes the use of an extracardiac valved conduit this is usually undertaken after the age of 4 years. In younger patients and in patients in whom the predicted right-to-left ventricular pressure ratio after repair will be greater than 0.8 a palliative operation is recommended.

The management of collateral arteries depends on their connection with the central pulmonary arteries. Collateral arteries connected to the central pulmonary arteries must be closed at the time of the surgical repair. Collaterals supplying a substantial volume of the pulmonary vascular bed should ideally be connected to the central pulmonary arteries.

The operations

PALLIATIVE PROCEDURES

These procedures are directed towards three goals: (1) to increase pulmonary blood flow in the cyanotic patient; (2) to decrease pulmonary blood flow in patients in heart failure; and (3) to prepare the pulmonary circulation of those patients with multifocal blood supply for a complete repair.

Cyanosis

Neonates presenting with ductus-dependent pulmonary circulation are treated with prostaglandin until pulmonary blood flow can be augmented surgically. Systemic-to-pulmonary artery shunt, right ventricular outflow tract enlargement and direct relief of peripheral stenoses are the available procedures.

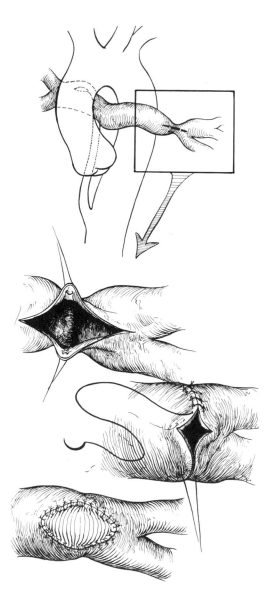

Systemic-to-pulmonary artery shunt. All commonly used shunts can be performed. We have found the modified Blalock-Taussig shunt, using a Gore-Tex prosthesis, particularly useful for patients with very small pulmonary arteries. This shunt is of particular value when the operation has to be performed on the side of the aortic arch.

Right ventricular outflow tract enlargement. This has been recommended for patients with hypoplastic confluent pulmonary arteries[8]. An outflow patch is inserted across the atretic segment on cardiopulmonary bypass and the ventricular septal defect is left open. A closed technique, consisting of sewing the patch in before the outflow tract is incised, using a thin wire, has been more recently reported[9, 10].

3

Relief of peripheral stenosis. Localized stenosis on a central pulmonary artery or a major aortopulmonary collateral artery can be relieved surgically. A longitudinal incision is made across the stenotic segment, which is then closed either transversely or with a patch.

3

Heart failure

Occasionally patients with pulmonary atresia with ventricular septal defect present in intractable heart failure due to an excessive pulmonary blood flow through bronchopulmonary segments perfused by major aortopulmonary collateral arteries or a persistent ductus arteriosus. If these segments have a duplicate source of pulmonary blood supply from collateral and central pulmonary arteries[11] the collaterals can be ligated if the blood source to the central pulmonary arteries is adequate. As pulmonary infarction following ligation of large collateral arteries has been reported[12] it is probably unwise to ligate collaterals which are the sole supply to some bronchopulmonary segments. For these cases banding of the collateral or its connection to the central pulmonary arteries with a shunt procedure are theoretical alternatives.

4a–c

Multifocal blood supply

Apart from cyanosis and heart failure, many infants with pulmonary atresia with ventricular septal defect have too little lung connected to the central pulmonary arteries. In the hope of an eventual connection of the right ventricle with as many bronchopulmonary segments as possible we have performed a number of 'unifocalizations'. These procedures are based on the observation that some collateral arteries connect with at least as many bronchopulmonary segments as does a central pulmonary artery and that the peripheral intrapulmonary arteries with which they connect appear at least as normal as do vessels connected to central pulmonary arteries[13].

Technically these operations have consisted in ligating major aortopulmonary collateral arteries at their aortic origin and: (1) connecting the central pulmonary arteries and a collateral to a subclavian artery with a bifurcated Gore-Tex graft (a); (2) performing a Blalock-Taussig or modified Blalock shunt on a collateral naturally connected to a central pulmonary artery (b); or (3) connecting the central pulmonary arteries with a collateral directly or by interposition of a Gore-Tex prosthesis (c).

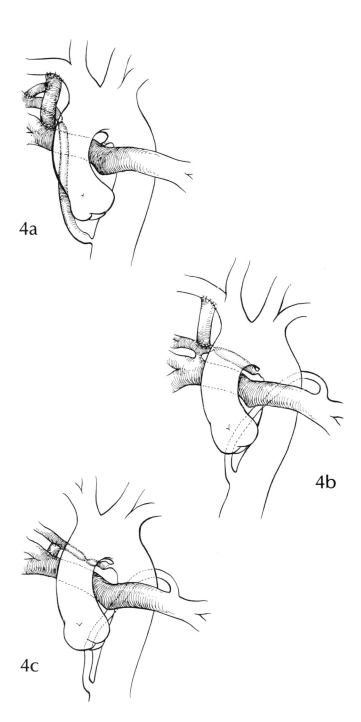

4a

4b

4c

CORRECTIVE PROCEDURES

The operative repair of pulmonary atresia with ventricular septal defect was poineered by Kirklin[14] and Ross and Somerville[15]. The repair consists in: (1) controlling the source of pulmonary blood flow, including the closure of major aortopulmonary collateral arteries in some cases; (2) closing the ventricular septal defect; and (3) connecting the right ventricle to the pulmonary arteries.

The operation is performed through a midline sternotomy incision on hypothermic cardiopulmonary bypass and with cold cardioplegia. The left side is vented through the left artium or left ventricle. Profound hypothermia is not used until all large systemic-to-pulmonary connections have been controlled in order to avoid overdistension of the heart as a result of ventricular fibrillation.

Control of pulmonary blood source

A persistent ductus arteriosus is dissected , encircled with a heavy ligature before the institution of extracorporeal circulation and ligated while on bypass. Various surgical anastomoses are controlled in the standard fashion.

Three possible approaches have to be considered for the exposure and ligation of major aortopulmonary collateral arteries[7].
1. If the target artery or arteries lie directly behind the posterior pericardium, cephalad to the left atrium, where they can be exposed by incising the posterior pericardium, one may approach them via the median sternotomy incision and pericardial space.

2. If the artery or arteries lie at or cephalad to the hilum of either lung they can often be exposed for ligation, again via the median sternotomy, by opening the anterior mediastinal pleura and dissecting the hilum while retracting the lung and mediastinum. This can sometimes be done before cardiopulmonary bypass is established if the haemodynamics and the arterial PO$_2$ remain stable. Ligation of the arteries is carried out while on bypass. If the descending aorta is on the side opposite to the heart even collateral arteries arising from the aorta caudal to the hilum can be exposed by retraction of the lung via an incision in the anterior mediastinal pleura.
3. When the descending aorta is on the side of the heart large collateral arteries arising caudal to the hilum are approached through a complementary lateral thoracotomy on the side of the descending aorta[16]. This is done, before the sternotomy incision is made, with the patient in the lateral decubitus position through the fourth intercostal space. The mediastinal pleura is incised over the upper descending aorta and suspended from the wound. The collateral vessels arising from the anteromedial surface of the aorta are dissected out and encircled with heavy braided silk ligatures which are left untied along the pericardial sac. These collaterals may be very thin-walled and must be handled as carefully as the enlarged intercostal arteries in patients with coarctation of the aorta. The pleural cavity is then drained, the thoracotomy incision closed and the patient placed in the supine position for the midline sternotomy incision. The ligatures are retrieved in the pleural space from the front and ligated after bypass has been instituted.

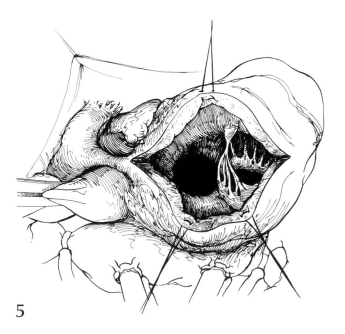

5

5

Closure of ventricular septal defect

A longitudinal right ventriculotomy incision is made, avoiding major coronary arteries. The defect is then exposed. This is often helped by mobilization and resection of the hypertrophied extensions of the infundibular septum.

6

As in tetralogy of Fallot, ventricular septal defects are of two types. The most common type is a perimembranous infundibular defect that extends to the area of aortic-mitral tricuspid continuity. This defect is closed with a patch of Dacron velour which is inserted with interrupted or continuous sutures. The inferior margin of the patch is attached to the base of the septal and anterior leaflets of the tricuspid valve to stay away from the conduction tissues.

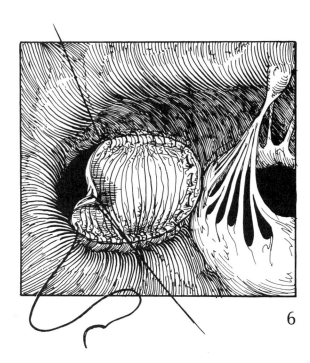

6

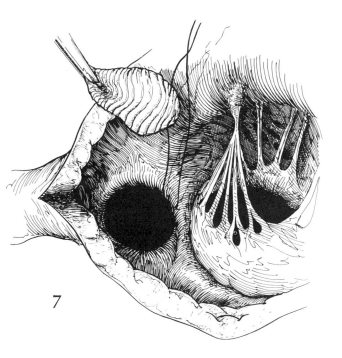

7

7

Less frequently the defect has a completely muscular rim which is formed posteriorly by the fusion of the posterior limb of the trabecula septomarginalis with the ventriculo-infundibular fold (infundibular muscular defect). The closure is effected by placing the sutures around the edge of the defect.

Establishment of continuity between right ventricle and pulmonary arteries

This may include the following procedures: (1) infundibular resection with patch enlargement of the right ventricular outflow tract; (2) extracardiac valved conduit; and (3) extensive pulmonary arterial reconstruction.

8 & 9

Infundibular resection with patch enlargement of right ventricular outflow tract

This can be done when the atretic segment is confined to the subpulmonary infundibulum and is short (no more than 1–1.5 cm). An incision is carried from the ventriculotomy site to the pulmonary artery, cutting into the fibrous core of the atretic segment. Then a wide and long patch of pericardium or a patch tailored from preclotted woven Dacron tube is sutured to the entire length of the combined ventriculotomy and arteriotomy, the stitches being placed through the epicardial edges of the incised fibrous core.

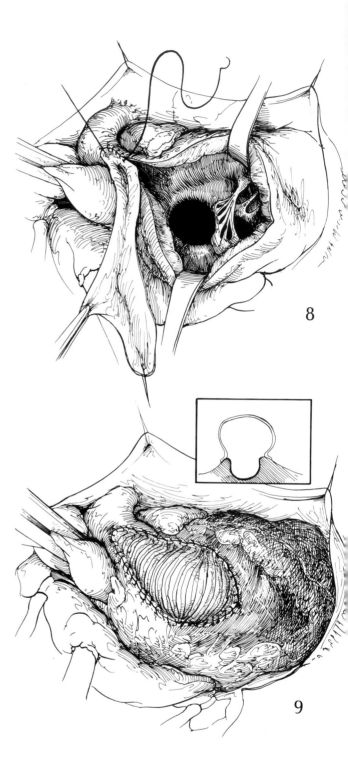

8

9

10

Extracardiac valved conduit

When there is discontinuity between the right ventricle and the pulmonary arteries or when a major coronary artery crosses the outflow tract of the right ventricle a conduit is anastomosed to the distal main pulmonary artery or its branches and the right ventriculotomy. For the conduit we use fresh antibiotic-preserved homografts as initially described by Ross and Somerville[15] or xenografts in Dacron tubes. Homografts are particularly useful when one is dealing with very thin-walled pulmonary arteries. Proximally the anterior mitral valve leaflet of the homograft can be used to close the ventriculotomy incision. If it is too short the homograft is extended proximally with a Dacron tube.

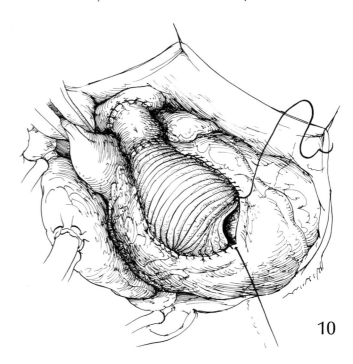

10

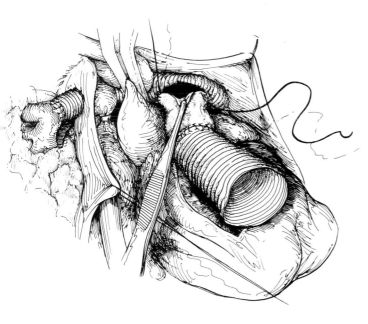

11

Extensive pulmonary arterial reconstruction

For patients with non-confluent pulmonary arteries or central hypoplasia of the right and left pulmonary arteries the first step of the pulmonary arterial reconstruction consists of establishing a wide confluence between both peripheral pulmonary arteries. This may require the use of a tube connecting both left and right pulmonary arteries in the hilum and an extracardiac valved conduit anastomosed to the first prosthesis. A patch enlargement of hypoplastic right and/or central pulmonary arteries may be facilitated by transection of the ascending aorta.

Results

PALLIATIVE PROCEDURES

The results of palliative surgery for this condition have been rather disappointing. Surgical treatment is often needed during the neonatal period and carries a not inconsiderable mortality but may be necessary if the anatomy is not suitable for repair. This applies particularly to those patients with multifocal pulmonary blood supply[17]. Between November 1963 and September 1981 125 palliative operations for pulmonary atresia with ventricular septal defect were performed on 98 patients in our unit. There were 17 early (within 30 days) and 10 late deaths (28 per cent). Three of the late deaths occurred at the time of complete repair. A total of 145 palliative procedures were performed (some in combination) to increase or decrease pulmonary blood flow or localize the source of pulmonary blood supply. Seventy-two patients had one palliative operation, 25 had two operations and one had three operations.

Unsuitability for complete repair after palliative surgery may result from an insufficient number of pulmonary segments connected to the central pulmonary arteries, severe hypoplasia of the central pulmonary arteries and/or uneven enlargement or growth of peripheral arteries after shunt procedures resulting in segmental stenoses[13, 18].

REPAIR

In a series of 103 patients who underwent definitive repair at the Mayo Clinic between 1967 and 1975 there were 10 hospital deaths (9.7 per cent)[12]. Alfieri et al.[6] reported a 16 per cent mortality in a group of 80 patients operated on at the University of Alabama Medical Center between 1967 and 1978. In that study the degree of immediate residual right ventricular hypertension was shown to be the most important determinant of hospital mortality. Both groups have recommended that a transannular patch should be used whenever possible rather than a valved external conduit.

References

1. Boyden, E. A. The time lag in the development of bronchial arteries. Anatomical Record 1970; 166: 611–614

2. Macartney, F., Deverall, P., Scott, O. Haemodynamic characteristics of systemic arterial blood supply to the lungs. British Heart Journal 1973; 35: 28–37

3. Macartney, F. J., Scott, O., Deverall, P. B. Haemodynamic and anatomical characteristics of pulmonary blood supply in pulmonary atresia with ventricular septal defect, including a case of persistent fifth aortic arch. British Heart Journal 1974; 36: 1049–1060

4. Nihill, M. R., Mullins, C. E., McNamara, D. G. Visualisation of the pulmonary arteries in pseudotruncus by pulmonary vein wedge angiography. Circulation 1978; 58: 140–147

5. Haworth, S. G., Macartney, F. J. Growth and development of pulmonary circulation in pulmonary atresia with ventricular septal defect and major aortopulmonary collateral arteries. British Heart Journal 1980; 44: 14–24

6. Alfieri, O., Blackstone, E. H., Kirklin, J. W., Pacifico, A. D., Bargeron, L. M. Surgical treatment of tetralogy of Fallot with pulmonary atresia. Journal of Thoracic and Cardiovascular Surgery 1978; 76: 321–335

7. McGoon, D. C., Baird, D. K., Davis, G. D. Surgical management of large bronchial collateral arteries with pulmonary stenosis or atresia. Circulation 1975; 52: 109–118

8. Gill, C. C., Moodie, D. S., McGoon, D. C. Staged surgical management of pulmonary atresia with diminutive pulmonary arteries. Journal of Thoracic and Cardiovascular Surgery 1977; 73: 436–442

9. Puga, F. J., Uretzky, G. Establishment of right ventricle: hypoplastic pulmonary artery continuity without the use of extracorporeal circulation. Journal of Thoracic and Cardiovascular Surgery 1982; 83: 74–80

10. Alvierez-Diaz, F. et al. Neuva tecnica serrado de ampliacion del tracto de salida de ventriculo derecho. Revista Espaniola de Cardiologia (Madrid) 1981; 34: 293

11. Faller, K., Haworth, S. G., Taylor, J. F. N., Macartney, F. J. Duplicate sources of pulmonary blood supply in pulmonary atresia with ventricular septal defect. British Heart Journal 1981; 46: 263–268

12. Olin, C. L., Ritter, D. G., McGoon, D. C., Wallace, R. B., Danielson, G. K. Pulmonary atresia: surgical considerations and results in 103 patients undergoing definitive repair. Circulation 1976; 54 (Suppl. III): 35–40

13. Haworth, S. G., Rees, P. G., Taylor, J. F. N., Macartney, F. J., de Leval, M. R., Stark, J. Pulmonary atresia with ventricular septal defect and major aortopulmonary collateral arteries; effect of systemic pulmonary anastomosis. British Heart Journal 1981; 45: 133–141

14. Rastelli, G. C., Ongley, P. A., Davis, G. D., Kirklin, J. W. Surgical repair for pulmonary valve atresia with coronary-pulmonary artery fistula: report of case. Mayo Clinic Proceedings 1965; 40: 521–527

15. Ross, D. N., Somerville, J. Correction of pulmonary atresia with a homograft aortic valve. Lancet 1966; ii: 1446–1449

16. Doty, D. B., Kouchoukos, N. T., Kirklin, J. W., Barcia, A., Bargeron, L. M. Surgery for pseudotruncus arteriosus with pulmonary blood flow originating from upper descending thoracic aorta. Circulation 1972; 45 (Suppl. I): 121–129

17. Macartney, F. J., Huhta, J. C., Douglas, J. M., Haworth, S. G., de Leval, M. R., Stark, J. Les résultats a long terme de la chirurgie de l'atrésie pulmonaire avec communication inter-ventriculaire. Coeur 1981; 13 (numero special) 747–753

18. McGoon, D. C., Fulton, R. E., Davis, G. D., Ritter, D. G., Neil, C. A., White, R. I. Systemic collateral and pulmonary artery stenosis in patients with congenital pulmonary valve atresia and ventricular septal defect. Circulation 1977; 56: 473–479

Right ventricular outflow tract obstruction with intact ventricular septum

Marc de Leval MD
Consultant Cardiothoracic Surgeon, The Hospital for Sick Children, Great Ormond Street, London, UK

Introduction

Obstructive lesions involving the right ventricular outflow tract and the pulmonary arteries are seen in about 25–30 per cent of all hearts with congenital defects. Anatomically the obstruction can occur at any level from the tricuspid valve to the branches of the pulmonary arteries. The obstruction may also exist at several levels simultaneously. Approximately half of these obstructions are seen in association with a ventricular septal defect.

This chapter is concerned only with obstructions in hearts with an intact ventricular septum. This includes an anatomical and clinical spectrum of anomalies from the hypoplastic right ventricle with pulmonary atresia in the neonate to mild pulmonary valve stenosis in adulthood. For practical purposes the patients can be divided into two groups: critical pulmonary stenosis and pulmonary atresia in infancy and pulmonary stenosis in childhood. Stenosis of pulmonary arterial branches will also be dealt with briefly.

CRITICAL PULMONARY STENOSIS AND PULMONARY ATRESIA IN INFANCY

Diagnosis

Cyanosis with severe right-sided failure within the first few days of life is the most common clinical presentation of this condition. If the pulmonary valve is completely atretic the pulmonary circulation is maintained only through the persistent ductus arteriosus and the patient becomes acutely ill when this structure is closing. Large A waves in the jugular venous pulse tracing and a presystolic pulsation of an enlarged liver are common findings. The heart size varies. There is only a single second sound. A ductus murmur may possibly be heard. The chest radiograph shows pulmonary ischaemia and the electrocardiogram shows a preponderance of left ventricular forces. The echocardiogram is helpful in showing the size of the right ventricular cavity and the degree of right ventricular hypertrophy. It has been our policy to perform cardiac catheterization with angiocardiography as a routine to confirm the diagnosis and decide on management.

Classification

We have proposed a revised classification of the right ventricular appearances of this condition[1] based on the tripartite approach to right ventricular morphology which was developed by Goor and Lillehei[2]. They defined a sinus (inlet) portion, a trabecular part and an infundibulum. These hearts can be classified anatomically and echographically into three groups.

In the first group all three portions of the right ventricular cavity are present and the anomaly consists of a greater or lesser degree of generalized hypoplasia. Most cases of critical pulmonary stenosis are in this group.

In the other two groups, besides the smallness of the cavity, at least one portion is missing. All cases by definition have a patent tricuspid valve and thus an inlet portion to the ventricle, but the trabecular portion, or both trabecular and infundibular components of the cavity, can be so overgrown by hypertrophic myocardium as to be effectively absent.

Preoperative

The aim of treatment in infancy is twofold: first to increase the arterial oxygen saturation and treat the acidosis and heart failure, and second, ideally, to prepare the right ventricle for complete repair.

An intravenous infusion of prostaglandin E_1 at a dosage up to 0.1 μ/kg/min is initiated as soon as the diagnosis is suspected so as to improve pulmonary blood flow. Metabolic acidosis and congestive heart failure are treated in the usual manner.

The operations

MODERATE RIGHT VENTRICULAR HYPOPLASIA

In the presence of a good-sized right ventricle with three components a complete repair consisting of relief of the right ventricular outflow tract obstruction and closure of the interatrial communication can be considered. In our experience this is an exceptional situation in the neonatal period since most of these patients have such a degree of right ventricular hypoplasia that the right ventricle is too small to provide a normal pulmonary blood flow.

A pulmonary valvotomy alone, leaving the interatrial communication open, is an alternative. This can be performed through a midline sternotomy incision either as a transventricular valvotomy (Brock procedure) or as an open valvotomy under inflow occlusion or on cardio-pulmonary bypass. The former has been our procedure of choice for several years.

1

The pericardium is opened longitudinally and traction sutures are placed at the junction of the trabecular and infudibular portions of the right ventricle, avoiding damage to the coronary arteries. A stab wound is made, blood loss being minimized by crossing traction on the sutures. The Brock knife is introduced into the right ventricular cavity and directed into the pulmonary outflow tract to the level of the obstruction and then forced into the main pulmonary artery. Several passes with the instrument are made to ensure an adequate valvotomy and progressively larger valvotomies are introduced. The diameter of the main pulmonary artery is a guide to the maximum size of knife that can be used. Care must be taken to keep the blade directed anteriorly to avoid posterior perforation.

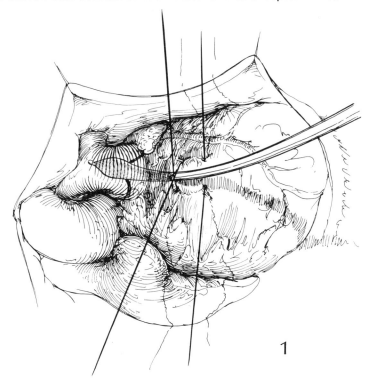

1

SEVERE RIGHT VENTRICULAR HYPOPLASIA

For patients with more than moderate hypoplasia of the right ventricle and for those in whom the trabecular portion is missing we now prefer a transpulmonary valvotomy with a modified left Blalock-Taussig shunt. The patient is positioned on the table on his right side and a left thoracotomy incision is made in the third or fourth intercostal space. The pericardium is opened in front of the phrenic nerve and the pulmonary artery dissected free of surrounding structures. Prostaglandin infusion is maintained.

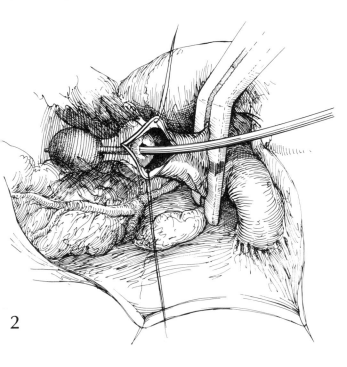

2

The main pulmonary artery is then clamped with a vascular clamp proximal to the bifurcation, care being taken not to distort the ductus arteriosus or to occlude the continuity of the left and right pulmonary arteries. A longitudinal incision is made in the main pulmonary artery. The atretic pulmonary valve appears as a membrane or, more frequently, as a tricuspid valve with complete fusion of the commissures. A stab wound is made in the valve and the incision is enlarged with artery forceps. Ideally a portion of the valve tissue should be excised to avoid restenosis. When the ventricular cavity is large enough a
Fogarty catheter can be introduced and threaded into the infundibular chamber to keep the surgical field dry of blood.

2

3

A valvotomy is then performed under direct vision (inset). Closure of the arteriotomy with a running monofilament suture is started inferiorly, the balloon is deflated and the catheter removed. The area of the arteriotomy is then grasped with a partial occlusion clamp so that the occluding vascular clamp on the pulmonary artery may be removed. Finally the left pulmonary artery is dissected as far as the hilum of the left lung and the origin of the left subclavian artery exposed. A Gore-Tex® prosthesis is anastomosed end-to-side from the subclavian artery to the pulmonary artery. It is important to ensure that the prosthesis lies straight along the mediastinum and does not kink.

For neonates without an infundibular portion to the right ventricular cavity the entire systemic venous return, with the exception of blood reaching the aorta via sinusoids, reaches the left atrium through the patent foramen ovale and pulmonary blood-flow depends entirely on systemic-to-pulmonary connections. Since pulmonary valvotomy is impracticable in these patients we recommend a right-sided systemic-to-pulmonary artery shunt to avoid intra-operative distortion of the persistent ductus arteriosus. Since the pulmonary atresia is not relieved and the patient's life still depends on an adequate interatrial communication, a balloon atrial septostomy after initial cardiac catheterization is recommended in these patients.

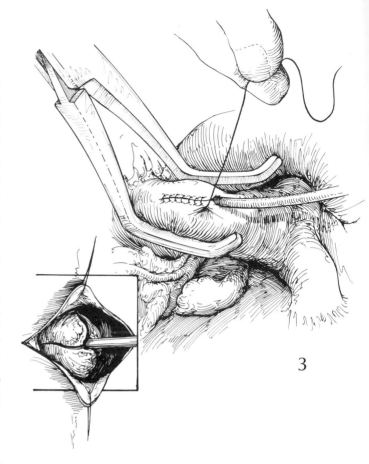

3

Results

The early mortality in neonates with pulmonary atresia and intact ventricular septum has fallen from 55 to 7 per cent since we adopted the techniques described above. The majority of the surviving patients, however, remain with major anatomical and haemodynamic abnormalities: a hypoplastic, hypertrophied right ventricle with residual right ventricular outflow tract obstruction and intra- and extracardiac shunts. Most require further surgery and a complete repair consisting of separation of the systemic and pulmonary circulations with right ventricular function. However, this can be achieved in only some of these patients.

PULMONARY STENOSIS IN CHILDHOOD

Pulmonary valve stenosis is the fourth most common congenital heart defect. Of these patients 50–80 per cent have pure pulmonary valve stenosis; the others have associated infundibular stenosis, presumed to be part of compensatory right ventricular hypertrophy. Though bicuspid and unicuspid valves may be seen, the most common form usually consists of three well formed leaflets which are fused in a domed shape with a central opening of varying diameter. The commissures are usually fairly well defined, but the leaflets are often adherent to the adjacent pulmonary arterial wall. The annulus is usually normal but may be hypoplastic. Post-stenotic dilatation of the pulmonary artery is common and often extends into the left pulmonary artery. A patent foramen ovale or an atrial septal defect is usually present.

Studies of the clinical course of uncomplicated pulmonary valve stenosis indicate that progression of the obstruction may occur, particularly in those patients presenting in infancy, though patients with trivial pulmonary valve stenosis (right ventricle-pulmonary artery gradient less than 25 mmHg) rarely show deterioration. A co-operative study group[3] recommended valvotomy in children with gradients greater than 50 mmHg. Those with mild obstruction (25–50 mmHg) may be treated surgically or followed conservatively for evidence of positive stenosis with equal safety.

We advocate surgery before school age (4–5 years). Early surgical relief of the stenosis is indicated whenever the patient becomes symptomatic (low exercise tolerance, right ventricular failure or cyanosis from shunting at atrial level) or whenever the right ventricular pressure is higher than the systemic pressure.

The operations

Repair of right ventricular outflow tract obstruction in childhood is performed on cardiopulmonary bypass with moderate hypothermia. Although induced ventricular fibrillation without clamping the aorta is sometimes used for short procedures, we prefer to clamp the aorta and induce cardioplegia. Left ventricular distension is avoided either by placing a vent through the patent foramen ovale (atrial septal defect) or by aspirating the pulmonary artery.

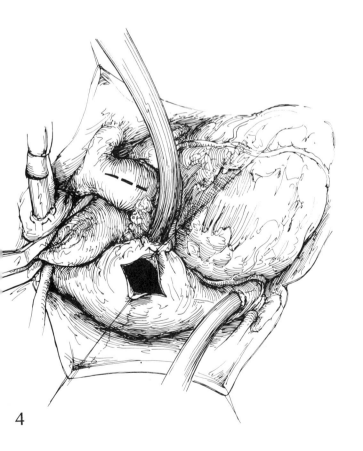

4

The patent foramen ovale or atrial septal defect is closed directly through a short right atriotomy incision made in front of the crista terminalis. A longitudinal incision is made in the main pulmonary artery and the pulmonary valve is examined.

4

5

The fused and vestigial commissures, either two or three, are identified and then incised with a scalpel. The adjacent cusps are held taut by the surgeon and an assistant as this incision is made and it may be carried deeply towards the pulmonary arterial wall. The aim here is to relieve the stenosis as completely as possible, even at the expense of creating some pulmonary insufficiency, which is the opposite to the guiding principle in the repair of aortic stenosis.

In the case of a bicuspid valve incision of the commissures may fail to relieve the stenosis adequately because the free edges of the cusps are of inadequate length. In that case some degree of insufficiency is deliberately produced by slightly disengaging the cusps from their lateral attachment to the pulmonary arterial wall. If the valve leaflets are rigid and dysplastic complete excision of the valve may become necessary to achieve relief of the obstruction. Visual and digital examination of the infundibular area can be carried out through the opened valve.

Spontaneous regression of infundibular stenosis can occur, but if the tissue is firm and unyielding regression is unlikely. The adequacy of the valvotomy and of the pulmonary valve annulus is then estimated by calibrating the Hegar dilators and referring to the tables of normal pulmonary annulus diameter. If too small, the pulmonary valve annulus is incised by extending the arteriotomy incision into the right ventricular outflow tract.

When the obstruction has been satisfactorily relieved the pulmonary artery is closed with a monofilament suture. The patient is then fully rewarmed and cardiopulmonary bypass discontinued. The right ventricular–left ventricular pressure ratio is measured. If this is greater than 0.75 the likelihood of reversibility of the gradient can be tested by the intravenous administration of propranolol at a dosage of 0.01–0.25 mg/kg. When the pressure difference between the right ventricle and the pulmonary artery is reduced by propranolol without changes in the systemic arterial pressure it can be assumed that the gradient is reversible and based on secondary muscular hypertrophy of the infundibulum. If the right ventricular pressure does not fall cardiopulmonary bypass is reinstituted and relief of the right ventricular outflow tract obstruction is performed[4].

6

A vertical incision is made in the right ventricular outlet chamber. This can be an extension of the pulmonary arteriotomy if the pulmonary annulus is small; otherwise the incision is limited to the outlet chambers. If grossly hypertrophied the septal and parietal extensions of the infundibular septum are excised in a manner similar to the one used to relieve right ventricular outflow tract obstruction in tetralogy of Fallot.

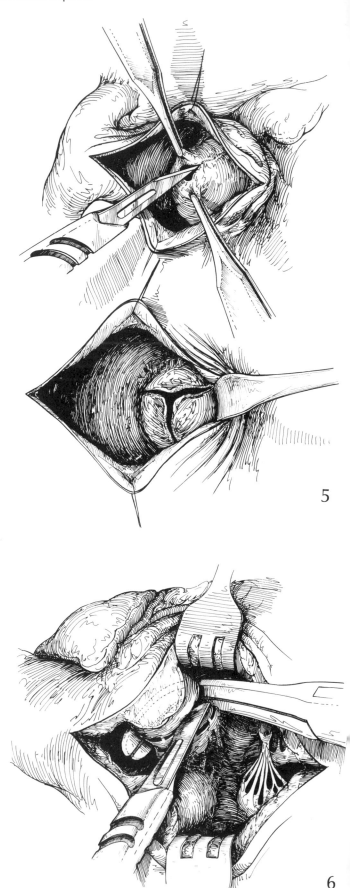

5

6

7

If the right ventricular outflow tract is hypoplastic, muscular resection is not possible and the obstruction is relieved by patch enlargement. The patch can be fashioned from pericardium or prosthetic tube. It should have enough length to relieve all levels of obstruction and adequate width to create an outflow tract of normal diameter for the body surface area. The patch should be tear-shaped or oval; diamond patches increase the risk of stenosis at the end of the patch.

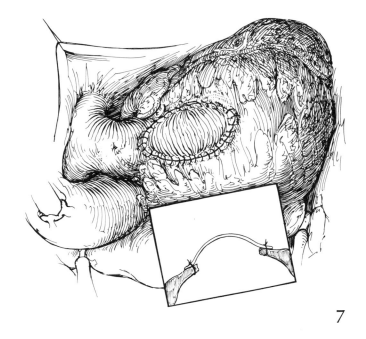

7

Results

In the co-operative natural history study published by Nugent et al.[3], 304 of 565 patients with isolated pulmonary valve stenosis were treated surgically. Open valvotomy under 2 years of age carried a 10 per cent mortality, but this was less than 0.5 per cent in those over 2 years.

Satisfactory gradient reduction (less than 50 mmHg) was achieved in 96 per cent of the patients, though right ventricular hypertrophy and cardiomegaly persisted in a significant number of patients.

STENOSIS OF PULMONARY ARTERIAL BRANCHES

Stenosis may occur at any level within the branches of the right or left pulmonary arteries. Most commonly these are seen in the main left or right pulmonary arteries.

The operations

Bypass is instituted. For left pulmonary artery stenosis a patch of pericardium may be sewn over an incision in the stenosis to provide a normal channel without clamping the aorta.

8

When the right main pulmonary artery is affected the aorta is clamped and divided. A longitudinal incision is made in the vessel over the stenotic area.

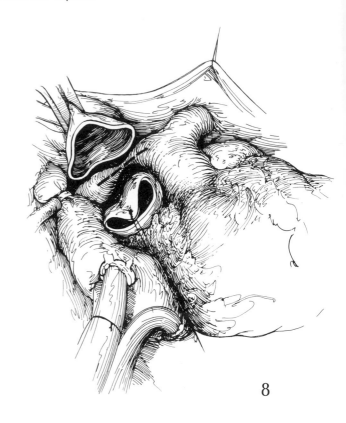

8

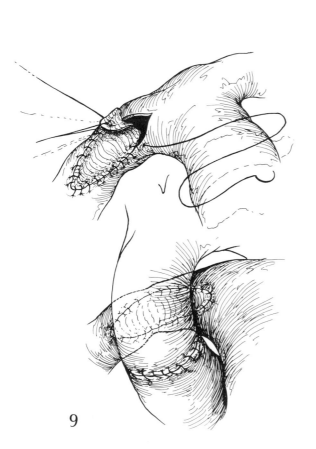

9

9

The vessel is widened with a patch of pericardium, though prosthetic material may be used if this is not available. After a haemostatic repair has been effected aortic continuity is restored and bypass discontinued.

References

1. Bull, C., de Leval, M. R., Mercanti, C., MaCartney, F. J., Anderson, R. H. Pulmonary atresia and intact ventricular septum: a revised classification. Circulation 1982; 66: 266–272

2. Goor, D. A., Lillehei, C. W. Congenital Malformations of the Heart. New York: Grune and Stratton, 1975; 11

3. Nugent, W. E., Freedom, R. M., Nora, J. J., Ellison, R. C., Rowe, R. D., Nadas, A. S. Clinical course in pulmonary stenosis. Circulation 1977; 56: (Suppl. 1) 38–47

4. Moulaert, A. J., Buis-Liem, T. N., Geldof, W. Ch., Rohmer, J. The postvalvotomy propranolol test to determine reversibility of the residual gradient in pulmonary stenosis. Journal of Thoracic and Cardiovascular Surgery 1976; 71: 865–868

Congenital aortic stenosis

Pietro A. Abbruzzese MD
Chief Resident, Division of Cardiopulmonary Surgery, Oregon Health Sciences University, Oregon, USA

Albert Starr MD
Professor of Surgery and Chief, Division of Cardiopulmonary Surgery, Oregon Health Sciences University, Oregon, USA

Introduction

With an incidence of approximately 5 per cent of all congenital cardiac abnormalities, aortic stenosis includes a range of left ventricular outflow tract obstructions at different levels and of unequal severity. Severe aortic stenosis in the newborn may be a variation of the more complex, surgically unresolved, hypoplastic left heart syndrome.

This chapter describes: (1) aortic commissurotomy as treatment for *valvular stenosis* (see Chapter on 'Treatment of aortic valve disease', pp. 446–453 for aortic valve replacement); (2) resection of *subvalvular fibrous stenosis* with or without concomitant myotomy or myectomy; (3) patch enlargement of the aortic root in the non-coronary sinus[1] for *discrete supravalvular stenosis*. The 'Morrow procedure'[2] for *idiopathic hypertrophic subaortic stenosis* is described in the Chapter on 'Hypertrophic subaortic stenosis', pp. 435–445. Optional surgical approaches are briefly considered. The controversial role of surgery for *diffuse supravalvular stenosis* is discussed, and procedures for a *narrow aortic root* and for obstruction at multiple levels are mentioned.

Indications

In the newborn and in infants severe stenosis presents with congestive heart failure and often with diminished cardiac output and cardiovascular instability, thus requiring urgent or emergency commissurotomy. In children, fatigue, angina and exertional dyspnoea are common symptoms and a gradient of at least 50 mmHg or a valve area index of $0.7 cm^2/m^2$ or less are commonly accepted indications for surgery. The well known risk of sudden death prompts surgical intervention in patients with a history of syncopal episodes or with a strain pattern on electrocardiography, even with lesser gradients across the left ventricular outflow tract.

Patients with diffuse supravalvular stenosis must be individually assessed and surgery, which has had disappointing results, must be considered with caution. Left and right heart catheterization is indicated in the evaluation of all patients to define the extent and the level(s) of obstruction as well as the often associated anomalies.

Preoperative

Stabilization of haemodynamic (prostaglandins, inotropic drugs), metabolic (sodium bicarbonate) and respiratory (mechanical ventilation) factors should be attempted in the ill infant, but surgery should not be delayed. Routine preoperative preparation of all patients includes administration of digitalis to decrease the incidence of postoperative arrhythmias (half the digitalizing dose is given during the 24 hours before surgery).

Anaesthesia

While the anaesthetic management of moderate aortic stenosis does not differ from that of other open heart procedures, critical aortic stenosis poses a serious challenge to the anaesthetist. A decrease in the perfusion pressure in the aortic root in these patients may impair coronary flow. Therefore induction is obtained with small doses of diazepam and ketamine, and anaesthesia is maintained with a light mixture of nitrous oxide and oxygen. If hypotension occurs a pure alpha-adrenergic drug such as phenylephrine is administered to increase peripheral vascular resistance and coronary blood flow rapidly. Opposite considerations apply to the management of idiopathic hypertrophic subaortic stenosis, in which the negative inotropic effect of barbiturates and halothane is used to lessen the severity of the dynamic obstruction.

The operations

The heart is approached through a standard median sternotomy incision. The ascending aorta is separated from the pulmonary artery with sharp dissection and is encircled with a Dacron tape. Cannulation of the transverse aortic arch or of the external iliac artery may be necessary in cases of diffuse supravalvular stenosis. Cardiopulmonary bypass is started and the patient's nasopharyngeal temperature is lowered to 26–28°C. An apical vent catheter is inserted, usually positioned beneath the aortic valve, and is connected to gentle suction. The ascending aorta is cross-clamped, the heart is electrically fibrillated and cardioplegic solution is given through the aortic root and drained into the heart-lung machine. We have found the frequently associated mild aortic regurgitation not to be a significant obstacle for root infusion of cardioplegics. The adipose tissue overlying the aortic root is sharply dissected and retracted inferiorly and the repair is begun.

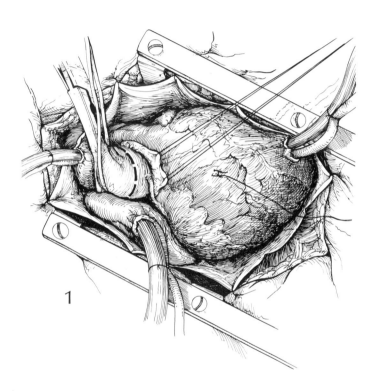

VALVULAR STENOSIS

1

A transverse aortotomy is started 1–2 cm above the ostium of the right coronary artery and is extended towards the commissure between the right and left cusps on the left and towards the centre of the non-coronary sinus on the right. Adequate exposure of the aortic valve is obtained with leaflet retractors held by the second assistant in the right and non-coronary sinuses. In infants, two fine forceps gently holding back the aortic adventitia provide the same exposure.

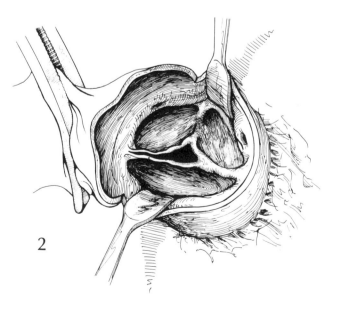

2

The valvular anatomy is assessed. Most frequently a bicuspid valve will be found, with the right coronary cusp fused to one of the other two. A primitive commissure (raphe) with various degrees of development will identify the two fused cusps. The commissure between the left and non-coronary cusps will be partially or completely open and the other well developed commissure will be fused.

3

Each well developed commissure is incised back to the annulus with a sawing motion of a No. 11 scalpel, the surgeon holding the leaflet closest to him and the first assistant the opposite one.

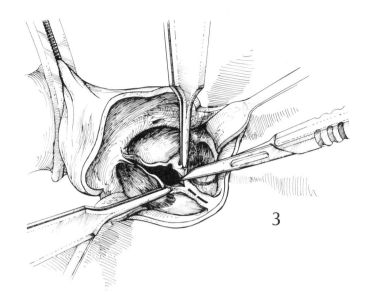

3

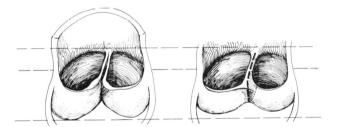

4a

4b

4a & b

The rudimentary commissure is then assessed and a decision whether or not to incise it is based on its degree of development and the depth of the corresponding sinuses. The commissure in the unicusp is usually vestigial (a). This should not be incised as aortic regurgitation will result. If the raphe is well developed (b) it may be incised safely.

Similar considerations will guide the incisions in the cases of monocuspid or tricuspid valves. A single incision should be made in the case of a diaphragm without recognizable commissures. After a satisfactory commissurotomy is obtained the subvalvular area is inspected to rule out the presence of subvalvular stenosis.

5

The aortotomy is closed with running 5/0 or 6/0 monofilament sutures started at each corner and tied in the mid portion of the incision. A closed aortic valvotomy has been used in very ill infants with satisfactory late results[3].

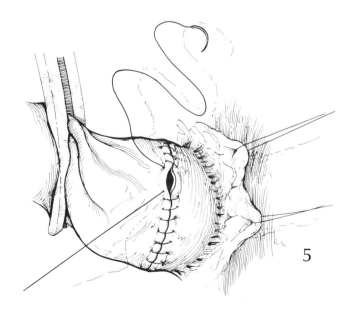

5

SUBVALVULAR FIBROUS STENOSIS

6

A transverse incision is made as previously described. After the valvular anatomy has been assessed the subvalvular structures are exposed with leaflet retractors holding back the right and non-coronary leaflets. The variable relationships of the 'membrane' to the surrounding structures – namely, the aortic valve, the anterior leaflet of the mitral valve and the ventricular septum in the area of the bundle of His – are assessed. The extent of fibromuscular septal hypertrophy is defined.

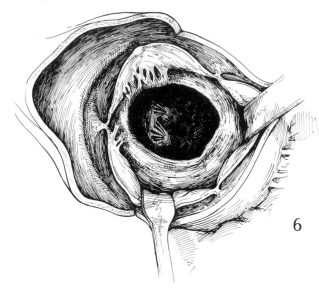

6

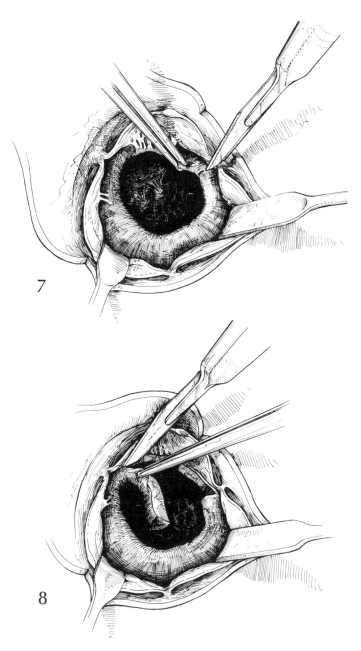

7

8

7 & 8

The 'membrane', or more precisely the fibrous collar, is grasped with toothed forceps anteriorly, next to the commissure between the right and left cusps, and is pulled inwards and downwards to define its insertion line. A No. 11 scalpel is used to incise it from its base to the free margin and then to start its excision counter-clockwise along the free wall of the ventricle to the anterior leaflet of the mitral valve and clockwise along the septum, carefully avoiding injury to the bundle of His. The excision is completed along the anterior leaflet of the mitral valve with scissors while gentle upward retraction on the membrane is exerted for better separation of the two structures. Frequently the membrane can be 'peeled off' partially or *in toto* as a natural cleavage plane exists between it and the surrounding structures.

9

When necessary a myotomy or a wedge myectomy is performed in the septal area underlying the left half of the right coronary cusp. The incision or excision is performed with a No. 15 scalpel, stabbing the septum at the desired depth (approximately 5 mm) and carrying the incision(s) towards the lumen. The aortotomy is closed as previously described.

Rare variations

The rare mitral webs, clefts and blebs as a cause of subvalvular aortic stenosis[4] need individual assessment and often require mitral valve replacement. The problem of subaortic tunnel stenosis and its surgical management is largely unresolved and will be discussed together with multiple level obstructions and narrow aortic root.

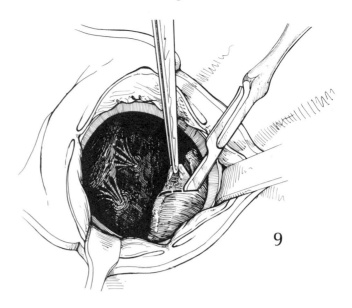

9

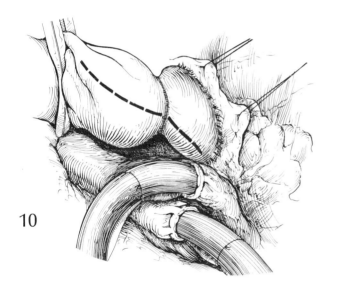

10

SUPRAVALVULAR STENOSIS

10

An oblique aortotomy incision is started 2 cm beyond the stenotic area and, through the narrowed segment, is extended into the non-coronary sinus to 1 cm from the line of insertion of the cusp. In most cases the stenosis is evident externally as a circumferential indentation that gives the ascending aorta an hourglass appearance.

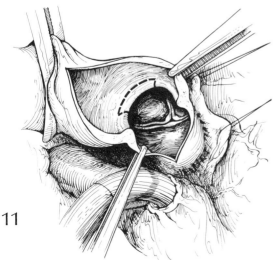

11

11

Internally a fibrous ridge is found just above the commissures and crowds them together, partially impairing valvular function and infrequently restricting coronary blood flow. When possible the ridge is partially excised with pointed scissors in the area above the left coronary cusp. This usually frees the commissures of that cusp, improving the leaflet's motion (and the left coronary blood flow).

12

An oval patch, previously tailored from a pre-clotted tubular woven Dacron prosthesis, is then sutured to the aortotomy with continuous 4/0 or 5/0 Prolene from the non-coronary sinus upwards along both edges. The width of the patch corresponding to the stenosed area is calculated by subtraction of the circumference of the stenosed segment from that of the normal aorta. Teflon strips may be required to reinforce the suture line if the aortic wall is very thin in the area of the non-coronary sinus.

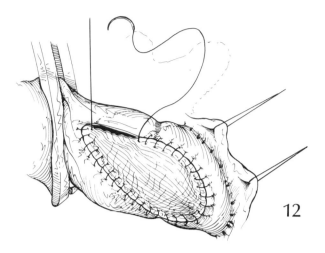

12

Alternative techniques

Patch enlargement of the aorta into both the right and the non-coronary sinuses is an alternative treatment[5]. Rarely a perforated diaphragm is found in an externally normal aorta and is easily resected with primary closure of the aortotomy. In the presence of the diffuse type of supravalvular stenosis the patch repair can be extended to the origin of the innominate artery or further, care being taken to protect the cerebral circulation[6]. A left ventricle-to-aorta conduit may be considered as an alternative method in this case [7].

NARROW AORTIC ROOT AND MULTIPLE LEVEL OBSTRUCTIONS

When a narrow aortic annulus significantly contributes to or is the main cause of the left ventricular outflow tract obstruction, or if a tunnel subaortic stenosis is present, we have employed aortoventriculoplasty[8,9] and mechanical valve replacement. Other methods of annular enlargement have been recommended[10-11]. A left ventricle-to-aortic conduit may be a satisfactory alternative in multiple level obstructions and in tunnel subaortic stenosis.

References

1. Starr, A., Dotter, C., Griswold, H. Supravalvular aortic stenosis: diagnosis and treatment. Journal of Thoracic and Cardiovascular Surgery 1961; 41: 134–140

2. Morrow, A. G., Reitz, B. A., Epstein, S. E. *et al.* Operative treatment in hypertrophic subaortic stenosis: techniques and the results of pre- and post operative assessments in 83 patients. Circulation, 1975; 52: 88–102

3. Trinkle, J. K., Grover, F. L., Arom, K. V. Closed aortic valvotomy in infants: late results. Journal of Thoracic and Cardiovascular Surgery 1978; 76: 198–201

4. Goor, D. A., Lillehei, C. W. Congenital Malformations of the Heart: Embryology, Anatomy and Operative Considerations. New York: Grune & Stratton, 1975

5. Doty, D. B., Polansky, D. B., Jenson, C. B. Supravalvular aortic stenosis: repair by extended aortoplasty. Journal of Thoracic and Cardiovascular Surgery 1977; 74: 362–371

6. Merin, G., Copperman, I. J., Borman, J. B. Surgical correction of diffuse supravalvular aortic stenosis involving the branches of the aortic arch. Chest, 1976; 70: 546–549

7. Cooley, D. A., Norman, J. C., Mullins, C. E., Grace, R. R. Left ventricle to abdominal aorta conduit for relief of aortic stenosis. Cardiovasc. Dis., Bull. Texas Heart Inst., 1975; 2: 367–383

8. Rastan, H., Koncz, J. Aortoventriculoplasty: a new technique for the treatment of left ventricular outflow tract obstruction. Journal of Thoracic and Cardiovascular Surgery 1976; 71: 920–927

9. Konno, S., Imai, Y., Lida, Y., Nakajima, M., Tetsuno, K. A new method for prosthetic valve replacement in congenital aortic stenosis associated with hypoplasia of the aortic valve ring. Journal of Thoracic and Cardiovascular Surgery 1975; 70: 909–917

10. Manouguian, S., Seybold-Epting, W. Patch enlargement of the aortic valve ring by extending the aortic incision into the anterior mitral leaflet: new operative technique. Journal of Thoracic and Cardiovascular Surgery 1979; 78: 402

11. Mori, T., Kawashima, Y., Kitamura, S., Nakano, S., Kawachi, K., Nakata, T. Results of aortic valve replacement in patients with a narrow arotic annulus: effects of enlargement of the aortic annulus. Annals of Thoracic Surgery 1981; 31: 111–116

Rashkind procedures

William J. Rashkind MD
Director, Cardiovascular Laboratories, The Children's Hospital of Philadelphia, One Children's Center, Philadelphia, Pennsylvania, USA

BALLOON ATRIOSEPTOSTOMY

The technique of balloon atrioseptostomy was first reported by Rashkind and Miller in 1966. The primary purpose of the procedure is to produce an atrial septal defect to increase intracardiac mixing or to decompress either atrial chamber. Thus it is used to increase mixing in transposition of the great arteries, to decompress the left atrium in mitral atresia or to decompress the right atrium in tricuspid atresia, pulmonary atresia with intact ventricular septum or total anomalous pulmonary venous return to the right side of the heart. It is of particular importance that the procedure can be performed as part of the diagnostic catheterization, thus minimizing delay in the treatment of critically ill infants.

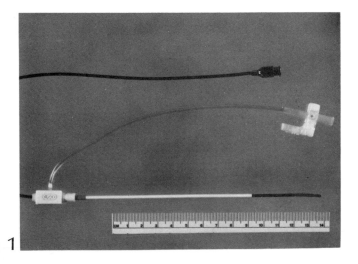

1

Equipment

A special balloon-tipped catheter is used for the procedure. Initially a double-lumen catheter was used to assist in localization of the balloon in the left atrium. However, the widespread availability of biplane fluoroscopy has obviated the need for a second lumen. The current equipment, therefore, is a single-lumen balloon-tipped catheter, generally 4.5–6F, which can be introduced via a 6F sheath.

The operation

Cardiac catherization is performed in the usual manner to achieve a complete diagnosis.

2 & 3

After the diagnosis has been established the balloon-tipped catheter is passed via the sheath into the inferior vena cava and the right atrium and then across the foramen ovale into the left atrium.

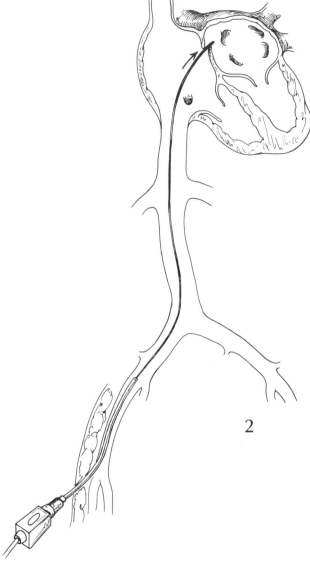

2

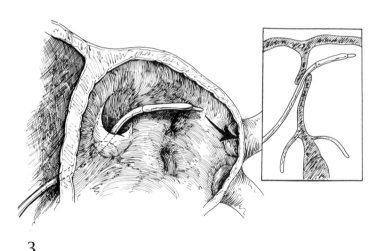

3

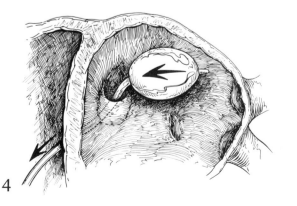

4

4

The balloon is then slowly dilated with dilute radio-opaque material. If the balloon happens to be in a pulmonary vein slow dilatation will result in the balloon being extruded to lie free in the left atrial chamber. Once it is certain that the catheter tip is in the left atrium the balloon is inflated to a volume of approximately 2 ml or to a diameter of approximately 15 mm.

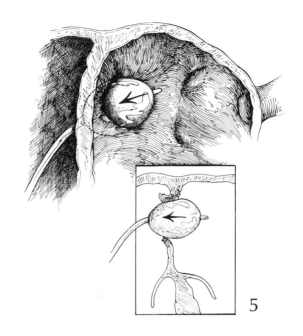

5 & 6

At this point the catheter is vigorously jerked through the atrial septum into the right atrium, care being taken not to wedge it into the inferior cava. It is allowed to float free in the right atrial chamber while the balloon is deflated. The success of the procedure is directly proportional to the strength of the jerk at the end of the catheter.

5

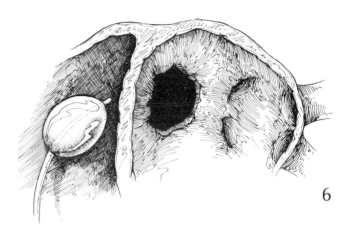

6

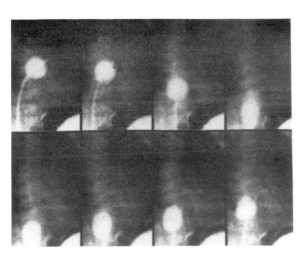

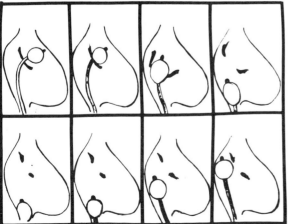

7

7

The upper half of this illustration shows a septostomy in consecutive frames from a 30/sec cineangiogram and the lower half represents the same frames shown diagramatically.

Adequacy of the atrial septal defect can be determined by sizing the defect with a balloon-tipped catheter (see below), measuring the change in atrial pressure gradient, determining the arterial oxygenation saturation or echocardiographic measurement of the size of the defect.

TRANSCATHETER CLOSURE OF ATRIAL SEPTAL DEFECTS

Equipment

The prosthesis consists of a six-rib skeleton. The ribs (or arms) are fashioned of 0.01-inch (0.25-mm) springs fastened to a stainless steel hub. The spring arms have helical turns at the hub band to permit proper recoil from a folded position. The other end of each alternate rib terminates in a small barbed hook. In addition, small eyes are formed at the terminal ends of all six ribs to permit anchoring the foam matrix. The hub is precisely machined to be an integral part of the delivery system. The spring arms are covered by a fine-mesh, open cell foam sheet sewn into place. The delivery system consists of a standard 6F catheter with a locking tip at its distal end. The locking tip mechanism consists of an expanding sleeve 0.05 inch (1.3 mm) in diameter which interlocks with the hub of the closure disc. The sleeve is expanded by means of a helical guide wire 0.035 inch (1 mm) in diameter. The catheter and closure disc, when threaded on to the guide wire, fix the disc hub to the locking tip while allowing free axial motion of the assembly along the guide wire. Removal of the guide wire allows the closure disc to be freed from the locking tip.

The current method of constraining the folded disc is to use a thin-walled catheter flared into a restraining pod at its distal end. This has the approximate calibre of 10–12F and will permit the entire prosthesis to be collapsed within it. The proximal end is fitted with a double 0 ring locking mechanism which surrounds the helical spring wire and a side arm with a Luer-Lock tip which permits flushing of the entire system before, during and after operation. This mechanism excludes air from the system and allows for flushing any blood that may come into the system without any blood loss from the distal end of the catheter. Thus the entire system is self-contained and prevents blood loss and the possibility of air embolization. There is a centring mechanism which is fashioned in a similar manner to the skeleton of the prosthesis. A central stainless steel hub is welded to the locking tip approximately 15 mm from the tip. It has five side arms bent into outward gentle curves. The portion near the hub is connected to the hub via a spring mechanism identical to that of the prosthesis. In operation the arms are collapsed inside the carrying pod catheter. When extruded from the pod they spring open and provide a funnel shape. On retraction of the entire system the centring device funnels the prosthesis (which is just distal to it) over the atrial septal defect and permits anchoring of the hooks in the proper portion of the atrial septum.

The operation

The procedure is performed in the cardiac catheterization laboratory. The patient is sedated with morphine (0.1 mg/kg) and pentobarbitone (pentobarbital) (4 mg/kg). Complete cardiac catheterization is performed to determine the accuracy of the diagnosis, the location of the defect and its size. In each patient selective cineangiograms are obtained with contrast injection into the left atrium with the patient in 30° left anterior oblique position. This view has proved satisfactory in placing the atrial septum on end and permits good visualization of the defect.

Sizing of the defect is performed in the following manner. A balloon-tipped catheter is passed across the atrial septal defect and inflated in the left atrium with a dilute contrast solution. Gentle traction is applied to the balloon until it is impacted in the defect. The balloon is then slowly deflated until it barely passes through the defect. The residual volume of the contrast material in the balloon is carefully measured and recorded. The balloon-tipped catheter is then removed from the patient, the balloon reinflated with the same volume of solution and its diameter measured. The use of this manoeuvre not only permits accurate sizing of the defect but also permits its accurate location since a strip of cineangiogram is recorded with the inflated balloon in place in the defect.

In addition a meticulous effort is made to preclude the possibility of anomalous pulmonary venous return to the right atrium. This is accomplished in two ways. First, both right and left pulmonary veins are explored with a catheter to be sure that they connect directly with the left atrium. If there is any residual question about this the balloon-tipped catheter is used to occlude the atrial septal defect and oxygen contents are measured in the superior vena cava, inferior vena cava and right atrium. If there is no elevation in oxygen content in the right atrium one may assume that anomalous pulmonary venous drainage into the right atrium has been excluded.

When the operator is satisfied that the defect is of appropriate size, shape and location to warrant transcatheter closure the entire system is introduced and delivered as described above. Heparinization (50 mg/kg) is started immediately before the procedure. The femoral vein is exposed, or a large sheath is placed percutaneously, and the entire delivery system is inserted. This consists of a carrying catheter with pod tip, collapsed prosthesis within the pod, collet-tipped carrying catheter and helical spring wire.

8

The tip of the device is passed across the atrial septal defect into the left atrium. With the tip of the system in the centre of the left atrium the prosthesis and its connecting system are held rigidly in place while the carrying sheath is retracted, thereby retracting the pod from the prosthesis.

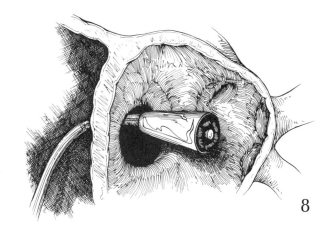

8

9

The prosthesis, still firmly anchored to the collet tip of the carrying catheter, springs open. The pod-tipped catheter is further retracted, allowing the centring mechanism to spring open. Rapid traction on the delivery catheter results in the centring mechanism funnelling the prosthesis into place directly over the defect.

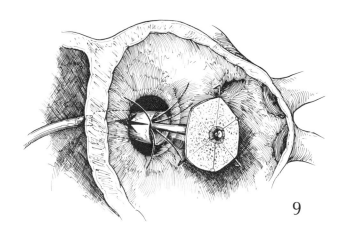

9

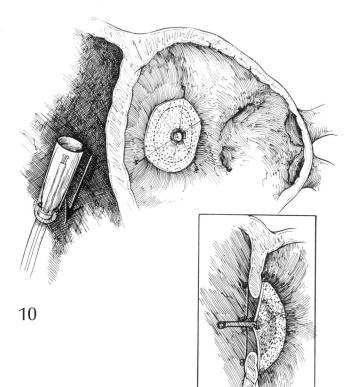

10

10

Firm traction on the delivery catheter imbeds the hooks of the prosthesis into the atrial septum. Retrograde pressure is exerted against the prosthesis by the carrying catheter to ensure that the hooks are firmly in place. When the anchoring of all three hooks is certain the helical spring wire is removed from the collet catheter. This permits the collet tip to collapse and allows it to be removed from the hub of the prosthesis, thus releasing the prosthesis. The entire delivery system is then removed.

TRANSCATHETER CLOSURE OF PERSISTENT DUCTUS ARTERIOSUS (HOOKED PROSTHESIS)

11

Equipment

The prosthesis consists of a stainless steel miniature grappling hook skeleton which is filled with a cone of medical grade foam. Each of the three limbs of the grappling hook connects to the central hub by a spring which permits the three arms to be collapsed against each other. Each arm also has a small joint near its hook end which permits the end of each arm to be folded upon itself. A loading device similar to that previously described for the atrial septal defect prosthesis enables the prosthesis to be collapsed so that it can be carried in a sheath of approximately 8F calibre. The apices of the three arms are welded together and terminate in a small loop.

This loop permits attachment to a pin-and-sleeve release mechanism. The pin is passed through the loop of the prosthesis and both are retracted into a sleeve which prevents release. The sleeve can be retracted only by a positive manoeuvre on the part of the operator; accidental release is impossible. The entire system is carried within a catheter sheath with a 15 mm thin-walled metal tube pod at the tip. This pod serves as a receptacle for the collapsed prosthesis. The opposite end of the carrying catheter is sealed by an 0 ring and has a side arm which permits flushing of the carrying catheter to prevent air embolization and accumulation of blood in the system.

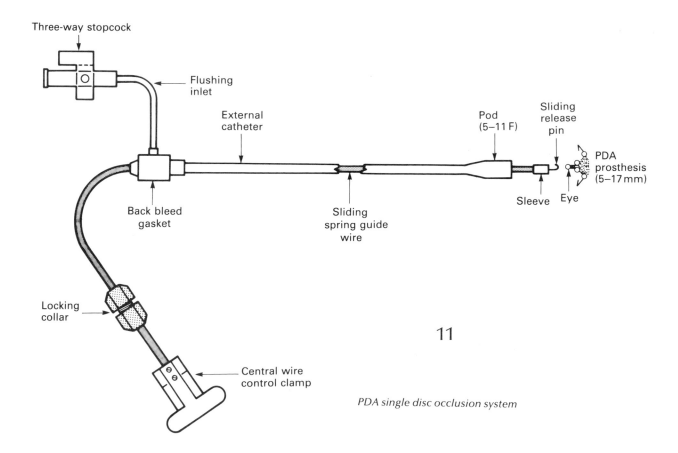

11

PDA single disc occlusion system

The operation

The procedure is performed in the cardiac catheterization laboratory. The patient is sedated with morphine (0.1 mg/kg) and pentobarbitone (pentobarbital) (4 mg/kg). General anaesthesia is *not* used. Biplane aortograms are obtained in the posteroanterior and lateral views to demonstrate the location, size and shape of the ductus. Heparinization (50 mg/kg) is started.

12, 13 & 14

The prosthesis, inside the delivery system, is introduced into the femoral artery, passed retrograde into the thoracic aorta and manipulated into the ductus arteriosus.

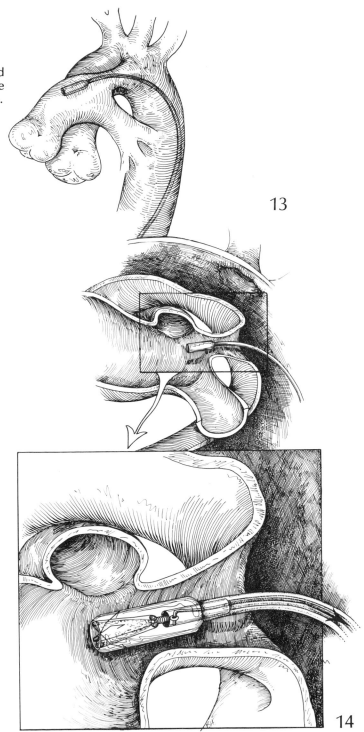

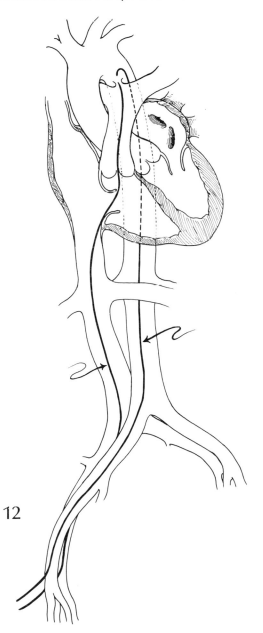

12

13

14

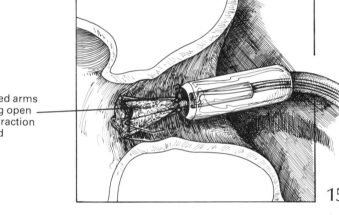

Outer pod only
is retracted

Hooked arms
spring open
on retraction
of pod

15

15

The prosthesis is extruded from the catheter and allowed
to expand in the ductus. Gentle but firm traction on the
carrying device is used to imbed the hooks into the wall of
the ductus.

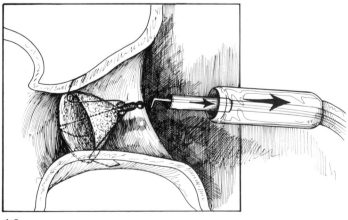

16

16

When the prosthesis is properly and firmly seated the
transporting catheter system is detached and removed
from the femoral artery.

TRANSCATHETER CLOSURE OF PERSISTENT DUCTUS ARTERIOSUS (DOUBLE-DISC PROSTHESIS)

Equipment

This persistent ductus occluder system consists of two major components, the delivery system and the occluder. The occluder is made up of two sets of spring-loaded parallel ribs and a capture eye bound together. Each set of ribs consists of three ribs spaced 120° apart. Two foam discs are positioned between the two sets of ribs and sutured, one to each set of ribs. The capture eye allows the prosthesis to be securely attached to the delivery system via the pin-and-sleeve release assembly.

The delivery system consists of several items. The wire control clamp serves to control the movement of the release pin and hence the release of the occluder after its extrusion from the pod into which it has been collapsed. The prosthesis is collapsed inside the pod with each set of ribs pointing in opposite directions. A locknut provides a fail-safe device which prohibits the inadvertent release of the occluder from its delivery pod. The backbleed gasket assembly prevents loss of blood through the delivery catheter. It also permits flushing of the system via the three-way stopcock to prevent air embolization and accumulation of blood. The catheter itself is made from polyethylene tubing with an internal sliding control guide wire.

The operation

The procedure is performed in the cardiac catheterization laboratory. The patient is premedicated as indicated above. Biplane aortograms are obtained in the postero-anterior and lateral views to demonstrate the location, size and shape of the ductus. Heparin 50–100 u/kg is administered to the patient.

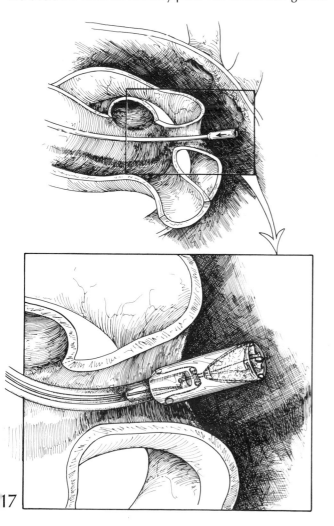

17

The prosthesis inside the delivery system is introduced into the femoral vein, passed antegrade into the pulmonary artery and manipulated across the ductus arteriosus.

18

The prosthesis is extruded from the catheter pod, allowing the distal set of ribs to expand in the aorta. Gentle traction is applied to the entire system until the distal set of ribs starts to funnel.

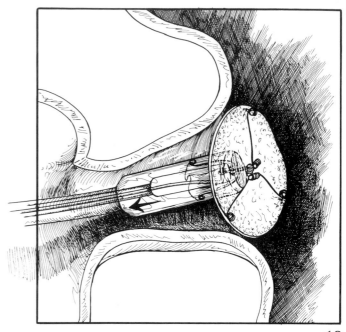

18

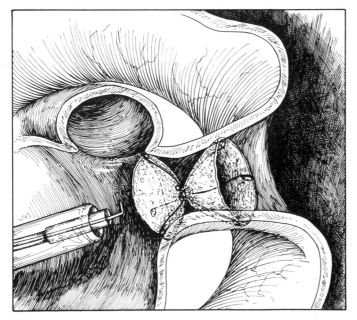

19

19

The system is fixed in that position and the pod is retracted from the proximal set of ribs. This anchors the entire prosthesis on both sides of the ductus. When the prosthesis is firmly seated the transporting catheter system is detached, the pin is retracted into the sleeve and the entire delivery system is removed from the femoral artery.

Complete transposition: surgical anatomy

Robert H. Anderson   BSc, MD, MRCPath
Joseph Levy Professor of Paediatric Cardiac Morphology, Cardiothoracic Institute, Brompton Hospital, London, UK

Introduction

Complete transposition of the great arteries is the congenital malformation which results from the abnormal chamber connections of atrioventricular concordance and ventriculoarterial discordance. Thus the morphologically right atrium connects to the morphologically right ventricle and thence to the aorta, while the morphologically left atrium is connected to the morphologically left ventricle and thence to the pulmonary trunk.

Since the lesion depends upon the presence of morphologically right and left atrial chambers it cannot by definition exist in the presence of atrial isomerism (visceral heterotaxy). Ventriculoarterial discordance ('transposition') can and does exist with visceral heterotaxy, but the picture is then dominated by the other associated malformations which characterize atrial isomerism. For this reason we consider it best to separate this type of ventriculoarterial discordance from that which we term *complete* transposition. Similarly, ventriculoarterial discordance can be found with atrioventricular discordance and this variant is distinguished as 'congenitally corrected transposition'. Ventriculoarterial discordance can also exist in the presence of a univentricular atrioventricular connection, particularly with either double-inlet left ventricle or·classical tricuspid atresia. Here it is the abnormal atrioventricular connections which predominate, so again we believe it best to separate these types of 'transposition' from the subject of this chapter.

It is also worthy of note that for many years the term 'transposition' was defined in terms of arterial relationship – namely, that in which the aorta was anterior to the 'crista' or its remnant[1]. When used in this fashion it was entirely logical to speak of 'double-outlet right ventricle with transposition' – that is, a heart with a double-outlet connection in which the aorta was in anterior position. This would clearly be a *non sequitur* in the convention as used at present, which places most emphasis on the connections of cardiac structures. It is for this reason that we choose not to define the discordant ventriculoarterial connection *itself* as a 'transposition' since we respect the logic which permits others to use the term for description of the arterial relationship. Nonetheless, we consider it entirely right and proper to define the combination of atrioventricular concordance and ventriculoarterial discordance as *complete transposition*.

Since this definition takes account only of the connections it is to be expected that there will be variability of relationships within this group of lesions, and this is indeed the case. Both this and the variation which exists in infundibular morphology will be described along with the significant associated lesions which colour so much the presentation of complete transposition. But we will start this section by accounting for the basic chamber connections which are the essence of the lesion.

Simple transposition

THE ATRIA, NODES AND CONDUCTION PATHWAYS

The atrial chambers are basically normal in complete transposition. In keeping with this the dispositions of the sinus node and atrioventricular node are also normal. It is significant in this respect, however, to keep in mind the variability of blood supply to the sinus node. As in the normal heart, the sinus node artery can arise from either the right or left coronary artery. Recent studies have shown that this origin can be very close to the origin of the coronary artery itself from the aorta, or in some instances the sinus node artery may have a separate origin from the aortic sinus[2].

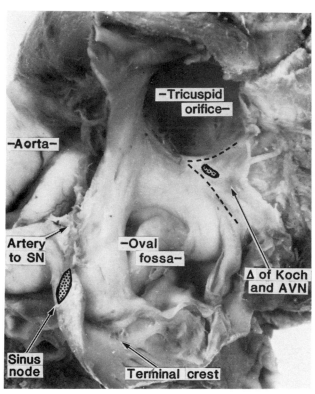

Figure 1. A dissection of the atrial septum showing the course of the sinus node artery through the superior margin of the oval fossa on its route to the node

1

Also of note is the fact that the sinus node (SN) artery often buries itself in the superior margin of the oval fossa as it courses towards the atriocaval junction (Figure 1) or alternatively crosses the lateral margin of the atrial appendage, then taking origin much more distally from the right coronary artery[3]. After the nodal artery has reached the cavoatrial junction there is then further variability in that it may cross the crest of the appendage to reach the terminal sulcus, may pass retrocavally or, alternatively, may divide to form an arterial circle around the cavoatrial junction (see chapter on 'Anatomy of congenital heart disease', pp. 88–106).

The sinus node (SN) itself almost always lies laterally within the terminal sulcus but may rarely be draped across the crest of the appendage in horseshoe fashion. All of this points to the major vulnerability of the entire cavoatrial junction in complete transposition.

There is now little doubt that it was trauma to the sinus node and/or its blood supply which underlay the numerous arrhythmias observed after atrial correction[4]. It has been shown that scrupulous attention to the preservation of these vital structures can more or less eradicate postoperative rhythm problems[5, 6], particularly when it is noted that some of the arrhythmias are present before the operation[7].

2

The disposition of the atrioventricular node (AVN) is entirely normal, lying within the confines of the triangle of Koch (*Figure 2*). It remains worthy of comment that there are no insulated 'specialized' conduction pathways extending through the atrial musculature between the cardiac nodes. Internodal conduction occurs preferentially through the thick muscle bundles of the atrial chambers, taking the shortest distance between the nodes. Thus the pathways of significance are the terminal crest and the superior margin of the oval fossa. The mapping studies of Wittig, de Leval and Stark[8] showed the advantages of preserving at least one of these pathways. The possible presence of the sinus node artery within the superior margin of the fossa suggests that this may be the better pathway to preserve, particularly since division of the terminal crest may be indicated in enlargement of the new pulmonary venous atrium during the Mustard procedure.

The oval fossa is almost always either patent or deficient in complete transposition, and nowadays the surgeon will usually find the floor of the fossa ruptured by balloon septostomy. Other types of atrial septal defect may be found, although they are rare, as are anomalies of venous connection[9].

A significant anomaly which occurs with some frequency is juxtaposition of the atrial apendages. This distorts the septal anatomy, displacing the oval fossa into posterior position, and also reduces the amount of atrial tissue available for use during a Senning procedure. It should also be noted that the atrial chambers are both of smaller capacity when left atrial isomerism is present. This is another good reason, along with the anomalous location of the sinus node, for distinguishing ventriculoarterial discordance in this setting from complete transposition[10]. Apart from the atrial septal deficiencies and the rare occurrence of total anomalous pulmonary venous connection the left atrium is anatomically normal in complete transposition.

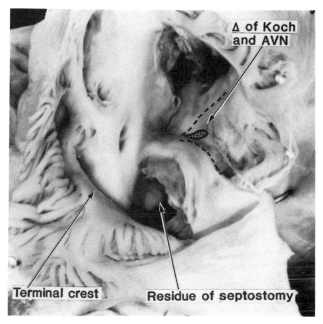

Figure 2. The opened right atrium photographed in surgical orientation to show the landmarks of the triangle of Koch and the site of the atrioventricular node

ATRIOVENTRICULAR JUNCTION

When one turns to the atrioventricular junction with a critical eye there are subtle differences between complete transposition and the normal heart. Thus the pulmonary valve in complete transposition is not as deeply wedged between the atrioventricular valves as is the aortic valve in the normal heart. As a consequence the tricuspid and mitral valves are attached to the septum at more or less the same level and over a greater distance so that the atrioventricular septum is less well formed or even absent[11]. However, these differences are unlikely to be of surgical significance. Neither are the minimal differences which exist in the morphology of the mitral and tricuspid valves and their tension apparatus when complete transposition is compared with the normal heart[12, 13].

THE VENTRICLES AND GREAT ARTERIES

3a & b

The major difference to be found in ventricular morphology is in the outlets. The aorta almost always arises from the morphologically right ventricle supported by a complete muscular infundibulum, while the pulmonary trunk arises from the morphologically left ventricle with fibrous continuity between its valve and the mitral valve (*Figure 3*). Rarely both valves may be supported by complete muscular outlet components. Even more rarely, particularly in the presence of a posterior aorta and a ventricular septal defect, there may be a complete subpulmonary infundibulum and aortic mitral fibrous continuity in the roof of the defect. The significant point of outlet morphology is that almost always the outlet part of the septum is in line with the rest of the septum. Consequently the entire ventricles are much more side by side than is found in the normal heart.

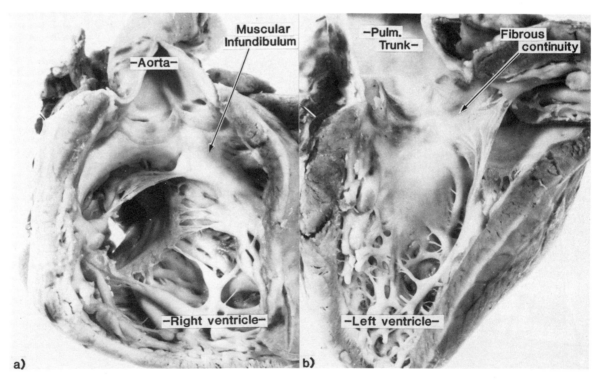

Figure 3. The aortic valve arising from the morphologically right ventricle (a) usually has a complete muscular infundibulum while the pulmonary valve, connected to the morphologically left ventricle (b), is usually in fibrous continuity with the mitral valve

4a & b

Considerable variability is found in the relationships of the great arteries. In about three-fifths of cases the aorta is anterior and to the right of the pulmonary trunk (PT) (*Figure 4a*). In about one-fifth it is anterior and to the left of the pulmonary trunk (*Figure 4b*)[14]. In rarer, isolated cases, almost always in the presence of a ventricular septal defect, the great arteries may be side by side with the aorta to the right or the aorta may be posterior and right-sided, the great arteries then spiralling round each other in 'normally related' fashion[15, 16].

It is this variability in arterial position which makes nonsense of the convention which attempts to describe complete transposition as 'D-transposition'. Apart from being a contravention of the originally intended usage of 'D-' and 'L-' as qualifiers of the abnormally connected aorta[17], the convention is scientifically inaccurate when used in the setting of complete transposition. Many examples of complete transposition possess a left-sided aorta – for example, the form which exists with mirror-image atrial arrangement. Many other anomalies which possess a right-sided aorta arising from the morphologically right ventricle are not examples of complete transposition. For all these reasons we cannot support the use of 'D-transposition' as a specific term for the group of hearts under discussion; the appropriate term is 'complete transposition'[18].

Although the general morphology of the ventricular mass is more or less comparable with that in the normal heart, the ventricular thicknesses deviate markedly from the normal and show quite different patterns of development. This is of considerable significance in relation to the timing of the arterial switch procedure should this be contemplated for correction of the anomaly in patients with an intact ventricular septum and no associated malformation such as persistent ductus arteriosus. The measurements of Smith *et al.*[19] showed that at birth the left ventricular wall was of equal thickness to or slightly thicker than that of the right ventricle in hearts with complete transposition. However, growth of the right ventricle in the first few months of life then rapidly outstripped that of the left ventricle in terms of wall thickness. Thus the optimal time for correction by arterial relocation in simple complete transposition is in the first days of life unless steps are taken to 'prepare' the left ventricle either by surgical procedures or by ensuring patency of the arterial duct with prostaglandins.

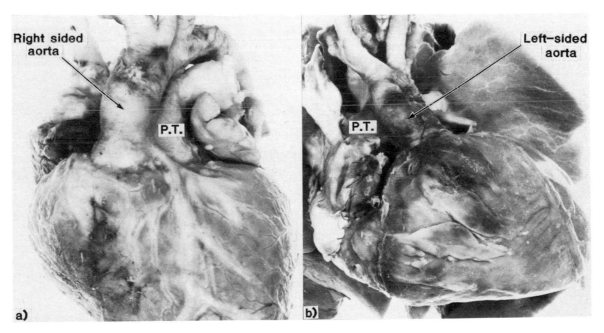

Figure 4. (a) shows the usual right-sided aortic position found in complete transposition. But, as seen in (b), the aorta can be unequivocally left-sided with this segmental combination

5

Also of note for potential arterial relocation is the arrangement of the coronary arteries. This is almost always favourable in the presence of an intact ventricular septum. Certain comparable patterns of this feature have been identified by various investigators[20-23]. Emerging from all these studies is the fact that almost without exception the coronary arteries emerge from the aortic sinuses which 'face' the pulmonary trunk as seen from the superior aspect in the dissection illustrated. This 'facing' may not be exact in terms of commissural position, but it is close enough readily to permit the transfer of the coronary arterial origins.

Difficulties may arise in the presence of origin of both coronary arteries from the same sinus or in the presence of a single coronary artery. These malformations seem to be found with most frequency when there is a ventricular septal defect and the great arteries are side by side[12]. The only other anatomical feature which may make transfer difficult is origin of the sinus node artery very close to the aortic sinus. To the best of our knowledge the possible dangers of this arrangement have yet to be evaluated.

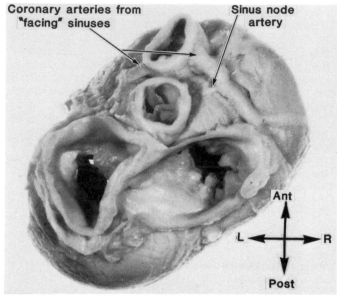

Figure 5. A dissection of the atrioventricular and ventriculoarterial junctions viewed from the superior aspect showing the origin of the coronary arteries from the aortic sinuses which face the pulmonary trunk

Complete transposition with ventricular spetal defect

6

The most significant lesion associated with complete transposition is a ventricular septal defect (VSD). Any of the types of defect encountered in other hearts (*see* chapter on 'Ventricular septal defect', pp. 215–221) can be found with this chamber combination. The anatomy is modified in complete transposition because the outlet septum is much more in line with the rest of the muscular septum. Thus the defect most frequently encountered is a malalignment defect, usually with the outlet septum to the right of the muscular septum (*Figure 6*). Such malalignment defects may have muscular posteroinferior rims, which protect the conduction tissue axis, or may extend to become perimembranous, when the axis is at risk in the posterioinferior fibrous margin. Often with these defects the tension apparatus of the tricuspid valve is attached across the defect, with anomalous papillary muscle attachments to the outlet septum. Also of note is the increasing divergence of the septal structures towards the anterior margin of the heart, making closure of the anterior quadrant of the defect more difficult.

Perimembranous defects may also extend into the inlet septum and then are hidden beneath the septal leaflet of the tricuspid valve. Equally significant inlet defects are those with overriding and straddling of the tricuspid valve together with those which are confined to the muscular inlet septum. Both of these have anomalous disposition of conduction tissue. With straddling tricuspid valve the node is displaced laterally to the point where the malaligned inlet septum joins the atrioventricular junction[24]. In muscular inlet defects the conduction axis runs anterior and cephalad[25]. Muscular defects may also be found in the apical trabecular septum, and these are often of the multiple 'Swiss cheese' type. The final defect to be found, particularly frequent in the presence of a left-sided aorta[26], is the doubly committed subarterial defect. The significance of this defect, roofed by the conjoined arterial valve rings, is the option it gives for direct connection of the aorta to the left ventricle, continuity between right ventricle and pulmonary trunk then being re-established with a conduit.

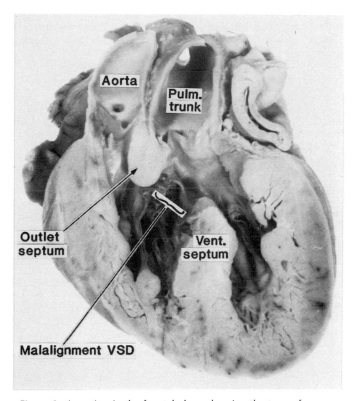

Figure 6. A section in the frontal plane showing the type of malalignment defect most typically found in complete transposition

Complete transposition with subpulmonary obstruction

7a & b

The second significant complicating lesion in complete transposition is stenosis of the subpulmonary outflow tract. Although this can occur at valve level, valvar obstruction is a very rare finding in isolation. Subpulmonary obstruction may occur in combination with a ventricular septal defect and is then most frequently due to posterior deviation of the outlet septum into the left ventricle (*Figure 7*). The defect in this situation can be found with a muscular inferior rim, which again protects

the conduction axis, or else can be perimembranous. This type of combination of ventricular septal defect and subpulmonary obstruction produces overriding of the left ventricle by the aorta and is the best anatomical combination for the Rastelli procedure. Usually the outflow to the aorta is sufficient in its native state, but if enlargement of the defect is necessary this can always be done safely by excising the outlet septum.

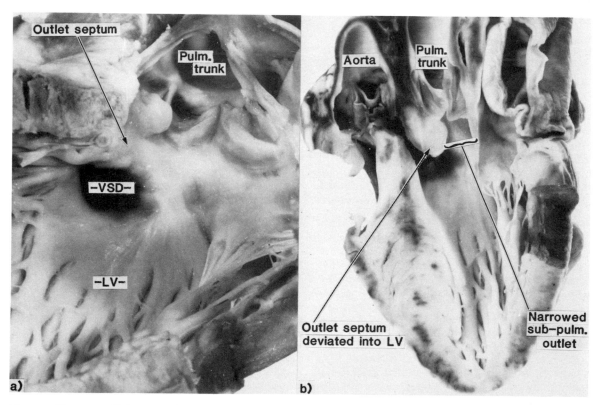

Figure 7. The opened left ventricular outflow tract in a specimen with subpulmonary obstruction due to a deviation of the outlet septum to the left. This is well shown in the long axis section of the same heart taken at right angles to the outlet septum

8

Subpulmonary obstruction with a ventricular septal defect can also be produced by any of the lesions which produce stenosis in isolation. These are a fibrous diaphragm, which in severe cases may become tunnel-like, fibrous tissue tags from the fibrous structures surrounding the outflow tract or anomalous attachment of papillary muscles across the tract (*Figure 8*). When relief of any of these lesions is contemplated the significant point to remember is the position of the left bundle branch on the septal surface of the outflow tract.

Also of note is the dynamic obstruction produced by bulging of the septum. Often this is more obvious in the autopsied heart and does not produce gradients during life. Nonetheless in some cases unequivocal obstruction may be present and the lesion then has all the features of hypertrophic cardiomyopathy. Dynamic obstruction of the outflow tract may be beneficial in the presence of an intact ventricular septum. This is because it may 'prepare' the ventricle and permit an arterial switch procedure, subsequently becoming inconsequential when the left ventricle assumes a systemic role. Yacoub has successfully operated on patients with this combination[27].

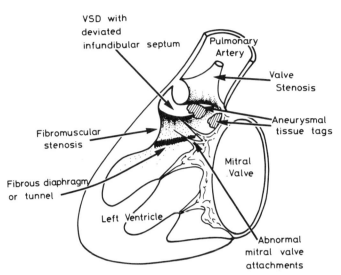

Figure 8. The different anatomical substrates of subpulmonary obstruction

Other associated malformations

Any other lesion can coexist with complete transposition when this is anatomically possible. Some are particularly important. Mention has already been made of juxtaposition of the atrial appendages and its significance for atrial redirection procedures. Persistent ductus arteriosus is important because it produces overload on the left ventricle and promotes its hypertrophy, thus producing natural 'preparation' of the ventricle and favouring an arterial switch procedure. Indeed, as discussed above, this combination may be so favourable as to make it worth while keeping the duct open with prostaglandins in the newborn period in preparation for arterial correction.

A lesion which has a much more deleterious effect on surgery is coarctation or interruption of the aortic arch.

This is usually associated with deviation of the outlet septum to the right, thus comprising the subaortic infundibulum[27]. As is so often the case with obstructive lesions of the aortic arch, the anatomical lesions indicate that most of the problem is within the ventricular mass. Repair of the arch lesion corrects only the tip of the iceberg. The other major problem in complete transposition which is of haemodynamic rather than anatomical origin is the development of pulmonary vascular disease. This is of great surgical significance particularly in the presence of a ventricular septal defect, when irreversible changes are frequently established by the age of 6 months.

References

1. Van Mierop, L. H. S. Transposition of the great arteries. I. clarification or further confusion? American Journal of Cardiology 1971; 28: 735–738

2. Arnold, R., Smith, A., Anderson, R. H., Wilkinson, J. L., Hamilton, D. I. Rhythm problems after Mustard's operation: the significance of nodal position and blood supply. Journal of Thoracic and Cardiovascular Surgery. In press

3. McAlpine, W. A. Heart and coronary arteries: an anatomical atlas for clinical diagnosis, radiological investigation and surgical treatment. New York: Springer-Verlag, 1975: 154–159

4. Gillette, P. C., Kugler, J. D., Garson, A. Jr., Gutgesell, H. P., Duff, D. F., McNamara, D. G. Mechanisms of cardiac arrhythmias after the Mustard operation for transposition of the great arteries. American Journal of Cardiology 1980; 45: 1225–1230

5. Turley, K., Ebert, P. A. Total correction of transposition of the great arteries: conduction disturbances in infants younger than three months of age. Journal of Thoracic and Cardiovascular Surgery 1978; 76: 312–320

6. Ullal, R. R., Anderson, R. H., Lincoln, C. Mustard's operation modified to avoid dysrhythmias and pulmonary and systemic venous obstruction. Journal of Thoracic and Cardiovascular Surgery 1979; 78: 431–439

7. Southall, D. P., Keeton, B. R., Leanage, R. et al. Cardiac rhythm and conduction before and after Mustard's operation for complete transposition of the great arteries. British Heart Journal 1980; 43: 21–30

8. Wittig, J. H., De Leval, M. R., Stark, J. Intraoperative mapping of atrial activation before, during and after Mustard operation. Journal of Thoracic and Cardiovascular Surgery 1977; 73: 1–13

9. Shaher, R. M. Complete Transposition of the Great Arteries. New York: Academic Press, 1973: 164–175

10. Pillai, R., Shinebourne, E. A., Anderson, R. H., Lincoln, C. Surgical correction in situs inversus and left atrial isomerism using a mirror-image Mustard procedure. Submitted for publication

11. Anderson, R. H. et al. Complete transposition. In: Anderson, R. H., Becker, A. E., Lucchese, F. E., et al. Morphology of Congenital Heart Disease. 1. Angiocardiographic, Echocardiographic and Surgical Correlates. Tunbridge Wells: Castle House Publications, 1983: 84–100

12. Smith, A., Anderson, R. H., Wilkinson, J. L., Arnold, R., Dickinson, D. F. The architecture of the ventricular mass and atrioventricular valves in complete transposition of the great arteries with intact septum: a comparison with the normal heart. Part 1. The left ventricle, mitral valve and interventricular septum. Pediatric Cardiology. In press

13. Smith, A., Wilkinson, J. L., Anderson, R. H., Arnold, R., Dickinson, D. F. The architecture of the ventricular mass and atrioventricular valves in complete transposition with intact septum: a comparison with the normal heart. Part II. The right ventricle and tricuspid valve. Pediatric Cardiology. In press

14. Carr, I., Tynan, M. J., Aberdeen, E., Bonham-Carter, R. E., Graham, G., Waterston, D. J. Predictive accuracy of the 'loop rule' in 109 children with classical complete transposition of the great arteries. (Abstract). Circulation 1968; 38 (Suppl. VI): 52

15. Van Praagh, R., Pèrez-Trevino, C., Lopez-Cuellar, M., et al. Transposition of the great arteries with posterior aorta, anterior pulmonary artery, subpulmonary conus and fibrous continuity between aortic and atrioventricular valves. American Journal of Cardiology 1971; 28: 621–631

16. Wilkinson, J. L., Arnold, R., Anderson, R. H., Acerete, F. 'Posterior' transposition reconsidered. British Heart Journal 1975; 37: 757–766

17. Van Praagh, R., Van Praagh, S., Vlad, P., Keith, J. D. Anatomic types of congenital dextrocardia: diagnostic and embryologic implications. American Journal of Cardiology 1964; 13: 510–531

18. Becker, A. E., Anderson, R. H. How should we describe hearts in which the aorta is connected to the right ventricle and the pulmonary trunk to the left ventricle? A matter for reason and logic. American Journal of Cardiology 1983; 51: 911–912

19. Smith, A., Wilkinson, J. L., Arnold, R., Dickinson, D. F., Anderson, R. H. Growth and development of ventricular walls in complete transposition of the great arteries with intact septum (simple transposition). American Journal of Cardiology 1982; 49: 362–368

20. Elliott, L. P., Neufeld, H. N., Anderson, R. C., Adams, P., Edwards, J. E. Complete transposition of the great vessels. I. An anatomic study of sixty cases. Circulation 1963; 27: 1105–1117

21. Rowlatt, U. F. Coronary artery distribution in complete transposition. Journal of the American Medical Association 1962; 179: 269–278

22. Shaher, R. M., Puddu, G. C. Coronary arterial anatomy in complete transposition of the great vessels. American Journal of Cardiology 1966; 17: 355–361

23. Yacoub, M. H., Radley-Smith, R. Anatomy of the coronary arteries in transposition of the great arteries and methods for their transfer in anatomical correction. Thorax 1978; 33: 418–424

24. Milo, S., Ho, S. Y., Macartney, F. J., et al. Straddling and overriding atrioventricular valves: morphology and classification. American Journal of Cardiology 1979; 44: 1122–1134

25. Milo, S., Ho, S. Y., Wilkinson, J. L., Anderson, R. H. The surgical anatomy and atrioventricular conduction tissues of hearts with isolated ventricular septal defects. Journal of Thoracic and Cardiovascular Surgery 1980; 79: 244–255

26. Lincoln, C., Hasse, J., Anderson, R. H., Shinebourne, E. Surgical correction in complete levotransposition of the great arteries with an unusual subaortic ventricular septal defect. American Journal of Cardiology 1976; 38: 344–351

27. Milanesi, O., Thiene, G., Bini, R. M., Pellegrino, P. A. Complete transposition of great arteries with coarctation of aorta. British Heart Journal 1982; 48: 566–571

Mustard's operation for transposition of the great arteries

J. Stark MD, FRCS, FACS
Consultant Cardiothoracic Surgeon, Thoracic Unit, The Hospital For Sick Children, Great Ormond Street, London, UK

Introduction

The natural history of infants with transposition of the great arteries is unfavourable. Without treatment 85 per cent die before their first birthday. The first milestone in the treatment of patients with transposition of the great arteries was atrial septectomy[1]. Physiological correction with redirection of blood flow at atrial level is based on Albert's work[2]. Two techniques are currently being used, one described by Senning[3] and the other suggested by Mustard[4].

Preoperative

Diagnosis

A complete cardiological investigation is mandatory. Real-time echocardiography can establish the initial diagnosis. Cardiac catheterization in a sick infant with transposition of the great arteries is limited to the performance of balloon atrial septostomy[5]. Complete catheterization and angiocardiography is performed before the Mustard operation. If non-invasive investigation excludes additional cardiac lesions and there is no reason to suspect raised pulmonary arteriolar resistance, operation is indicated without prior cardiac catheterization.

Indications

At the present time all children with transposition of the great arteries can be offered surgical treatment. Those with atrial septal defect or previous balloon atrial septostomy are operated on with a low risk at the age of 6–8 months. Should balloon atrial septostomy prove ineffective an early inflow repair is preferable to septectomy. Currently a Senning-type repair is favoured. The indications for operation depend largely on the presence or absence of associated cardiac anomalies[6].

The operation

1

The incision

Midline sternotomy is used. The sternum is opened with an electric saw; in young infants heavy scissors may be used. The anterior surface of the pericardium is cleaned by sharp and blunt dissection. The thymic lobes are dissected and freed from the pericardium. The pleura is pushed to each side and care is taken not to open either pleural space.

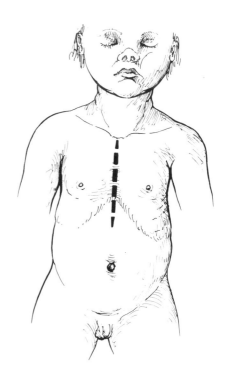

1

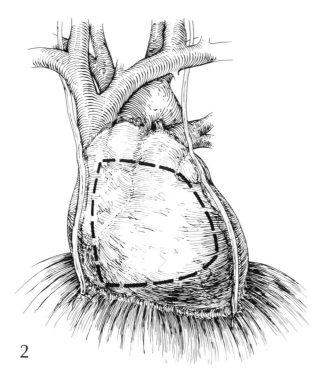

2

2

Pericardial patch

The pericardium is incised vertically on the right side parallel with the phrenic nerve and about 15–20 mm in front of it. Stay stitches are placed at the upper and lower ends. Incisions are then continued to the left, across the heart. An adequate pocket of pericardium should be left at the apex of the heart as otherwise the heart can dislocate easily. The pericardial patch is bathed in heparinized saline. If a previous intrapericardial operation has been performed dissection of the pericardium may be tedious and the pericardium may not be suitable for the baffle. In this situation a 'weaveknit' patch (Thackeray's No. MT44) or a patch of Gore-Tex can be used.

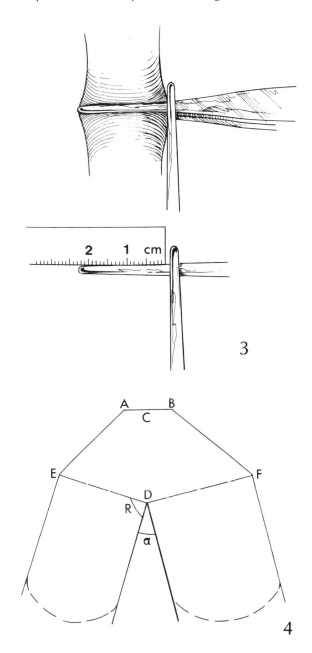

3

4

3 & 4

Calculating the size of the patch

The technique described by Brom[7] is used. The flat diameters of the superior and inferior venae cavae are measured. The patch is then cut according to these measurements. A–B is the distance between the left upper and lower pulmonary veins. It is not measured but estimated at about 1 cm for a 1-year-old child; it can be a few millimetres shorter for a neonate and about 1.5 cm for a 3–4-year-old. E–D is, in practice, twice the flat diameter of the superior vena cava and D–F is twice the flat diameter of the inferior vena cava. Then

$$C{-}D = \frac{(E{-}D) + (D{-}F)}{2}$$

The angle α is about 30° and R is a right angle. The legs of the patch are trimmed to the appropriate length when the patch is being inserted. These measurements are helpful, but adjustments are sometimes necessary because the anatomy of each atrium differs slightly.

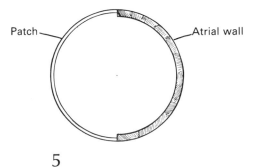

5

5

The fundamental reason for these measurements is to construct adequate pathways without excessive ballooning of the patch. When the pericardium shrinks the atrial wall should form at least 40–50 per cent of the circumference of the pathway.

6

Dissection of the inferior and superior venae cavae

The pericardium is freed from the lower portion of the superior vena cava. Care must be taken not to injure the phrenic nerve, especially with electrocautery. A purse-string suture is then placed directly on the superior vena cava, starting about 15 mm above its junction with the right atrium. It should be more oblong than circular so as to avoid superior vena caval constriction when it is tied. The inferior vena cava cannulation site lies posteriorly at the junction of the right atrium with the inferior vena cava. Intracardiac pressures are then measured and heparin is given.

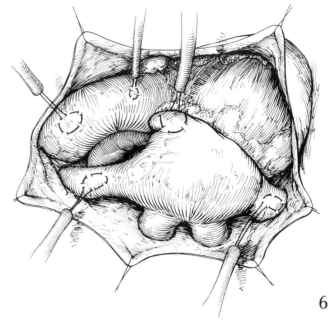

6

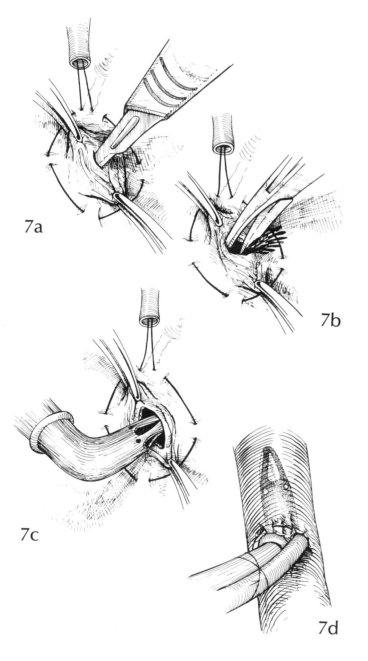

7a

7b

7c

7d

7a–d

Aortic and caval cannulation

Standard aortic cannulation with a right-angled cannula is used. For caval cannulation a technique avoiding partial occlusion clamps is preferred. Fine artery forceps grasp the atrial wall within the purse-string suture (a). An incision is made and enlarged with another artery forceps (b). A right-angled Rygg cannula is then inserted without difficulty (c). The purse-string suture is tightened and secured to the cannula (d). The inferior vena cava is cannulated in the same way. In very small infants special metal venous cannulae* are used.

* Genito Urinary Manufacturing Co., Plimpton Street, London W8

8

Cardiopulmonary bypass and atriotomy

Care is taken not to let any air into the right atrium during cannulation because the tricuspid valve is the systemic atrioventricular valve and systemic embolization can occur. A small vent may be placed through the right atrial appendage. Perfusion is started and when the calculated flow is achieved (2.4 l/m²/min) the caval snares are tightened and ventilation discontinued. The perfusate is cooled to 20°C and at this temperature the aorta is cross-clamped. Cardioplegic solution is infused to the root of the aorta. The right atrium is opened and the cardioplegic solution is aspirated with a discard sucker. When the pulmonary venous return is excessive a small vent can be placed in the pulmonary artery to improve visualization of the left atrium. Alternatively a short period of reduced flow or circulatory arrest can be employed.

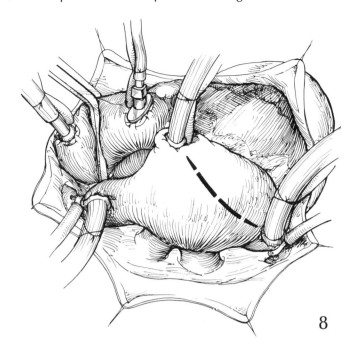

8

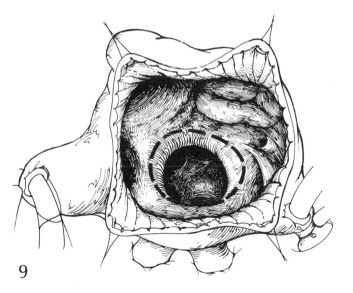

9

9

Atrial stay sutures and excision of the atrial septum

Stay sutures are placed anteriorly close to the tricuspid valve and posteriorly on the crista terminalis. These bring both atrial cavities into view without the excessive use of retractors. After careful inspection of the right atrium, tricuspid valve, atrial septal defect, left atrium and orifices of all pulmonary veins, the remnant of the atrial septum is excised. It is carefully detached from the lateral and superior wall of the atrium. Care must be taken not to cut through the wall of the atrium. This can happen, but if recognized and repaired properly it is of no great importance.

10

Placement of pericardial baffle

The raw surfaces remaining after the excision of the atrial septum are oversewn with a few single stitches. The baffle is inserted with a double-needled suture of 5/0 polypropylene. The suture line starts at the point 'C' on the patch (*see* Illustration 4), which is attached between the left pulmonary veins and the base of the left atrial appendage.

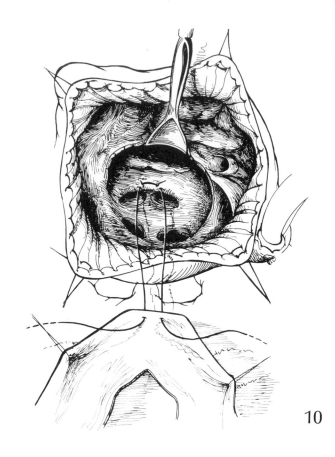

10

Correct

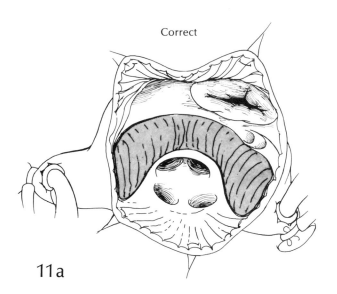

11a

Incorrect

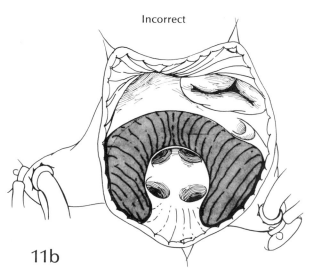

11b

11a & b

The suture line then runs superiorly around the orifice of the pulmonary veins, then across the posterior wall of the left atrium towards the upper margin of the right upper pulmonary vein (*a*). The lower part of the patch encircles the lower left pulmonary vein and runs across to between the right lower pulmonary vein and the orifice of the inferior vena cava (*b*). Care is taken not to bring the two suture lines too close together on the lateral wall of the right atrium because a constricting ring may thus be formed.

12

Anterior part of the baffle

Point 'D' on the baffle (see Illustration 4) is then sutured with a second double-needled suture to the remnant of the atrial septum. The suture line continues upwards and then around the superior vena caval pathway. If the trabeculations here are numerous the suture is brought through the wall of the right atrium as a continuous mattress stitch to avoid any leaks behind the trabeculations.

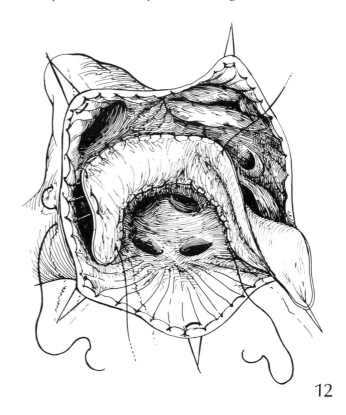

12

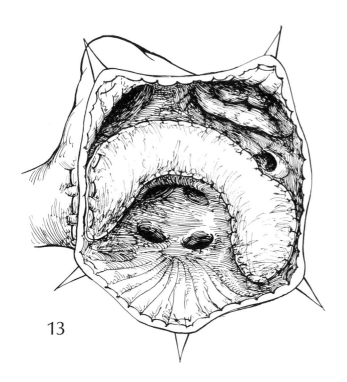

13

13

Completion of the baffle

The lower part of the baffle is sutured to the cut edge of the septum, then behind the coronary sinus. This leaves the coronary sinus to drain into the pulmonary venous atrium; it has no serious physiological consequences. The length of the patch is trimmed for both the superior and inferior venae cavae to allow adequate ballooning; the two pathways should not meet when filled with blood.

14

Enlargement of the pulmonary venous atrium

In some infants the distance between the superior and inferior venae cavae is rather short. Placement of the baffle may compromise either the pulmonary venous or systemic venous return. In such cases the pulmonary venous atrium can be enlarged with a patch[8]. We now prefer to enlarge the pulmonary venous atrium in all infants younger than 6 months. If enlargement of the pulmonary venous atrium is planned the right atrium is opened from the base of the right atrial appendage, across the crista terminalis and down to between the right upper and right lower pulmonary veins (*see* insert).

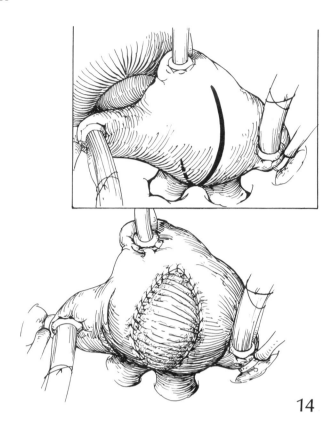

14

Atrial closure and termination of bypass

Before the completion of the atrial suture line the cardioplegia needle is connected to suction of the vent line. Caval snares are released and the aortic clamp removed. When the heart regains its tone the aorta is again cross-clamped, the lungs inflated and air carefully removed from the right ventricle and aortic root. A monitoring line is then inserted through the right atrial appendage into the right (physiologically left) atrium. One venous cannula may be clamped and removed on partial bypass. Perfusion is then discontinued at an atrial pressure of 10–12 mmHg.

COMPLICATIONS

Obstruction of the systemic venous or pulmonary venous pathway has been observed by several authors. With the technique described above it has become a very rare complication. Arrythmias still occur after the Mustard operation. However, both incidence and severity have diminished in recent years[9–11]. Better knowledge of the conduction mechanism and more meticulous operative technique are undoubtedly responsible for this improvement.

Tricuspid valve incompetence is a rare but severe complication which may require valve replacement.

Right ventricular dysfunction has been observed in some patients. The long-term results of inflow-type operations (Mustard or Senning) will undoubtedly depend upon the ability of this ventricle to support the systemic circulation.

Results

Our current operative mortality for children with transposition of the great arteries without additional lesions (simple transposition) is less than 3 per cent for both Mustard and Senning operations. The long-term results[12] show that between 70 and 90 per cent of patients can lead normal lives.

Reoperation

Obstruction of the pulmonary veins should be treated surgically. Isolated narrowing or even complete obstruction of the superior vena cava often does not require treatment because if the azygos vein remains patent and the inferior vena caval channel is adequate the patient may not show any symptoms of obstruction. If symptoms persist the superior vena caval channel can be enlarged with a patch.

15

For all reoperations in patients with transposition of the great arteries we prefer a right thoracotomy through the fifth intercostal space, extending it across the sternum if necessary[13] (see insert), making cannulation of the superior and inferior venae cavae easier; the aorta is usually anterior and right-sided and thus is also easily reached from this approach. As the operation is performed in the right atrium one can avoid dissection underneath the sternum where the right ventricle and the coronary arteries are no longer protected by pericardium. The atrial incision runs from the atrioventricular groove down to between the right upper and lower pulmonary veins.

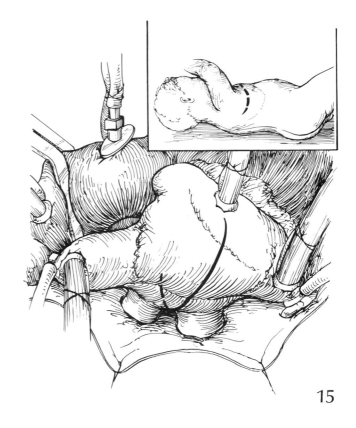

15

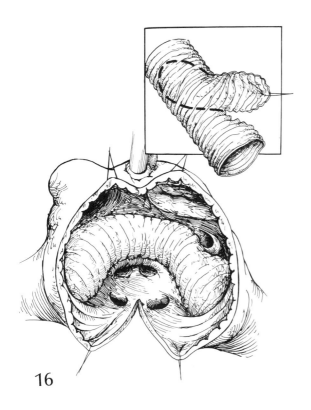

16

16

If a localized superior vena caval obstruction is present the pathway is incised and a patch is inserted. If both the superior and inferior venae cavae are obstructed the original patch is removed and a new one fashioned from a tube of woven Dacron or Gore-Tex is inserted.

17

The pulmonary venous atrium is then enlarged with a patch.

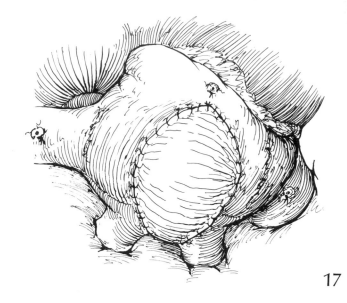

17

Additional lesions

PERSISTENT DUCTUS ARTERIOSUS

This should be ligated before establishment of cardiopulmonary bypass from the anterior approach. Isolated ligation of the ductus in patients with transposition of the great arteries should be approached with caution. It may suddenly decrease the arterial oxygen saturation so that the patient becomes acutely hypoxic. For this reason, early repair (Mustard or Senning operation) plus ligation of the ductus is recommended.

COARCTATION OF THE AORTA

This is preferably repaired before correction through a left thoractomy (see chapter on 'Coarctation of the aorta', pp. 364–370).

VENTRICULAR SEPTAL DEFECT

Patients with a large ventricular septal defect can be offered several operations. They can have an early inflow repair (Mustard or Senning) with closure of the ventricular septal defect. Alternatively they can have pulmonary artery banding followed by a Rastelli operation, arterial switch operation[14], external conduit repair operation[15] or delayed Mustard or Senning operation. In all these two-stage operations the pulmonary artery has to be reconstructed.

When ventricular septal defect closure is indicated it is best performed from the right atrium through the tricuspid valve. The right ventricle functions as a systemic ventricle; therefore right ventriculotomy should be avoided. Occasionally a ventricular septal defect can be closed through the pulmonary artery or through the left ventricle.

In the presence of a ventricular septal defect pulmonary vascular obstructive disease may develop at an early stage. For this reason operation, either palliative or corrective, is recommended at the age of 3–6 months. If pulmonary arteriolar resistance is already elevated above $8\,u/m^2$ inflow repair can be performed, but the ventricular septal defect should be left open. This so-called 'palliative' Mustard or 'palliative' Senning operation can improve arterial oxygen saturation[16]. Similarly a 'palliative' arterial switch operation can be performed under such circumstances. Patients with transposition of the great arteries, intact ventricular septum and pulmonary vascular obstructive disease can also be treated by an inflow-type repair and creation of a ventricular septal defect[17].

LEFT VENTRICULAR OUTFLOW TRACT OBSTRUCTION

Pulmonary valve stenosis can be easily relieved by valvotomy. Severe fibromuscular obstruction is sometimes difficult to relieve, as is the obstruction caused by an abnormal insertion of the mitral valve. A conduit from the left ventricle to the pulmonary artery may bypass this obstruction[18]. If the ventricular septal defect and left ventricular outflow tract obstruction are associated with transposition of the great arteries a Rastelli operation is the treatment of choice.

Acknowledgement

Illustrations 3, 4, 5, 10, 16 and 17 were modified from illustrations by M. Courtney in Stark, J. Concordant transposition: Mustard operation. In: Stark, J., de Leval, M. R., eds. Surgery for Congenital Heart Defects. London, New York, Academic Press, 1983: 331–344

References

1. Blalock, A., Hanlon, C. R. Surgical treatment of complete transposition of the aorta and pulmonary artery. Surgery, Gynecology and Obstetrics 1950; 90: 1–15

2. Albert, H. M. Surgical correction of transposition of the great vessels. Surgical Forum 1955; 5: 74

3. Senning, A. Surgical correction of transposition of the great vessels. Surgery 1959; 45: 966–980

4. Mustard, W. T. Successful two-stage correction of transposition of the great vessels. Surgery 1964; 55: 469–472

5. Rashkind, W. J., Miller, W. W. Creation of an atrial septal defect without thoracotomy: a palliative approach to complete transposition of the great arteries. Journal of the American Medical Association 1966; 196: 991–992

6. Stark, J. Concordant transposition: Mustard operation. In: Surgery for Congenital Heart Defects. Eds. Stark, J., de Leval, M. London: Grune & Stratton, pp. 331–344

7. Brom, B. A. Technique of Mustard operation. In: Hahn, C. ed. Thorax Chirurgie, Leiden, Neederlands Drukkerij Bedrijf, 1975: 194

8. Replogle, R. L., Lin, C. Y. Surgical correction of transposition of the great vessels: a technical suggestion. Journal of Thoracic and Cardiovascular Surgery 1972; 63: 196–198

9. Turley, K., Ebert, P. A. Total correction of transposition of the great arteries: conduction disturbances in infants younger than three months of age. Journal of Thoracic and Cardiovascular Surgery 1978; 76: 312–320

10. Ullal, R. R., Anderson, R. H., Lincoln, C. Mustard's operation modified to avoid dysrhythmias and pulmonary and systemic venous obstruction. Journal of Thoracic and Cardiovascular Surgery 1979; 78: 431–439

11. Stark, J. et al. Late results of surgical treatment of transposition of the great arteries. Advances in Cardiology; 1980; 27: 254–265

12. Champsaur, G. L., Sokol, D. M., Trusler, G. A., Mustard, W. T. Repair of transposition of the great arteries in 123 pediatric patients: early and long-term results. Circulation 1973; 47: 1032–1041

13. Szarnicki, R. J., Stark, J., de Leval, M. Reoperation for complications after inflow correction of transposition of the great arteries: technical considerations. Annals of Thoracic Surgery 1978; 25: 150–154

14. Jatene, A. D. et al. Successful anatomic correction of transposition of the great vessels: a preliminary report. Arquivos Brasileiros de Cardiologia 1975; 28: 461–464

15. Stansel, H. C. Jr. A new operation for d-loop transposition of the great vessels. Annals of Thoracic Surgery 1975; 19: 565–567

16 Dhasmana, J. P. et al. Long-term results of the 'palliative' Mustard operation. Journal of the American College of Cardiology 1985; 6: 1138–1141

17. Stark, J., de Leval, M., Taylor, J. F. N. Mustard operation and creation of ventricular septal defect in two patients with transposition of the great arteries, intact ventricular septum and pulmonary disease. American Journal of Cardiology 1976; 38: 524–527

18. Singh, A. K., Stark, J., Taylor, J. F. N. Left ventricle to pulmonary artery conduit in the treatment of transposition of the great arteries, restrictive ventricular septal defect and acquired pulmonary atresia. British Heart Journal 1976; 38: 1213–1216

The Senning operation for transposition of the great arteries

A. Gerard Brom MD
Head of Cardiac Surgery, Mafraq Hospital, Abu Dhabi, United Arab Emirates

Jan M. Quaegebeur MD
Assistant Professor, Department of Thoracic Surgery, University Hospital, Leiden, The Netherlands

John Rohmer MD
Head, Department of Pediatric Cardiology, University Hospital, Leiden, The Netherlands

Introduction

Arterial reversal implies an anatomical correction of transposition of the great vessels, and indications for this operation are therefore likely to increase in the future. However, the pressure in the left ventricle is too low in most cases to permit this operation and consequently one must either prepare the left ventricle for an arterial switch operation by banding the pulmonary artery[1] or perform a venous inflow correction.

The two operations most commonly used for transposition are the Mustard procedure and the Senning I operation[2]. The latter was first described by Senning in 1959 and until 1964 remained the only operation used in the treatment of transposition. It was associated with a high mortality, which was unjustly attributed to the procedure itself. Consequently nearly all surgeons adopted the technique described by Mustard in 1964[3].

In our unit we performed eight Senning I operations between 1960 and 1964. The good clinical condition of the two surviving patients (born 1959 and 1960 respectively) prompted us to make a critical reappraisal of the Senning procedure, as a result of which we reintroduced this operation in December 1975. The advantages of the Senning over the Mustard procedure can be summarized as follows:

(1) The Mustard procedure calls for the use of a fairly large patch, whereas none or only a small patch is required for the Senning procedure (slightly larger after a Blalock-Hanlon operation). In the classical Senning operation the entire repair is made with the aid of atrial tissue, which is not a free graft but remains in contact with adjacent tissue.

(2) By using vital atrial tissue one ensures a contracting new right and left atrium, as demonstrated by postopera-tive angiography and function studies (Parenzan, L., personal communication)[4,5].

(3) In order to obtain an optimal effect with the Mustard procedure the size of the patch to be used has to be calculated exactly in order to prevent obstruction of systemic or pulmonary veins. This problem is much more serious when the patient is very small. Unlike the Mustard procedure the Senning operation makes use of the fact that Nature has already made the calculations and presents us with the necessary material of the proper dimensions for the patient's age. This is particularly important in the treatment of patients under 6 months of age. It is justifiable to state that the smaller the patient, the easier the Senning technique as compared with the Mustard technique.

(4) So far arrhythmias have been less frequent after Senning operations than after Mustard operations. This could be due to our improved knowledge of the conduction system in the atrium. It should be borne in mind, however, that during a Mustard procedure it is necessary to place many sutures around the inlet of the superior vena cava; this involves the risk of causing a lesion of the sinus node or its arteries.

(5) Stenosis, both of the caval and of the pulmonary veins, is still being reported after Mustard operations. Pulmonary vein stenoses are probably due to shrinking of tissue at the site of resection of the atrial septum and consequently they are rarely (if ever) described in association with a Mustard operation after a Blalock-Hanlon procedure. Caval vein stenoses (especially of the superior vena cava), however, are still being mentioned in most published results. We have so far seen no such stenoses after a Senning operation and believe that they can be avoided by proper technique.

Indication for operation

Since arterial reversal is an anatomical correction in the treatment of transposition of the great vessels we always consider this operation first for patients with or without a ventricular septal defect (VSD) whose left ventricular pressure exceeds 50 mmHg and who show no outflow obstruction of this ventricle. We even consider this procedure as palliative treatment for patients with VSD and fixed high pulmonary resistance. If there is severe pulmonary stenosis as well as a VSD a Rastelli-type operation merits consideration.

In the majority of cases, however, venous reversal will be required. In our department this is nearly always effected by a Senning procedure, with the exception of the rare cases in which a previous Blalock-Hanlon procedure has caused so many adhesions that the right phrenic nerve might be endangered during dissection. For this reason we have performed a Mustard operation after a Blalock-Hanlon procedure on three patients since 1975, though a Senning procedure was feasible in five similar cases.

In the event of juxtaposition of the atrial appendages the part of the right artrial wall localized between the terminal line and the transition from right atrium to right ventricle is only a few centimetres wide and this is insufficient for construction of the ('left') pulmonary atrium. In this situation we perform the first part of the Senning operation but use a prosthesis (dura mater) for construction of the ('left') pulmonary atrium.

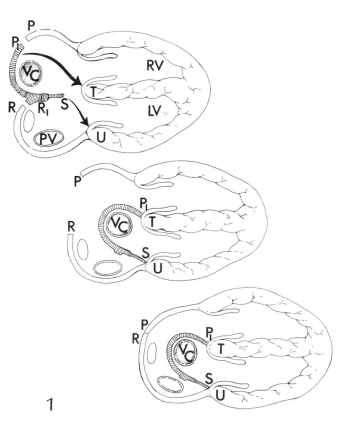

1

Principles of the Senning operation

As in the Mustard operation, it is necessary to construct a new right atrium-to-be and two conduits through which the blood is guided from the caval veins to the new atrium. The dimensions of this new right wall should be at least as large as those of the opposite side of the new right atrium. This opposite side consists of the mitral orifice and part of the left atrial wall between the mitral orifice and left pulmonary veins.

1

This new right wall is made up of two adjoining parts, part of the right atrium (P_1–R_1) plus the atrial septum (R_1–S). It is unnecessary to use a patch to 'extend' the septum as is often the case in Mustard's procedure. The caval veins and the new right atrium are moved to the left, thus ensuring that the new orifice for the pulmonary veins becomes circular instead of slit-shaped so that the blood flow is in no way obstructed – the same reasoning as in the Mustard procedure. If, however, the septum is 'extended' a less perfect orifice for the pulmonary veins may result, with consequent flow obstruction.

Since the atriotomy is located in front of the terminal sulcus, and therefore in front of the superior vena cava, stenosis of that vein during suture of the terminal sulcus to the septal remnant above the valves is practically impossible. Also, since the Eustachian valve is used for the inferior vena cava, stenosis of this vein is also impossible.

Unobstructed outflow from the pulmonary veins is ensured by the following measures: (1) The superior aspect of the mobilized septum is sutured above the two left pulmonary veins. After balloon septostomy this superior aspect is too narrow and a patch must be used to bring it up to size. The correct size is found by measuring the veins (for example, if the diameter of one vein is 6 mm, then the two left veins measure 12 mm together and, taking sutures into account, the superior aspect should be slightly larger (15 mm)). (2) The dimensions of the base of the mobilized septum are determined by the heart itself. It is the site at which the anterior aspect of the pulmonary veins merges with their posterior aspect (cranial for the right superior, caudal for the right inferior pulmonary vein). The atrial septum now constitutes the roof of the channel which guides the blood from the two left pulmonary veins to the right. The base of this septum becomes the wall of the confluence of the right and left pulmonary veins. (3) The confluence of all pulmonary veins should be in wide communication with the new left atrium. This is ensured by dissecting the intra-atrial groove, whereupon the left atrium is opened by a craniocaudal incision made as medially as possible. The opening in the left atrium is further enlarged by a transverse incision between the two right pulmonary veins. Because the caval veins and the new right atrium have been luxated to the left a large oval-to-round opening in the left atrium results.

The operation

A midline sternotomy is used.

2

Extracorporeal circulation

Three venous cannulae are used. The ascending aorta and right atrium are cannulated after heparinization. The caval veins are cannulated after extracorporeal circulation is started with cannulae with curved tips, the superior caval vein high in the mediastinum and the inferior caval vein as far caudally as possible and on its right side, keeping the cannula distal and to the left of the Eustachian valve. The patient is cooled to 20°C and during this cooling the intra-atrial groove is dissected free. When the temperature reaches 20°C the caval veins are tied around the cannulae, the third cannula is removed from the right atrium, the aorta is clamped proximal to the cannula and cardioplegic solution is administered.

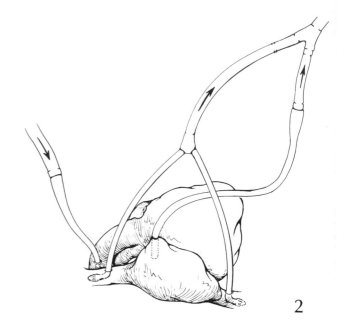

2

Incision in the atrium

3

An incision (A-B) is made in the right atrium less than 5 mm ventral to the terminal sulcus. This incision is extended cranially around the base of the right auricle of the heart. The sinus node is situated in the cranial part of the terminal sulcus, covered only by epicardium. The area of the sinus node should not be touched with instruments during the operation. The incision extends caudally over a distance equal to approximately three-quarters of that between the venae cavae. At a later stage the incision is extended in the direction of the lateral end of the valve of the inferior vena cava (Eustachian valve) (B_1).

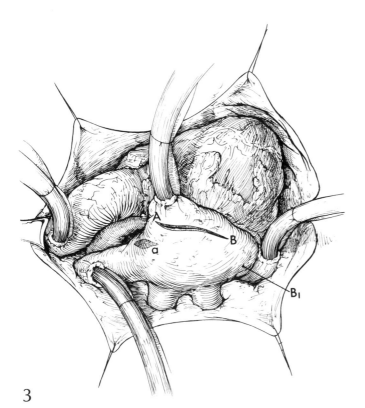

3

Mobilization of the atrial septum and formation of a flap

4

After the right atrium has been opened the septum is carefully inspected. After a balloon septostomy only the fossa ovalis is missing. However, after a Blalock-Hanlon procedure the septum is largely absent. In either case a trapeziform roof must be constructed to be sutured above the left pulmonary veins (comparable to the trapeziform midportion of the Mustard patch). Thus after a Rashkind procedure the incision is started in the foramen ovale and extended parallel to the tricuspid valve ring in a caudocranial direction for a distance of about 7 mm (C-D). From point D the incision extends to the junction of the superior vena cava with the atrial septum. The same is repeated for the inferior vena cava, starting at the lower corner of the fossa ovalis. At this site tissue is sometimes absent, making the incision (F-G) unnecessary.

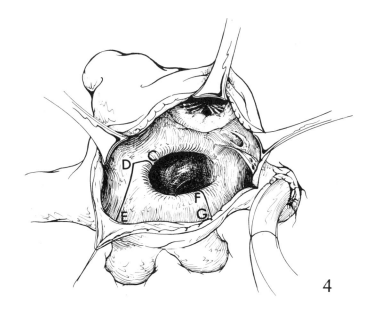

4

5

The resulting flap has nearly always the same dimensions in infants aged 6–12 months. Its base is formed by the atrial wall between the two venae cavae and is about 2–3 cm in length. Its height is about 2 cm. The dimensions of the pulmonary veins are then measured with Hegar's dilators (usually size 6 or 8 mm) which indicate that the distance above the top side of the trapeziform roof must therefore be the same length. This is achieved by suturing a small patch to the septal remnant, slightly larger to allow for the suture line. After a Blalock-Hanlon operation the absent atrial septum is replaced by a trapeziform Dacron patch to achieve the same dimensions.

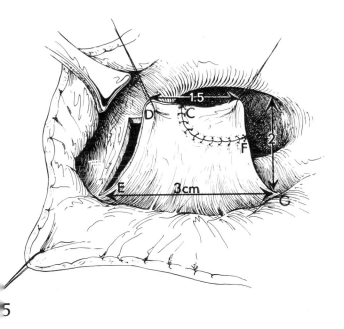

5

6

Formation of a left atrial outlet

The interatrial groove is dissected in front of the right pulmonary veins, thus slightly separating the two atria. The left atrium is then opened by a craniocaudal incision as close to the midline as possible (E_1–G_1). These two points, situated on the outside of the heart, correspond to points E and G (see illustration 5) inside the heart. The length of the left atrial incision is therefore likewise about 3 cm. The left atrial outlet is further enlarged by a small transverse incision between the two pulmonary veins or a separate incision in both veins.

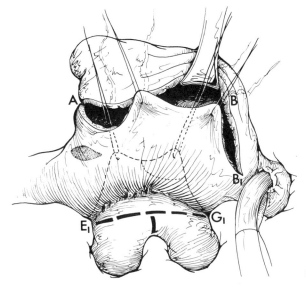

6

7

Fixing the atrial septal flap inside the left atrium

The atrial flap (like the central part of the patch in the Mustard procedure) is sutured in front of the left pulmonary veins and along the posterior wall of the left atrium.

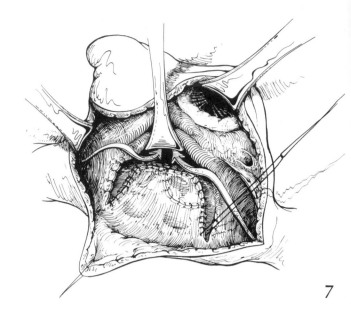

7

7

8

Creation of a new systemic 'right' atrium

In order to ensure that no inferior caval vein stenosis can develop we make use of the Eustachian valve (if available) in constructing the new systemic atrium. This valve marks the ventral delimitation of the inferior caval vein. As already mentioned, this vein must be cannulated far caudally and via its right side in order to keep the valve intact and visible. The original right atrial incision is now extended to the lateral end of the Eustachian valve. The posterior part of the right atrial wall is then sutured to the remnant of the atrial septum between the atrioventricular valves, use being made caudally of the Eustachian valve. During this part of the operation it is often necessary to remove the cannula temporarily from the inferior caval vein and resort to total circulatory arrest. Once the distal part of the A-B suture is in position the cannula is reinserted and the extracorporeal circulation restored. Cranially the sutures are placed in the endocardial layers of the atrial wall to avoid the sinoatrial node, which is located immediately below the epicardium.

9

Creation of a new pulmonary 'left' atrium

The original incision in the right atrium extends from the insertion of the Eustachian valve in a caudal direction to the base of the right atrial appendage. The tissue along this incision is divided into three portions for separate covering of the inferior and superior venae cavae, and finally the midportion of the flap is sutured to the boundary of the incision in the left atrium

Since the insertion of the Eustachian valve is located on the extreme right lateral aspect of the inferior caval vein there is no risk of stenosis as the flap is being sutured over this vein. This part of the operation therefore requires but little tissue, and the suture from B_1 to G_1 (see *illustration 8*) can be placed continuously without any tension so that very little tissue is used.

The covering and crossing of the superior vena cava is more difficult. If in this part of the procedure an error is made by using an insufficient amount of atrial tissue or by applying too much tension to the continuous suture, then stenosis of the superior vena cava is possible (and has in fact been described). We try to avoid this by first measuring the circumference of the superior vena cava and, for crossing this vein, using a flap portion which has a length of about three-quarters of this circumference. In addition, the cannula in the caval vein is repeatedly clamped briefly during the placing of the continuous suture from A to E_1 (see *illustration 10*). During these brief periods of clamping the superior caval vein fills optimally so that constriction (purse-string) is prevented.

Since this part of the operation involves work near the sinus node, the A-E_1 suture must be placed far cranially and, until the danger zone has been passed, in purely anteroposterior direction.

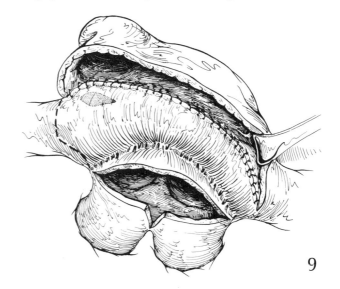

9

10

The remaining midportion of the flap is now sutured to the right of the E_1-G_1 incision. The transverse incision has made the opening in the left atrium as large as possible. The total length of the midportion of the flap *must* exceed the length of the incision in the left atrium. If it does not it should likewise be enlarged by one or several transverse incisions (see *illustration 6*). The appropriate diameter of the opening between the old and the new left atrium is determined by measuring the pulmonary veins.

The surface area of the pulmonary veins is related to the flow. For example, given Hegar 6 (surface area $27\,mm^2$), the space for the two left pulmonary veins should amount to Hegar 9 (surface area $61\,mm^2 > 2 \times 27$), while the anastomosis (E_1-G_1) should amount to at least Hegar 13 (surface area $127\,mm^2 > 4 \times 27$). When these dimensions are borne in mind, stenosis is virtually impossible; in all our patients the anastomosis was substantially larger than necessary.

The anastomosis is established with knotted sutures of 6/0 polypropylene, both with a view to stretching of the anastomosis during growth and to preventing a purse-string effect.

In one patient with juxtaposition of the heart auricles in addition to transposition we had to make use of dura mater for construction of a new left atrium. In all other cases we obtained an ample superior caval vein lumen as well as a spacious new left atrium without using foreign material.

Completion of the operation

As the patient is being rewarmed the single cannula is reinserted into the new 'left' atrium via the appendage of the atrium, whereupon the cannula in the superior vena cava and that in the inferior vena cava are removed in succession. Finally the cannula in the left atrium is removed and replaced by a small catheter for postoperative pressure measurements. Two pacemaker electrodes are placed on the atrium and one on the ventricle.

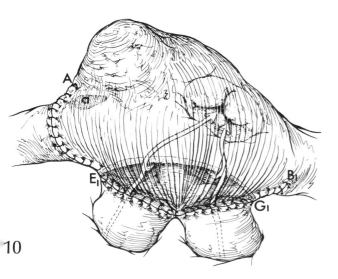

10

References

1. Yacoub, M. H. The case for anatomic correction of transposition of the great arteries. Journal of Thoracic and Cardiovascular Surgery 1979; 78: 3–6

2. Senning, A. Surgical correction of transposition of the great vessels. Surgery 1959; 45: 966–980

3. Mustard, W. T. Successful two-stage correction of transposition of the great vessels. Surgery 1964; 55: 469–472

4. Wyse, R. K. H., Macartney, F. J., Rohmer, J., Ottenkamp, J., Brom, A. G. Differential atrial filling after Mustard and Senning repairs. British Heart Journal 1980; 44: 692–698

5. Bjornstad, P. G., Semb, B. K. H. Echocardiographic comparison of atrial function after Mustard and Senning repair for transposition of the great arteries (Abs). Circulation 1981; 64 (Suppl. IV): 226

Transposition of the great arteries with left ventricular outflow tract obstruction

J. Stark MD, FRCS, FACS
Consultant Cardiothoracic Surgeon, Thoracic Unit, The Hospital for Sick Children, Great Ormond Street, London, UK

Introduction

Left ventricular outflow tract obstruction may be caused by different anatomical abnormalities. Some, like pulmonary valve stenosis, subvalvar fibrous shelf, aneurysms of the membranous portion of the interventricular septum or redundant tricuspid valve tissue, can be easily relieved. Hypertrophy of the interventricular septum or fibromuscular tunnel presents more difficult surgical problems. A long and narrow fibromuscular tunnel and abnormal insertion of the mitral valve cannot be relieved but only bypassed. The surgical technique depends on the severity of the obstruction and on the presence and position of the ventricular septal defect. In patients with severe obstruction and ventricular septal defect located in the subaortic area a Rastelli operation is our first choice[1]. In patients with intact ventricular septum and severe left ventricular outflow tract obstruction a Mustard or Senning operation is performed and a left ventricle-to-pulmonary artery conduit inserted[2]. If severe left ventricular outflow tract obstruction is associated with a subpulmonary or uncommitted ventricular septal defect the ventricular septal defect is closed, a Mustard or Senning operation is performed and a left ventricle-to-pulmonary artery conduit placed.

Preoperative

Diagnosis

Complete cardiac catheterization and angiography are essential. The size, position and number of ventricular septal defects and the size of the main pulmonary artery are assessed. Additional lesions such as persistent ductus arteriosus, large aortopulmonary collateral arteries and patency of previous shunts have to be diagnosed with certainty. The nature of left ventricular outflow tract obstruction is assessed by real-time echocardiography and high-quality angiocardiography. It is important to distinguish the patient with simple transposition of the great arteries who only have flow gradients from those with true anatomical obstruction.

Indications

Severe cyanosis, polycythaemia and/or cyanotic spells are indications for the operation. If symptoms occur in infancy a systemic pulmonary shunt is the treatment of choice. The author prefers a Blalock-Taussig shunt on the side opposite to the aortic arch (see chapter on 'Shunt procedures', pp. 107–116). A Rastelli operation is better deferred until the age of 3–4 years. At this age an adult-size homograft or heterograft can be used. Patients with intact ventricular septum may be treated as those with simple transposition if the left ventricular outflow tract obstruction is not severe or if it can be relieved. Pressures are measured after completion of the Mustard or Senning operation. If the left ventricular pressure is at or above right ventricular pressure and the pulmonary artery pressure is less than normal a left ventricle-to-pulmonary artery conduit is inserted.

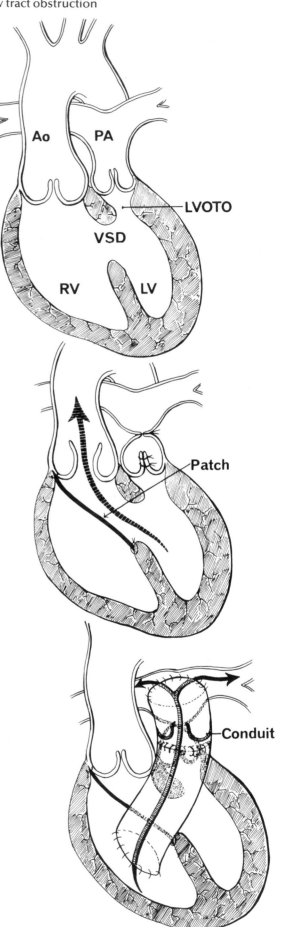

The operations

PATIENTS WITH VENTRICULAR SEPTAL DEFECT

1, 2, & 3

The principle of the Rastelli operation is shown in the accompanying illustrations. Left ventricular outflow obstruction (LVOTO) is not resected and the ventricular septal defect (VSD) is not closed, but the left ventricle (LV) is connected to the aorta (Ao) with a large intraventricular patch. Exit from the left ventricle to the pulmonary artery (PA) is closed by suture of the pulmonary valve through the ventricular septal defect and ligation of the pulmonary artery above the valve. Continuity between the right ventricle (RV) and the pulmonary artery is then established with a valved conduit.

4

Cannulation, perfusion and ventriculotomy

The pulmonary artery and aorta are completely dissected and separated. This is particularly important when there are adhesions after previous operations. Dissection should be completed before the patient is heparinized. Intracardiac pressures are then measured, heparin given and the arterial cannula inserted high into the ascending aorta. The superior vena cava is cannulated through a separate purse-string in the low right atrium. A vent is inserted into the left atrium through the right upper pulmonary vein. Perfusion is started with a perfusate temperature of 25°C and further cooling to 20°C follows. The aorta is cross-clamped and cardioplegic infusion is then repeated every 30 minutes or if the myocardial temperature rises over 20°C or electrical activity appears on the electrocardiogram. The right atrium is opened and the cardioplegic solution is recovered from the coronary sinus and discarded.

The atrial and ventricular anatomy is first assessed. If an atrial septal defect (natural or previous Blalock-Hanlon septectomy) is present it is closed. The position of the papillary muscles is checked through the tricuspid valve before the ventriculotomy is performed. The right ventriculotomy is a vertical incision directed towards the main pulmonary artery. As the pulmonary artery is usually posterior and to the left of the aorta the ventriculotomy is usually directed towards the left side.

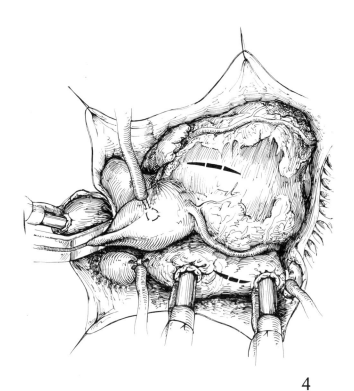

4

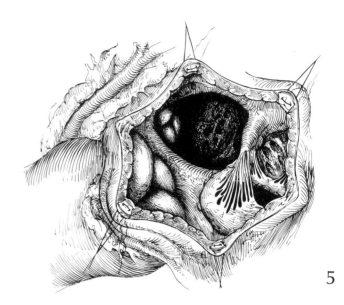

5

5, 6 & 7

Connection of left ventricle to aorta

Stay stitches buttressed with Teflon pledgets are placed at the edges of the ventriculotomy. When it is established that the left ventricle can be connected to the aorta through the ventricular septal defect the pulmonary valve is inspected through the ventricular septal defect and carefully oversewn in two layers with 4/0 polypropylene. The main pulmonary artery is then doubly ligated just outside the heart. In this way transection of the pulmonary artery is avoided.

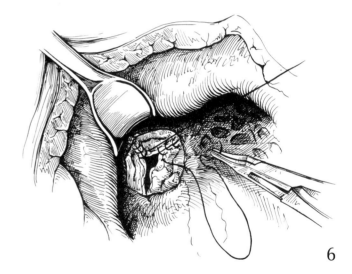

6

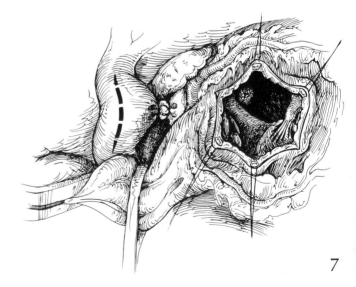

7

8

If it is decided to divide the pulmonary artery its ventricular end is oversewn with a continuous mattress stitch and then over-and-over polypropylene stitches. This suture line must be meticulous because it is very difficult to deal with any leaks once the conduit is inserted.

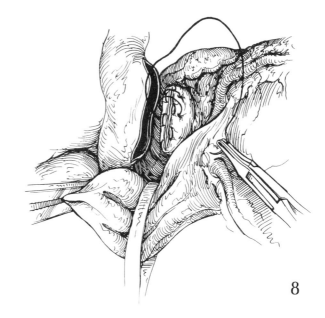

8

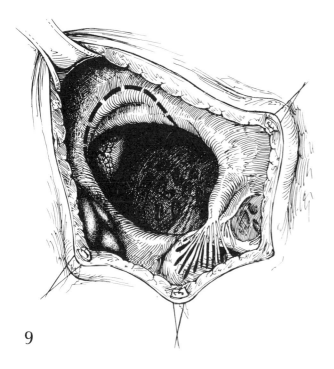

9

9

The ventricular septal defect is checked and if it is smaller than the aortic valve ring it is enlarged in the lateral superior margin either by a simple incision or by excision of a wedge of the muscle.

10

The length and width of the channel from the left ventricle to the aorta is then measured and a generous patch of Dacron velour is prepared. The suture line of the patch is started from the lower corner of the ventricular septal defect close to the tricuspid valve. On the left side it runs around the ventricular septal defect and up to the anterior wall of the right ventricle and the edge of the ventriculotomy. On the other side the suture line runs to the edge of the ventriculotomy. At present we use mattress sutures of 3/0 Ethibond buttressed with Teflon pledgets. The upper part of the suture line can be completed with a running stitch of 4/0 polypropylene. Anteriorly the suture line is left incomplete to allow access to the aortic valve. When the aortic clamp is removed an instrument can be passed between the stitches through the aortic valve to evacuate air from the ascending aorta. When the ventricular septal defect has been closed the pulmonary artery is opened. This can either be with a longitudinal incision in the main pulmonary artery or the incision can be horizontal into both left and right pulmonary arteries.

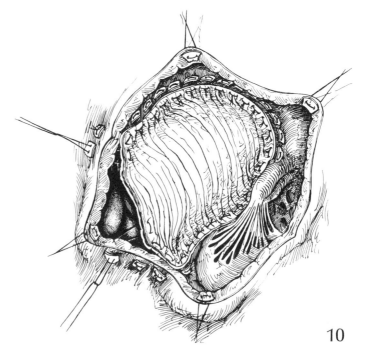

10

11

Insertion of conduit between right ventricle and pulmonary artery

Fresh antibiotic-sterilized homograft is preferred for the conduit. The coronary ostia of the homograft are oversewn and the distal aorta trimmed and sutured to the pulmonary artery. The posterior anastomosis is first performed, starting from the left side. A sucker or sump is left in the right pulmonary artery during this procedure. If the pulmonary venous return is excessive a short period of reduced flow or even circulatory arrest may be used. The homograft valve is placed distally close to the pulmonary artery. In this position the valve is protected by the ascending aorta and compression of the valve is avoided.

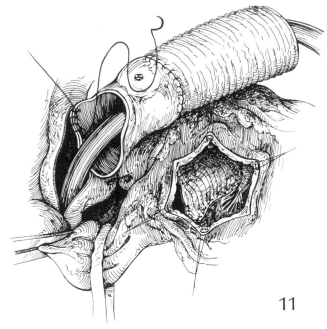

11

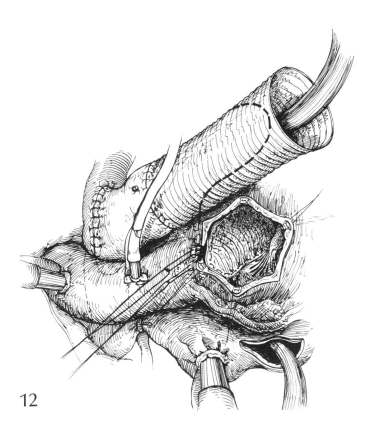

12

12

The largest conduit which will fit the pulmonary artery is selected. After the age of 3 years a 22 mm valve can usually be inserted.

It is often possible to use the anterior cusp of the mitral valve to attach the homograft to the right ventricle. If this is not possible, homograft can be extended with a Dacron tube. Several complications related to build-up of neo-intima involved in Dacron conduits have been described[3]. Pretreatment of knitted prostheses with fibrin seal[4,5] is currently considered a better alternative.

If an aortic homograft is not available, a conduit incorporating one of the heterograft valves can be used instead[6]. Because of the early calcification of the heterograft valves, we would prefer a valveless conduit should the homograft be unavailable.

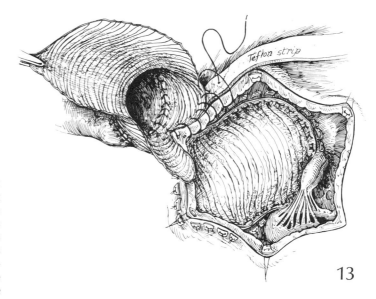

13

13 & 14

When the distal anastomosis is completed the aortic clamp is removed and the patient rewarmed. The last stitches on the ventricular septal defect patch are tied. The needle used for infusion of cardioplegic solution is connected to the vent suction. The length of the conduit is then assessed on the beating heart. The conduit is trimmed obliquely and anastomosed to the right ventriculotomy with 4/0 polypropylene on a large needle. The upper part of the conduit is sutured to the edge of the ventricular septal defect patch. To improve haemostasis the ventricular suture line may be buttressed with two strips of Teflon felt. After the completion of bypass intracardiac pressures are measured before the cannulae are removed from the heart.

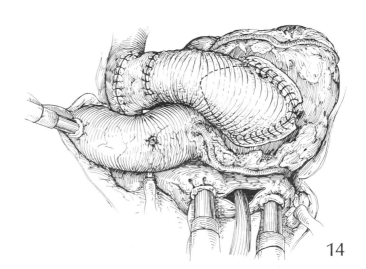

14

Complications

Numerous suture lines and a long conduit increase the risk of postoperative bleeding and tamponade. Haemostasis must therefore be meticulous. Preclotting of the conduit is helpful. Compression of the conduit by the sternum occurred in earlier years in several series; this can be avoided by placing the conduit away from the midline. It is usually placed to the left of the aorta.

Residual ventricular septal defect, pseudoaneurysm of the right ventricle, stenosis of the conduit, obstruction between the left ventricle and aorta and late infections have been described. The long-term fate of the valve and conduit remains to be evaluated. To date the fresh antibiotic-sterilized homograft aortic valve is considered to be the optimal conduit.

15

PATIENTS WITH INTACT VENTRICULAR SEPTUM

In these cases a Mustard or Senning operation is performed. After the aorta has been cross-clamped the left ventricular outflow tract obstruction is examined. This can be done from above after opening the pulmonary artery and inspecting the valve and subvalvar region. A modified nasal speculum[7] facilitates visualization of the subvalvar region. Alternative approaches to the left ventricular outflow tract obstruction are through the mitral valve after excision of the interatrial septum or from the apical left ventriculotomy[8].

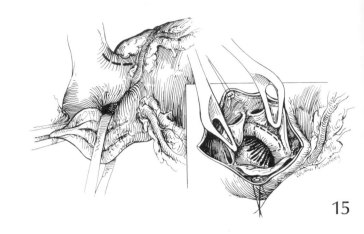

15

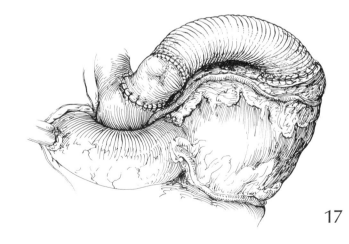

16

16

If relief of the obstruction is inadequate or impossible a left ventricle-to-pulmonary artery valved conduit is inserted. A short ventriculotomy is performed at the apex of the left ventricle. Care is taken not to damage any coronary arteries. A preclotted valved conduit is sutured to the edges of the ventriculotomy. The suture line is buttressed with two strips of Teflon felt. We do not excise a button of myocardium before insertion of the conduit, nor do we use a metal extension of the conduit into the left ventricular cavity in patients with transposition of the great arteries.

17

The left pleural space is opened and the length of the conduit is estimated. It is important that the conduit assumes a gentle curve· so that it is not compressed or kinked. Distally the conduit is anastomosed to the side of the main or left pulmonary artery with 5/0 polypropylene. Residual gradients between the left ventricle and pulmonary artery are well tolerated in patients with transposition of the great arteries for a number of years.

17

References

1. Rastelli, G. C., McGoon, D. C., Wallace, R. B. Anatomic correction of transposition of the great arteries with ventricular septal defect and subpulmonary stenosis. Journal of Thoracic and Cardiovascular Surgery 1969; 58: 545–552

2. Singh, A. K., Stark, J., Taylor, J. F. N. Left ventricle to pulmonary artery conduit in treatment of transposition of great arteries, restrictive ventricular septal defect and acquired pulmonary atresia. British Heart Journal 1976; 38: 1213–1216

3. Agarwal, K. C., Edwards, W. D., Feldt, R. H., Danielson, G. K., Puga, F. J., McGoon, D. C. Clinicopathological correlates of obstructed right sided porcine-valved extracardiac conduits. Journal of Thoracic and Cardiovascular Surgery 1981; 81: 591–601

4. Haverich, A., Waltherbusch, G., Borst, H. G. The use of fibrin glue for sealing vascular prostheses of high porosity. Thoracic and Cardiovascular Surgery 1981; 29: 252–254

5. Stark, J., de Leval, M. Experience with fibrin seal (Tisseel) in operations for congenital heart defects. Annals of Thoracic Surgery 1984; 38: 411–413

6. Moulton, A. L., de Leval, M. R., Macartney, F. J., Taylor, J. F. N., Stark, J. Rastelli procedure for transposition of the great arteries, ventricular septal defect, and left ventricular outflow tract obstruction. British Heart Journal 1981; 45: 20

7. Alfieri, O., Subramanian, S. A new instrument for surgical exposure of subaortic and subpulmonic stenosis. Annals of Thoracic Surgery 1975; 19: 589–591

8. Stark, J. Primary definitive intracardiac operations in infants: transposition of the great arteries. In: Advances in Cardiovascular Surgery. Kirklin, J. W., ed. New York: Grune and Stratton, 1973: 101

Anatomical correction of transposition of the great arteries

Magdi H. Yacoub FRCS, DSc (Hon)
Consultant Cardiac Surgeon, Harefield Hospital, Harefield, Middlesex;
National Heart Hospital, London, UK

Preoperative

Indications

Anatomical correction of transposition at the arterial level is the only operation which offers hope for complete cure of this anomaly by normalizing both anatomical and physiological aspects of the disease. However, as the operation entails extensive surgical manoeuvres, usually at a very young age, and because of the fact that the long-term results are still unknown, it is advisable that it should only be attempted in specialized centres with wide experience in open heart surgery in infants and children. The operation can be applied to all patients with complete transposition, except those with *organic* obstruction of the left ventricular outflow tract, usually involving the pulmonary valve.

Prior to considering the child for anatomical correction, it is essential to define accurately the state of the atrioventricular valves, particularly with reference to the presence or absence of straddling tricuspid or mitral valves. The presence, size and number of ventricular septal defects and the degree of development of the right and left ventricles must be assessed, as well as the state of the left ventricular outflow. This information can be obtained by a high-quality two-dimensional echocardiogram, thus obviating the necessity for invasive investigations, particularly in neonates.

The correction can be performed as a one-stage procedure in patients with additional lesions which maintain a high peak systolic pressure in the left ventricle (at least two-thirds of that in the systemic ventricle), such as large ventricular septal defects, persistent ductus arteriosus, or significant dynamic subpulmonary stenosis.

In patients with intact ventricular septum regression of pulmonary vascular resistance and systolic pressure in the pulmonary artery following birth leads to a fall in systolic pressure in the left ventricle which, in turn, results in lack of development of the left ventricle. This eventually leads to the ventricle being incapable of supporting the systemic circulation. There is a time during the neonatal period when it is possible to perform anatomical correction. In my experience, this period varies from 12 to 35 days.

In infants presenting during the first few days of life, after confirming the diagnosis non-invasively, the clinical state of the child is assessed, and if there is no ventricular septal defect, but there is adequate mixing through a patent foramen ovale and a persistent ductus arteriosus, prostaglandins are given to keep the ductus open while preparations are made for anatomical correction within the next few days. The state of the left ventricle can be accurately assessed from day to day by frank vectocardiogram, monitoring the direction of the initial forces in the horizontal loop. If this is counter-clockwise, it indicates a well-developed ventricle capable of supporting the systemic circulation. In addition, if a short axis subcostal view of a high-quality two-dimensional echogram shows the left ventricular cavity to be circular this confirms the suitability of the patient for a one-stage procedure.

After the first few weeks of life, when the ventricle is judged to be incapable of supporting the systemic circulation, it is possible to redevelop the left ventricle by banding the pulmonary artery in combination with a systemic to pulmonary artery shunt[1].

The operation

PREPARATION OF THE LEFT VENTRICLE BY A FIRST-STAGE OPERATION

1

A right anterolateral thoracotomy is performed through the lower border of the fourth rib, the child being placed in a semi-lateral position.

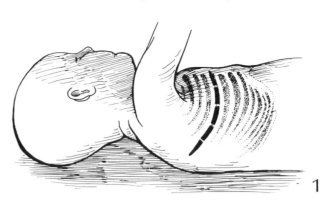

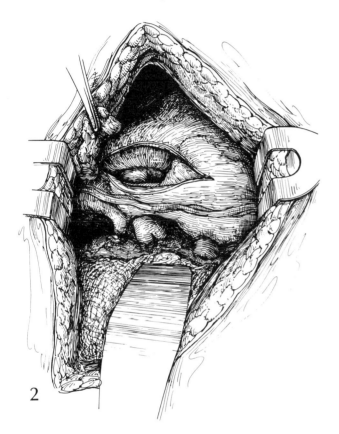

2

The thymus is dissected off the pericardium in front of the phrenic nerve, to expose the uppermost part of the pericardium. A limited longitudinal incision is then performed about 4 mm in front of and parallel to the phrenic nerve, thus exposing the two great arteries. In addition the junction of the right and main pulmonary arteries and junction between the right atrium and superior vena cava are exposed.

The diagnosis is confirmed. The type of coronary anatomy is noted, and pressures in the main pulmonary artery and ascending aorta are measured.

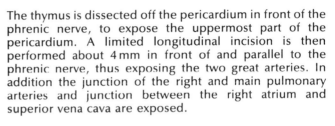

3

A systemic to pulmonary artery shunt is performed, with interposition of a Goretex graft. The azygos vein is doubly ligated and divided.

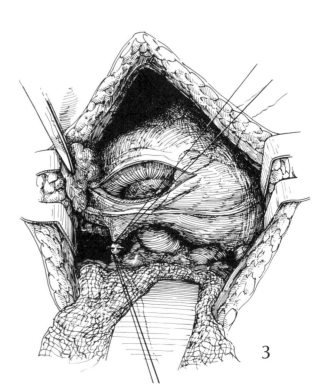

4

The subclavian artery is dissected at the apex of the pleural cavity, exposing the right vagus nerve and the origin of the recurrent laryngeal nerve. An area for the anastomosis is then chosen, either proximal to (as in the diagram) or, more commonly, distal to the vagus nerve.

The patient is heparinized using 1.5 mg/kg. A side occluding clamp is applied to the subclavian artery at the chosen point. A 4 mm Goretex tube is then cut off obliquely and anastomosed to the artery using a 6/0 polypropylene suture.

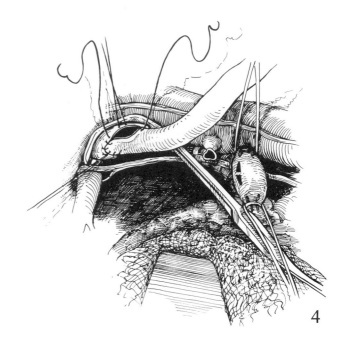

4

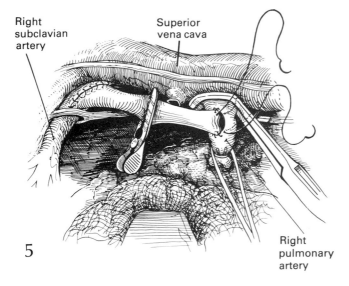

Right subclavian artery

Superior vena cava

Right pulmonary artery

5

5

The proximal part of the right pulmonary artery is dissected freely, identifying its point of origin, as well as the point of origin of its first upper lobe branch. This is facilitated by dividing the azygos vein, preparing a bed for the Goretex tube. The site for the peripheral anastomosis, between the Goretex shunt and the pulmonary artery, is then chosen. This should be as near as possible to the bifurcation of the pulmonary artery and as far removed as possible from the first branch of the right pulmonary artery. This is to facilitate control of the shunt at the second-stage operation and to distribute blood evenly to the two pulmonary arteries.

The proximal pulmonary artery is then controlled using a Cooley-type clamp and the distal artery controlled using a loop of 1/0 linen thread. The incision is then made in the pulmonary artery at the selected point which should be at the junction of the anterior and superior walls of the artery.

The incision itself should be slightly smaller than the envisaged anastomosis, as the elastic pulmonary artery usually stretches to the desired size. The length of the shunt should be adjusted by cutting any excess length of the Goretex, dividing the artery exactly transversely.

The anastomosis is then performed using 6/0 sutures, starting at the posterior end. A shunt larger than 4 mm should never be used for this operation as, unlike patients with Fallot's tetralogy who have relatively small pulmonary arteries, the pulmonary arteries in simple transposition are extremely large, and the use of a larger shunt can result in severe pulmonary oedema. Arterial saturation is measured both before and after releasing the shunt. Usually, there is an increase of about 10 per cent.

6

The position of the band is of crucial importance, as it should not be too close to the commissures of the pulmonary valve (the future aortic valve) and not too near the bifurcation of the pulmonary artery so as to encroach on the pulmonary artery branches.

The appropriate site is chosen and a very limited dissection between the two great arteries is made sharply and developed in a plane exactly perpendicular to the axis of the great arteries. The tunnel so created should measure only 2 mm in width. This should prevent migration of the band distally, which can be produced by the high pressure proximal to the band. A 2.5 mm nylon band is usually used for this operation.

Passage of the band around the pulmonary artery can be performed in two stages.

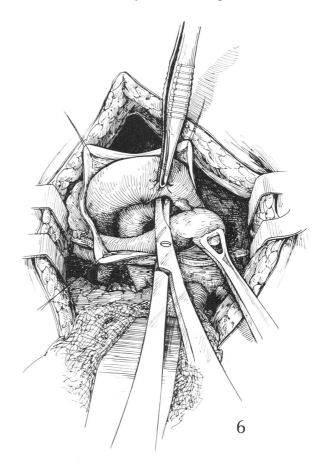

6

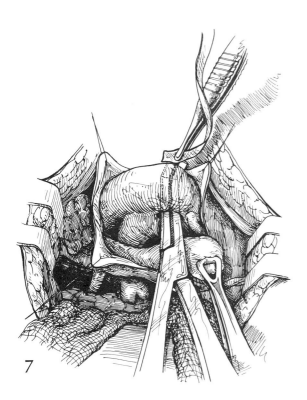

7

7

First, a right-angled forcep is passed around the aorta and the band threaded around that vessel.

8

The far end of the band is then drawn behind the pulmonary artery through the transverse sinus, thus placing the band around the pulmonary artery at the desired position.

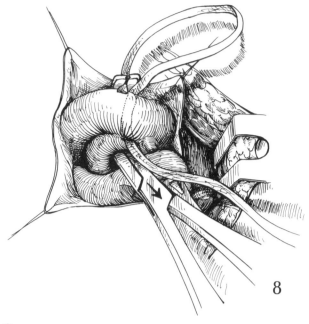

8

9

The band is then tightened by placing tension on the two limbs of the band and suturing the band, creating a constricting ring measuring between 7 and 8 mm in circumference. Finally, 4/0 sutures are used to stitch the sides of the band to each other.

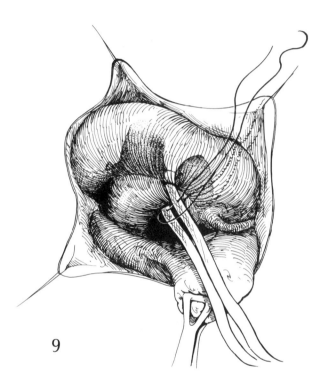

9

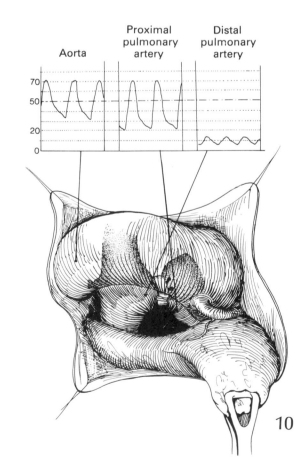

10

10

The degree of tightness is of crucial importance and might need to be readjusted several times. The objectives are to obtain a systolic pressure equal to or just under that in the aorta while maintaining a pulsatile pressure tracing distal to the band and arterial oxygen saturation equal to or more than 45 per cent. The heart rate should not drop. The arterial acid-base status should be repeatedly monitored after placing the band. Progressive acidosis indicates that the band is too tight.

ANATOMICAL CORRECTION OF THE GREAT ARTERIES

The incision and preparation for bypass

A median sternotomy is performed. The position and relative size of the great arteries, as well as the site of origin and exact distribution of the coronary arteries, is determined. All four chambers are inspected and pressures recorded. The relationship between the peak systolic pressure in the right and left ventricles, as well as the presence or absence of a gradient across the left ventricular outflow tract, is noted.

A cannula is inserted in the aortic arch for arterial return. For neonates a metal cannula measuring 2 mm in diameter is used. The superior and inferior venae cavae are separately cannulated through the right atrial wall. The patient is then cooled to a nasopharyngeal temperature of 16°C.

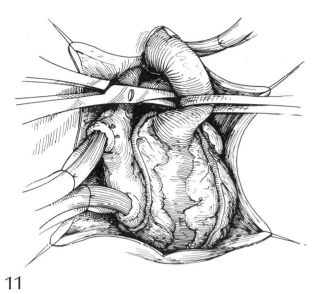

11

11

Mobilization of aorta and pulmonary arteries

The two great arteries are separated by dividing the pericardial reflection and adventitial tissue between them, starting from the level at the top of the commissures and pulmonary artery, and extending to the level of the ductus or ligamentum arteriosum. The latter is doubly ligated and divided.

12

Inspection of the pulmonary valve

The pulmonary valve is inspected through a transverse incision in the pulmonary artery at the level chosen for transecting that vessel. This should be about 3 mm above the top of the commissures of the pulmonary valve. In patients who have had previous banding, this incision should be immediately below the site of the band. Any organic stenosis of the pulmonary valve constitutes an absolute contraindication to anatomical correction. In these patients, a Mustard or Senning operation is performed. The presence of a bicuspid, functionally normal, pulmonary valve is a relative contraindication.

The subpulmonary regions are carefully inspected. The presence of functional subpulmonary stenosis is usually accompanied by subendocardial fibrous thickening at the level of the tip of the mitral valve. In these patients, the left ventricular outflow tract is very wide in a relaxed heart, and no surgical excision of any tissue in this region is necessary.

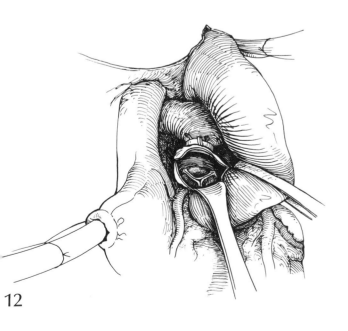

12

13

Transection of the aorta and pulmonary arteries

The level of transection of the aorta depends on whether the Le Compte manoeuvre or a non-valved conduit is going to be used for bridging the gap between the proximal aorta and distal pulmonary artery. If the Le Compte manoeuvre is to be used, the incision should be performed as high as possible (level A in the diagram), leaving about 4 mm of aortic tissue below the aortic clamp, which is applied as near as possible to the arterial return cannula. However, if a non-valved conduit is to be used, the incision is performed 4 mm above the top of the aortic valve commissures (level B in the diagram).

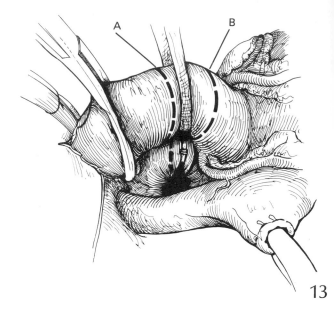

13

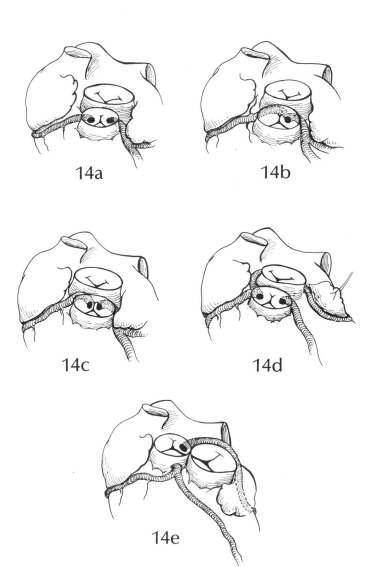

14a

14b

14c

14d

14e

14a–e

Identification of coronary artery

The position of the coronary ostia and their relation to the sinuses of Valsalva of the aortic and pulmonary valves are then determined. In addition, the course and mode of branching of the proximal 5 mm of each artery is carefully inspected.

In all patients with transposition of the great arteries, the coronary ostia are situated in the two sinuses facing the pulmonary artery and therefore lend themselves to coronary transfer. Most commonly, the right and left coronary arteries arise from the right and left posterior sinuses, respectively[2]. Occasionally, both arteries arise by common trunk or by two orifices adjoining each other, very closely related to the commissure between the two coronary sinuses b and c respectively). Not uncommonly, the right coronary artery gives rise to the circumflex branch which passes behind the pulmonary artery to reach to atrioventricular groove (d). When the two great arteries are situated side by side, the right coronary artery arises from the anterior left sinus and passes in front of the right ventricular outflow tract. In these patients, the right coronary gives origin to the anterior descending or a right ventricular branch, which runs parallel to the anterior descending. The circumflex arises from the left posterior sinus and passes behind the pulmonary artery to reach the atrioventricular groove (e).

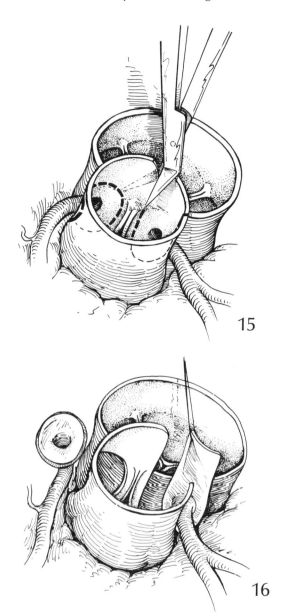

15

16

15 & 16

Mobilization of coronary ostia

The ostia are mobilized with a surrounding rim of aortic wall, which should include almost the whole of the wall of the sinus of Valsalva. This process is started at the edge of the transected aortic wall for the left coronary ostium. The right ostium is, however, mobilized with a circular surrounding rim of aortic wall.

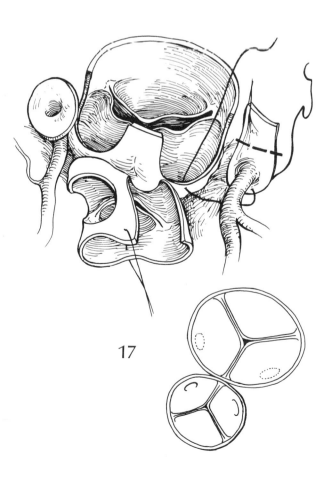

17

17

Preparation for coronary anastomosis

A site on the pulmonary artery for the coronary anastomosis is chosen. This should be higher than the top of the sinus of Valsalva, to avoid distorting the aortic valve or producing tension or kinking of the coronary artery. The site chosen should allow for rotation of the mobilized disc through an angle of not more than 30°. A disc of pulmonary artery wall is excised.

Coronary anastomosis

18

The coronary anastomosis is performed using 6/0 absorbable suture, taking care not to produce any torsion of the mobilized disc.

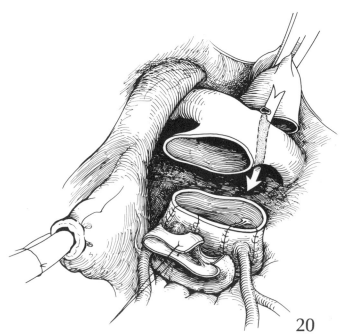

18

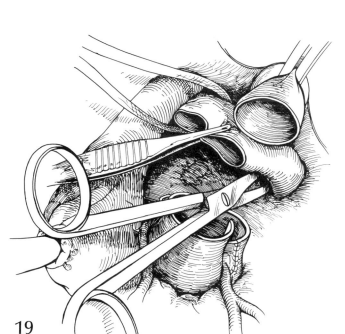

19

19

The Le Compte manoeuvre entails threading the top end of the aorta behind the mobilized pulmonary artery bifurcation.

For this purpose, the bifurcation of the pulmonary artery is dissected freely. The dissection is extended beyond the site of the divided ductus into the pulmonary hilum on the left side and behind the superior vena cava to the branching of the right pulmonary artery on the right.

20

The top end of the ascending aorta is then threaded behind the pulmonary artery and the controlling clamp transferred onto the aorta at its new site behind the pulmonary artery bifurcation.

20

21

The small distal end of the aorta is matched to the usually larger proximal pulmonary artery for anastomosis by making a longitudinal incision in the posterior wall of the distal aorta. The two vessels are then anastomosed using either continuous 5/0 absorbable sutures or interrupted 5/0 prolene sutures. The aortic clamp is then released, thus allowing perfusion of the coronary arteries.

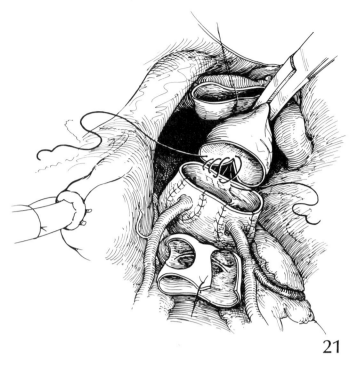

21

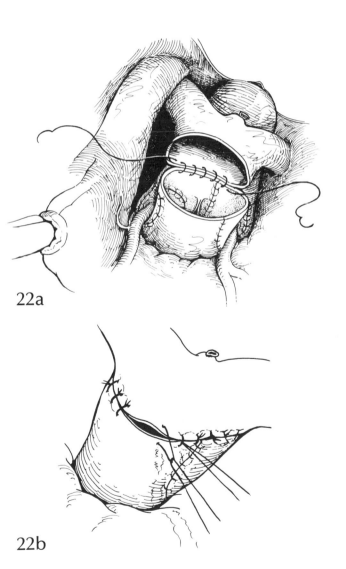

22a

22b

22a & b

Following transfer of the coronary ostia, two defects are produced in the facing sinuses of the aortic root. These are repaired by inserting two patches of homologous dura mater or calf pericardium. The size of each patch should be approximately one and a half times the size of the defect, thus enlarging the diameter of the proximal aorta to match the size of the distal pulmonary artery.

The last stage of the Le Compte manoeuvre consists of direct anastomosis between the reconstructed proximal aorta and the distal pulmonary artery using a 6/0 absorbable suture (a). The long stump of the proximal aorta allows this anastomosis to be performed without stretching the newly-constructed main pulmonary artery or compressing the proximal parts of the coronary arteries.

23

An alternative method for bridging the gap between the proximal aorta and distal pulmonary artery is to use a non-valved conduit. If this alternative method is to be used, the aorta should be divided at a lower level, as mentioned earlier.

A tube of homologous dura, previously sterilized by antibiotics and preserved in glycerin, is fashioned.

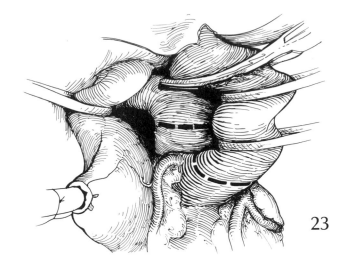

23

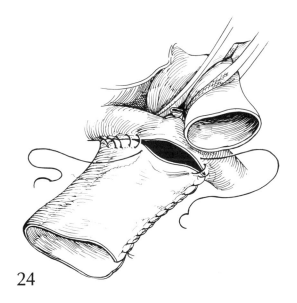

24

24

The tube should measure 7.5 cm in circumference or 2.5 cm in diameter, and should be about 8 cm in length. The dura tube is anastomosed to the distal pulmonary artery using 5/0 continuous prolene. This anastomosis is performed before anastomosing the distal aorta to the proximal pulmonary artery.

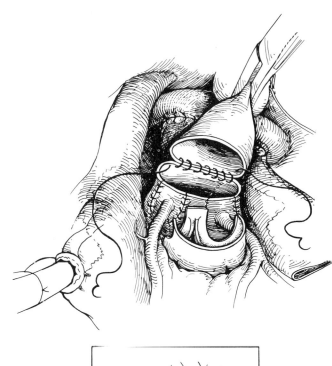

25

In this alternative technique, the long segment of distal aorta is then anastomosed to the proximal pulmonary artery using 5/0 absorbable suture. The excess length of the distal aorta allows the newly-constructed ascending aorta to arch forwards, thus preventing compression of the anastomosis between the dura tube and the distal pulmonary artery.

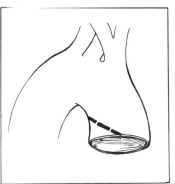

25

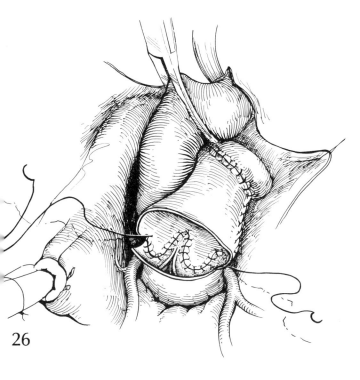

26

26

The dura tube is then placed to the left of the newly constructed ascending aorta. The length of the tube is adjusted, allowing for expansion of the ascending aorta after releasing the aortic clamp, thus preventing any future compression of the coronary ostia. A posterior slit is then performed in the tube to accommodate the intercoronary commissure and allow the tube to fill the gaps created by excision of the coronary ostia.

27

Completion of the anastomosis between the dura tube and the proximal pulmonary artery is achieved by continuing the same suture, anastomosing the anterior wall of the tube to the proximal aorta.

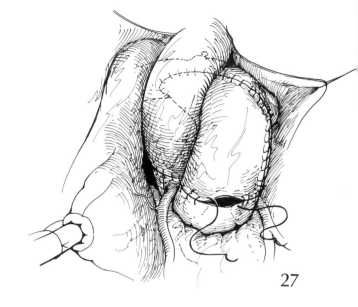

27

Postoperative management

In patients who had a peak systolic left ventricular pressure lower than systemic preoperatively, an afterload reducing agent is used for the first 48 hours. Any signs of a low cardiac output state, e.g., fall in peripheral temperature, low urinary output, poor peripheral perfusion, fall in blood pressure, is treated by increasing preload by plasma or blood transfusion, depending on the result of the packed cell volume at the time and not allowing the mean left atrial pressure to rise above 18 mmHg. Inotropic agents (such as dopamine or isoprenaline) may be administered as a slow drip. Intravenous clear fluids in the form of one-fifth normal dextrose saline are limited to 3 ml/kg per hour. Blood sugar is measured every 3 hours, and any tendency to hypoglycaemia is corrected by administering 5–15 ml of 50 per cent dextrose.

References

1. Yacoub, M., Radley-Smith, R., Maclaurin, R. Two-stage operation for anatomical correction of the great arteries with intact interventricular septum. Lancet 1977; 1: 1275

2. Yacoub, M., Radley-Smith, R. Anatomy of the coronary arteries in transposition of the great arteries and methods for their transfer in anatomical correction. Thorax 1978; 33: 418

Persistent truncus arteriosus: surgical anatomy

Robert H. Anderson BSc, MD, MRCPath
Joseph Levy Professor of Paediatric Cardiac Morphology, Cardiothoracic Institute, Brompton Hospital, London, UK

Benson R. Wilcox MD
Professor and Chief of Cardiothoracic Surgery, University of North Carolina, Chapel Hill, North Carolina, USA

Introduction

Persistent truncus arteriosus ('truncus') is one of the anomalous ventriculoarterial connections which provide the heart of the newborn infant with a single outlet. It is defined as a single arterial trunk directly supplying the systemic, pulmonary and coronary arteries. In this way truncus is distinguished from the other types of single outlet – namely, a solitary aortic trunk with pulmonary atresia or a solitary pulmonary trunk with aortic atresia, both of these being appropriately described as single outlet when it is not possible to determine the ventricular origin of the atretic great artery.

For the purposes of definition it is also our convention to define truncus only when the solitary trunk is guarded by a common arterial valve[1]. In this we follow common practice, although some authorities[2,3] have suggested that truncus can exist with two discrete outflow tracts and two separate aortic and pulmonary valves. We believe that, from a surgical viewpoint, these latter lesions are best regarded as large aortopulmonary windows. They certainly pose far less severe problems for repair than those malformations with a common outflow tract which are to be discussed here.

It is worth while to consider one further anomaly before leaving the vexatious realm of definitions. That is the lesion characterized by a solitary arterial trunk with no evidence whatsoever of intrapericardial pulmonary arteries, the intrapulmonary circulation being supplied by way of major aortopulmonary collateral arteries. The controversy as to whether the solitary great vessel is a truncus ('Truncus Type IV') or an aorta is readily solved by the simple expedient of describing it as a solitary arterial trunk[4,5]. From the surgical viewpoint the treatment is more akin to that for pulmonary atresia than for truncus.

Anatomy in relation to surgical correction

The anatomical features of truncus which determine the success of surgical treatment are its precise connection to the ventricular mass, the state of the truncal valve, the morphology of the ventricular septal defect and the arrangement of the great arteries. Although truncus can exist with any atrioventricular connection, it is exceedingly rare to find it other than with a concordant atrioventricular connection.

1

The truncus usually overrides the ventricular septum and is connected more or less equally to the right and left ventricles. The septal defect is present because of complete lack of the infundibular septum, so it is directly subarterial. The illustration is of a long-axis section at right angles to the ventricular septum showing the salient features of a typical truncus.

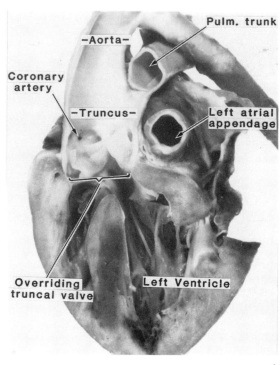

1

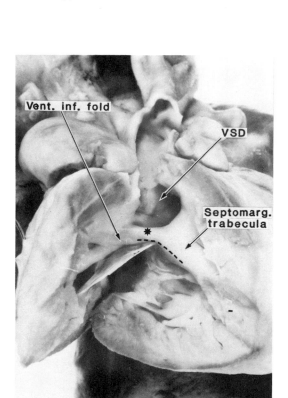

2

2

Usually the defect is cradled between the limbs of the septomarginal trabecula and the posterior limb fuses with the ventriculoinfundibular fold. As with other defects of this type, the muscle bundle thus formed between the truncal and tricuspid valves (*asterisk in illustration*) serves to buttress the conduction tissue axis (*dotted line in illustration*) away from the septal crest.

3

More rarely there can be truncal-tricuspid continuity, and then the conduction axis is much more at risk during closure of the defect when the truncus is being connected to the left ventricle since it is much closer to the defect edge (see *illustration*).

4

In the rare case in which the defect is found to be restrictive it is usually because the truncus is connected exclusively or mostly to the right ventricle, often with a subtruncal infundibulum.

If the defect is to be enlarged this can safely be done along its anterocephalad margins[6]. After surgical repair of truncus following the Rastelli technique[7] the truncal valve effectively becomes the aortic valve. Valvar incompetence or stenosis, if present, is therefore of considerable significance. Although dysplastic truncal valves have been encountered with some frequency in autopsy studies of infant hearts[8], they do not seem to pose a major problem in surgical repair in infancy. Predominant connection of the truncus to the left ventricle can also occur, but this variation is working in the surgeon's favour and does not pose any additional problems.

Variation in great arterial morphology occurs in both the pulmonary and the aortic pathways. Following the classical studies of Collett and Edwards[9] truncus is usually classified according to the mode of origin of the pulmonary arteries. The most common patterns are either for the two pulmonary arteries to arise from a short confluent channel ('Type I') or for them to arise separately but directly from the left posterior aspect of the trunk ('Type II'). The presence of a short pulmonary confluence would certainly facilitate banding, but this procedure is now rarely performed in specialized centres. Either of the two patterns permits easy connection to a right ventricular conduit during complete repair.

The much rarer variant in which each pulmonary artery arises from the side of the trunk ('Type III') makes complete repair more difficult but not impossible.

As stated above, we believe that so-called 'truncus Type IV' with no evidence of intrapericardial pulmonary arteries is best described as a solitary arterial trunk. The possibility of successful surgical treatment is dictated by the pattern of pulmonary arterial supply via the major aortopulmonary collateral arteries. If these arise together from the descending aorta it may be possible to isolate this segment together with the collateral arteries and effect 'complete' repair.

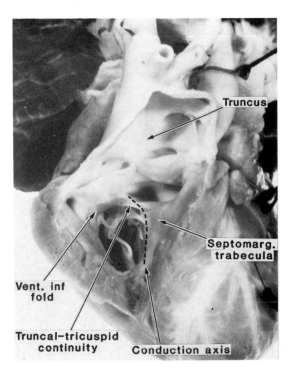

3

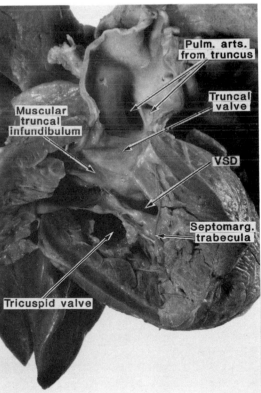

4

Although categorization of truncus tends to concentrate on the pulmonary arteries, the pattern of the aortic arch is of equal if not greater surgical significance. Usually the aorta arises in its anticipated position, or more rarely anteriorly[10], but continues to supply the head and neck arteries and the descending aorta.

5

The variant in which the aortic arch is interrupted is the pattern which will give the surgeon problems. In this arrangement the ascending aorta supplies only the head and neck arteries or even only part of this supply[3]. Usually the interruption is at the isthmus, but it can occur proximal to the origin of the left subclavian artery. In either pattern the descending aorta is supplied by the ductus. It is therefore imperative to recognize this arrangement and make appropriate modifications if surgical repair is contemplated[11].

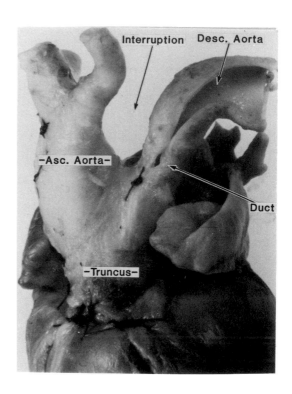

5

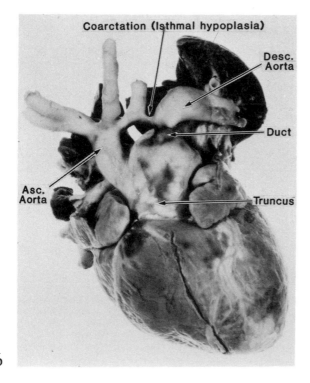

6

6

Interruption with truncus is by no means infrequent, being found in up to one-fifth of autopsy series[1-3,12]. Coarctation can also occur, though rarely, with hypoplasia rather than interruption of the arch (see *illustration*). Again the supply to the descending aorta will be primarily duct-dependent.

References

1. Crupi, G., Macartney, F. J., Anderson, R. H. Persistent truncus arteriosus: a study of 66 autopsy cases with special reference to definition and morphogenesis. American Journal of Cardiology 1977; 40: 569–578

2. Van Praagh, R., Van Praagh, S. The anatomy of common aorticopulmonary trunk (truncus arteriosus communis) and its embryologic implications: A study of 57 necroscopy cases. American Journal of Cardiology 1965; 16: 406–425

3. Calder, L., Van Praagh, R., Van Praagh, S. Truncus arteriosus communis: clinical, angiocardiographic, and pathologic findings in 100 patients. American Heart Journal 1976; 92: 23–38

4. Thiene, G., Anderson, R. H. Pulmonary atresia with ventricular septal defect: anatomy. In: Anderson R. H., Macartney, F. J., Shinebourne, E. A., Tynan, M., eds. *Paediatric Cardiology*, Volume 5. Edinburgh: Churchill Livingstone, 1983: 80–101

5. Anderson, R. H. Truncus Type IV: does it exist? (Invited introduction). In: Moulton, A. L., ed. Current Controversies in Techniques in Congenital Heart Disease. Pasadena: Appleton Davis Inc, 1984: 101–105

6. Thiene, G., Cucchini, F., Pellegrino, P. A. Truncus arteriosus communis associated with underdevelopment of the aortic arch. British Heart Journal 1975; 37: 1268–1272

7. Rastelli, G. C., Titus, J. L., McGoon, D. C. Homograft of ascending aorta and aortic valve as a right ventricular outflow: an experimental approach to the repair of truncus arteriosus. Archives of Surgery 1967; 95: 698–708

8. Becker, A. E., Becker, M. J., Edwards, J. E. Pathology of the semilunar valve in persistent truncus arteriosus. Journal of Thoracic and Cardiovascular Surgery 1971; 62: 16–26

9. Collett, R. W., Edwards, J. E. Persistent truncus arteriosus: a classification according to anatomic types. Surgical Clinics of North America 1949; 29: 1245–1270

10. Angelini, P., Verdugo, A. L., Illera, J. P., Leachman, R. D. Truncus arteriosus communis: unusual case associated with transposition. Circulation 1977; 56: 1107–1110

11. Gomes, M. M. R., McGoon, D. C. Truncus arteriosus with Interruption of the aortic arch: report of a case successfully repaired. Mayo Clinic Proceedings 1971; 46: 40–43

12. Bharati, S., McAllister, H. A. Jr., Rosenquist, G. C., Miller, R. A., Tatooles, C. J., Lev, M. The surgical anatomy of truncus arteriosus communis. Journal of Thoracic and Cardiovascular Surgery 1974; 67: 501–510

Persistent truncus arteriosus

Marc de Leval MD
Consultant Cardiothoracic Surgeon, The Hospital for Sick Children, Great Ormond Street, London, UK

Introduction

INCIDENCE AND DEFINITION

Persistent truncus arteriosus ('truncus') is a rare condition which accounts for less than 3 per cent of all congenital heart defects. It is characterized by: (1) the presence of a single arterial trunk emerging from the bases of both ventricles by way of a single semilunar valve; (2) a high ventricular septal defect (VSD) subjacent to the valve; and (3) origin of the pulmonary arteries from the truncus.

1

In Type I the pulmonary trunk connects the left and right pulmonary arteries to the truncus, in Type II the arteries originate from a common orifice of the truncus and in Type III the right and left pulmonary arteries originate separately from the lateral aspect of the truncus. Patients with Collett and Edwards's Type IV truncus arteriosus[1], in whom the lungs are supplied by way of systemic arteries, should be grouped with patients having pulmonary atresia.

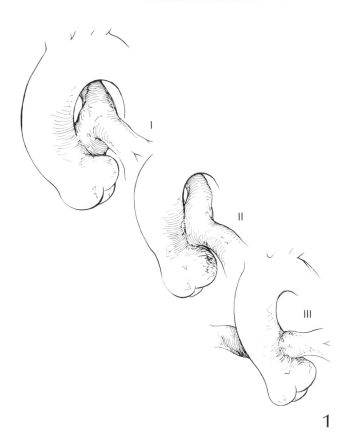

1

NATURAL HISTORY

The median age of death reported in autopsy series varies from a few weeks to a few months. Congestive heart failure secondary to large pulmonary blood flow with or without associated truncal valve regurgitation is the major cause of death in early infancy. Progressive pulmonary vascular obstructive disease is likely to occur in patients who survive beyond the age of 1 year.

INDICATIONS FOR SURGERY

Banding of the pulmonary artery or arteries as palliative treatment of heart failure in young infants carries a very high mortality and there is now a tendency to consider performing complete repair even in infancy when the patient is in intractable congestive heart failure. In older patients surgical repair should be undertaken before irreversible pulmonary vascular obstructive disease develops and probably before the age of 2 years.

PREOPERATIVE INVESTIGATIONS

Complete cardiac catheterization and angiocardiography are necessary to delineate the exact anatomy and to evaluate the haemodynamic status. The latter includes an assessment of the pulmonary arteriolar resistance and the competence of the truncal valve.

The operations

The heart is approached through a midline sternotomy incision. The anatomy is defined and the aorta and pulmonary arteries are dissected free. The ascending aorta is cannulated high above the origin of the pulmonary arteries. If the heart is large enough both venae cavae are cannulated and the operation is performed with hypothermic cardiopulmonary bypass and cold cardioplegia. In the small infant we have used the technique of hypothermia and total circulatory arrest. In order to limit the length of arrest time we now prefer to use a single right atrial venous cannula so as to maintain cardiopulmonary bypass for most of the operation. A short period of circulatory arrest may be required during closure of the inferior part of the VSD and the atrial septal defect, if present, as these procedures may otherwise produce an air lock in the venous line.

The left atrium or the left ventricle (in the case of truncal valve incompetence) is vented as a routine.

During the cooling period and before the aorta is clamped the pulmonary arteries must be occluded to prevent flooding of the lungs when the contractions of the heart become less effective. This can be done with clamps or snares. The pulmonary arteries must remain occluded during infusion of the cardioplegic solution. In cases of severe truncal valve incompetence the cardioplegic solution may have to be infused by direct cannulation of the coronary arteries.

SURGICAL REPAIR

Surgical repair of persistent truncus arteriosus consists of three steps: (1) detachment of the pulmonary artery or arteries from the truncus and repair of the aorta; (2) closure of the VSD; (3) establishment of continuity between the right ventricle and pulmonary artery or arteries.

2

In Type I truncus arteriosus the discrete main pulmonary artery is excised from the left posterolateral aspect of the truncus and the defect closed by direct suture in the transverse direction.

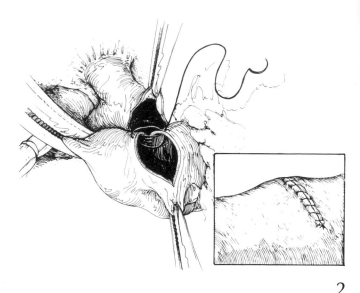

2

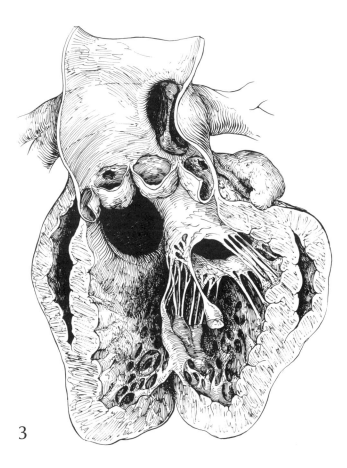

3

3

The anatomy of the condition, with the relation of the pulmonary artery to the aortic cusps, is shown in the illustration.

4

An incision is first made anteriorly at the base of insertion of the pulmonary arteries. The artery is then detached inferiorly and posteriorly, care being taken to avoid damaging the left coronary ostium and the truncal valve. The defect in the aorta is closed by double running mattress and over-and-over sutures.

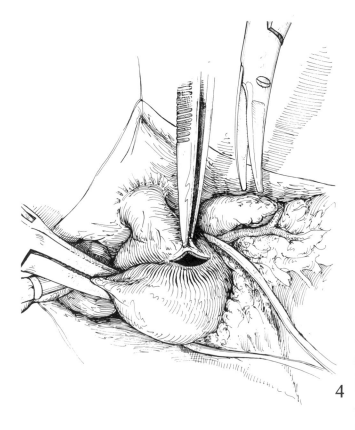

4

5

If the two pulmonary arteries arise from a common orifice on the left dorsal aspect of the truncus without a common pulmonary trunk (Type II) an oval defect is formed in the back of the truncus after their excision. This can often be closed directly, but sometimes a more satisfactory repair is obtained with a small patch of Dacron. Great care must be exercised to obtain a watertight closure of this defect as the suture line becomes inaccessible when the aorta is under tension after release of the clamp.

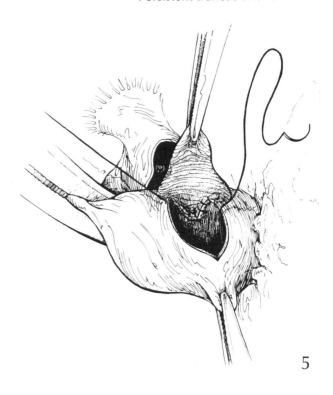

5

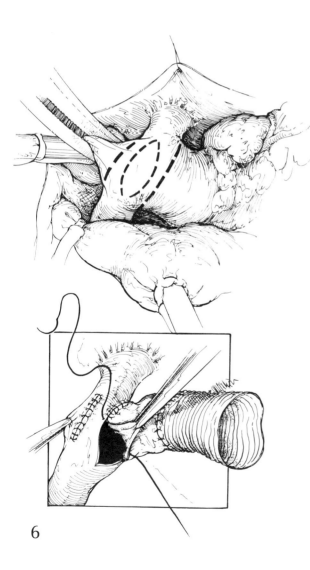

6

6

If the pulmonary arteries arise separately from the truncus (Type III) a segment of aorta containing the orifices of both pulmonary arteries is excised from the truncus so as to make a cuff of tissue containing the two pulmonary arteries. After closure of the distal defect a valved conduit is anastomosed to the proximal portion. Aortic homograft conduits are preferable, extended if necessary with Dacron.

7

Aortic continuity is restored by direct suture or by interposing a pre-clotted graft of woven Dacron.

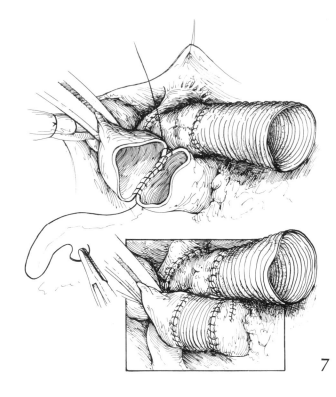

7

8

A vertical right ventriculotomy incision is then made from about the midpoint of the anterior right ventricular wall to the base near the left aspect of the annulus of the truncal valve. Some prefer a transverse ventriculotomy. The VSD is then closed so as to direct the left ventricular blood flow through the aorta as described below.

8

9

In truncus arteriosus the infundibular septum is absent and the semilunar valve constitutes the roof of the defect. Usually the trunk overrides the septum. Sometimes, however, it arises predominately from the right or left ventricle. Anteriorly the defect is limited by the superior limb of the trabecula septomarginalis. Posteriorly two types of arrangement can be seen[2]. In approximately 80 per cent of cases the posterior margin of the defect is muscular, completely separated from the anterior leaflet of the tricuspid valve and made by the posterior limb of the trabecula septomarginalis fusing with the ventriculo-infundibular fold. These are, therefore, infundibular subarterial defects.

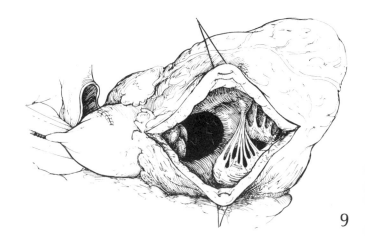

9

10

The remaining patients have a perimembranous infundibular defect in which the posterior margin goes back to the anterior leaflet of the tricuspid valve. In some of these cases the effacement of the ventriculoinfundibular fold is such that there is wide truncal triscupid continuity.

The defect is closed with a patch of Dacron velour inserted with continous or interrupted sutures.

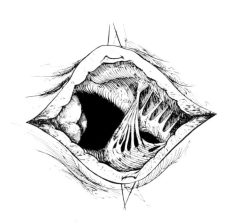

10

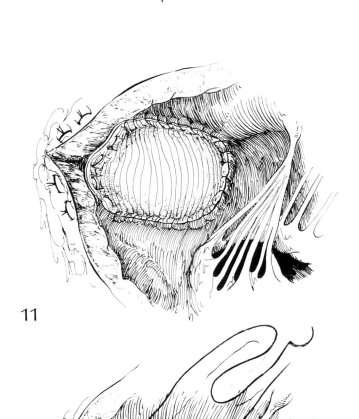

11

11

For the infundibular type of defect the muscular margin is devoid of conduction tissue and can be used to anchor the patch.

12

For the perimembranous type of defect some of the sutures must be placed through the tricuspid valve in order to avoid the penetrating bundle. The patch is then brought up to the anterior wall of the right ventricle to provide a large ventricular outflow to the aorta and to reinforce the attachment of the conduit to the right ventricle later.

12

13

Distal anastomosis of the extracardiac valved conduit can be performed either before or after closure of the defect. The conduit is placed alongside the left border of the heart into the pericardial sac while the posterior aspect of the anastomosis is being performed. In infants we usually use 5/0 polypropylene.

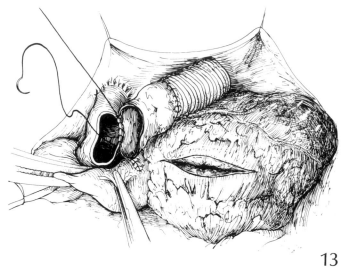

13

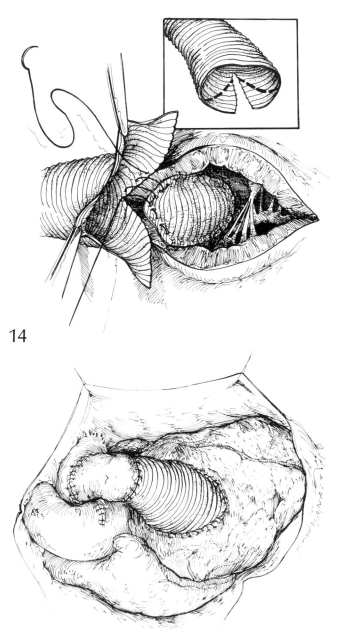

14

14 & 15

Proximally the conduit is cut obliquely to obtain a wide opening without a gradient. This anastomosis is performed with a continuous suture of 4/0 polypropylene and can be done with the aorta unclamped while the patient is being rewarmed. We prefer to use aortic homograft conduits when available. If these are too short they can be extended proximally with a pre-clotted Dacron tube. If homografts are not available we use heterograft conduits (12–16 mm in diameter in infants and 20–25 mm in children). The advantages of homograft over heterograft conduits are that it is easier to achieve a haemostatic suture line, larger conduits can be accommodated even in small infants and late obstructions have been less frequently seen.

In small infants the conduits may be accommodated by routine excision of the thymus and opening the pericardium posteriorly behind the left phrenic nerve to allow the heart to rotate to the left and posteriorly. This avoids compression of the conduit by the sternum[3].

15

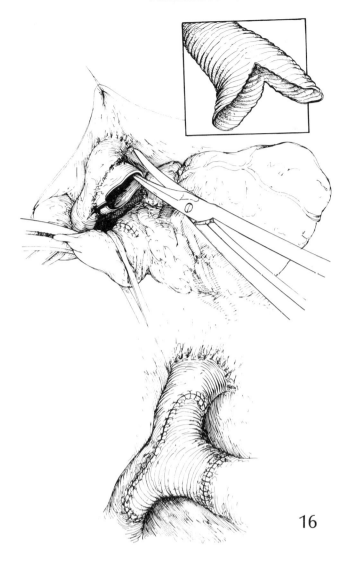

SURGICAL REPAIR IN SPECIAL CIRCUMSTANCES

Repair of truncus arteriosus with prior banding of the pulmonary arteries

16

The pulmonary arteries are detached from the truncus and the resulting aortic defect closed as previously described. The pulmonary arterial orifice is then enlarged by lateral incisions into the right and left pulmonary arteries through and well beyond the fibrotic banded zone. If the pulmonary arterial wall is of good quality a pre-clotted Dacron conduit can be trimmed in fishmouth fashion so that the resulting flap-like extension can be sutured as a gusset to enlarge the proximal banded and fibrotic pulmonary arteries[4].

16

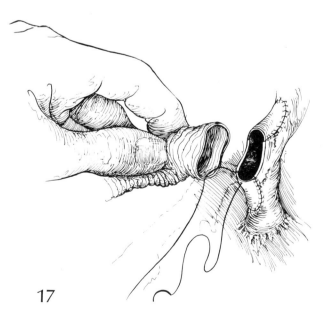

17

17

The pulmonary arteries beyond the band are sometimes so thin and friable that direct anastomosis of a stiff Dacron prosthesis would tear the vessels. We have found it useful in these cases to sew a patch of pericardium across the banded area of both pulmonary arteries and to anchor the conduit to this stronger tissue.

Repair of truncus arteriosus with interruption of the aortic arch

Persistent truncus arteriosus may be associated with interruption of the aortic arch of all three types. Surgical repair of truncus arteriosus with interrupted aortic arch consists in leaving the ductus arteriosus in continuity with the truncus as a substitute aortic arch[5].

Arterial cannulation for cardiopulmonary bypass is accomplished by using two cannulae, one in the descending aorta and the other in an external iliac artery. When the patient's temperature has been lowered to the appropriate level the ascending aorta and the ductus arteriosus are both occluded. The truncus is incised anteriorly and the pulmonary arteries excised so as to leave the ductus arteriosus superiorly connected to the ascending aorta. A valved conduit is anastomosed to the pulmonary arteries and aortic continuity is re-established by direct anastomosis or interposition of a vascular prosthesis. In infancy a single arterial cannula in the descending aorta is used to cool the patient and the reconstruction of the great vessels is performed under circulatory arrest.

Repair of truncus arteriosus with truncal valve regurgitation

Since no technique of repair of an incompetent truncal valve has provided satisfactory long-term results and in view of the poor late results of valvular replacement in children, a conservative policy is advisable for patients with mild to moderate truncal valve regurgitation.

The technical implications of truncal valve regurgitation are twofold. The cardioplegic solution cannot be infused adequately through the root of the aorta since most of it will escape to the left ventricular cavity. In older children the coronary arteries can be directly perfused, but this is often not feasible in the very small infant. Here temporary approximation of the truncal valve cusps by placing a stitch in their centre through the ventriculotomy incision is an alternative[6]. This stitch, which keeps the valve competent, is also useful to deal with the second technical aspect of the truncal valve regurgitation – namely, the combination of poor cardiac output and cardiac distension which can occur as the aortic clamp is released. The tacking suture is led through the VSD, which is left unclosed along its superior aspect. The aortic clamp is released after completion of the distal anastomosis of the conduit and the perfusate is rewarmed.

After cardiac action has returned to normal a short additional period of aortic cross-clamping is instituted. During this period the tacking suture in the aortic valve is removed, the closure of the VSD completed and the aortic clamp released. The beating heart should be capable of ejecting the regurgitation volume of blood. The proximal anastomosis of the conduit to the right ventricle is then performed on the beating heart.

Conduit replacement

Small extracardiac valved conduits (12–16 mm) are inserted in infants; replacement of the prosthesis is required at a later stage. This often becomes necessary 2–4 years after the original operation, depending on the size of the conduit. The operation is performed on cardiopulmonary bypass. The ascending aorta is cannulated in most patients. If, however, the heart is surrounded by very dense adhesions the arterial blood is returned from the pump oxygenator into an iliac artery. A single cannula is inserted into the right atrium for venous drainage and hypothermic cardiopulmonary bypass is instituted. Removal of the conduit is facilitated by opening it longitudinally. The pulmonary arteriotomy is then extended to accommodate the new prosthesis, which ideally should have a diameter of at least 20 mm. For the proximal anastomosis the sutures must be placed on the margin of the previous ventriculotomy incision, injury to the left anterior descending coronary artery being avoided.

Results

After initial single case reports of successful primary repair of persistent truncus arteriosus in infancy larger series have now been reported. Among them Ebert has undoubtedly produced the most remarkable results. He recently reported (Ebert, P., personal communication) a series of 112 infants with 13 deaths (11.6 per cent). The mortality rate was lower for patients treated under the age of 6 months (84 patients), with 8 deaths (9.5 per cent), than for patients operated on between 6 and 12 months (28 patients), with 5 deaths (17.8 per cent). This was attributed by Stanger et al.[7] from the same institution to the early development of severe pulmonary vascular disease in some patients aged 6–12 months; in their opinion patients with persistent truncus arteriosus should be electively treated before the age of 6 months.

When we reviewed our early experience of primary repair in infancy[8] the poor preoperative condition of the patients was an important risk factor. Among 13 infants there were 3 deaths in patients under 4 weeks of age treated on an emergency basis. Pulmonary vascular obstructive disease was another determinant factor in 2 patients, aged 9 and 11 months respectively, who died. Histological examination showed Grade III pulmonary vascular changes.

In patients not operated on in infancy and who remained operable according to the criteria outlined above, operative mortality was 25 per cent in a series of 92 patients reported by Marcelletti et al.[9]. The overall late mortality in that group of patients was 9 per cent. Early and late results were related to the degree of pulmonary vascular obstructive disease at the time of the operation.

References

1. Collett, R. W., Edwards, J. E. Persistent truncus arteriosus: a classification according to anatomic types. Surgical Clinics of North America 1949; 29: 1245–1270

2. Crupi, G., Macartney, F., Anderson, R. H. Persistent truncus arteriosus: a study of 66 autopsy cases with special reference to definition and morphologenesis. American Journal of Cardiology 1977; 40: 569–578

3. Dunn, J., Stark, J., de Leval, M. Avoiding compression of extracardiac valved conduits. Paediatric Cardiology, in press

4. Parker, R. K., McGoon, D. C., Danielson, G. K., Wallace, R. B., Mair, D. D. Repair of truncus arteriosus in patients with prior banding of the pulmonary artery. Surgery 1975; 78: 761–767

5. Gomes, M. M. R., McGoon, D. C. Truncus arteriosus with interruption of the aortic arch: report of a case successfully repaired. Mayo Clinic Proceedings 1971; 46: 40–43

6. de Leval, M., McGoon, D., Wallace, R. B., Danielson, G. K., Mair, D. D. Management of truncal valvular regurgitation. Annals of Surgery 1974; 180: 427–432

7. Stanger, P., Robinson, S. J., Engle, M. A., Ebert, P. A. 'Corrective' surgery for truncus arteriosus in the first year of life (Abstract). American Journal of Cardiology 1977; 39: 293

8. Stark, J., Gandhi, D., de Leval, M., Macartney, F., Taylor, J. F. N. Surgical treatment of persistent truncus arteriosus in the first year of life. British Heart Journal 1978; 40: 1280–1287

9. Marcelletti, C., McGoon, D. C., Danielson, G. K., Wallace, R. B., Mair, D. D. Early and late results of surgical repair of truncus arteriosus. Circulation 1977; 55: 636–641

Persistent ductus arteriosus: surgical anatomy

Robert H. Anderson   BSc, MD, MRCPath
Joseph Levy Professor of Paediatric Cardiac Morphology, Cardiothoracic Institute, Brompton Hospital, London, UK

Benson R. Wilcox   MD
Professor and Chief of Cardiothoracic Surgery, University of North Carolina, Chapel Hill, North Carolina, USA

Persistent patency of the arterial duct occupies a special place in the study of congenital cardiovascular disease since it was the first lesion to be cured by surgical intervention[1]. Recently it has become popular to promote ductal closure by medical manipulation[2,3], but this cannot always be achieved. Ductal interruption by surgery remains an example of the best of surgical science since the anatomy is almost invariably predictable and the surgical results are uniformly excellent.

Since the arterial system develops in bilaterally symmetrical fashion a duct can persist in either right- or left-sided position, though the latter is overwhelmingly more common. Because the duct can persist on either side, or bilaterally, its presence is significant in vascular ring anomalies (see Chapter on 'Anomalies of the aortic arch', pp. 381–392). Ductal patency also plays an important physiological role when it accompanies other complex congenital cardiovascular anomalies such as interrupted arch, aortic or pulmonary valve atresia or complete transposition of the great vessels. The morphology of the ductus in those settings has been described with the primary lesion. Here we are concerned with the isolated left-sided persistently patent duct.

The arterial duct arises from the posterior superior aspect of the junction of the pulmonary trunk and left pulmonary artery. It courses posteriorly and slightly leftwards to join the junction of the aortic arch and descending aorta just distal to and opposite the left subclavian orifice (Figure 1). Its pulmonary end is covered by a fold of pericardium and its aortic end by parietal

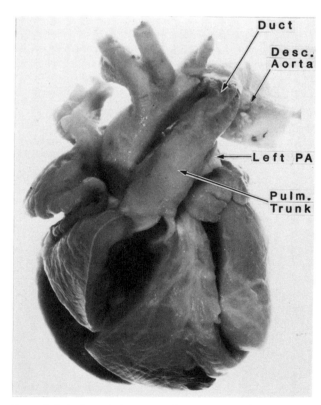

Figure 1 A ductus arteriosus seen in an anatomical specimen.

pleura. Care must be taken, particularly in the infant, not to confuse the duct with the aortic isthmus or even the left pulmonary artery. Even in the best regulated households other structures may be mistakenly ligated instead of the duct. The caveats of this procedure have recently been elegantly reviewed by Pontius et al.[4]. The best anatomical guide to the duct is the vagus nerve and its recurrent laryngeal branch. The vagus nerve passes along the subclavian artery and over the arch before heading in a posterior direction to disappear behind the hilum. Just at the level of the duct it gives off the recurrent nerve (Figure 2), which curves beneath the inferomedial wall of the duct before ascending along the posteromedial aspect of the aorta into the groove between the trachea and oesophagus.

The fold of pericardium at the pulmonary end of the duct has been alluded to above. In its posteromedial wall the duct is firmly attached by another, more fibrous, pericardial extension to the left mainstem bronchus. This firm fibrous fold prevents the easy circumscription of the duct with a right-angle clamp. To minimize the risk of tearing the ductal wall this tissue is best divided by sharp dissection. During this procedure small but potentially troublesome bronchial vessels may be encountered arising from the posterior wall of the aorta. Another structure of anatomical note in the ductal environs is the thoracic duct and its tributaries in the area of the origin of the subclavian artery. Division of any of these major lymph vessels is liable to lead to chylothorax and its attendant difficulties. Should such lymphatic trunks be divided they must be ligated to prevent this complication.

The duct in an infant or small child measures between 2 and 15 mm in length and diameter; rarely it may become aneurysmally dilated[5]. The anatomy of the short and 'fat' duct favours cross-clamping, division and oversewing of both ends to minimize the chances of incomplete closure or tearing of the vessel wall. The longer 'thin' duct is adequately dealt with by a triple ligation technique[6].

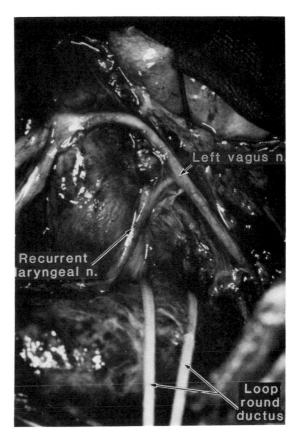

Figure 2 The duct as seen at surgery through a left thoracotomy. Note the relationship of the vagus and recurrent laryngeal nerves.

References

1. Gross, R. E. Surgical management of patent ductus arteriosus with summary of four surgically treated cases. Annals of Surgery 1939; 110: 321–356

2. Starling, M. B., Elliott, R. B. The effect of prostaglandins, prostaglandin inhibitors, and oxygen on the closure of the ductus arteriosus, pulmonary arteries, and umbilical vessels in vitro. Prostaglandins 1974; 8: 187–203

3. Heymann, M. A., Rudolph, A. M., Silverman, N. H. Closure of the ductus arteriosus in premature infants by inhibition of prostaglandin synthesis. New England Journal of Medicine 1976; 295: 530–533

4. Pontius, R. G., Danielson, G. K., Noonan, J. A., Judson, J. P. Illusions leading to surgical closure of the distal left pulmonary artery instead of the ductus arteriosus. Journal of Thoracic and Cardiovascular Surgery 1981; 82: 107–113

5. Mendel, V., Luhmer, J., Oelert, H. Aneurysma des Ductus arteriosus bei einem Neugeborenen. Herz 1980; 5: 320–323

6. Wilcox, B. R., Peters, R. M. The surgery of patent ductus arteriosus: a clinical report of 14 years' experience without an operative death. Annals of Thoracic Surgery 1967; 3: 126–131

Surgery of persistent ductus arteriosus

J. D. Wisheart MCh, FRCS
Cardiothoracic Surgeon, Bristol Royal Infirmary, Bristol, UK

J. P. Dhasmana FRCS
Senior Registrar in Cardiac and Thoracic Surgery, United Bristol Hospitals and Frenchay Hospital, Bristol, UK

Introduction

Isolated persistent ductus arteriosus is the second most common congenital cardiac anomaly, accounting for 12 per cent of the total. Spontaneous closure is usual in the first few days of life but is rare after the third month.

Bloodflow along the ductus is determined by the relative resistances, and hence pressures, in the pulmonary and systemic vascular beds. Patients may present for surgery at any time in the natural history of the abnormality. As neonatal pulmonary vascular resistance falls the left-to-right shunt increases and left ventricular failure may develop. Later, as pulmonary vascular resistance slowly increases, shunt flow moderates, the threat of left ventricular failure recedes and the patient is usually free of symptoms. Eventually, in about 5–7 per cent of cases, pulmonary vascular resistance will rise sufficiently to cause reversal of the shunt and the development of the Eisenmenger complex. In those who survive without shunt reversal aneurysmal dilatation or calcification of the duct may occur in adult life. At any time the small threat (probably about 1 per cent) of bacterial endocarditis is present.

The presence of a persistent ductus arteriosus in a premature neonate with the respiratory distress syndrome may contribute to pulmonary dysfunction and thus threaten life; surgical ligation of the ductus is performed in these circumstances. A persistent ductus may coexist with any other congenital cardiac abnormality. Of particular interest are those conditions in which pulmonary atresia is also present so that the ductus is the only source of blood flow to the lungs; in these 'ductus-dependent' conditions spontaneous closure of the ductus may be prevented or delayed by the use of prostaglandin E.

Optimally, operation is carried out between the second and fifth years of life or at the time of diagnosis if complications are present. Surgery is contraindicated in the presence of severe pulmonary hypertension with shunt reversal. When associated with other congenital cardiac anomalies the persistent ductus should not usually be surgically treated in isolation but should be closed at the time of definitive corrective operation and before the institution of bypass.

The aim of surgery is to interrupt the communication between the pulmonary and systemic circuits, either by division or ligation of the duct. Panagopoulos et al.[1] have shown that ligation is a safe and satisfactory technique in most cases, while division may be reserved for the short, wide or high-pressure duct. The operative mortality in uncomplicated cases is less than 0.5 per cent but is higher in infancy, when associated with other abnormalities or in the presence of pulmonary hypertension.

Preoperative

Special investigations are not required for the classical clinical picture of persistent ductus arteriosus in childhood. Cardiac catheterization will help to elucidate any unusual clinical finding or associated abnormalities, will permit measurement of the level of pulmonary vascular resistance and is often helpful in infants or in adults.

In the uncomplicated case preoperative bacteriological screening and blood count should be carried out and 2 units of blood should be cross-matched; prophylactic antibiotic treatment should be started before surgery. An arterial cannula should be inserted in infants; they may also require postoperative mechanical ventilation. When left ventricular failure is present it should be treated with digoxin and diuretics: subacute bacterial endocarditis should be treated with appropriate antibiotics for at least 6 weeks and some authorities advise a further delay of up to 3 months before surgery.

The operation

1

The incision

Left posterolateral thoracotomy is carried out through the third or fourth intercostal space.

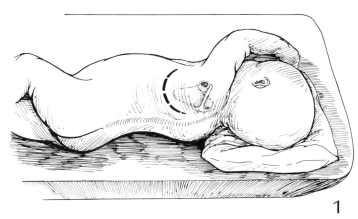

2

Surgical anatomy

When the left lung is retracted forwards and downwards the aortic arch, the left subclavian artery, the pulmonary artery and the vagus and phrenic nerves can be seen. A thrill is palpable, but it is not usual to see the ductus clearly at this stage. The aortic sheath is opened by a vertical incision extending from the left subclavian artery to below the ductus.

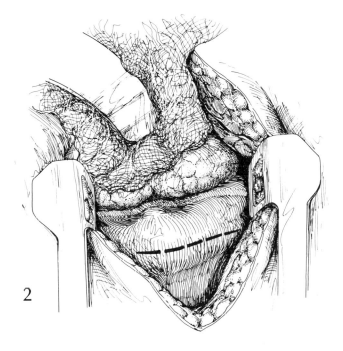

3

Dissection of the aortic sheath

After the aortic sheath has been reflected forwards, sharp and blunt dissection being used to maintain the correct plane, it is retracted by stay sutures which also serve to keep the left lung out of the immediate operative field. If it is necessary to pass tapes around the aorta above and below the ductus the posterior part of the aortic sheath is dissected next and care taken to avoid damaging the intercostal arteries.

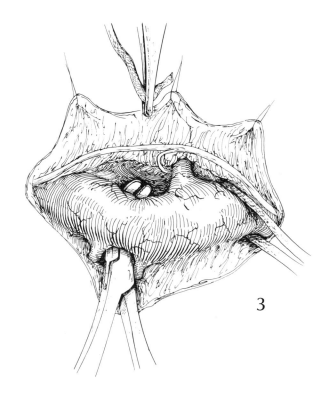

Identification of the ductus

The aortic end of the ductus can now be seen and the anatomy of the arch of the aorta is confirmed by identification of the left common carotid artery proximal to the left subclavian artery. Further reflection of the aortic sheath anteriorly permits dissection of the anterior, superior and inferior aspects of the ductus, still in the same tissue plane. The vagus and recurrent laryngeal nerves are reflected safely with the pleura and sheath.

4 & 5

Dissection of the ductus

Development of the same plane usually permits a right-angled dissecting instrument to be passed around the back of the ductus. If it is difficult to free the back of the ductus the aorta may be lifted forwards with the tapes and the dissection completed under direct vision. Gentle lateral retraction of the aorta facilitates dissection of the pulmonary end of the ductus; in particular it may be freed from the pouch of overlying pericardium.

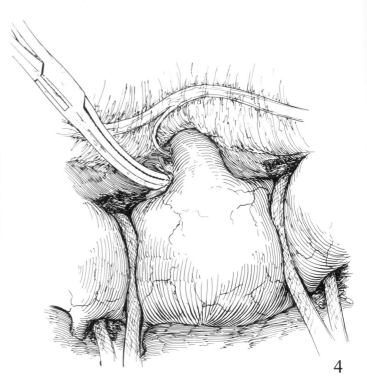

4

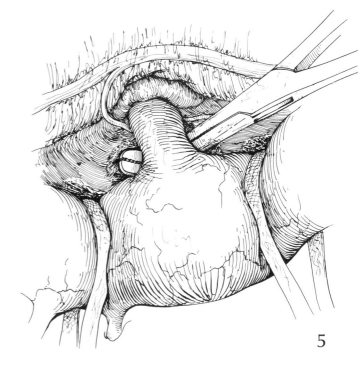

5

Ligation of the ductus

The effects of occluding the ductus should now be observed by 'test-clamping' with a vascular clamp. It is usually sufficient to observe arterial pressure and heart rate. Should the arterial pressure fall and the heart rate rise, especially in the presence of known pulmonary vascular disease, the pulmonary artery pressure should be measured before and after clamping. Failure of the pulmonary artery pressure to fall indicates that the operation should not be carried further.

6

Two ligatures of 1/0 linen or plaited silk are now passed around the ductus and the aortic end ligated first. Temporary reduction in aortic pressure makes this safe and is most easily achieved by cross-clamping the aorta above the ductus for the 20 seconds needed to apply the first two throws to the knot, which is then completed with the aorta released. The second ligature is applied to the pulmonary end of the ductus, which has now been decompressed. It is important that the two ligatures should be separated.

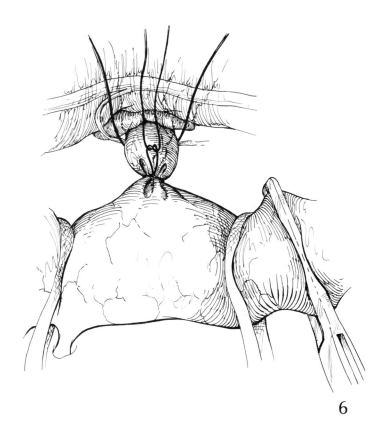

6

7

Closure

When haemostasis has been secured the pleura should be reconstituted over the aorta, a basal intercostal drain inserted, the lung carefully reinflated and the chest closed.

7

8a & b

Division of the ductus

When the ductus is to be divided two clamps should be applied to the aortic and pulmonary ends. Traditionally a pair of Potts clamps has been used, but if a side-biting clamp is applied to the aorta at the origin of the ductus more secure control is achieved and more room provided for suturing (a). A straight or angled vascular clamp is applied at the pulmonary end of the ductus, which is now divided and its two ends secured with running sutures of 3/0, 4/0 or 5/0 Prolene mounted on an atraumatic needle (b).

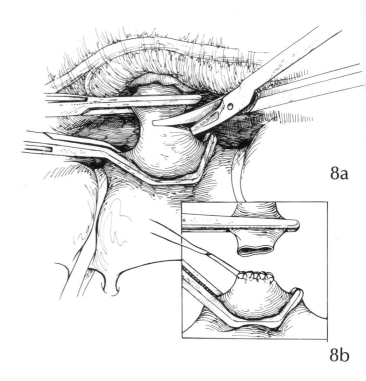

8a

8b

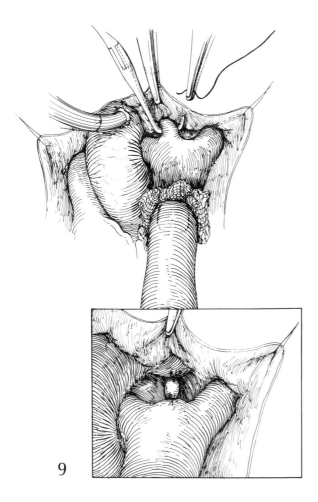

9

9

Closure of a persistent ductus associated with intracardiac abnormalities

In these circumstances the ductus should be closed at the time of correction of the intracardiac anomaly[2]. Control of the ductus should be achieved first so that when cardiopulmonary bypass is instituted loss of pump flow from the systemic vascular compartment to the lungs may be avoided. The most widely used method is that described by Kirklin and Silver[3], in which the bifurcation of the pulmonary artery is brought into view by digital retraction of the main trunk. The pericardial reflection at the bifurcation is opened, permitting the ductus to be identified and dissected out (a). Ligatures are passed around it and after cardiopulmonary bypass has been established the ductus is closed by multiple ligation (b).

Alternative techniques describe suture closure of the ductus from within the pulmonary artery after cardio-pulmonary bypass has been established; in these circumstances control of ductal flow may be achieved by digital pressure while bypass is being established followed by a short period of very low flow when the pulmonary artery has been opened. Alternatively, maintaining normal flow a Fogarty catheter may be placed in the ductus and the balloon inflated to prevent flow from the aorta to the pulmonary artery. The catheter should be removed as the suture is being tied, which will secure the pulmonary arterial orifice of the ductus.

10

Closure of a calcified or aneurysmal ductus

None of the above techniques is appropriate when closing a complicated ductus in an older patient as any direct approach is very hazardous. Pifarre, Rice and Nemickas in 1973[4] described a technique in which the aortic end of the ductus is exposed by opening the descending aorta between clamps and the orifice closed by a patch applied under direct vision. The distal circulation may be supported by left atriofemoral bypass or by aortoaortic bypass using a 'Gott' shunt, which has the advantage of avoiding heparinization. Flow through the ductus from the pulmonary end may be controlled when the aorta is opened either by applying a side-clamp to the pulmonary artery at the origin of the ductus or by inflating the balloon of a Fogarty catheter placed in the ductus. Alternatively, full cardiopulmonary bypass may be used with both proximal and distal arterial cannulation as described by Morrow and Clark in 1966[5]. With this technique the distal circulation is supported and flow through the ductus is satisfactorily reduced.

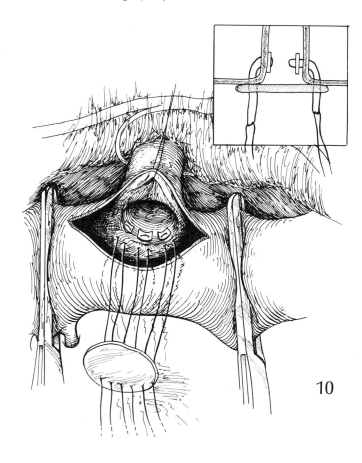

10

Postoperative care

Most children have an uneventful postoperative course. Antibiotic treatment should be maintained for 48 hours. The intercostal drain may usually be removed on the day after surgery and the patient mobilized as soon as possible. Hoarseness due to recurrent laryngeal nerve damage is uncommon and is usually temporary. Chylothorax has been described following surgery for a persistent ductus.

References

1. Panagopoulos, Ph. G., Tatooles, C. J., Aberdeen, E., Waterston, D. J., Bonham-Carter, R. E. Patent ductus arteriosus in infants and children: a review of 936 operations (1964–69). Thorax 1971; 26: 137–144

2. McGoon, D. C. Closure of patent ductus during open heart surgery. Journal of Thoracic and Cardiovascular Surgery 1964; 48: 456–464

3. Kirklin, J. W., Silver, A. W. Technic of exposing the ductus arteriosus prior to establishing extracorporeal circulation. Proceedings of the Staff Meetings of the Mayo Clinic 1958; 33: 423–425

4. Pifarre, R., Rice, P. L., Nemickas, R. Surgical treatment of calcified patent ductus arteriosus. Journal of Thoracic and Cardiovascular Surgery 1973; 65: 635–638

5. Morrow, A. D., Clark, W. D. Closure of calcified patent ductus: a new operative method utilising cardiopulmonary bypass. Journal of Thoracic and Cardiovascular Surgery 1966; 51: 534–538

Coarctation of the aorta: surgical anatomy

Robert H. Anderson   BSc, MD, MRCPath
Joseph Levy Professor of Paediatric Cardiac Morphology, Cardiothoracic Institute, Brompton Hospital, London, UK

Introduction

Coarctation, literally meaning 'a drawing together', can occur in any artery. For the surgeon specializing in congenital heart disease, however, coarctation without further qualification describes lesions of the arch of the aorta, almost always in the immediate environs of the isthmus and the duct or ligament.

The restrictive lesions which produce coarctation take several forms. Usually there is a discrete shelf within the lumen (*Figure 1a*), and this often coexists with a waist-like narrowing and hypoplasia of the isthmus, although the waist can be found without any luminal shelf (*Figure 1b*). A more extensive narrowing than just at the waist can also be found. The more severe lesion affects a segment of the arch, narrowing it in uniform fashion (*Figure 1c*), and was

termed tubular hypoplasia by Edwards[1]. The tubular lesion can affect segments of the arch other than the isthmus, almost invariably in association with a duct. A series of lesions may then be encountered in the arch segments of the isthmus, the area between left common carotid and left subclavian arteries and between brachiocephalic and left common arteries respectively (*Figure 2*). This series extends from tubular hypoplasia (*Figure 1c*) through atresia of the arch segment, the atretic segment being represented by a fibrous cord (*Figure 1d*), to complete interruption of the aortic arch (*Figure 1e*). The more severe lesions are much less frequent than simple coarctation, but the anatomical principles have much in common and will be discussed briefly.

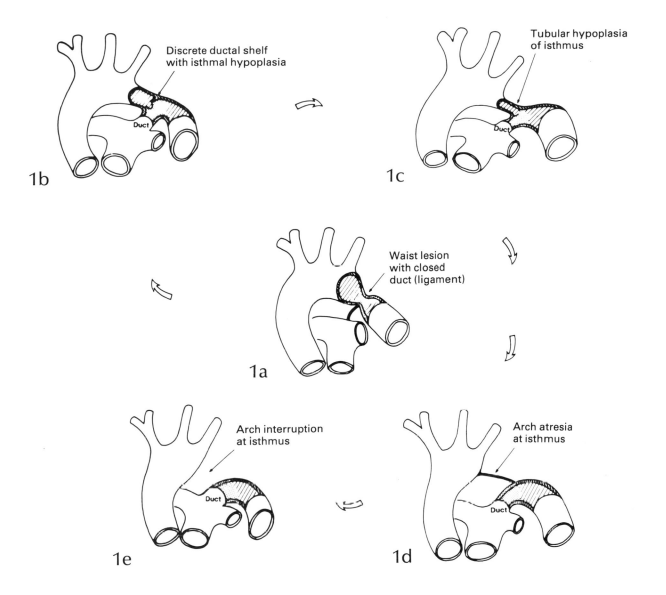

Discrete ductal shelf
with isthmal hypoplasia

1b

Tubular hypoplasia
of isthmus

1c

Waist lesion
with closed
duct (ligament)

1a

Arch interruption
at isthmus

1e

Arch atresia
at isthmus

1d

Figure 1. *The series of lesions ranging from simple discrete coarctation with a closed duct (a) to complete interruption of the aortic arch (e)*

between brachiocephalic artery
and left common carotid artery

Between left common carotid artery
and left subclavian artery

At isthmus

Asc-ending Aorta

Pulmonary Trunk

Duct

Des-cending Aorta

2

Figure 2. *The steps of tubular hypoplasia through to interruption (see Figure 1 c–d) can be found in each of three different segments of the aortic arch*

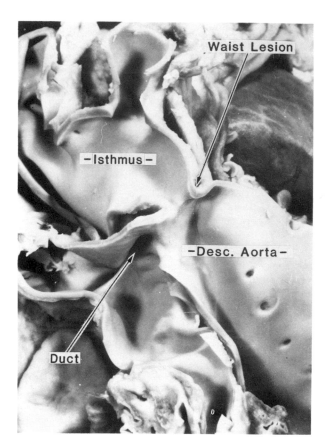

Figure 3. *The discrete waist-like coarctation lesion found with an open duct*

Isthmic coarctation

The shelf and waist-like coarctation lesions are, almost without exception, found in the isthmic segment of the arch. The significant differentiating feature of these lesions is the presence or absence of a duct.

Those found with a ligament are much simpler lesions. They tend to be of waist-like type and to be associated with a well-formed collateral circulation. They are found in older patients, and make up the 'adult' form of the old classification of Bonnet[2]. This will be the type found in those who present with coarctation in adult life, although they can be found in children. They tend not to be associated with other congenital lesions within the heart apart from a high frequency of bicuspid aortic valve. The waist-like lesion is the infolded aortic wall with a fibrous cap on its luminal aspect[1].

Coarctation in the presence of a duct is a much more complex lesion. This type can be simply of the waist pattern (*Figure 3*) but most usually it is found with a shelf lesion in preductal position (*Figure 4*). Much has been written recently concerning the 'juxtaductal' nature of isthmic coarctation[3, 4]. Whether the shelf is juxtaductal depends entirely upon definition. All the shelves found in association with a duct are in its immediate environs, and in that respect are self-evidently juxtaductal, but the position of the shelf varies relative to the mouth of the duct[5]. In the great majority of cases the major flow pathway in this type of coarctation is from the pulmonary trunk via the duct to the descending aorta. The coarctation lesions at the isthmus-ductal junction are upstream of this pathway and therefore in preductal position (*Figure 4*). More rarely the shelf lesion can be found directly opposite the ductal junction, or even more rarely in postductal position[5].

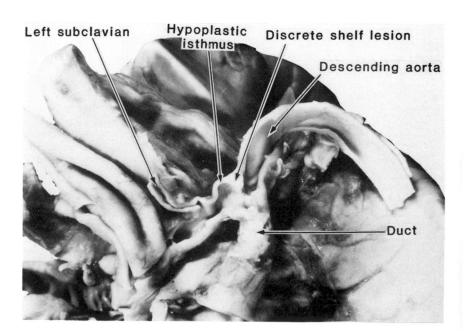

Figure 4. *The shelf-like coarctation lesion. Note the coexisting tapering hypoplasia of the isthmus. This is particularly variable, as is the distance to the left subclavian artery*

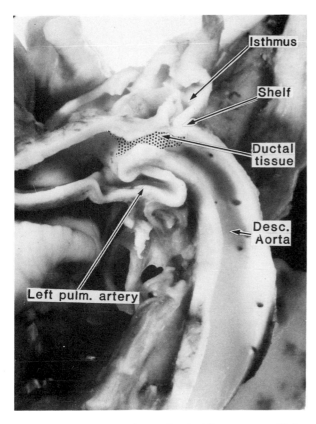

Figure 5. *In autopsy specimens the duct tissue can readily be indentified and distinguished from the arterial wall*

In the usual arrangement, with the shelf in preductal position, there is no doubt that the shelf is composed of a ring of ductal tissue[6,7] which encircles the isthmus-aortic junction on its luminal aspect (*Figures 4–6*). With increasing age the ductal tissue becomes fibrotic[8], and presumably the fibrous cap of 'adult' type represents fibrosed ductal tissue in cases in which the duct has closed. In autopsied hearts from neonates it is easy to observe the extent of the ductal tissue with the naked eye (*Figure 5*). It does not make up the full thickness of the arterial wall: instead it is a luminal hoop which encircles the isthmic orifice (*Figure 6*).

The relationship of coarctation and ductal tissue has long been controversial. Some[9,10] have denied the presence of the ductal sling, despite the carefully conducted studies of Wielanga and Dankmeijer[6] and their endorsement by Brom[11]. Equally, the presence of the ductal sling should not detract from the significance of lesions which potentiate reduced aortic flow during the fetal life of those who have coarctation. It was this flow hypothesis[3,4] that was promoted by those who questioned the significance of ductal tissue[9,10]. Thus, there is no doubt that it is exceedingly rare for patients with reduced pulmonary flow to have aortic coarctation. Nevertheless, in the majority of those with coarctation presenting in the neonatal period of infancy there is some lesion which reduces aortic flow. In the more severe cases, such as those with univentricular connection to the left ventricle or double outlet right ventricle with subpulmonary defect, the cardiac lesion is the major problem, although this in itself may not become manifest until the coarctation is surgically repaired. In other cases the lesion will simply be a ventricular septal defect. Recent studies in an autopsy

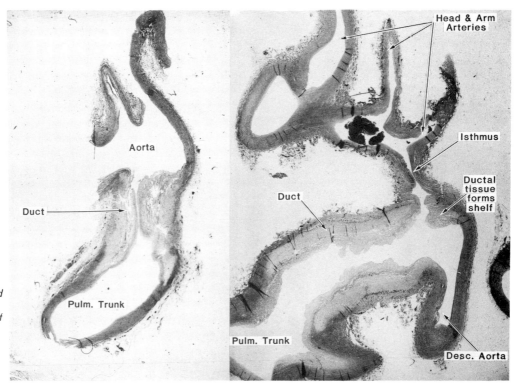

Figure 6. *A histological section through the normal duct (left-hand panel) and a coarctation lesion with a duct, showing how the shelf is composed of a luminal hoop of pale-staining ductal tissue (right-hand panel). (Photographs reproduced by courtesy of Dr Siew Yen Ho)*

series[12] endorsed by echocardiography[13] suggest that the ventricular septal defect in these circumstances may be of unusual morphology. In some cases, the defect is of malalignment type, as found in interruption (see below). More frequently it is a confluent perimembranous defect over-ridden by the aortic valve and partially closed on its right ventricular aspect by tricuspid valve tissue tags (Figure 7). Whether this type of defect will close spontaneously after treatment of the coarctation remains to be established. In some other cases the duct may be the only associated lesion. In this circumstance care must be taken to assess the significance of a shelf-like coarctation lesion, since this may not become clinically manifest until the duct is surgically closed[10].

Anatomy of the isthmus and the arch vessels varies most in coarctation with a duct and other associated lesions. Tubular hypoplasia can coexist with a discrete coarctation, but more frequently there is extensive tapering hypoplasia of the isthmus. The proximity of the left subclavian artery to the isthmus-aortic junction also varies, and in some instances there may be a retro-oesophageal origin of the right subclavian artery. This anatomy must be carefully evaluated when judging the merits of the subclavian flap versus end-to-end anastomosis following resection. The anatomy suggests that different cases may be particularly amenable to one or other of these procedures, and the procedure should be chosen appropriately for each case according to its anatomy.

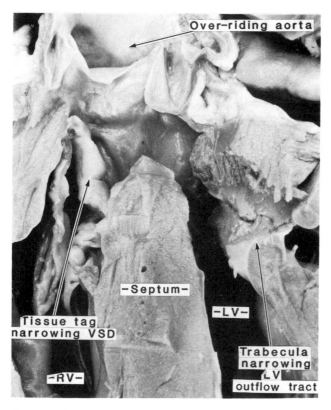

Figure 7. The unusual ventricular septal defect found in a good proportion of cases of coarctation. Illustrated by a 'four-chamber' long axis section, it shows the over-riding aortic valve and the tricuspid valve tissue tag closing the right ventricular aspect. LV = left ventricle; RV = right ventricle; VSD = ventricular septal defect. Specimen photographed and reproduced by courtesy of Dr J. R. Zuberbuhler, University of Pittsburgh)

Aortic interruption

As indicated, in anatomical terms interruption of the aortic arch is the end point of a series of lesions which starts with simple coarctation. However, the anatomy of the associated lesions which coexist with interruption (including atresia for this purpose) are so surgically significant that they warrant discussion. It is well known that interruption usually occurs at the isthmus or between the left common carotid and left subclavian arteries and rarely between the brachiocephalic and left common carotid arteries. Retro-oesophageal origin of the right subclavian can occur with any of these variants, and the whole series must be anticipated in mirror-image pattern with a right arch. These features, while important, are less significant than the associated lesions.

Very rarely interruption can be found with an intact ventricular septum and closed duct[14]. Treatment then consists of anastomosis of the interrupted arch segments. In the overwhelming majority of cases there are associated lesions. Where these lesions include abnormal ventriculo-arterial connections, such as truncus or double outlet right ventricle, the abnormal connections will dominate. Most cases will have atrioventricular and ventriculoarterial concordance. Then the significant associated lesion will be the defect permitting left-to-right shunting. Less frequently this will be an aortopulmonary window. The major problem in this combination is precise diagnosis. More usually there is a ventricular septal defect. Autopsy studies[15-18], confirmed by echocardiography[19], have shown that this defect is of particular morphology in the majority of cases. Whether the defect involves the perimembranous muscular outlet or area, or is of doubly committed subarterial type, there is obstruction of the subaortic outflow tract. In cases with a muscular outlet septum (perimembranous and muscular outlet defect), the outlet septum is deviated posteriorly so that the pulmonary valve overrides the rest of the septum and there is narrowing of the subaortic region (Figure 8). In cases with doubly committed defects (Figure 9a), there is gross disproportion between the sizes of the aortic and pulmonary valves, and the raphe between them narrows the subaortic outlet (Figure 9b). Study of autopsied hearts suggests that, in these cases, repair of the interruption is only part of the necessary treatment, since the subaortic obstruction remains. This may explain the poor surgical prognosis of most cases of aortic interruption.

Since the outlet septum never contains conduction tissue it is tempting from the anatomical evidence to suggest that it be removed surgically at the time of closure of the ventricular septal defect. However, other patients do well after surgical repair of interruption and simple closure of the ventricular septal defect[20]. Do these patients have more favourable anatomy without subaortic obstruction? Only prospective studies using echocardiography and knowing the anatomical possibilities will resolve this question and point to the optimal surgical management of aortic interruption.

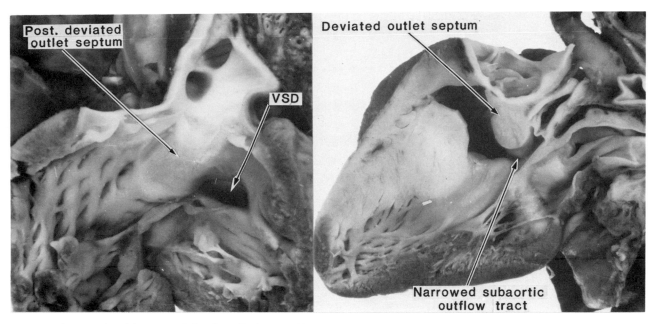

Figure 8. *The typical malalignment defect found in hearts with interrupted aortic arch. In this case the defect is perimembranous. It is shown (a) as seen from the right ventricle and (b) as seen in long axis section parallel to the outlet septum*

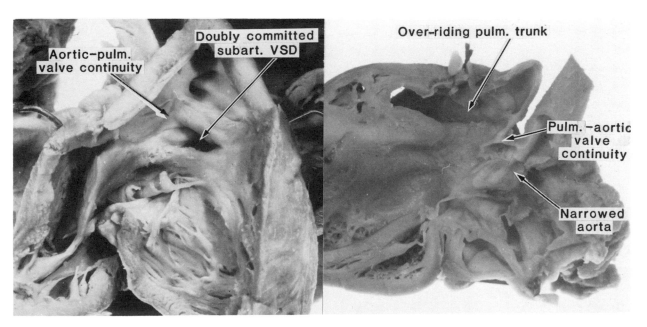

Figure 9. *A doubly committed subarterial defect found with interrupted aortic arch. The pulmonary valve is huge compared to the aortic valve. The heart is seen (a) from the right ventricle and (b) in long axis section. Compare with* Figure 8

References

1. Edwards, J. E. Aortic arch system. In: Gould, S. E., ed. Pathology of the heart and blood vessels, 3rd edn. Springfield, Ill.: Charles C. Thomas, 1968: 416–454

2. Bonnet, L. M. Sur la lésion dite sténose congénitale de l'aorte dans la region de l'isthme. Revue de Médecine Paris 1903; 23: 108–126

3. Rudolph, A. M., Heymann, M. A., Spitznas, U. Haemodynamic considerations in the development of narrowing of the aorta. American Journal of Cardiology 1972; 30: 514–525

4. Rudolph, A. M. Congenital diseases of the heart. Chicago: Year Book Medical Publishers, 1974

5. Becker, A. E., Becker, M. J., Edwards, J. E. Anomalies associated with coarctation of aorta: particular reference to infancy. Circulation 1970; 41: 1067–1075

6. Wielanga, G., Dankmeijer, J. Coarctation of the aorta. Journal of Pathology and Bacteriology 1968; 95: 265–274

7. Ho, S. Y., Anderson, R. H. Coarctation, tubular hypoplasia and the ductus arteriosus: histological study of 35 specimens. British Heart Journal 1979; 41: 268–274

8. Elzenga, N. J., Gittenberger-de-Groot, A. C. Localized coarctation of the aorta. An age dependent spectrum. British Heart Journal 1983; 49: 317–323

9. Shinebourne, E. A., Elseed, A. M. Relation between fetal flow patterns, coarctation of the aorta and pulmonary blood flow. British Heart Journal 1974; 36: 492–498

10. Elseed, A. M., Shinebourne, E. A., Paneth, M. Manifestation of juxtaductal coarctation after surgical ligation of persistent ductus arteriosus in infancy. British Heart Journal 1974; 36: 687–692

11. Brom, A. G. Narrowing of the aortic isthmus and enlargement of the mind. Journal of Thoracic and Cardiovascular Surgery 1965; 50: 166–180

12. Anderson, R. H., Lenox, C. C., Zuberbuhler, J. R. Morphology of ventricular septal defect associated with coarctation of aorta. British Heart Journal 1983; 50: 176–181

13. Smallhorn, J. F., Anderson, R. H., Macartney, F. J. Morphological characterization of ventricular septal defects associated with coarctation of aorta by cross-sectional echocardiography. British Heart Journal 1983; 49: 485–494

14. Milo, S., Massini, C., Goor, D. A. Isolated atresia of the aortic arch in a 65-year old man. Surgical treatment and review of published reports. British Heart Journal 1982; 47: 294–297

15. Van Praagh, R., Bernhard, W. F., Rosenthal, A., Parisi, L. F., Fyler, D. C. Interrupted aortic arch: surgical treatment. American Journal of Cardiology 1971; 27: 200–211

16. Moulaert, A., Bruins, C. C., Oppenheimer-Dekker, A. Anomalies of the aortic arch and ventricular septal defects. Circulation 1976; 53: 1011–1015

17. Freedom, R. M., Dische, M. R., Rowe, R. D. Conal anatomy in aortic atresia, ventricular septal defect, and normally developed left ventricle. American Heart Journal 1977; 94: 689–698

18. Ho, S. Y., Wilcox, B. R., Anderson, R. H., Lincoln, J. C. R. Interrupted aortic arch – anatomical features of surgical significance. Thoracic and Cardiovascular Surgeon 1983; 31: 199–205

19. Smallhorn, J. F., Anderson, R. H., Macartney, F. J. Cross-sectional echocardiographic recognition of interruption of aortic arch between left carotid and subclavian arteries. British Heart Journal 1982; 48: 229–235

20. Moulton, A. L., Bowman, F. O. Jr. Primary definitive repair of type B interrupted apiac arch, ventricular septal defect, and patent ductus arteriosus. Journal of Thoracic and Cardiovascular Surgery 1981; 82: 501–510

Repair of coarctation of the aorta

John A. Waldhausen MD
John W. Oswald Professor of Surgery, Chairman, Department of Surgery,
The Pennsylvania State University College of Medicine, Pennsylvania, USA

David B. Campbell MD
Assistant Professor of Surgery, Division of Cardiothoracic Surgery, The Pennsylvania State University College of Medicine,
The Milton S. Hershey Medical Center, Hershey, Pennsylvania, USA

Introduction

Indications for operative intervention in coarctation of the aorta differ. Infants usually present with life-threatening congestive heart failure, while children have few, if any, symptoms and the operation is performed for the treatment or prevention of hypertension. The latter is clearly the most common problem in children and adults, although infection and aneurysm formation distal to the stenosis or in the intercostal arteries are also indications for operative intervention.

Coarctation was first successfully treated by Crafoord and Nylin[1] and by Gross[2] independently by resection of the coarctation and end-to-end anastomosis.

The choice of operation is influenced by the size of the patient and the underlying anatomical abnormality. At the Hershey Medical Center the operation of choice for neonates and infants is the subclavian flap angioplasty. In older children, adolescents and adults the options are more numerous and include resection with end-to-end anastomosis or insertion of a tubular prosthesis, patch aortoplasy, Vosschulte-type aortoplasty and insertion of a bypass prosthesis.

Resection and end-to-end anastomosis was first successfully applied to critically ill infants by Kirklin[3]. Initially, operative mortality was very high[4], and those infants who survived had a 30–60 per cent incidence of restenosis[5]. With modern intensive perioperative therapy, including the preoperative use of prostaglandin E_1 to maintain patency of the ductus[6], operative mortality has markedly declined[7]. The introduction of the subclavian flap angioplasty in 1966[8] has reduced the recurrence rate to close to zero[9, 10].

The operations

SUBCLAVIAN FLAP ANGIOPLASTY

1

After the usual exposure of the aortic isthmus and subclavian artery, the vertebral artery, which is usually the first branch of the subclavian artery and originates behind it, is exposed and ligated to prevent possible 'subclavian steal' syndrome. The persistent ductus arteriosus is ligated with a single heavy silk ligature.

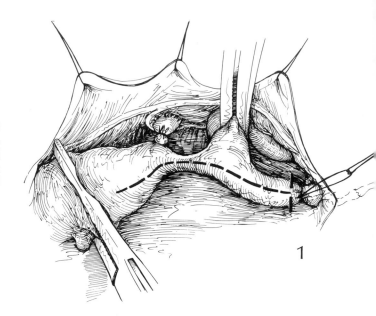

2

An anterolateral incision from the descending aorta is extended across the isthmus and along the lateral border of the subclavian artery and the shelf-like intimal thickening is excised.

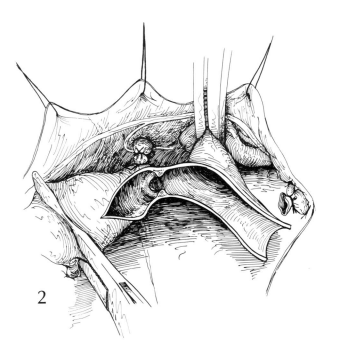

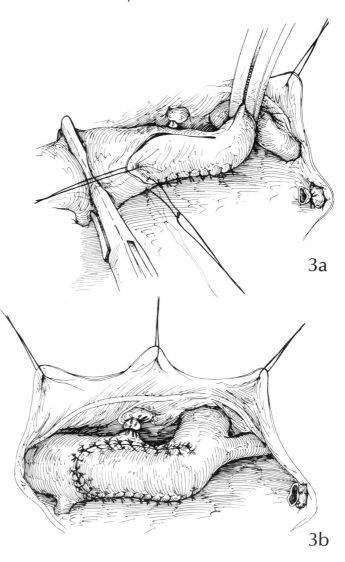

3a

3b

3

The subclavian flap is then sutured with 6/0 interrupted sutures to the aortic incision. This results in a widely patent isthmus often larger than the transverse arch, which with time and increased blood flow will enlarge to normal.

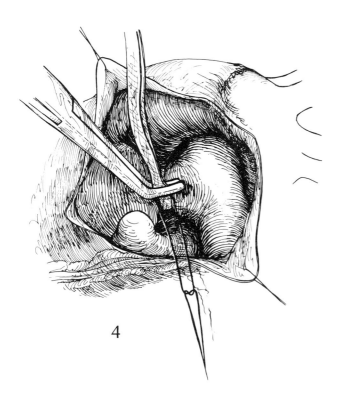

4

4

Controversy exists as to whether or not to band the pulmonary artery at the same operation when there is a large ventricular septal defect. In patients with very large shunts, pulmonary artery banding is best performed prior to the application of aortic crossclamps so that the increased systemic resistance does not cause massive pulmonary hyperperfusion. Some authorities do not recommend concomitant pulmonary artery banding and believe that prolonged ventilator dependency or right heart failure are indications for either closure of the ventricular septal defect or pulmonary artery banding at a second operation.

RESECTION WITH END-TO-END ANASTOMOSIS

This operation is the standard one for children and adults for the repair of coarctation of the aorta. The excellent results achieved by most centres justify its continued use, particularly since prosthetic material with its potentially adverse properties is excluded and the normal anatomy of the aortic arch and its branches remains intact.

5

The aorta is exposed through a fourth interspace left lateral thoracotomy. The lungs are retracted anteriorly and inferiorly. The pleura is incised at the distal left subclavian artery and upper descending aorta and retracted anteriorly, exposing the area of coarctation. Tapes are placed around the subclavian artery, distal aortic arch and descending aorta. The aorta is mobilized by careful dissection distally so that it may be readily brought up to the arch after resection of the area of narrowing.

The ligamentum arteriosum is ligated since occasionally it is still patent. Intercostal arteries are not sacrificed unless absolutely necessary to achieve an adequate resection. More often they can be temporarily occluded with Potts' ties. Application of the aortic clamps may acutely increase the afterload on the heart with proximal aortic hypertension. Blood pressure should therefore be monitored with a right radial artery catheter and if excessive hypertension develops the blood pressure should be controlled with an intravenous infusion of nitroprusside. The aorta-to-aorta anastomosis should be at least as large as the aortic arch. Additional orifice size can be achieved by incising the subclavian artery laterally, creating a 'fish mouth'. The distal orifice must be equally large to the proximal one, but this is readily achieved since the distal aorta usually shows poststenotic dilatation.

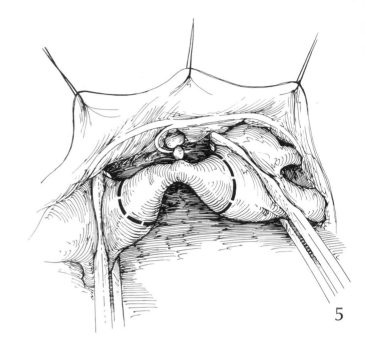

6 & 7

The anastomosis is constructed by placing a continuous posterior row of everting mattress sutures using a 4/0 or 5/0 synthetic monofilament suture. Each end is then tied to a single similar interrupted suture. The anterior portion of the anastomosis is completed with simple interrupted sutures. Before the aortic clamps are released sodium bicarbonate solution (1 mmol/kg) is given intravenously for correction of the acidosis after reperfusion of the distal body. After release of the distal clamp the suture line is inspected and any significant bleeding stopped with additional sutures. The proximal clamp is then released in stages. Partial occlusion will dampen the pulse pressure and reduce the sudden tension otherwise exerted on the suture line. When haemostasis appears adequate the clamp is removed completely. The pleura is closed with a 4/0 continuous absorbable synthetic suture. The lungs are re-expanded and the chest closed in routine manner after insertion of a chest tube.

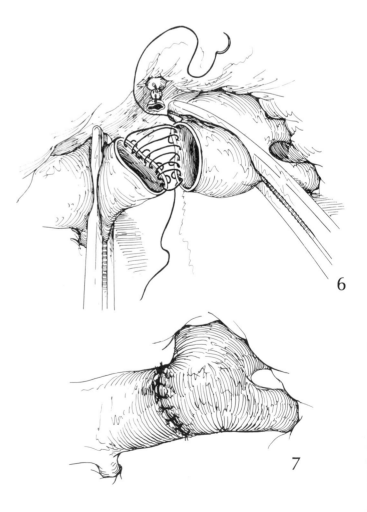

RESECTION WITH INSERTION OF TUBULAR DACRON PROSTHESIS

8

In some patients (5 per cent) the area of coarctation is too long for a primary anastomosis to be performed without undue tension[11]. In these cases insertion of a tubular woven Dacron prosthesis will give excellent results. After excision of the area of narrowing an appropriately sized prosthesis is sutured to the proximal aorta. The prosthesis should be at least as large as the transverse aortic arch. The suture material is 4/0 or 5/0 Dacron. Preclotting the woven prosthesis can be helpful in preventing bleeding from the cloth interstices.

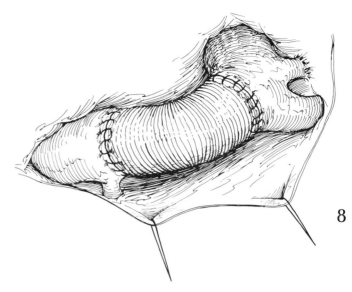

8

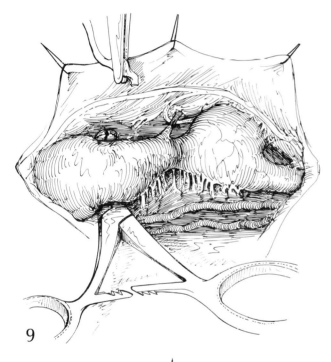

9

AORTOPLASTY WITH DACRON PATCH

In older patients whose aorta has undergone sclerotic changes mobilization and end-to-end anastomosis may be hazardous and the use of a diamond shaped Dacron patch can be very helpful[12–14].

9

After the usual exposure of the aortic isthmus and area of coarctation tapes are placed around the subclavian artery, transverse arch and descending aorta. The vessels are mobilized. Appropriate intercostal arteries are occluded temporarily with Pott's ties.

10

An incision is extended from the base of the subclavian artery across the area of coarctation into the proximal descending aorta.

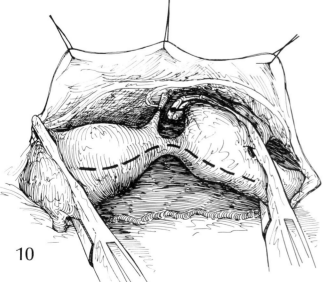

10

11a, b

The coarctation membrane is excised with fine scissors. This membrane is generally a thickening of the intima and does not involve the media.

A large diamond-shaped Dacron patch is now cut appropriately. The diameter of the patch (D) is likely to be underestimated unless the material is so cut as to add adequate width to provide the desired circumference (C). By measuring the flattened remaining posterior wall of the aorta (A) the maximum width (W) of the patch can be calculated thus: $C = D \times \pi$; $W = C - A$. (Example: when A = 10 mm and D = 20 mm, $C = 20 \times \pi = 63$ mm and $W = 63 - 10 = 53$ mm.) A slight excess of graft material to allow for loss in the suture line is added to the measured prosthesis.

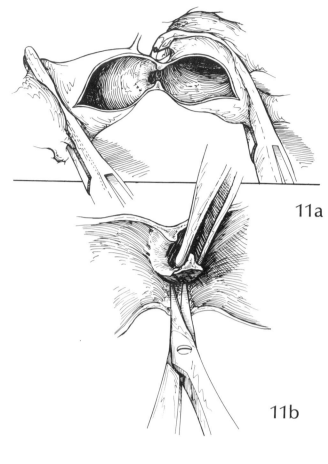

11a

11b

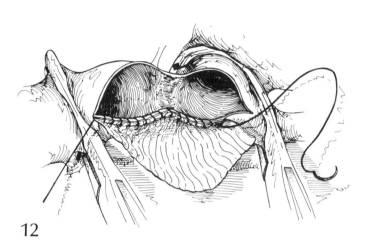

12

12 & 13

The patch is then sewn in place using continuous polypropylene sutures and beginning on the lateral aspect of the aorta. The lateral side of the anastomosis is conveniently performed from inside, and the two ends of the suture are then brought around on the medial aspect of the incision to where they meet. They are then cut and tied.

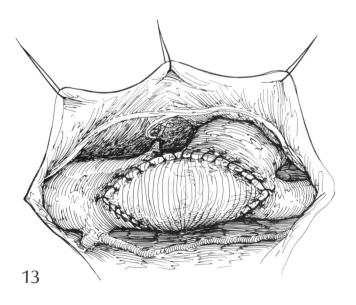

13

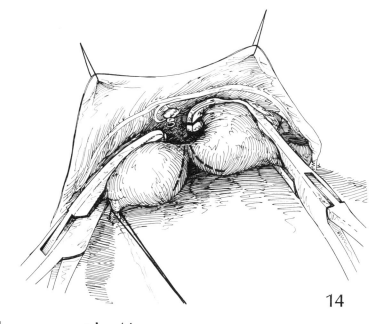

14

VOSSCHULTE AORTOPLASTY

In some patients the coarctation consists only of a lateral shelf and the proximal and distal ends of the aorta are in close proximity.

14–16

In such cases a lateral incision across the area of narrowing and a transverse closure with interrupted sutures[15] will produce a widely patent anastomosis. This operation is particularly applicable in young children.

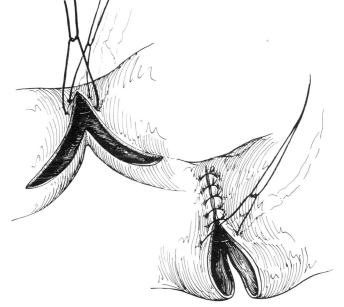

15

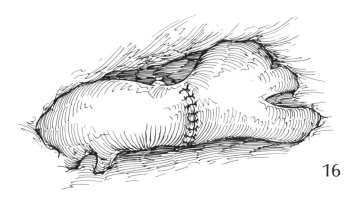

16

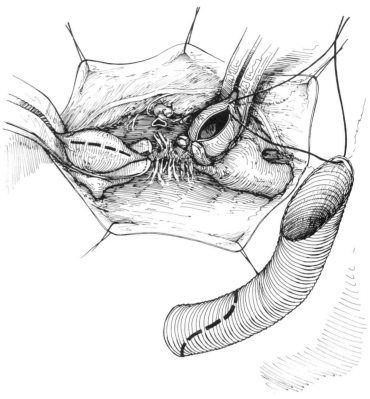

INSERTION OF BYPASS PROSTHESIS

Occasionally patients present with recurrent stenosis, most often after resection of the coarctation and end-to-end anastomosis in infancy. Rather than dissect out the often heavily scarred area of the previous anastomosis a bypass Dacron prosthesis can be inserted. The prosthesis should be of adequate size, preferably 18–20mm in diameter.

17 & 18

The prosthesis is sutured proximally to that portion of aorta previously unexposed, such as the transverse arch or ascending aorta. Distally it is inserted into the descending aorta.

17

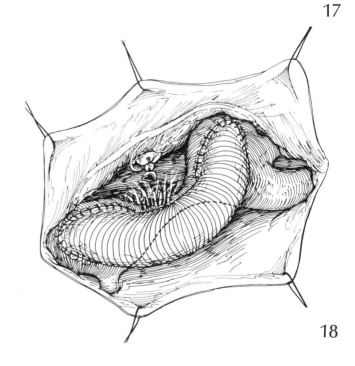

18

19

Occasionally it may be inserted proximally into the side of the aorta and subclavian artery.

Rarely patients have coarctation of the aorta in locations other than the isthmus. Thus it has been described in the distal thoracic aorta as well as the abdominal aorta[16]. Adequate preoperative aortographic localization of the area involved is essential in these patients. They are best managed by insertion of an adequately sized Dacron bypass prosthesis extending from the proximal to the distal aorta[17]. Renal artery involvement often requires separate bypass grafts.

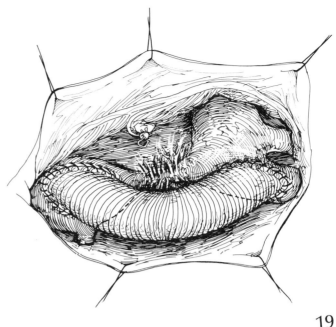

19

Postoperative management

Postoperative management is generally straightforward, with the removal of the chest tube the day after operation. Occasional paradoxical hypertension becomes a significant problem and may require the use of an antihypertensive drug[18]. Reserpine has been especially effective. Some of these patients also develop severe abdominal pain and even signs of an acute abdomen with intestinal gangrene and perforation. This is due to intense vasospasm of the mesenteric arteries and in its early phase may also be relieved by reserpine[19].

Results

The results of the subclavian flaps procedure in infants have been excellent at a number of centres[9, 10, 20, 21]. In a recent report, operative mortality at the Hershey Medical Center was 4 per cent, due, in part, to aggressive perioperative therapy which included the infusion of prostaglandin E_1 to maintain ductal patency, the correction of acidosis, and mechanical ventilation. A late follow-up showed normal exercise haemodynamics in several children, aged 5–6 years, who had undergone flap angioplasty in infancy[23]. The senior author's experience includes 100 cases of resection of coarctation and end-to-end anastomosis in children over one year of age. There was one death due to dehiscence of the suture line 8 hours after completion of the operation.

Untreated coarctation of the aorta is associated with premature death and late cardiovascular morbidity which includes sustained hypertension, coronary artery disease, and aortic rupture[24]. Long-term results suggest that early repair of coarctation is optimal as long as a pressure gradient does not persist or develop later. Our group advocates that the coarctation be repaired at the time of diagnosis, regardless of the symptomatic state of the patient. Residual gradients following the subclavian flap repair in infancy have been minimal in our experience, and resection with primary anastomosis has given excellent results in older patients.

Although in all of these procedures the aorta is clamped, collateral circulation is usually sufficient to avoid spinal cord injury. Brewer et al.[23] reviewed this problem in 1200 patients from many centres and found a 0.4 per cent incidence of spinal cord injury. This serious complication appears to be related to the anatomy of the anterior spinal artery, the magnitude of collateral circulation around the coarctation and the presence of severe operative hypotension.

References

1. Crafoord, C., Nylin, G. Congenital coarctation of the aorta and its surgical treatment. Journal of Thoracic Surgery 1945; 14: 347–361

2. Gross, R. E. Surgical correction for coarctation of the aorta. Surgery 1945; 18: 673–678

3. Kirklin, J. W., Burchell, H. B., Pugh, D. G., Burke, E. C., Mills, S. D. Surgical treatment of coarctation of the aorta in a ten week old infant: report of a case. Circulation 1952; 6: 411–414

4. Waldhausen, J. A., King, H., Nahrwold, D. L., Lurie, P. R., Shumacker, H. B., Jr. Management of coarctation in infancy. Journal of the American Medical Association 1964; 187: 270–275

5. Eshaghpour, E., Olley, P. M. Recoarctation of the aorta following coarctectomy in the first year of life: a follow-up study. Journal of Pediatrics 1972; 80: 809–814

6. Heymann, M. A., Berman, W., Jr, Rudolph, A. M., Whitman, V. Dilation of the ductus arteriosus by prostaglandin E_1 in aortic arch abnormalities. Circulation 1979; 59: 169–173

7. Waldhausen, J. A., Parr, G. V. S. Coarctation of the aorta interrupted aortic arch, hypoplastic left heart. In: Glenn W. L., ed. Thoracic and cardiovascular surgery 4th ed. East Norwalk C. T. Appleton-Century-Crofts), 1983, 813–828

8. Waldhausen J. A., Nahrwold, D. L. Repair of coarctation of the aorta with a subclavian flap. Journal of Thoracic and Cardiovascular Surgery 1966; 51: 532–533

9. Pierce, W. S., Waldhausen, J. A., Berman, W., Jr, Whitman, V. Late results of the subclavian flap procedure in infants with coarctation of the thoracic aorta. Circulation 1978; 57–58 (Suppl.I): 78–82

10. Hamilton, D. I., DiEusanio, G., Sandrasagra, F. A., Donnelly, R. J. Early and late results of aortoplasty with a left subclavian flap for coarctation of the aorta in infancy. Journal of Thoracic and Cardiovascular Surgery 1978; 75: 699–704

11. Shumacker, H. B., Nahrwold, D. L., King, H., Waldhausen, J. A. Coarctation of the aorta. Current Problems in Surgery 1968; February: 1–64

12. King, H., Kaiser, G., King, R. Repair of coarctation of the aorta by patch grafting. Journal of Thoracic and Cardiovascular Surgery 1962; 43: 792–795

13. Reul, G. J., Kabbani, S. S., Sandiford, F. M., Wukasch, D. C., Cooley, D. A. Repair of coarctation of the aorta by patch graft aortoplasty. Journal of Thoracic and Cardiovascular Surgery 1974; 68: 696–704

14. Moor, G. F., Ionescu, M. I., Ross, D. N. Surgical repair of coarctation of the aorta by patch grafting. Annals of Thoracic Surgery 1972; 14: 626–630

15. Vosschulte, K. Surgical correction of coarctation of the aorta by an 'isthmusplastic' operation. Thorax 1961; 16: 338–345

16. Pierce, W. S., Vincent, W. R., Fitzgerald, E., Miller, F. J. Coarctation of the abdominal aorta with multiple aneurysms: Operative correction. Annals of Thoracic Surgery 1975; 20: 687–693

17. Nantor, M. A., Olley, P. M. Residual hypertension after coarctectomy in children. American Journal of Cardiology 1976; 37: 769–772

18. Fox, S., Pierce, W. S., Waldhausen, J. A. Pathogenesis of paradoxical hypertension after coarctation repair. Annals of Thoracic Surgery 1980; 29: 135–141

19. Ho, E. C., Moss, A. J. The syndrome of 'mesenteric arteritis' following repair of aortic coarctation: Report of nine cases and reviews of the literature. Pediatrics 1972; 49: 40–45

20. Bergdahl, L. A., Blackstone, E. H., Kirklin, J. W., Pacifico, A. D., Bargeron, L. M. Determinants of early success in repair of coarctation in infants. Journal of Thoracic and Cardiovascular Surgery 1982; 83: 736–742

21. Moulton, A. L., Brenner, J. I., Roberts, G., Tavares, S., Ali, S., Nordenberg, A., Burns, J. E., Ringel, R., Bermann, M. A., McLaughlin, J. S. Subclavian flap repair of coarctation of the aorta in neonates. Realization of growth potential. Journal of Cardiovascular and Thoracic Surgery 1984; 87: 220–235

22. Campbell, D. B., Waldhausen, J. A., Pierce, W. S., Fripp, R., Whitman, V. Should elective repair of coarctation be done in infancy? Journal of Thoracic and Cardiovascular Surgery 1984; 88: 929–938

23. Fripp, R. R., Whitman, V., Werner, J. C., Nicholas, G. G., Waldhausen, J. A. Blood pressure response to exercise in children following the subclavian flap procedure for coarctation of the aorta. Journal of Thoracic and Cardiovascular Surgery 1983; 85: 682–685

24. Maron, B. J., Humphries, J. O., Rowe, R. D., Mellits, E. D. Prognosis of surgically corrected coarctation of the aorta: a 20-year postoperative appraisal. Circulation 1973; 47: 119–126

25. Brewer, L. A., Fosburg, R. G., Mulder, G. A., Verska, J. J. Spinal cord complications following surgery for coarctation of the aorta. A study of 66 cases. Journal of Thoracic and Cardiovascular Surgery 1972; 64: 368–381

Congenital abnormalities of the aortic arch

David I. Hamilton FRCS
Cardiac Surgeon, Royal Liverpool Children's Hospital, Liverpool, UK

Developmental considerations

During fetal development six pairs of aortic arch vessels connect the dorsal and ventral aortas, but all of these structures are never present at the same time. The first, second and fifth pairs regress. The third pair forms the carotid arteries. Usually the fourth right arch vessel is absorbed, leaving the left to form the normal left aortic arch. The sixth pair is involved in the formation of the pulmonary arteries and the ductus arteriosus. Developmental abnormalities result from unusual persistence or absorption of these vessels.

The Edwards[1] classification is based on this embryological symmetrical double aortic arch system.

1

The ascending (ventral) aorta gives rise to the anterior left aortic arch, which gives origin to the left common carotid and subclavian arteries, and the right aortic arch, which gives origin to the right common carotid and subclavian arteries. Both arches, which are of similar calibre in this case, join the dorsal descending thoracic aorta posteriorly. This system persists in fishes.

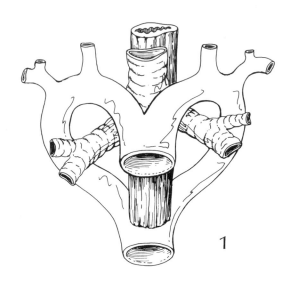

2

A dominant right aortic arch system with absorption of the distal portion of the minor left arch is seen in the bird kingdom. The anterior portion of the minor left aortic arch forms the innominate artery, giving rise to the left common carotid and subclavian arteries.

3

A dominant left aortic arch system with absorption of the distal portion of the minor right arch persists in mammals, including man. The anterior portion of the minor right aortic arch forms the innominate artery, giving rise to the right common carotid and subclavian arteries.

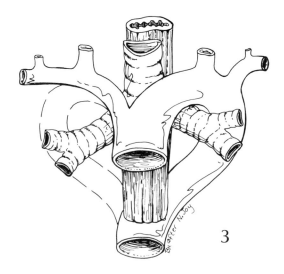

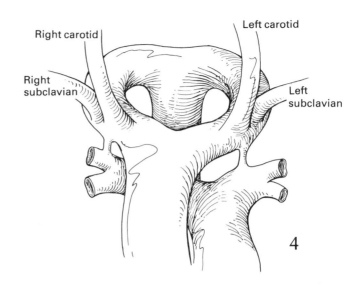

4

A complete symmetrical double aortic arch system (complete vascular ring) with bilateral ductus arteriosus communicating with the branch pulmonary arteries was first described in man by Hommel[2] in 1737 and was first operated on by Gross[3] in 1946.

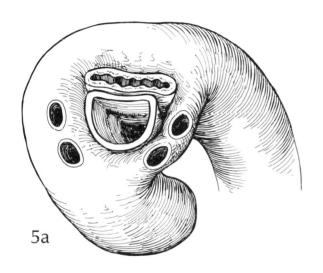

5a

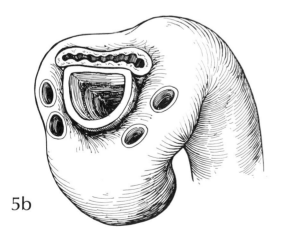

5b

5a & b

Persistence of both fourth arch vessels produces a complete vascular ring which encircles the trachea and oesophagus usually causing constriction of both of these structures. The right arch vessel, which passes behind the oesophagus, and trachea, is the dominant vessel in 75 per cent of cases (*a*), the left being larger in 15 per cent (*b*) and the two components being approximately equal in calibre in 10 per cent. Portions of the minor arch system may be hypoplastic or even atretic, often between the left subclavian artery and descending thoracic aorta or between the carotid and subclavian arteries. The integrity of the vascular ring is not broken in such cases and compression of midline structures may still be present.

6

In 70 per cent of cases the descending thoracic aorta lies in the left chest (as shown here) but it may descend in the thorax in the midline (*as in Illustration 2*) or, rarely, remain on the right of the vertebral column.

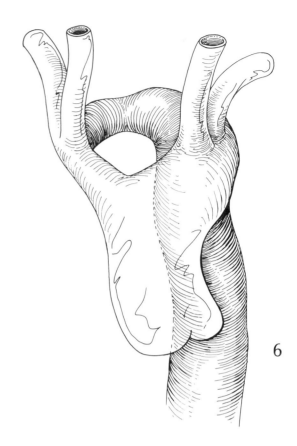

6

Symptomatology

Symptoms result from tracheal and/or oesophageal compression and depend upon the degree of tension exerted by the vascular ring or an aberrant vessel, though in some cases there are no symptoms. Presentation is common in infancy but can be delayed until the second year of life or later. The usual symptoms are stridor, wheezing, cough or recurrent chest infections causing an increase in respiratory rate. Intercostal recession and cervical extension are present in severe cases. Moist sounds may be heard on auscultation of the chest. Dysphagia can occur early or may be delayed until solid food is taken.

Preoperative

Investigation

Chest radiography An abnormal vascular shadow is seen in the presence of a right aortic arch. The trachea may be displaced or compressed.

Barium swallow The swallow is observed during fluoroscopy with the patient in the postero-anterior, lateral and oblique positions to assess the degree of indentation of the oesophagus and trachea.

Aortography Studies of the aortic arch or aberrant vessel are obtained either by retrograde aortic or left ventricular injection. Pulmonary artery injection may also be required.

Endoscopy Oesophagoscopy may be performed under general anaesthesia. The site and nature of any narrowing is noted. Palpation of the upper limb and femoral pulses is performed during manipulation of the oesophagoscope. Obliteration of any pulse, for example in the right upper limb, may be produced by pressure on the aberrant artery with the endoscope.

Considerations in surgical management

Before surgery is undertaken three questions must be answered: Is a vascular anomaly present? Is it causing symptoms? Has the anomaly been demonstrated clearly so that surgical correction can be planned?

As stated above 75 per cent of patients with a double aortic arch have a dominant right arch passing behind the oesophagus posteriorly and a left arch of minor calibre passing in front of the trachea.

Up to 80 per cent of the patients with a dominant left arch will have the descending aorta on the left side of the chest. Thus approximately 95 per cent of patients with a double aortic arch can be treated surgically through a left thoracotomy.

Preoperative management

Respiratory infection should be treated and controlled by physiotherapy, antibiotics and humidity. Surgery may be indicated as an emergency measure.

The operations

At intubation the endotracheal tube will have to be passed though any tracheal obstruction, usually 2–3 cm above the carina.

In the majority of patients satisfactory access is obtained through a left posterolateral thoracotomy with the patient on his right side. The third or fourth intercostal space is opened.

EXPOSURE OF THE AORTIC ARCHES IN COMPLETE VASCULAR RING

7

The mediastinal pleura is opened posterior to the vagus nerve from above the lung hilum towards the apex of the chest. The pleura is reflected off the underlying vessels, which are dissected out carefully and isolated in tape slings. It may be helpful to pass a stomach tube into the oesophagus to assist in identifying this structure.

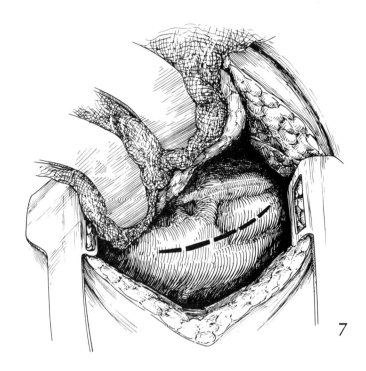

7

8

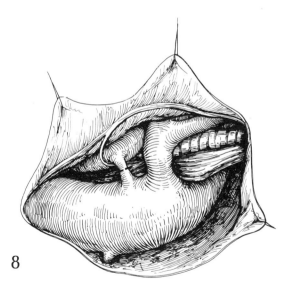

8

A careful inspection and identification of the anatomical disposition of the normal and anomalous vessels is made and the minor anterior left aortic arch dissected out. The ligamentum arteriosum or persistent ductus arteriosus is divided; the recurrent laryngeal nerve is a faithful landmark to this structure. The major persistent right aortic arch lies behind the oesophagus.

DIVISION OF A VASCULAR RING (DOUBLE AORTIC ARCH)

9

In the usual situation with a minor left arch this should be divided distal to the right subclavian artery or between the left subclavian and common carotid arteries. The correct site for division is selected after trial clamping of the anomalous vessels. An assessment is made of the pulsation in all the vessels arising from the anomalous artery and in the descending aorta itself. Only when it is clear that blood flow in them will not be impeded is the division made. The divided vessel ends are either ligated or sutured. It is usual for the separated ends of the anomalous artery to spring apart quite widely after division, thus reflecting the degree of tension previously present.

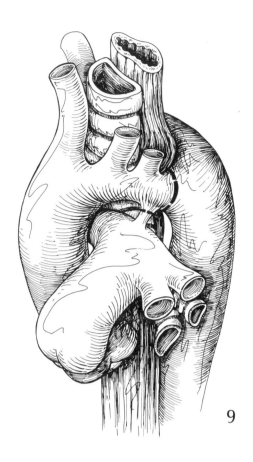

9

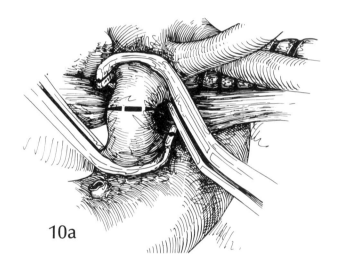

10a

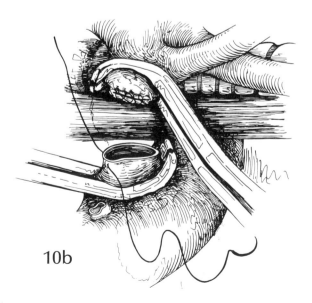

10b

10a & b

The anomalous minor anterior aortic arch is controlled in vascular clamps (a) leaving a sufficient length of vessel for safe suturing. After division the compression of the midline structures is completely relieved (b).

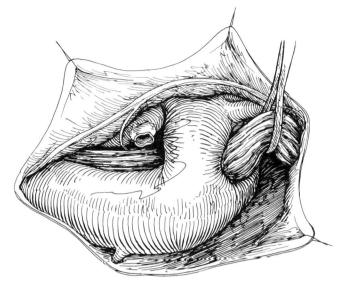

11a

11a, b & c

In the less common situation of a minor right posterior component to the double aortic arch this vessel is exposed behind the oesophagus, which may be displaced in a tape sling (a). The compression of the midline structures (b) is completely relieved after division (c).

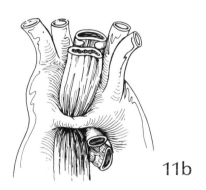

11b

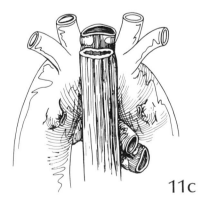

11c

THE RIGHT AORTIC ARCH

12a & b

Usually there are no symptoms associated with this anomaly unless a left-sided ductus arteriosus or ligamentum arteriosum connects with the left pulmonary artery by passing behind the oesophagus (a). This virtually completes a vascular ring and compression of the oesophagus and trachea may result which is relieved by division of the ductus (b).

A right aortic arch is frequently associated with tetralogy of Fallot, truncus arteriosus and tricuspid atresia. The condition is noted on the chest radiograph as there is absence of the aortic knuckle in the usual site, and the aortic arch is seen to the right of the trachea above the right main bronchus. It frequently indents and narrows the trachea.

Rarely a right aortic arch is associated with a right-sided descending aorta, in which case the ductus arteriosus arises from the underside of the arch and enters the right pulmonary artery. A very few cases of right aortic arch with coarctation of the aorta have been described. The surgical approach chosen should probably be governed by the site of the descending thoracic aorta in these cases (left, midline or right-sided).

Normally 'mirror image' branching of the brachiocephalic vessels is present in association with right aortic arch. The first branch, which arises from the junction of the ascending aorta with its transverse arch, is the left-sided innominate artery. The second branch is the right common carotid artery and the third branch is the right subclavian artery.

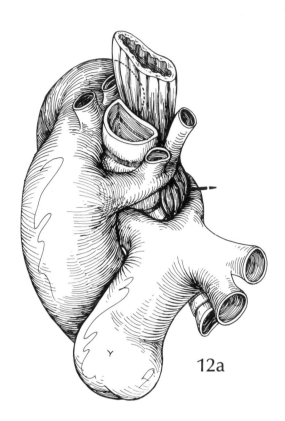

12a

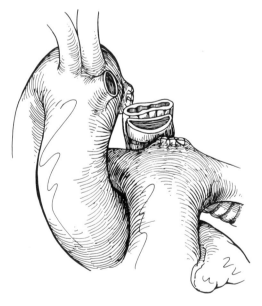

12b

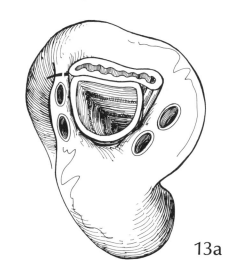

13a

13a–d

Double aortic arch or complete vascular ring is rarely associated with a right aortic arch (also shown in *Illustrations 10a* and *10b*)

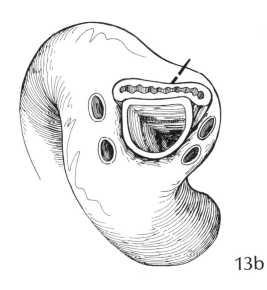

13b

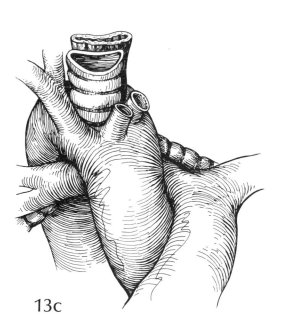

13c

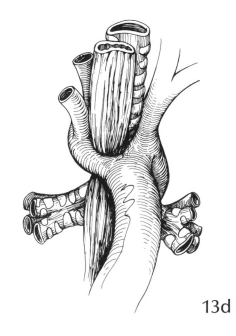

13d

ABERRANT RIGHT SUBCLAVIAN ARTERY

An anomalous (aberrant) right subclavian artery arising from a left descending thoracic aorta is a relatively common finding on routine radiological and postmortem examination and is the most common aortic arch abnormality. The right subclavian artery arises from the descending thoracic aorta distal to the left subclavian artery and passes upwards and behind the oesophagus to the right upper limb. There may be no symptoms and signs, but compression of the oesophagus is quite common. This is demonstrated as a posterior indentation during the barium swallow. Bayford[4] used the term 'dysphagia lusoria' in describing this condition in 1789. The mirror image situation is present when a right aortic arch gives origin to an aberrant left subclavian artery.

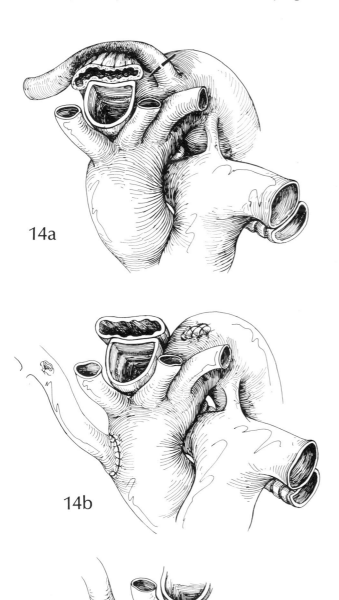

14a

14b

14c

14a–d

The right vertebral artery may arise from the right common carotid artery. This aberrant vessel does not form a vascular ring. If symptoms are troublesome the aberrant vessel can be divided close to its origin from the upper descending thoracic aorta through a left thoracotomy. The point of division is shown for an aberrant right subclavian artery (a) arising from the upper thoracic aorta in the left chest and (d) arising from the left aortic arch with normal left-sided aorta. An alternative technique is to divide the vessel close to its origin and reimplant it into the aortic arch to the right of the midline structures (b) with an interposition graft if necessary to relieve tension (c). This is best approached from a right thoracotomy or a low right cervical incision. Other symptoms which may arise from aberrant right (or left) subclavian arteries which pass behind the oesophagus are rupture into the gullet following prolonged intubation or oesophageal ulceration. This can lead to sudden and catastrophic haemorrhage.

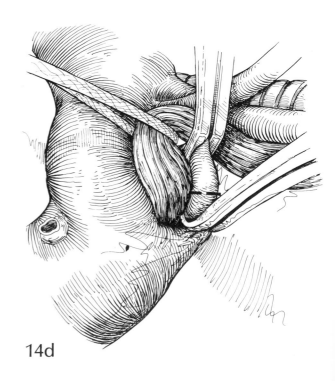

14d

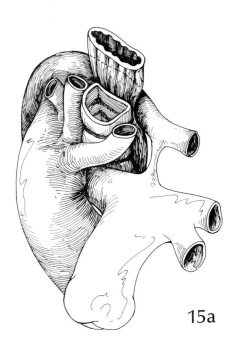

15a

ABERRANT LEFT SUBCLAVIAN ARTERY

15a & b

An aberrant left subclavian artery may arise as the fourth branch from the distal portion of a right aortic arch rather than from the innominate artery (a). It crosses behind the oesophagus to reach the left axilla but only causes constriction in association with a left-sided ligamentum arteriosum or persistent ductus arteriosus. This condition is a mirror image of the aberrrant right subclavian artery arising from a left aortic arch. If necessary it can be treated by division and reimplantation into the aortic arch (b).

In right-sided aortic arch the right recurrent laryngeal nerve passes around the aortic arch and the left around the left-sided ductus arteriosus. When a right-sided ductus is present the nerve relates to this structure in the usual way.

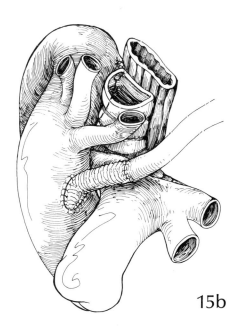

15b

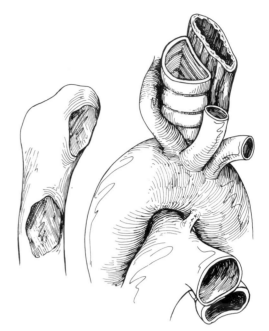

16a

ANOMALOUS INNOMINATE ARTERY

16a & b

The origin of this vessel is situated further to the left of the transverse aortic arch than is usual and therefore the artery must spiral across the trachea to reach the right side of the neck (a). If the vessel is short tracheal obstruction is likely. The anomalous vessel may be displaced anteriorly by suturing its outer adventitial coat to the retrosternal tissues (b). This may alleviate tracheal compression very satisfactorily.

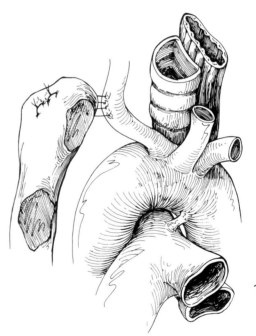

16b

References

1. Edwards, J. E. Anomalies of the derivatives of the aortic arch system. Medical Clinics of North America 1948, 32: 925–949

2. Molz, G., Burri, B. Aberrant subclavian artery (arteria lusoria): sex differences and prevalence of various forms of malformation: evaluation of 1378 observations. Virchows Archiv. Series. A Pathological Anatomy and History. 1978, 380: 303–315

3. Gross, R. E. Surgical relief of tracheal obstruction from a vascular ring. New England Journal of Medicine 1945, 233: 586

4. Bayford, D. An account of a singular case of obstructed deglutination. Memoirs of the Medical Society of London 1794, 2: 275–286

Pericardiectomy and pericardiotomy

Sir Keith Ross MS, FRCS
Consultant Cardiac Surgeon, Wessex Regional Cardiothoracic Centre, Southampton, Hampshire, UK

PERICARDIECTOMY

History

In 1920 Rehn[1] reported four pericardial resections for constrictive pericarditis and is generally credited with the first successful case of surgical intervention, although interest in the condition dates back to the time of Galen. Following the early work of authors such as Churchill[2], and Beck and Griswold[3], pericardiectomy had become an established procedure by the 1930s and the technique remained essentially unchanged in practice until cardiopulmonary bypass was introduced as an adjunct.

Preoperative

Indications

Pericardiectomy is indicated when objective evidence of cardiac restriction is accompanied by subjective disability. Clinical signs of impaired filling of the heart with raised systemic venous pressure, ascites, pleural effusions and peripheral oedema are often associated with radiological evidence of pulmonary venous hypertension and biochemical evidence of impaired liver and kidney function. An overlay of impaired ventricular function due to the low fixed cardiac output and reduced coronary blood flow may be further aggravated by the onset of atrial fibrillation and loss of atrial transport.

The principle of the operation is to remove the thickened and often fused parietal and visceral layers of pericardium; particular attention should be paid to the latter, which may alone be responsible for the patient's disability, particularly when the space between the thickened parietal layer and the epicardium is filled with fluid. Particular care must be taken to remove localized constricting bands in the atrioventricular groove and in relation to the entry of the great veins.

Preoperative preparation

Fluid retention may be partly relieved by appropriate diuretic therapy and pericardial aspiration may be useful if there is a tense effusion. The patient should be digitalized if in atrial fibrillation.

Whether or not tuberculous infection has been identified, antituberculosis drug therapy should be started before and continued after the operation until it has been shown to be unnecessary by bacteriological and histological examination of the material removed at operation.

Anaesthesia

Anaesthetic techniques are governed by the fact that profound hypotension may result from anaesthetic-induced falls in preload, myocardial contractility or arterial impedance. Adequate cardiovascular monitoring, including direct measurement of arterial and venous pressure, is essential. Expert choice of the many anaesthetic agents available for cardiac surgery and their use in appropriate dosage will ensure that marked changes in the circulation are avoided.

The operation

Operative approach

1

The classical approach for pericardiectomy is by *left anterolateral thoracotomy* (Incision A), with the patient tilted slightly to the right. The submammary incision, with entry into the chest by way of the fourth or fifth intercostal space, gives good access to the left ventricle and left atrium and makes identification and preservation of the left phrenic nerve easy. Access to the right ventricle, right atrium and great veins can be achieved with certainty and safety only by extending the incision across the midline, with ligation and division of both sets of internal mammary vessels and transverse division of the sternum. If one of the cardiac chambers is breached during pericardial resection by this approach and cardiopulmonary bypass be needed to regain control of the situation conventional intrathoracic venous and arterial cannulations may be impossible. If it is decided to use this approach it is wise to have the drapes arranged for easy access to the left femoral vessels so that femorofemoral supportive bypass can be provided quickly should the need arise.

A *midline approach* (Incision B) is more satisfactory. Median sternotomy gives good access to the right ventricle, right atrium and great vessels but less good access to the left side of the heart. This disadvantage is overcome by the use of cardiopulmonary bypass, which allows safe dislocation of the heart and rotation to the right so that the left ventricle and atrioventricular groove may be properly freed.

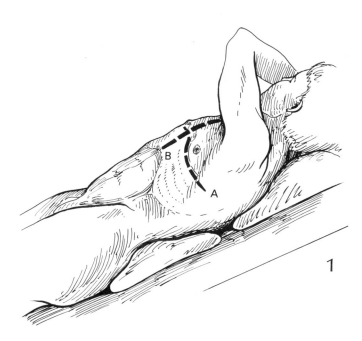

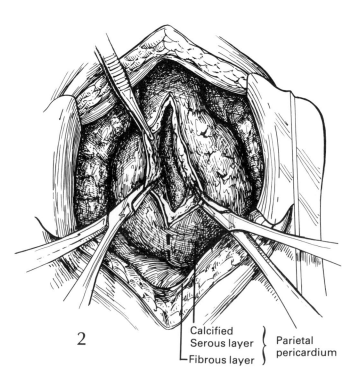

2

Calcified
Serous layer } Parietal
Fibrous layer } pericardium

2

The thickened pericardium is opened longitudinally in the midline and the incision extended to right and left in cruciform fashion. Loculated pus may be encountered at this or subsequent stages in the dissection; specimens should be sent for culture for pyogenic and acid fast organisms although they are almost invariably sterile.

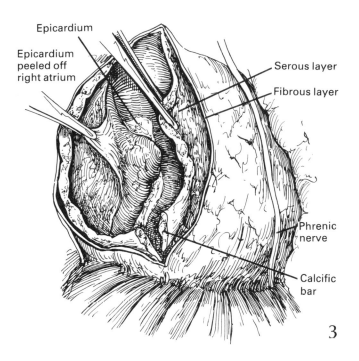

3

The incision is then deepened to include the constricting epicardial layer, which is peeled off the right atrium and other structures.

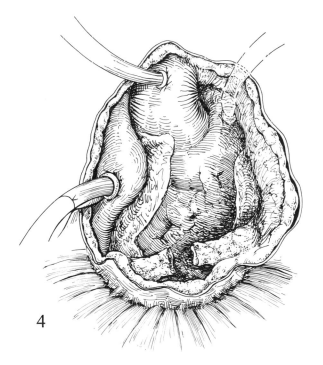

4

Once the ascending aorta, pulmonary artery and right atrium have been freed and the patient has been heparinized the necessary cannulations for cardiopulmonary bypass may be made. A single venous cannula in the right atrium is sufficient, and venous return may be supplemented by the insertion of a pulmonary artery vent. This also keeps the right ventricle decompressed and helps to prevent left ventricular distension when the heart is dislocated to permit work on its posterior aspect. Perfusion with moderate hypothermia (30–32°C) provides ideal operating conditions, making for safe sharp dissection and decreased risk of muscle and coronary artery damage.

Calcific plates and bars must be mobilized and if necessary divided with bone-cutting instruments and removed piecemeal. Isolated calcific deposits burrowing deeply into ventricular muscle may be safely left *in situ*.

5

The dissection is then carried downwards towards the lower end of the right atrium and inferior vena cava, the right ventricle having been completely decorticated.

Injury to major coronary arteries may be avoided by leaving strips of adherent pericardium on the surface of the ventricles and in the atrioventricular and interventricular grooves, but care must be taken not to leave important constricting bands in the former (*see also illustrations 6 and 7*).

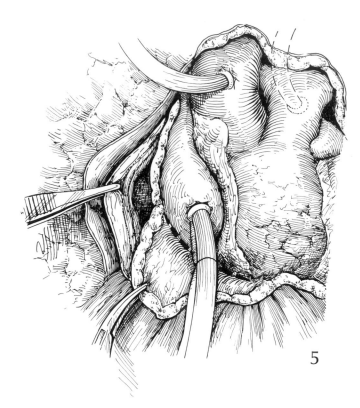

5

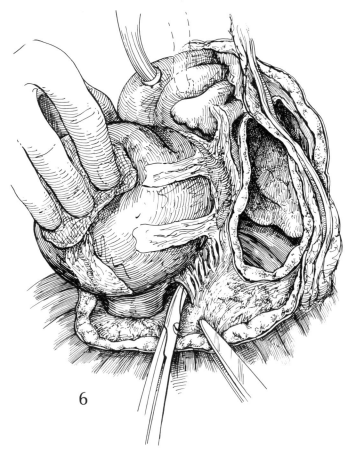

6

6

The use of cardiopulmonary bypass allows unhurried and accurate decortication of the back of the left ventricle, left atrioventricular grove and inferior vena cava. The left phrenic nerve is identified and preserved, leaving an underlying strip of pericardium.

7

Finally, all readily available parietal pericardium is trimmed away and the heart allowed to drop back into its normal position.

The chest is closed in layers in routine fashion with drains to both pleural cavities and the mediastinum. The opportunity should be taken to suck out large pleural effusions before closure is completed. It is doubtful whether ascitic fluid should be aspirated, but if the quantity is large enough to embarrass respiration this may be indicated.

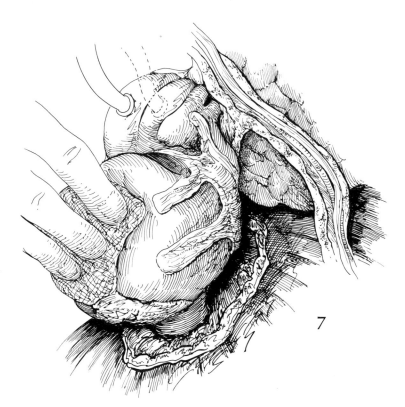

7

Hazards of pericardiectomy

Breaching of a cardiac chamber   The cardiac muscle is degenerate and infiltrated with fat and the right ventricle particularly thin-walled. Teflon-reinforced mattress sutures of 3/0 or 4/0 polypropylene should be used to close holes in the walls of the cardiac chambers.

Injury to superficial coronary arteries   This may be anticipated and prevented as described above. If serious injury to a major artery occurs and the vessel has to be ligated venous bypass grafting may be needed.

Phrenic nerve injury   The phrenic nerves are not always easy to identify and diathermy must be used with caution in their vicinity.

Incomplete epicardial decortication   It is essential to remove the epicardial layer as well as the thickened parietal pericardium.

PERICARDIOTOMY

Recurrent pericardial effusions, managed with difficulty and distress to the patient by repeated aspiration, may demand pericardiotomy. This may apply to effusions due to malignant disease, uraemia and other serious systemic disease processes as well as to idiopathic recurrent effusions.

The operation

8

The approach is by standard left lateral thoracotomy (or, if preferred, by an anterolateral approach) by way of the fifth or sixth intercostal space.

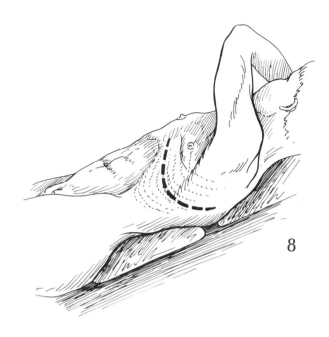

8

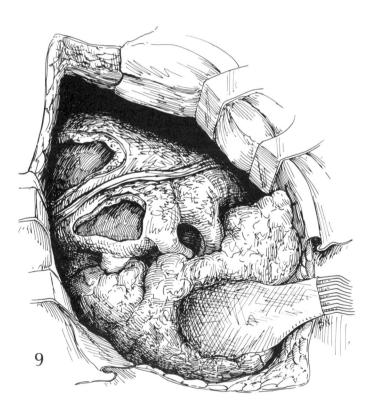

9

9

Large windows are cut in the pericardium on either side of the phrenic nerve. The opportunity may be taken for lymph-node or other biopsy inside the chest. The portions of pericardium removed should be sent for histological examination.

The chest is closed in layers in routine fashion with a single pleural drain.

References

1. Rehn, L. Neben Perikardiale Verwachsungen. Medizinische Klinik 1920; 16: 999

2. Churchill, E. D. Decortication of the heart (Delorme) for adhesive pericarditis. Archives of Surgery 1929; 19: 1457–1469

3. Beck, C. S., Griswold, R. A. Pericardiectomy in the treatment of the Pick syndrome: experimental and clinical observations. Archives of Surgery 1930; 21: 1064–1113

Closed mitral commissurotomy

Avenilo P. Aventura MD
Director, Philippine Heart Center for Asia, Quezon City, The Philippines

Introduction

Closed mitral commissurotomy should be considered in young patients (often female) with tight mitral stenosis and without significant mitral regurgitation or mitral calcification, especially when atrial fibrillation is not present and there has been no history of embolization.

The operation

1

The patient is prepared for left posterolateral thoracotomy. Endobronchial anaesthesia is used in order to achieve collapse of the left lung. The chest is entered through the bed of the fifth rib.

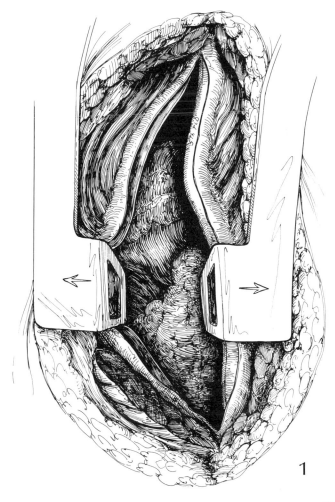

1

2 & 3

After thoracotomy the pericardium is exposed. A full-length longitudinal incision is made in the pericardium anterior to the phrenic nerve. Stay sutures are then placed in the pericardium to achieve exposure. The atrial appendage is inspected; gentle palpation occasionally reveals this to be thrombosed. If intra-atrial thrombosis is suspected the appendage is opened and allowed to flush with blood from the atrial cavity before a side-biting clamp is placed. If excessive thrombosis is present the institution of cardiopulmonary bypass with open mitral commissurotomy is probably wisest as cerebral and peripheral embolization is a major hazard of mitral commissurotomy in these circumstances. Preoperative echocardiography should be used when possible to determine the presence of clots.

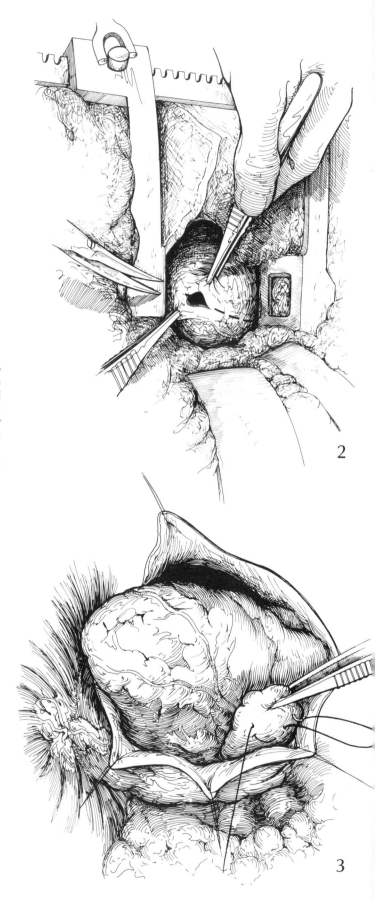

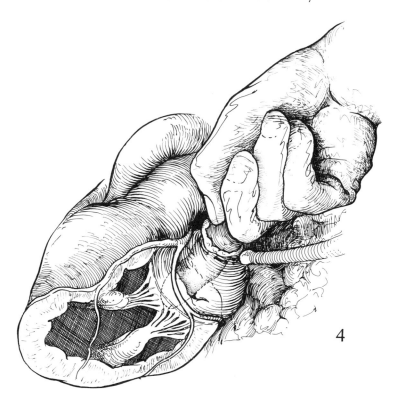

4 & 5

If it is decided to proceed with closed mitral commissurotomy an incision is made in the atrial appendage just large enough to admit the index finger of the right hand. The finger is slowly advanced through the opening and the mitral valve palpated. Care should be taken not to occlude the residual opening of the mitral valve for more than a few seconds during this palpation. Often commissurotomy can be readily effected with the finger alone.

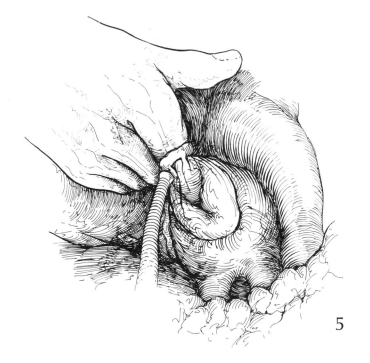

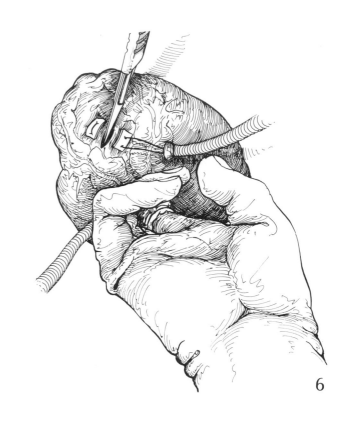

6

6 & 7

If difficulty is encountered in performing commissurotomy with the finger alone the apex of the heart is lifted and a purse-string suture placed at the apex of the left ventricle by an assistant and a small stab wound made through it. A Tubbs transventricular dilator is then passed from the apex to the mitral valve orifice.

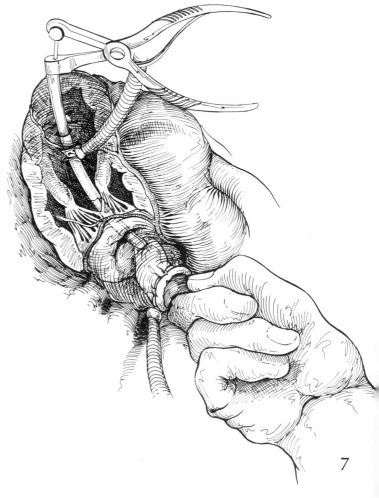

7

8

The open size of the dilator can be altered, and a suitable size is selected with the aid of a ruler before insertion of the dilator into the ventricle.

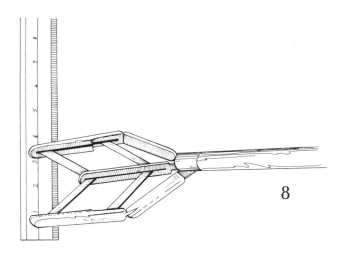

8

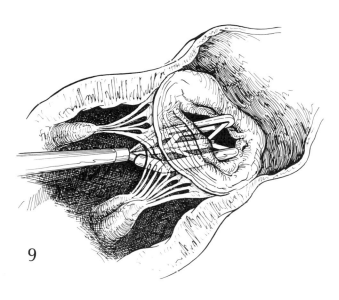

9

9

Occasionally after initial commissurotomy with the dilator the index finger in the left atrium completes the commissurotomy. Generally, however, with the trans-ventricular dilator both anterolateral and posteromedial commissures are readily dilated.

10a & b

After commissurotomy the dilator is withdrawn and the valve reassessed to determine any residual regurgitation (a). If no or minimal regurgitation is found the index finger is withdrawn and the side-biting clamp reapplied to the left atrial appendage. Care must be taken during the application of this instrument not to interfere with the passage of the circumflex coronary artery. Major mitral regurgitation necessitates repair or replacement of the valve using cardiopulmonary bypass. The transventricular dilator is slowly withdrawn and the purse-string suture tightened over Teflon pledgets (b). This suture is then reinforced by a further suture.

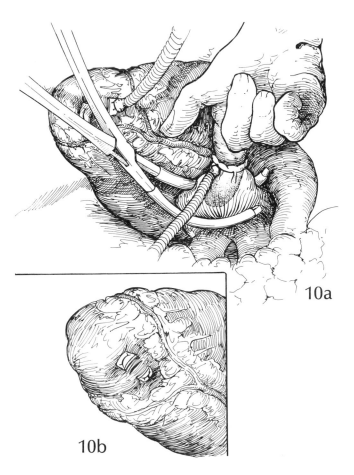

10a

10b

11

The left atrial appendage is closed with polypropylene. Any excessive atrial appendage is excised.

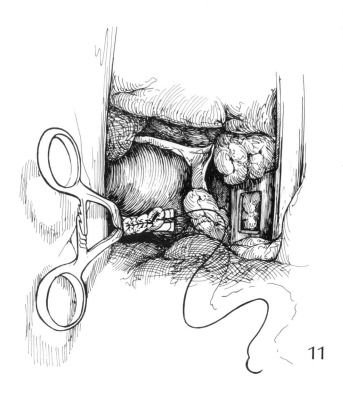

11

12

12

After confirmation of haemostasis the pericardium is reapproximated with interrupted sutures, though the inferior aspect of the pericardium should be left open as a drain. The chest is then routinely closed in layers.

Reoperation

For repeat commissurotomy, the atrial appendage is commonly fibrotic or too small to admit the index finger, and the purse-string suture can be placed in the atrial wall itself. Should there be difficulty in controlling bleeding within the atrium or atrial appendage, control may be obtained with a 20 ml Foley catheter while the atrial wall is being sutured.

Mitral valve reconstructive surgery

Alain Carpentier MD, PhD
Professor of Cardiovascular Surgery, University of Paris;
Chief, Department of Cardiovascular Surgery, Hôpital Broussais, Paris, France

Introduction

Mitral valve reconstruction is still a subject of controversy, largely because the techniques of annuloplasty developed at the beginning of cardiac surgery were associated with disappointing and unpredictable results. The reason for this was a lack of comprehension of the causes of mitral regurgitation: dilatation of the annulus was thought to be the primary lesion and annular plication the treatment of choice. The recognition that mitral regurgitation could result from several lesions affecting the various structures of the valvular apparatus – annulus, leaflets, chordae tendineae and papillary muscles – led to the development of appropriate techniques of valve reconstruction with more predictable results.

Indications for valve repair

Mitral regurgitation

Mitral regurgitation may result from the following conditions

1. Primary valvular disease
   (a) Congenital malformations
   (b) Inflammatory diseases: rheumatic fever; lupus; others
   (c) Degenerative diseases: fibroelastic deficiency; Barlow's syndrome; Marfan's disease; others
   (d) Trauma
   (e) Bacterial endocarditis
   (f) Calcification
2. Primary cardiac disease
   (a) Ischaemic heart disease
   (b) Obstructive cardiomyopathy
   (c) Non-obstructive cardiomyopathy
   (d) Endocardial fibroelastosis

Whatever their origin, all cases of non-calcified mitral valve regurgitation should be considered for valve reconstruction. The decision to operate should be taken as soon as possible after the onset of atrial fibrillation since early correction is then more likely to be followed by successful conversion to sinus rhythm, thus avoiding the need for anticoagulation.

In children, since atrial fibrillation is exceptional even in advanced disease, the indications for mitral valve repair are based on repeated episodes of heart failure or continuous and significant increase in heart size.

Mitral stenosis

Mitral stenosis results from either a congenital malformation or rheumatic valvular disease. Established mitral stenosis alone usually merits early surgical relief; again, operation should not be delayed after the onset of atrial fibrillation. Pulmonary oedema and systemic embolization are additional urgent indications. Long-standing disease and the presence of calcification make the valve less suitable for reconstruction.

The operation

A midline sternotomy is preferred. On investigation of the heart with mitral regurgitation, increased pulmonary artery pressure, atrial fibrillation and an enlarged left atrium with a systolic thrill are common findings. In mitral stenosis a small left atrium may be found, raising the question of the appropriate approach to the valve. An enlarged right atrium suggests associated tricuspid disease, but false right atrial enlargement may occur as a result of distension by a very large left atrium. They can be differentiated by intra-atrial palpation.

1

The venae cavae are cannulated separately and surrounded by tapes. Aortic cannulation is carried out in routine fashion. A needle for removing air and preventing air embolism is also inserted into the ascending aorta 1 cm below the aortic cannula and connected to suction. The patient is cooled to 22°C. Myocardial protection is achieved either by intermittent revascularization (2 minutes every 12 minutes) or by cardioplegia instituted after analysis of the lesion of the valve.

The left atrial incision is carried out between the posterior interatrial groove and the pulmonary veins. A biatrial trans-septal incision is preferred when the left atrium is small. With the latter approach both atria are opened by an incision from the right atrial appendage to the right superior pulmonary vein and the septum is incised forwards towards the tricuspid valve.

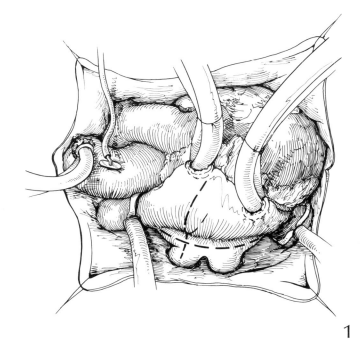

1

2

2

Pericardial adhesions, whenever present, must be divided in order to mobilize the heart fully and to facilitate exposure of the subvalvular apparatus. Two medium-sized retractors are used to expose the mitral valve. Exposure of the posterior papillary muscle, if necessary, can be achieved by placing a sponge in the pericardial cavity between the pericardium and the diaphragmatic surface of the heart.

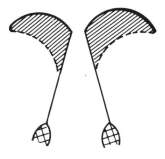

Type I : Normal leaflet motion

3

Each structure of the mitral apparatus must be systematically and critically inspected – annulus, leaflets, commissures, chordae tendineae and papillary muscles. Leaflet dysfunction is recognized by mobilizing the two leaflets successively. Leaflet prolapse is present when the free edge of one leaflet overrides the plane of the orifice when the edge is pulled towards the atrium with a nerve hook. Restricted leaflet motion is present when a leaflet does not fully and/or easily open. The causes of leaflet dysfunction (*Table 1*) are usually easy to recognize.

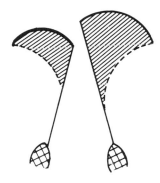

Type II : Leaflet prolapse

Table 1 Pathology of valvular lesions

Type	Acquired valvular disease	Congenital valvular disease
I	Pure annulus dilatation Leaflet perforation Leaflet defect	Pure annulus dilatation Leaflet perforation Leaflet defect
II	Chordal rupture Chordal elongation Papillary muscle rupture Papillary muscle elongation	Chordal rupture Chordal elongation Capillary muscle elongation
III	*(a) Valvular lesions* Commissure fusion Leaflet thickening	*(a) Valvular malformations* Commissure fusion Excess valvular tissue Supravalvular ring
	(b) Subvalvular lesions Chordal fusion Chordae thickening Absent papillary muscle	*(b) Subvalvular* *malformations* Papillary muscle- commissure fusion Parachute valve Hammock valve Absent papillary muscle

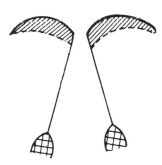

Type III : Restricted leaflet motion   3

REPAIR OF ANNULUS DILATATION

4a & b

In the normal mitral valve (a) the transverse diameter (tt′) of the annulus exceeds the anteroposterior diameter (ap). The annulus is deformed (b) when its transverse diameter is found to be smaller than the anteroposterior diameter. The deformity may be symmetrical (tp = t′p) or asymmetrical (tp ≠ t′p). Dilatation of the orifice is usually associated with the deformation. The dilatation affects the posterior leaflet and the commissures but not the anterior leaflet portion of the annulus.

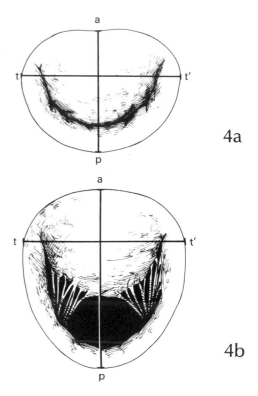

4a

4b

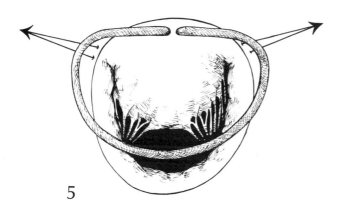

5

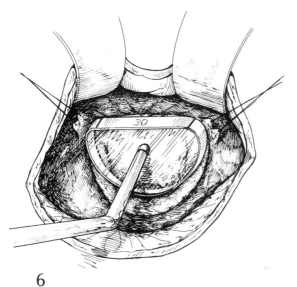

6

ANNULUS REMODELLING

Annulus remodelling with a prosthetic ring, unlike annulus narrowing by commissure plication or circular sutures, restores the normal shape and therefore the normal function of the valve.

5 & 6

Ring selection is based on measurement of the base of the anterior leaflet, which is not affected by dilatation. One pilot suture is placed at each commissure and the distance between these two points is measured with obturators specifically designed for this purpose. The appropriate-sized prosthetic ring is then selected.

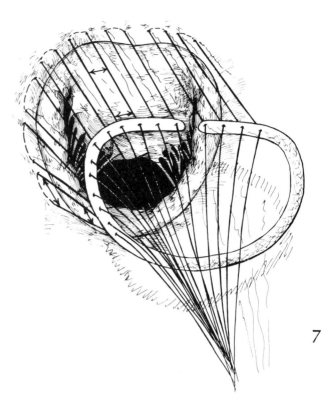

7 & 8

Approximately 12 sutures are placed through the annulus around the whole periphery of the mitral ring. These sutures are evenly and equally spaced between the base of the anterior leaflet and the corresponding portion of the prosthetic ring. Elsewhere spacing of sutures is so arranged as to achieve remodelling of the natural valve ring to conform to the size and shape of the prosthesis. If there is an asymmetrical dilatation of the annulus with a predominant enlargement of one commissure, the distribution of the sutures is adapted by reducing the spacing of the sutures in the corresponding area of the prosthetic ring.

The ring is then slid into position and the sutures tied, thus repositioning the different annular structures without reducing the normal orifice area or affecting leaflet motion.

7

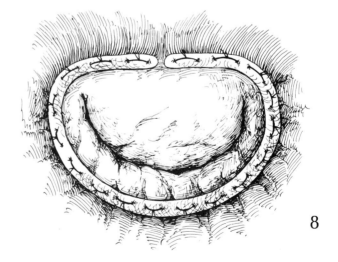

8

REPAIR OF LEAFLET PERFORATION

9a & b

Leaflet perforation is the result of bacterial endocarditis and may involve either the anterior or the posterior leaflet. Valve repair can be attempted only after a minimum of 15 days of antibiotic therapy.

Posterior leaflet perforations are treated by resection of the affected area and repair of the resulting gap with interrupted stitches (5/0 polypropylene). Anterior leaflet perforations may be treated by oval resection and closure by suture if the hole is less than 5 mm in diameter. Larger holes should be closed with a glutaraldehyde-fixed autologous pericardial patch (0.6 per cent glutaralhehyde for 5 minutes, then washing in saline + 5 per cent magnesium chloride) (b). Glutaraldehyde fixation of pericardium has been shown to prevent shrinkage or distension.

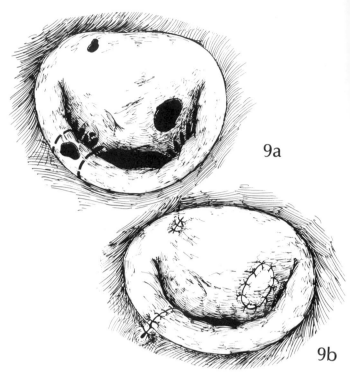

9a

9b

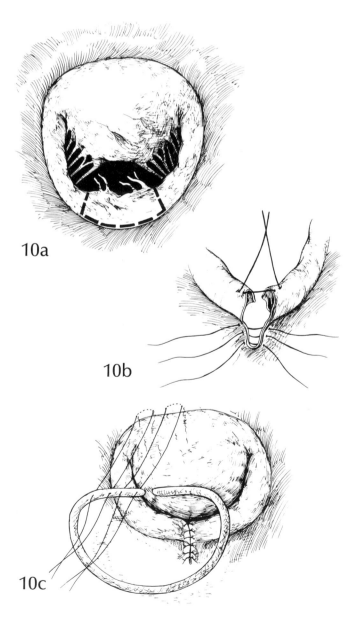

10a

10b

10c

REPAIR OF LEAFLET PROLAPSE

Leaflet prolapse must be systematically searched for in all cases of mitral regurgitation. The leaflet is pulled towards the atrium with a nerve hook. Prolapse is present if the free edge of the leaflet overrides the plane of the orifice. Leaflet prolapse may result from ruptured chordae, chordal elongation or a ruptured papillary muscle. Comparison of the position of the edges of the two leaflets may be of great help since prolapse of the two leaflets is rare (with the exception of Barlow's syndrome).

Repair of ruptured chordae

10a, b & c

Only ruptured chordae of the posterior leaflet are suitable for repair. Two stay sutures are placed around the normal chordae at the limits of the prolapsed part of the leaflet. The distance between these two chordae is projected down to the annulus so that a rectangle is formed which corresponds to the prolapsed portion of the leaflet (a). This tissue is removed. A 'U' suture is placed in the annulus in order to approximate the free edges of the leaflet, which are then sutured with interrupted 5/0 polypropylene sutures (b). A quadrangular resection is preferred to the usual triangular plication or resection since it avoids excessive tension on the free edge of the leaflet. A prosthetic ring is placed to reinforce the repair and to remodel the annulus (c). A valve replacement is necessary if the rupture affects more than one half of the posterior leaflet or the main chordae of the anterior leaflet.

Repair of chordal elongation

11a–d

Chordal elongation (a) has only recently been recognized and was previously responsible for many cases of residual regurgitation after valve repair.

Moderate (<4 mm) elongation of two or three chordae of the anterior leaflet is treated by a sliding plasty of the corresponding papillary muscle. The portion of the papillary muscle corresponding to the elongated chordae is split longitudinally (b) and is resutured at a lower level (c, d). The length of the sliding displacement should correspond to the excess length of the chordae, which is judged by the degree of leaflet overriding.

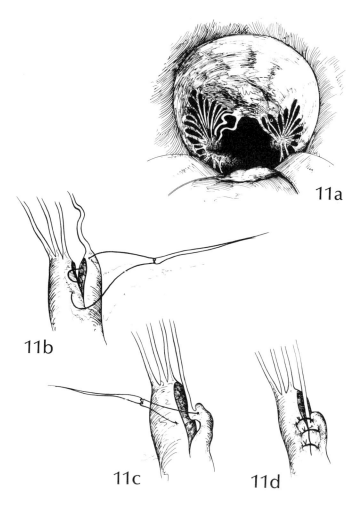

12a–c

Severe (>4 mm) elongation of the chordae is treated by a shortening plasty of the chordae. The anterior aspect of the tip of the papillary muscle is incised longitudinally. A 5/0 suture is passed through one half of the trench, then around the chordae to be shortened and then through the other half of the trench at a distance from the tip of the papillary muscle equal to half of the excess length of the chordae (a). Traction on the ends of the suture buries the excess length of the chordae (b). The papillary muscle is then closed around the buried portion of the chordae (c).

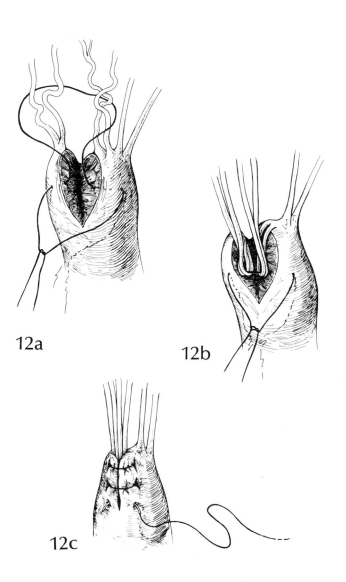

REPAIR OF RESTRICTED LEAFLET MOTION AND VALVULAR STENOSIS

13a–e

The motion of the leaflets may be restricted by commissure fusion, short chordae, hypertrophied chordae, fused chordae and/or leaflet thickening.

Fusion of the commissure may be classified into three grades according to the severity of the lesions. In Grade I there is partial fusion of the commissures with preservation of commissural chordae (a and b). In Grade II there is complete fusion of the commissures with a well-defined border between the anterior and posterior leaflets (c). In Grade III there is complete fusion of the commissures with no delineation between the anterior and posterior leaflets and fused commissural chordae (d). In Grades I and II commissurotomy is easily performed and should not extend further than 3 mm from the annulus (b). In Grade III it is difficult to determine the correct site for commissurotomy. This can be achieved by traction on the main chordae of the anterior leaflet opposite to the commissure (e). This manoeuvre creates a furrow indicating the delineation between the anterior and posterior leaflets.

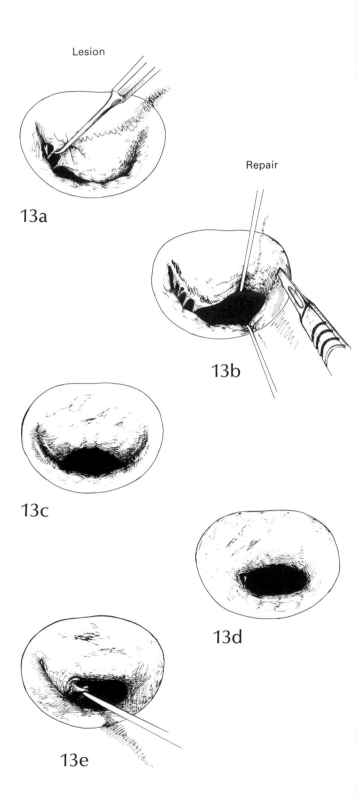

Lesion

13a

Repair

13b

13c

13d

13e

14a–c

Short chordae and hypertrophied chordae inserted on the inferior surface of the leaflet (intermediate chordae) or at the base of the leaflet (basal chordae) are responsible for thickening and restricted movement of the leaflets (*a* and *b*). Extensive resection of these chordae allows mobilization of the leaflet (*c*). All secondary and basal chordae can be removed, care being taken to leave in place marginal chordae (those attached to the free margin of the leaflet), which prevent leaflet prolapse.

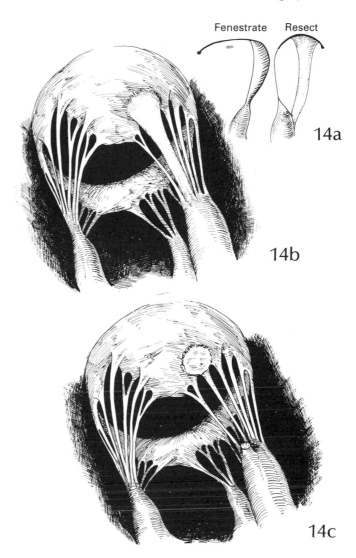

14a

14b

14c

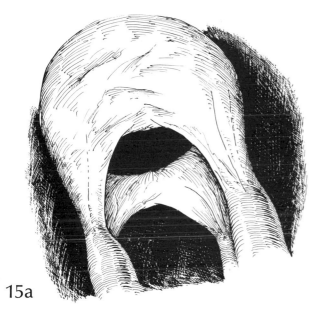

15a

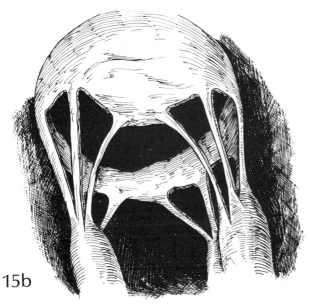

15b

15a & b

Fused marginal chordae (*a*) should be fenestrated by resection of triangular portions of the fibrous tissues (*b*). The resection can be extended to the papillary muscle.

In almost every case of mitral valve disease there are several distinct abnormalities which should be separately assessed and then treated. The sequence to follow in the correction of these lesions is as follows: commissurotomy, quadrangular leaflet resection, repair of subvalvular lesions, sutures of leaflet edges and annulus remodelling.

ASSESSMENT OF THE REPAIR

16

The competence of the valve should be tested after the ring has been pulled down into position but before the sutures are tied so that the ring can be pulled out should an additional minor correction prove to be necessary at the subvalvular level. The competence of the valve is tested after suction has been established through the needle in the ascending aorta in order to prevent air embolism to the coronary arteries. Saline is injected through the mitral valve into the left ventricle under pressure from a 250 ml bulb syringe.

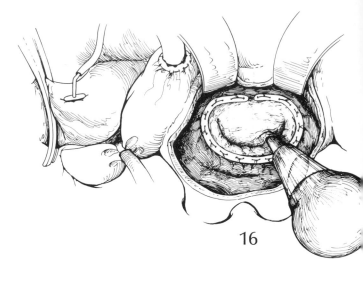

16

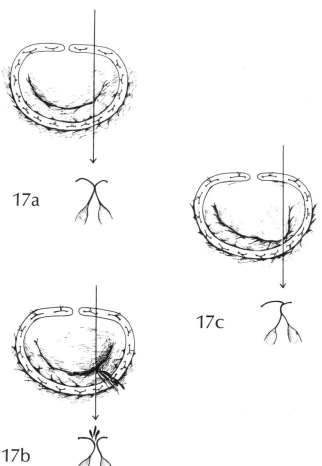

17a

17b

17c

17a–c

The quality of the repair is judged from the morphology of the line of closure of the leaflets. A line of closure parallel to the posterior leaflet attachment (a) indicates a satisfactory repair even if a small leak persists (b), since it means that good coaptation has been restored. An asymmetrical line of closure (c) indicates a certain degree of persistent prolapse or excessively restricted leaflet motion. Slight asymmetry with good approximation is acceptable. Important asymmetry with the edge of one leaflet overriding the other (c) is not acceptable. In this case the ring should be pulled out and correction of the residual prolapse by either chordal shortening or limited triangular resection should be carried out. The ring is then pulled down into position and another injection is made. Any unsatisfactory result, i.e. poor leaflet mobilization or significant residual leak in areas of no leaflet coaptation, should lead to a valve replacement. However, this is rarely necessary if one has carefully followed the steps and guidelines outlined above.

Postoperative care

Heparinization is started as soon as significant pericardial drainage has ceased and there is no other evidence of major bleeding. Anticoagulation should be maintained for 2 months in all cases, at which time it can be discontinued in those patients who are in sinus rhythm. In the remaining patients electrical cardioversion should be attempted 2–4 months after the operation. If sinus rhythm is established and maintained anticoagulants may then be stopped. Anticoagulation may be discontinued after 6 months in patients with irreversible atrial fibrillation if the atrium is only moderately enlarged and the cardiac output is fairly good. In this situation treatment with aspirin is recommended.

Valve prostheses

David J. Wheatley MD, ChM, FRCS (Ed. and Glas.)
Professor of Cardiac Surgery, University of Glasgow;
Honorary Consultant Cardiac Surgeon to Greater Glasgow Health Board, Glasgow, UK

Introduction

Removal of a diseased heart valve and its replacement with a prosthesis is commonly the only practical option in the surgical management of valvular heart disease. Prosthetic valves have been improved considerably since their introduction in the early 1960s. The present commercially available prosthetic heart valves all offer acceptable performance and have transformed the management of valvular heart disease[1,2]. However, problems and uncertainties remain and account for the wide choice of prostheses and differing practices[3]. Procedures which restore good valve function and conserve the patient's own valve (*see* Chapter on 'Mitral valve repair', pp. 405–414) should always be considered before excision of the valve as satisfactory valve repair, when feasible, avoids the problems of valve prostheses.

Throughout the development of valve prostheses the major problems have been the need to provide reasonably physiological valve function (minimal obstruction to forward flow and minimal regurgitation) without major risk of thromboembolism and haemolysis, together with satisfactory durability.

Two broad groups of valve prostheses can be distinguished – biological valves and mechanical valves.

Biological valves are constructed principally from human or animal tissue and usually mimic the natural aortic valve. They are relatively free from thromboembolic complications, but their durability has been disappointing in the past and remains uncertain, even for current valves.

Mechanical valves are manufactured from a variety of materials (alloy, silicone rubber, pyrolytic carbon) and do not resemble natural valves. The majority consist of a circular valve seat with a restrained ball occluder or tilting disc occluder. Durability is not a problem with current models, but thromboembolism remains a risk. Permanent oral anticoagulation is required and there is a small risk of sudden valve dysfunction or systemic embolism.

Biological valves

ALLOGRAFT (OR HOMOGRAFT) AORTIC VALVE

1

Transplantation of the human aortic valve, obtained from a cadaver, into the aortic valve position was pioneered independently by Ross in London[4] in 1962 and Barratt-Boyes et al. in New Zealand[5] in 1962. The valve is transplanted with a small amount of aortic valve tissue around the donor annulus. Several methods of sterilization and storage have been used, including exposure to ethylene oxide or betapropriolactone and gamma irradiation with freeze-drying.

Once the valve has been sewn into place the end result looks much like the natural valve. Function is usually excellent, technical difficulty in precise insertion being occasionally responsible for valve distortion and regurgitation. Thromboembolism is not a problem and anticoagulation is not required. The major problem has been late valve dysfunction due to tearing or disruption of leaflets, often with calcification. Gradually increasing regurgitation is the usual manifestation; sudden onset of regurgitation or stenosis is rare. This deterioration has been reduced by the adoption of methods of antibiotic sterilization and storage in cell nutrient media at 4°C, with undoubted improvement in valve durability[6]. However, the continuing late failure rate and the problems of acquiring and preparing the valves, as well as the relative difficulty of accurate insertion, have severely restricted the use of the allograft valve.

The allograft aortic valve retained in its donor aorta has been used for a valved conduit for reconstruction in congenital cardiac anomalies. For small children this probably offers the best currently available valved conduit. Calcification occurs early in the donor aortic wall, but valve function continues for many years without thromboembolism.

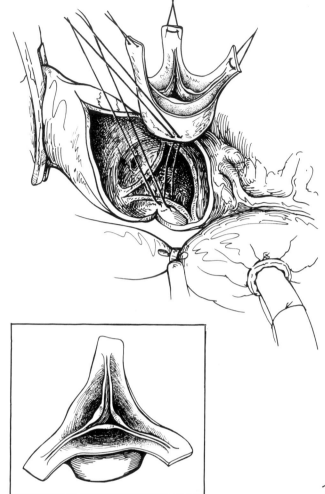

1

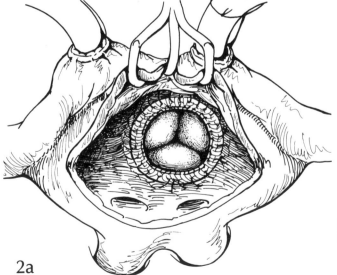

2a

2a, b & c

The allograft aortic valve has been used in the mitral position (a), mounted on a three-pronged frame (b) or in a tube of Dacron (c). The problems of late deterioration have been greater in this position and this valve is no longer considered suitable for use.

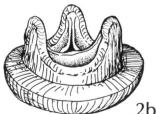

2b

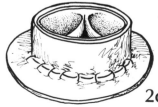

2c

BIOPROSTHETIC VALVES

Bioprosthetic valves are derived from living tissue and treated, usually with glutaraldehyde, to increase the strength of the collagen framework of the tissue, thus providing added durability and also reducing tissue antigenicity. Two groups of glutaraldehyde-treated bioprosthetic valves are currently popular. These are: (1) glutaraldehyde-treated porcine aortic valves mounted on a supporting frame, and (2) glutaraldehyde-treated bovine pericardium wrapped around a three-pronged frame to form a three-leaflet valve mimicking the naturally occurring aortic valve.

3

Hancock valve

Available since 1970, the Hancock porcine bioprosthesis consists of the aortic valve of the pig secured to a flexible polypropylene support which has a stellite ring at the annulus to prevent distortion. The tissue is treated with a stabilized glutaraldehyde process to cross-link the collagen of the valve and increase tissue strength. The frame is covered with fabric and there is a sewing ring to enable the valve to be secured to the patient's tissues.

The inherent stiffness of the glutaraldehyde-fixed leaflets, together with the septal myocardial bar at the base of the right coronary leaflet, creates a fall in pressure across the valve equivalent to that of mild stenosis. Most reports, however, indicate satisfactory haemodynamic performance in the larger sizes of prosthesis, but several centres advocate avoiding the smaller prostheses in the aortic position. In 1976 a modified-orifice bioprosthesis was introduced. In this valve the right coronary leaflet is replaced with a muscle-free leaflet from another valve. The resultant composite valve has an improved haemodynamic performance and is intended for use in the small aortic root[7,8].

The Hancock valve is relatively free from thromboembolism[9]. A short period of oral anticoagulation is recommended for the initial 6–12 week postoperative period. After this most patients with aortic valve replacements do not require long-term anticoagulation. A significant number of those with mitral valve replacement, however, remain in atrial fibrillation, the presence of which or of left atrial dilatation may be regarded as an indication for long-term anticoagulation[10,11].

The likelihood of sudden valve failure is minimal. However, accelerated onset of valve calcification has been reported in children and in patients on chronic haemodialysis, and the Hancock valve is not recommended in these circumstances[12,13]. Long-term integrity and function remain uncertain in adults and, although satisfactory durability is reported for 6 years of follow-up, repeat surgery to replace the bioprosthesis must be regarded as a possibility in all patients[14].

The Hancock prosthesis should be stored and handled with care, according to the manufacturer's instructions. Thorough rinsing before insertion is essential and drying of the leaflets should be avoided. Sizing obturators are available to aid the choice of correct size of prosthesis. Valve insertion technique will further influence the choice of valve size; a larger valve size can usually be accommodated if the prosthesis is seated above the aortic annulus or on to the left atrial floor rather than within the valve annulus. In mitral valve replacement the prongs of the supporting frame may damage the myocardium if the ventricular cavity is small and, if this is anticipated, a low-profile mechanical valve may be more appropriate. The prongs of a mitral prosthesis should be orientated to lie on either side of the left ventricular outflow tract. The greatest technical danger during insertion is looping of a suture over a prong. This is less of a risk with a continuous suture technique, but with interrupted sutures the valve should be lowered into place with the sutures under tension, particular note being taken of the valve prongs and the open valve being checked after the sutures have been tied; a dental mirror may aid in this. Vigorous massage of the ventricle or lifting of the apex may cause laceration of the myocardium by the prongs of a mitral prosthesis and these manoeuvres should therefore be avoided. With aortic valve replacement the prongs should be orientated to avoid obscuring the coronary ostia and, although it is less of a hazard, there is still a possibility of looping a suture around a prong, either during valve insertion or during closure of the aortotomy, and due care is required to avoid this.

Every effort should be made to avoid injury to the leaflet tissue and it should be kept moist with saline during insertion. Where it is necessary to open the valve to check on valve seating a smooth instrument should be gently inserted between the leaflets to retract them with care.

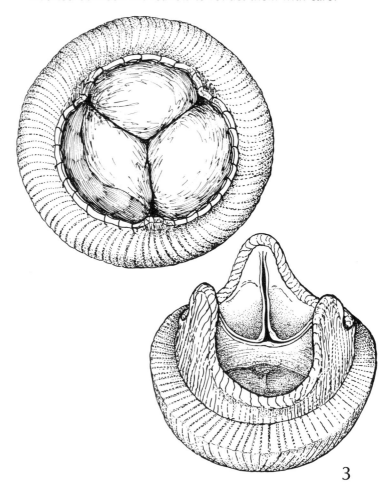

3

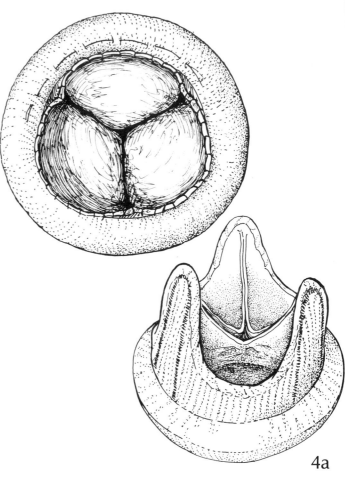

4a & b

Carpentier-Edwards valve

The Carpentier-Edwards valve is a porcine bioprosthesis which has been available since 1976. It consists of the aortic valve of the pig treated in a buffered glutaraldehyde solution and sewn into a flexible support made of a cobalt and nickel alloy (a). The aortic frame has a slightly scalloped lower margin to faciliatate its fit into the host annulus (b). The support is covered with polytetra-fluoroethylene fabric and there is a sewing ring for securing the valve to the patient.

Haemodynamic performance is satisfactory, except possibly in the smaller sizes[15]. The valve is relatively free from thromboemboli and after the initial 6–12 week period of anticoagulation which is recommended, long-term anticoagulation is not required unless other indications exist. The technical aspects of insertion of the valve are similar to those mentioned for the Hancock prosthesis and the manufacturer's instructions must be followed with care. The risk of looping a suture round a supporting prong has been reduced by provision of an integral valve holder with an easily removed suture linking the tips of the prongs. The Carpentier-Edwards valve should not be used in children under the age of 15 or in patients on chronic renal dialysis. Long term integrity and function remain uncertain, as with all bioprosthetic valves.

4a

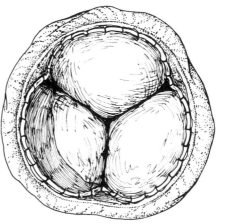

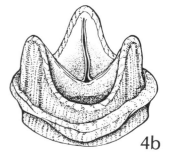

4b

5

Ionescu-Shiley valve

The Ionescu-Shiley valve is a bioprosthetic valve consisting of three leaflets of bovine pericardium attached to a symmetrical titanium support covered with Dacron fabric. Purified glutaraldehyde is used for treatment of the pericardium. The valve resembles the natural aortic valve and has been in use since 1971

Haemodynamic function is probably superior to that of glutaraldehyde-prepared porcine aortic valves and is comparable to that of most mechanical prostheses. Haemodynamic performance in the smaller sizes is significantly better than for similar-sized porcine bioprostheses. The Ionescu-Shiley valve is therefore suitable for use in the small aortic root or in a small mitral annulus. The valve is relatively free from thromboembolic complications, enabling it to be used without long-term anticoagulation. Long term integrity and function, however, remain uncertain, as with other bioprosthetic valves[16,17].

Valve preparation should follow the manufacturer's instructions to remove excess glutaraldehyde from the tissues. Care must be taken to avoid drying of the valve and injury to the leaflet tissue, which is more vulnerable than in the porcine valves. It is particularly easy to damage leaflet tissue with a continuous suture technique, and care is required to avoid this. The hazard of looping a suture round a prong with this valve is similar to that with other bioprosthetic valves, and great care is required with suture techniques during valve insertion. The length of the prongs does increase the risk of impingement on left ventricular muscle with mitral valve prostheses and makes aortic prosthesis insertion a little difficult. A new 'low-profile' model with shorter prongs is under evaluation.

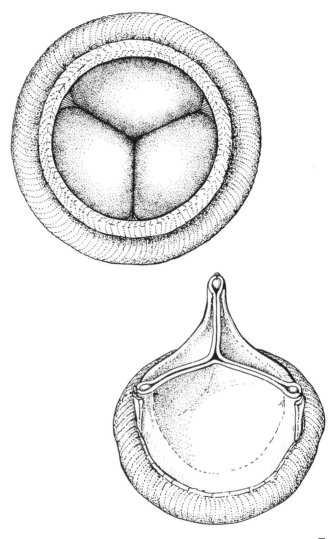

5

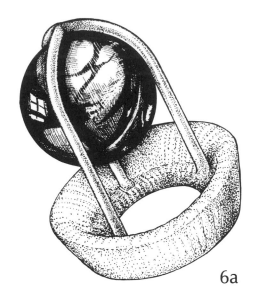

6a

Mechanical valves

6

Starr-Edwards valve

The Starr-Edwards valve consists of a circular valve seat with a surrounding sewing collar and a cage to restrain a ball occluder, originally made of chrome steel (*a*). There have been many modifications of design in an attempt to reduce complications and improve haemodynamic performance. However, the Model 1260 aortic prosthesis (*b*), introduced in 1968, and Model 6120 mitral prosthesis (*c*), introduced in 1965, which have a silicone rubber ball occluder and an uncovered, polished stellite alloy cage, have given good long-term results and probably represent the best choice in this type of valve. Haemodynamic performance is satisfactory although, as with most prostheses, the smaller prostheses are relatively obstructive. The cage may impinge on the walls of a small left ventricle and, in these circumstances, this valve may be unsatisfactory. With a small aortic root the cage may produce obstruction requiring the use of a corrective enlarging patch in the aortic root. There is a risk of thromboembolism, as with all mechanical valves, and long-term anticoagulation is required. Long-term durability is well-established for the Starr-Edwards valve[18].

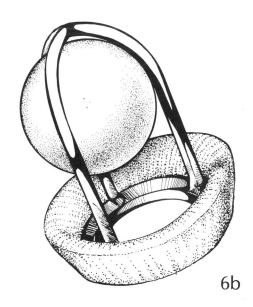

6b

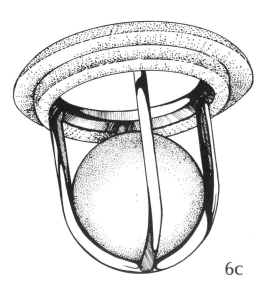

6c

7

Smeloff-Cutter prothesis

The Smeloff-Cutter prosthesis, introduced in 1964, is a caged ball prosthesis with a silicone rubber ball occluder and a titanium retaining cage on each side of the valve seat. The valve has given satisfactory clinical results and, as with other prostheses, requires long-term anticoagulation[19].

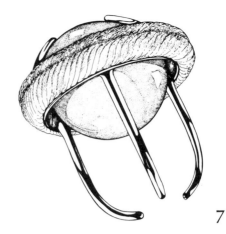

7

8

Bjork-Shiley valve

The Bjork-Shiley prosthesis was introduced in 1968. It consists of a circular valve seat and a pyrolytic carbon disc which is restrained by two struts. Recently the valve has been slightly modified by making the disc convex-concave and this has given wider opening and better flow characteristics. The haemodynamic performance of the valve is good and the transvalve pressure gradient is insignificant in the aortic position; for the mitral position the function appears similar to other tilting disc prostheses[2]. Good long-term clinical performance is reported[20,21]. Thromboembolism is a risk with this valve, as with other mechanical valves, and it requires long-term anticoagulation. There is a small risk of thrombus building up on the valve and interfering with valve function. Any patient who appears to develop heart failure suddenly with a Bjork-Shiley valve should be suspected of this complication. The valve is usually readily audible and loss of valve sounds is an indication of valve thrombosis. A radio-opaque marker in the disc enables its movement to be readily confirmed on screening.

The major technical problem in insertion is the avoidance of impingement of the disc on surrounding tissue or prolapse of excessive tissue into the valve orifice interfering with disc closure. Thus all excess chordae should be trimmed from the mitral annulus and valve orientation should take account of tissue impingement on the disc. Once seated, the free opening of the disc should be confirmed. The valve can be reorientated once inserted by use of the valve holder. Grasping of the disc occluder with surgical instruments should be avoided.

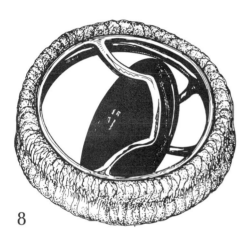

8

9

Omniscience valve

The Omniscience valve is a tilting disc prosthesis with a pyrolytic carbon occluder in a titanium housing. Haemodynamic performance is satisfactory and the risk of thromboembolism requires the use of long-term anti-coagulation. Techniques of insertion are similar to those for the Bjork-Shiley prosthesis[2].

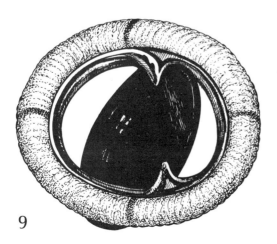

9

10

Lillehei-Kaster valve

This is a tilting disc prosthesis with a pyrolytic carbon occluder, giving good haemodynamic performance but still carrying the risk of thromboembolism and having the need for long-term anticoagulation.

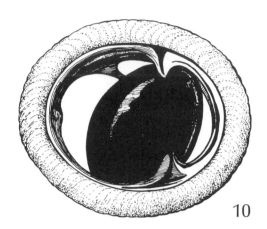

10

11

Hall-Kaster (Medtronic Hall) valve

This prosthesis has a pyrolytic carbon disc occluder in a titanium valve housing. The disc is restrained by sliding along a central bar. The valve has been used since 1977 and good haemodynamic and clinical results are reported. Long-term anticoagulation is required for the reduction of thromboembolism risk.

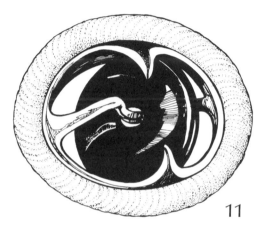

11

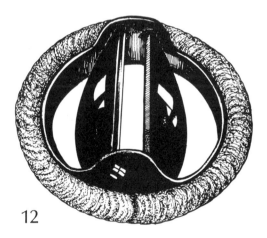

12

12

St Jude Medical valve

The St Jude Medical prosthesis consists of a circular orifice with two pyrolytic carbon leaflets which open to give central flow. The haemodynamic performance of this valve is good, and satisfactory clinical performance has been reported [22,23]. Long-term anticoagulation is required with this valve. During insertion care must be taken to avoid handling the leaflets. The valve has given good results in the small aortic root.

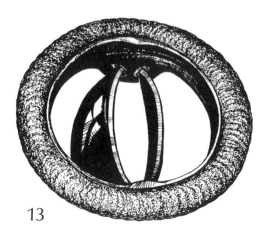

13

13

Duromedics (Hemex) prosthesis

The Duromedics prosthesis is a recently introduced pyrolytic carbon bileaflet valve which has good flow characteristics but long-term clinical experience is lacking at present.

General considerations in choice of valve prosthesis

The number of valve prostheses currently available indicates the lack of obvious superiority of any one type. Individual surgical practice varies considerably and greater experience must be awaited before further guidelines can be given.

The surgeon is confronted with the problem of using either established valves with known long-term performance or the newest prostheses to become available, which may offer significant improvements but which may have as yet unrecognized hazards. Surgeons undertaking valve replacement should maintain familiarity with current literature relating to late results of valve replacement, and when newer types of valves are used careful follow-up and early reporting of any undue incidence of complications are required.

In general, the biological valves that have been described offer satisfactory haemodynamic performance and reasonable freedom from thromboembolism, although the mitral prostheses in patients with atrial fibrillation or left atrial enlargement probably require long-term anticoagulation. Uncertainty regarding long-term durability is the chief drawback to these valves, and it must be assumed that there will be an increasing number of valve failures with them. For this reason many surgeons have advocated the use of biological valves in those patients whose natural life expectancy is anticipated to be less than the likely period of valve function. For women of childbearing age most surgeons advocate the use of a biological valve to avoid the problems of thromboembolism and anticoagulation with pregnancy. Those patients in whom anticoagulation is impractical or specifically contraindicated should have a biological valve. Biological valves should be avoided in children. When a biological valve is inserted in a young adult it must be assumed that valve replacement will be a possibility in the future, and this should be explained to the patient.

The particular types of valve prosthesis illustrated indicate examples of the range available at present, but there are other types, and technical improvements are continuing. Further experience and developments must be awaited before the goal of a truly durable valve, devoid of the complications of thromboembolism, is achieved.

References

1. Carpentier, A., Dubost, C., Lane, E., *et al.* Continuing improvements in valvular bioprostheses. Journal of Thoracic and Cardiovascular Surgery 1982; 83: 27–42

2. Scotten, L. N., Racca, R. G., Nugent, A. H., Walker, D. K., Brownlee, R. T. New tilting disc cardiac valve prostheses: *In vitro* comparison of their hydrodynamic performance in the mitral position. Journal of Thoracic and Cardiovascular Surgery 1981; 82: 136–146

3. Bonchek, L. I. Current status of cardiac valve replacement: selection of a prosthesis and indications for operation. American Heart Journal 1981; 101: 96–106

4. Ross, D. N. Homograft replacement of the aortic valve. Lancet 1962; 2: 487

5. Barratt-Boyes, B. G., Lowe, J. B., Cole, D. S., Kelly, D. T. Homograft replacement for aortic valve disease. Thorax 1965; 20: 495–504

6. Thompson, R., Yacoub, M., Ahmed, M., Somerville, W., Towers, M. The use of 'fresh' unstented homograft valves for replacement of the aortic valve analysis of 8 years experience. Journal of Thoracic and Cardiovascular Surgery 1980; 79: 896–903

7. Borkon, A. M., McIntosh, C. L., Jones, M., Lipson, L. C., Kent, K. M., Morrow, A. G. Haemodynamic function of the Hancock standard orifice aortic valve bioprosthesis. Journal of Thoracic and Cardiovascular Surgery 1981; 82: 601–607

8. Rossiter, S. J., Miller, D. C., Stinson, E. B. *et al.* Haemodynamic and clinical comparison of the Hancock modified orifice and standard orifice bioprosthesis in the aortic position. Journal of Thoracic and Cardiovascular Surgery 1980; 80: 54–60

9. Oyer, P. E., Stinson, E. D., Reitz, B. A., Miller, D. C., Rossiter, S. J., Shumway, N. E. Long-term evaluation of the porcine xenograft bioprosthesis. Journal of Thoracic and Cardiovascular Surgery 1979; 78: 343–350

10. Fleming, H. A., Bailey, S. M. Mitral valve disease, systemic embolism and anticoagulants. Postgraduate Medical Journal 1971; 47: 599–604

11. Jamieson, W. R. E., Janusz, M. T., Miyagishima, R. T. *et al.* Embolic complications of porcine heterograft cardiac valves. Journal of Thoracic and Cardiovascular Surgery 1981; 81: 626–631

12. Curcio, C. A., Commerford, P. J., Rose, A. G., Stevens, J. E., Barnard, M. S. Calcification of glutaraldehyde-preserved porcine xenografts in young patients. Journal of Thoracic and Cardiovascular Surgery 1981; 81: 621–625

13. Geha, A. S., Laks, H., Stansel, H. C. *et al.* Late failure of porcine valve heterografts in children. Journal of Thoracic and Cardiovascular Surgery 1979; 78: 351–364

14. Oyer, P. E., Miller, D. C., Stinson, E. B., Reitz, B. A., Moreno-Cabral, R. J., Shumway, N. E. Clinical durability of the Hancock porcine bioprosthetic valve. Journal of Thoracic and Cardiovascular Surgery 1980; 80: 824–833

15. Levine, F. H., Carter, J. E., Buckley, M. J., Daggett, W. M., Akins, C. W., Austen, W. G. Haemodynamic evaluation of Hancock and Carpentier-Edwards bioprostheses. Circulation 1981; 64 (Suppl. II): 192–195

16. Becker, R. M., Strom, J., Frishman, W. *et al.* Haemodynamic performance of the Ionescu-Shiley valve prosthesis. Journal of Thoracic and Cardiovascular Surgery 1980; 80: 613–620

17. Becker, R. M., Sandor, L., Tindel, M., Frater, R. W. Medium-term follow-up of the Ionescu-Shiley heterograft valve. Annals of Thoracic Surgery 1981; 32: 120–126

18. Macmanus, Q., Grunkemeier, G. L., Lambert, L. E., Teply, J. F., Harlan, B. J., Starr, A. Year of operation as a risk factor in the late results of valve replacement. Journal of Thoracic and Cardiovascular Surgery 1980; 80: 834–841

19. Starr, D. S., Lawrie, G. M., Howell, J. F., Morris, G. C. Clinical experience with the Smeloff-Cutter prosthesis: 1 to 12 year follow-up. Annals of Thoracic Surgery 1980; 30: 448–454

20. Bjork, V. O., Henze, A. Ten years' experience with the Bjork-Shiley tilting disc valve. Journal of Thoracic and Cardiovascular Surgery 1979; 78: 331–342

21. Karp, R. B., Cyrus, R. J., Blackstone, E. H., Kirklin, J. W., Kouchoukos, N. T., Pacifico, A. D. The Bjork-Shiley valve. Intermediate-term follow-up. Journal of Thoracic and Cardiovascular Surgery 1981; 81: 602–614

22. Nicoloff, D. M., Emery, R. W., Arom, K. V. *et al*. Clinical and haemodynamic results with the St Jude Medical cardiac valve prosthesis: a three year experience. Journal of Thoracic and Cardiovascular Surgery 1981; 82: 674–683

23. Horstkotte, D., Haerten, K., Herzer, J. A., Serpel, L., Bircks, W., Loogen, F. Preliminary results in mitral valve replacement with the St Jude Medical prosthesis: comparison with the Bjork-Shiley valve. Circulation 1981; 64 (Suppl. II): 203–209

Mitral valve replacement

Magdi H. Yacoub, FRCS, DSc (Hon)
Consultant Cardiac Surgeon, Harefield Hospital, Harefield, Middlesex;
National Heart Hospital, London, UK

Preoperative

Indications

Mitral valve replacement is indicated in patients with severe symptomatic mitral valve disease, in whom valve conserving procedures are judged not to be feasible. With increasing experience in applying restorative operations for the treatment of mitral stenosis and/or regurgitation, the number of patients requiring replacement should constitute approximately 20–30 per cent of all patients undergoing operations on the mitral valve. The choice of a valve substitute depends on the experience of the surgeon and needs of the patient. Currently, there is no agreement as to what constitutes the best available mitral valve substitute.

Prosthetic valves offer the advantages of ready availability and, in general, very good durability, however, they all require long-term anti-coagulation. In contrast, tissue valves do not require anti-coagulation, but almost invariably will require re-replacement at periods varying from 7 to 15 years. The choice of a valve substitute in children is of crucial importance, as it should allow for growth, preferably avoiding anti-coagulation and the need for relatively frequent valve replacement. In this age group, every attempt should be made to repair the valve, accepting less than perfect results. Unlike homograft valves, xenografts have been shown to degenerate very rapidly in children.

Except when 'unstented' homografts are used, the operative technique of mitral valve replacement is very much the same, regardless of the type of valve selected. This is because all these valves have a cloth margin which can be sutured to the mitral annulus.

The operation

A median sternotomy is used. All four chambers are inspected and pressures recorded. A cannula is inserted into the ascending aorta for arterial return. The superior and inferior venae cavae are separately cannulated through the right atrial wall. To facilitated retraction, the lateral aspect of the superior vena cava and the posterior aspect of the inferior vena cava are separated from the pericardium.

1

Left atrial incision

The ascending aorta is clamped and the left atrium opened by an incision which starts in the right upper pulmonary vein immediately behind the interatrial groove and extends upwards towards the roof of the left atrium and downwards into the oblique sinus. This lies behind the pericardial reflection, close the interatrial groove, thus avoiding the thin-walled inferior pulmonary vein.

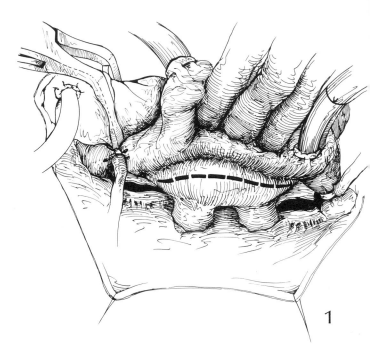

Inspection of the left atrium and mitral valve

2

Firm retraction of the anterior wall of the incision enables thorough inspection of the left atrium and mitral valve. Any clots are removed.

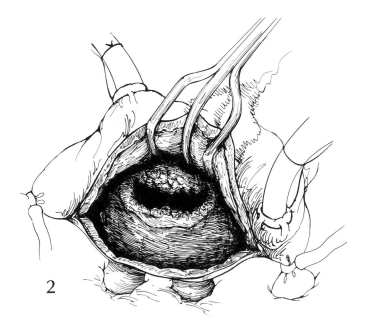

3

In patients with a massive clot, a plane of cleavage is developed between the organized clot and left atrial wall. This enables complete decortication of the left atrium. The mitral valve is carefully inspected, and the suitability for repair is considered.

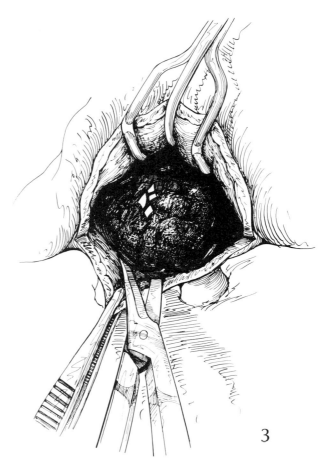

3

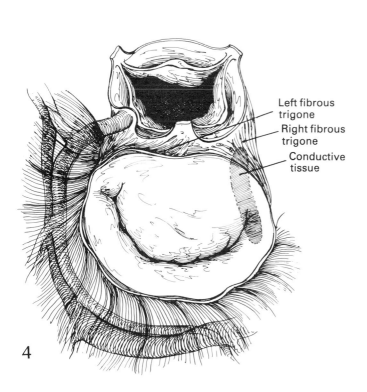

Left fibrous trigone

Right fibrous trigone

Conductive tissue

4

4

Surgical anatomy of the mitral valve

A thorough knowledge of the exact relationship between the mitral annulus and the surrounding structures is of extreme importance. These structures include the conducting tissue, the right and left fibrous trigones, the aortic valve and subaortic curtain, circumflex coronary artery, and the coronary sinus.

Excision of the mitral valve

5

The mitral valve is brought into view by pulling on the posterior cusp, using a Vulsalum forceps. Excision is started by incising the anterior cusp 2 mm distal to its junction with the left atrial wall, which is generally well-defined.

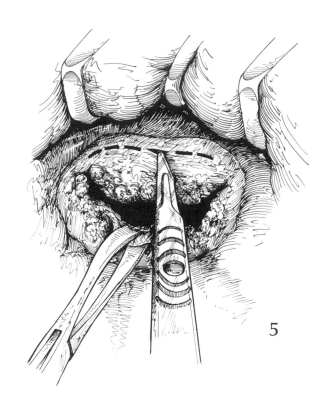

6

The incision is extended in both direction around the area of the commissures, using a pair of scissors.

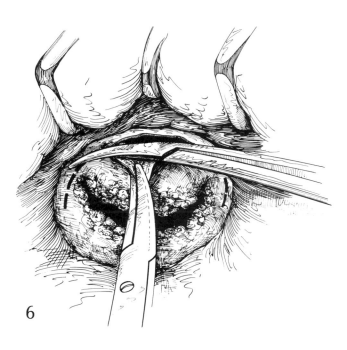

7

Traction on the cut edge of the anterior cusp brings the attachment of the papillary muscles into view. Both papillary muscles are then divided near their bases, taking care not to include parts of the surrounding free left ventricular wall.

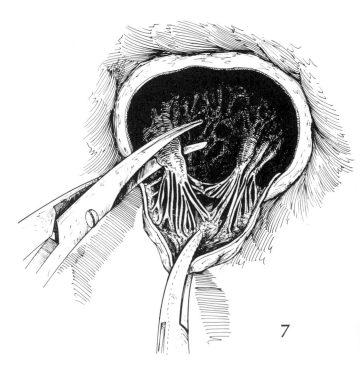

8

Further traction on the valve brings the ventricular aspect of the junction between the posterior cusp and myocardium into view. This aspect is always well-defined and easy to identify, in contrast to the junction between the atrial aspect of the posterior cusp and the atrial wall which is often obscured by calcium deposition.

Excision of the mitral valve is completed by dividing the remaining attachments of the posterior cusp.

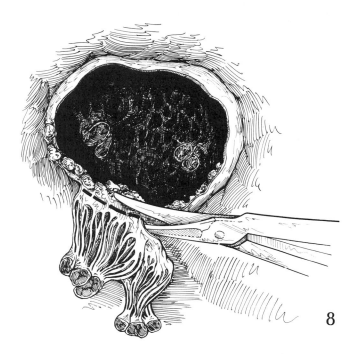

8

9

Any remnants of calcification of the mitral annulus are carefully removed, taking care not to detach the fibrous annulus and atrial wall from the ventricular myocardium. Postoperative rupture of this junction constitutes a very serious complication.

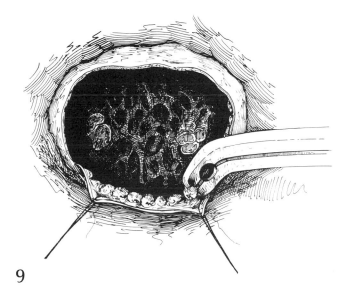

9

10

The insertion of valve sutures is achieved with a series of multiple interrupted 'figure of 8' 2/0 synthetic sutures, starting from the mid-point of the posterior cusp and proceeding in a counter-clockwise direction.

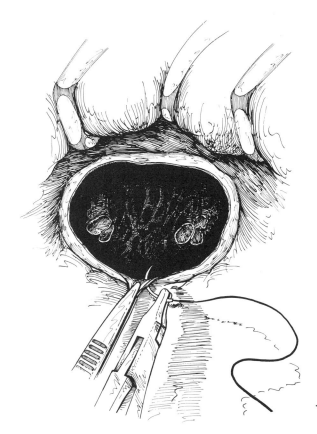

10

11a, b & c

Valve orientation

This is not important if a ball valve is used. If a mounted tissue valve is used, the location of the struts should be away from the left ventricular outflow tract (LVOT) (*a & b*). If a Bjork-Shiley prosthesis is used, the major orifice should face the posterior ventricular wall (*c*).

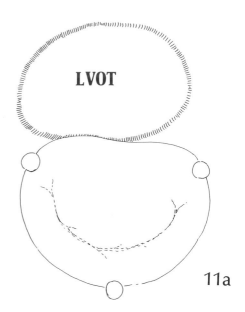

11a

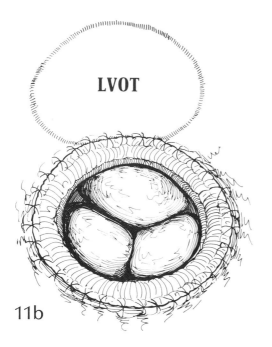

11b

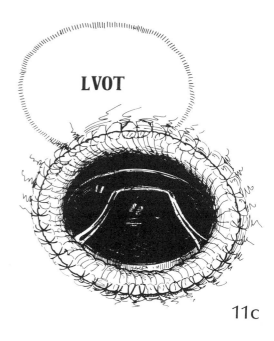

11c

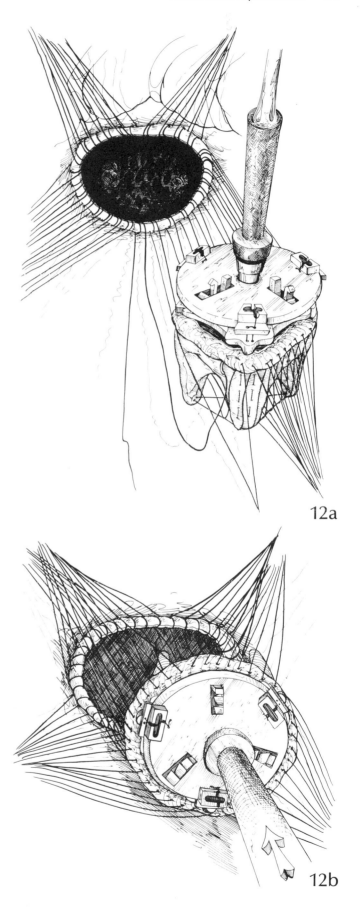

12a

12b

Positioning of bioprosthetic valve

12a & b

When a bioprosthetic valve is inserted using interrupted sutures, extreme care should be taken to avoid one of the prongs catching on a suture. Most valves have temporary sutures between the tips of the three prongs to avoid this complication. Repeated inspection of the prongs is essential to avoid damage to one of the cusps.

13

The appearance of the seated valve after tying and cutting the sutures is shown.

If a homograft valve is to be used, the technique of insertion is somewhat different. Homografts are obtained from routine post-mortem material, sterilized by antibiotics, and stored in tissue culture medium. The largest available aortic homograft (2.4–3 cm in diameter) is selected.

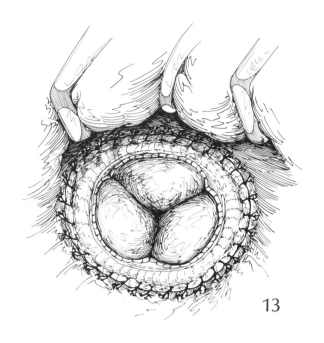

13

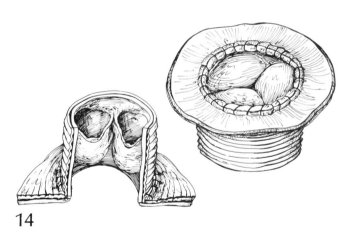

14

14

The graft is trimmed in a circular fashion 1 mm above the top of the commissures at one end and 1 mm below the lowest point of the attachment of the cusps at the other. The coronary ostia are sutured and the valve fixed inside a segment of woven dacron tube (35 mm in diameter, measuring about 4 cm in length, which has a collar of 2-way stretch dacron previously sutured to it). The 'ventricular' end of the graft is sutured to the tube by a 5/0 taper-cut synthetic suture, taking care not to evert the attachment of the right coronary cusp. The dacron collar is then covered by autogenous pericardium. The width of the collar depends on the size of the left atrium and should be trimmed accordingly.

15

The first suture line consists of a series of interrupted everting mattress sutures (2/0 synthetic suture) placed in the mitral annulus with the loop on the atrial side of the remnants of the cusp. The sutures are then passed through the aortic wall of the homograft and the surrounding dacron tube.

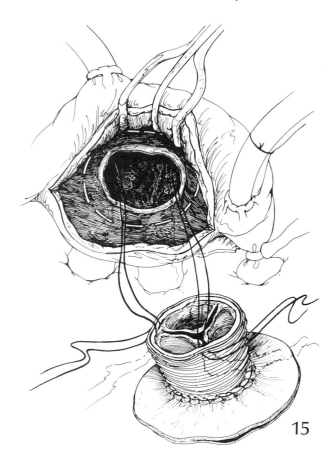

15

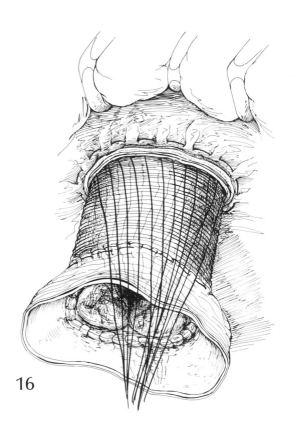

16

16

The valve is then lowered into the left atrium and the sutures are tied. The edge of the homograft is compressed between the everted mitral annulus and the dacron sleeve.

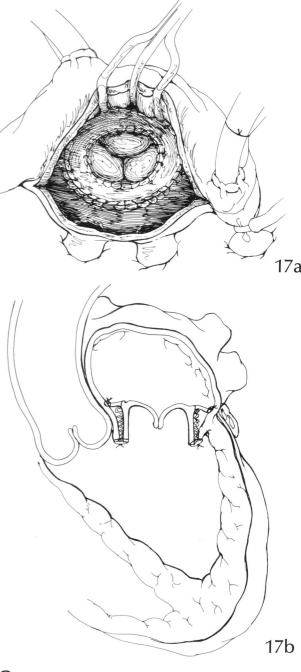

17a

17b

17

Special care is taken to ensure that there is no torsion between the upper and lower suture lines. The pericardial and dacron collars are fixed to the left atrial wall using continuous 3/0 sutures, starting at the ridge between the left pulmonary veins and the left atrial appendage, and progressing upwards to the roof of the left atrium onto the atrial septum in one direction and the posterior left atrial wall, towards the septum in the other. This suture line excludes from the circulation the knots of the first suture line, all prosthetic material, and the cavity of the left atrial appendage.

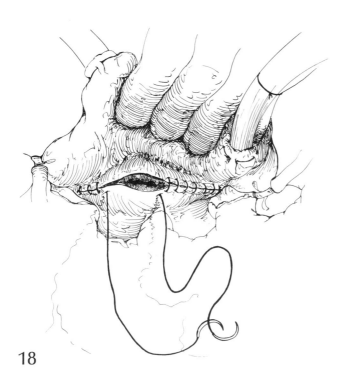

18

18

The left atrium is closed, using 3/0 sutures. During this period, the left ventricle is decompressed by suction through a left ventricular vent. Trapped air in the left side of the heart is removed, and the heart is defibrillated.

A 15 minute period of supportive bypass is utilized to ensure vigorous contraction of the heart with return of the ST segment to the prebypass configuration. This period also serves to position the homograft cusps appropriately in relation to the dacron tube.

Bypass is then discontinued in routine fashion. Postoperative care is as outlined for other operations.

Hypertrophic subaortic stenosis

Andrew G. Morrow MD
acknowledged to be the world's authority on the surgical relief of this condition, died shortly after the completion of this chapter. This was his last work.

Introduction

Hypertrophic subaortic stenosis first emerged as a discrete disease entity in the early 1960s. Since that time it has been the subject of intense study, and a vast number of reports have appeared concerning its clinical, haemodynamic, electrocardiographic, pathological and echocardiographic features. An extensive bibliography detailing many of these studies carried out at the National Heart Institute is appended to a recent publication[1]. The disease has been described under a bewildering variety of names (more than 60 have appeared in the literature), but here the term idiopathic hypertrophic subaortic stenosis (IHSS) will be used.

The anatomical hallmark of IHSS is left ventricular hypertrophy, usually asymmetrical so that the interventricular septum is considerably thicker than the left ventricular free wall. In many patients the enlarged septum bulges so far into the basal portion of the left ventricular cavity that during systole it severely reduces the lumen of the left ventricular outflow tract. This change, in association with the typical systolic anterior motion of the mitral leaflet, causes apposition of the septum and mitral leaflet, which leads to obstruction of left ventricular outflow. The presence of obstruction can easily be detected by echocardiography and its severity accurately determined at left heart catheterization. The operation to be described was designed to relieve outflow obstruction in IHSS and is almost always effective. Thus, it is often indicated in the severely symptomatic patient with obstruction in whom pharmacological treatment has proved ineffective.

Preoperative

The usual indications for operation

Since 1960, 1312 patients with IHSS have been examined and treated at the National Heart Institute. (This number does not include additional individuals with the disease who were seen only in the course of family surveys.) Operation has been carried out in 342 (26 per cent) of these 1312 patients. These statistics emphasize the fact that operation is necessary in a relatively small proportion of patients with IHSS.

The patient with IHSS is usually referred to the surgeon because he has been shown to have severe outflow obstruction and has remained symptomatic in spite of optimal pharmacological therapy. Symptoms in IHSS are similar to those associated with the discrete forms of aortic stenosis: dizziness, syncope, angina pectoris, dyspnoea, heart failure and arrhythmias. Virtually every patient I see has been treated for a prolonged period with propranolol, and, in recent years, a large number have had therapeutic trials with verapamil as well. A peak systolic gradient within the left ventricle of 50 mmHg or more, either under resting conditions or following provocative interventions, must be shown at left heart catheterization; the gradient is usually much larger. In all operative candidates the interventricular septum is thickened, and the ratio of the thickness of the septum to that of the posterior free wall of the ventricle is usually 1.3 or greater (asymmetric septal hypertrophy; ASH). I am reluctant to operate upon a patient in whom M-mode or two-dimensional echocardiography indicates that the septum is less than 14 or 15 mm thick; in most patients it is more than 20 mm thick.

Thus, the usual patient with IHSS who comes to operation is (1) severely symptomatic; (2) has not improved with optimal pharmacological treatment; (3) has asymmetrical septal hypertrophy; (4) has severe left ventricular outflow obstruction at rest or with provocative interventions; and (5) has no intercurrent disease which makes the risk of operation unacceptable.

Some special indications for operation

Prior cardiac arrest

I have resected the interventricular septum in 14 patients who had IHSS and severe obstruction and who also had had documented ventricular fibrillation from which they were successfully resuscitated. In 3 of the patients the diagnosis of IHSS was first made after sudden death; 7 of the 14 patients were asymptomatic. Eleven patients are still living 1½ to 7½ years after operation. One patient died in the perioperative period of obscure causes (not arrhythmia) and 2 others have died later, one of arrhythmia and the other following aortic valve replacement. All patients have been treated with antiarrhythmic drugs postoperatively.

There is no proof that relief of obstruction and lowering of left ventricular systolic pressure in patients with IHSS and severe obstruction will offer protection against subsequent sudden death. On the other hand, it is difficult to conceive that relief of obstruction will *increase* the risk of death from arrhythmia. Only continued follow-up of these and other patients will permit a definitive conclusion as to the role of operation in the management of this subgroup of patients.

IHSS and Valvular Disease

In any large group of patients with IHSS some will be found to have significant associated mitral or aortic valve disease which must also be treated; but first it must be appreciated that mitral regurgitation, mild to severe, is present in about 75 per cent of patients with IHSS who are operated upon. In these patients the mitral valve is structurally normal except for some thickening, and immediately after resection of the septum it becomes competent – a sequence confirmed many times by palpation of the valve before and after myectomy. Rarely, however, regurgitation may result from intrinsic valve disease and mitral valve replacement will be necessary. I have seen 3 such patients: in one there were numerous ruptured chordae tendineae and in the others the valves seemed congenitally deformed. In each, the mitral valve was replaced after resection of the septum. I have not seen a patient with IHSS and mitral stenosis. Two patients had valvular aortic stenosis in addition to IHSS. In each the valve was amenable to commissurotomy and debridement, and afterward the valve could be retracted to provide adequate exposure of the septum. Four patients have had IHSS and aortic regurgitation, in 2 of whom the

valve had been damaged by infective endocarditis. All 4 patients had aortic valve replacement after septal resection; all are living and have good symptomatic and haemodynamic improvement.

IHSS and Coronary Artery Obstruction

Early in the operative experience it was considered that patients with IHSS seldom had severe coronary atherosclerosis. In fact, some physicians held the opinion that by an obscure mechanism the presence of IHSS afforded protection against the development of coronary artery disease. This belief has been proved false, principally because coronary arteriography is now carried out in the course of preoperative study in most patients. If coronary arteriograms reveal obstructive disease of the type and severity usually indicating the need for coronary artery bypass, *and* if angina pectoris is a prominent symptom, bypass grafts are constructed at the time of operation. The septal myotomy/myectomy is carried out first, the aorta is closed and appropriate grafts are then placed. The incision in the aorta does not interfere significantly with the aorta-to-vein anastomoses. This combined operation has been utilized in 9 patients.

Preoperative preparation

Most patients operated upon for IHSS are receiving propranolol. It is my practice to continue this drug in the required dose until 48h before operation. The dose is then gradually reduced to about 20mg four times daily, and the drug is given in this amount until 8h before operation. In patients in chronic atrial fibrillation, digoxin is continued until 24h before operation. Prophylactic antibiotics are administered, beginning 12h preoperatively.

Anaesthesia

An intravenous infusion of phenylephrine is always prepared before the induction of anaesthesia and is readily available to treat hypotension; pressor agents with significant positive inotropic actions are specifically contraindicated in patients with IHSS. Anaesthesia is induced with morphine (0.5mg/kg) and sodium thiopental. For tracheal intubation, succinylcholine is administered. Anaesthesia is maintained with nitrous oxide, oxygen, and either halothane or enflurane. During maintenance, relaxation is effected by an infusion of succinylcholine or small intermittent doses of pancuronium. Experience has shown that *d*-tubocurarine is to be avoided in patients with IHSS. The histamine release and ganglionic blockage which it causes will almost invariably result in significant hypotension. Also, a large dose of pancuronium, given as a bolus injection will cause undesirable tachycardia and hypotension.

The operation

1

A median sternotomy is employed. A single venous cannula (40 Fr) is introduced from the right atrium into the mouth of the inferior vena cava. I prefer femoral arterial cannulation for arterial return. A drainage cannula is passed into the left ventricle through an apical stab wound. The coronary perfusion lines originate from the arterial return line distal to the arterial pump. A 'Y' in the left ventricular drainage line permits the return to enter the pump-oxygenator (clamp position A) or to be discarded (clamp position B).

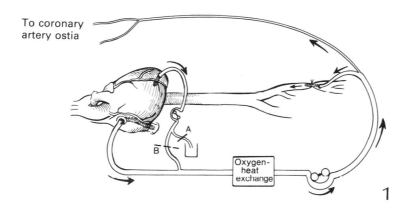

2

The heart and great vessels are exposed in preparation for left ventriculomyotomy and myectomy. The pericardium is opened widely as is the left pleural space. The apical left ventricular drainage catheter passes through a stab wound in the chest wall, and this site is after used for the introduction of an intrapleural drainage tube. The site of the incision to be made in the ascending aorta is indicated by the broken line.

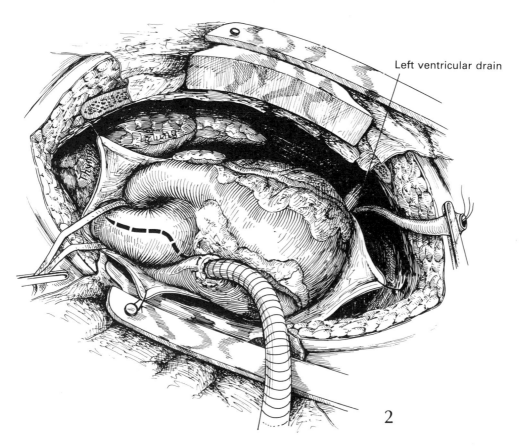

3

After the institution of cardiopulmonary bypass, general body hypothermia is induced (25–30°C), and the aorta is clamped and opened. The heart is allowed to go into flaccid arrest. I do not employ chemical cardioplegia. The aortic incision is carried down to within 1–2mm of the aortic valve ring in the centre of the non-coronary sinus of Valsalva. The aortic valve leaflets may be diffusely thickened but are otherwise normal. The hypertrophied interventricular septum can be seen and felt to protrude well to the right of the anterior descending coronary artery when the heart is decompressed.

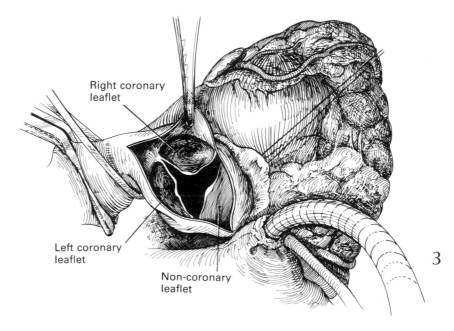

Right coronary leaflet

Left coronary leaflet

Non-coronary leaflet

3

4

The thickness of the interventricular septum determines the depth of the resection. The thickness will have been measured preoperatively by M-mode and/or sector scan echocardiography, but it should also be estimated at operation by bimanual palpation. As illustrated the mass of muscle is grasped between the two index fingers, the left in the ventricular cavity and the right on the exterior surface of the septum over the left anterior descending coronary artery.

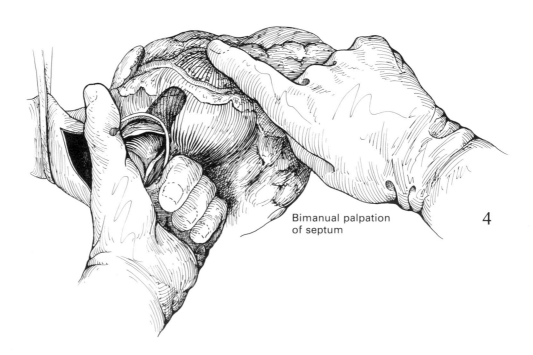

Bimanual palpation of septum

4

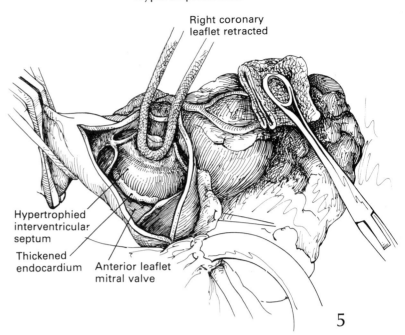

Right coronary
leaflet retracted

Hypertrophied
interventricular
septum

Thickened
endocardium

Anterior leaflet
mitral valve

5

5

Exposure in the flaccid heart is facilitated by upward traction on the right coronary valve leaflet with a cloth-covered wire retractor and is improved by counter-pressure on the external left ventricular wall, applied via a stick sponge by the second assistant (at the surgeon's right). Posteriorly the anterior mitral leaflet is visible; it is usually thickened and opaque. Opposite the mitral valve the most prominent part of the bulging septum is covered with thick, opaque, white endocardium, where it is contacted by the anterior mitral leaflet during systole; this is the site of outflow obstruction.

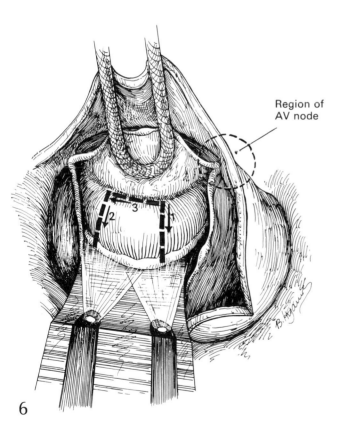

Region of
AV node

6

6

A lighted ribbon retractor is passed through the valve ring to the apex of the ventricle where it displaces posteriorly and protects the mitral valve and papillary muscles. Retractors 18, 20 and 22 mm in width are available; 20 mm width is usually employed in the adult patient. The sites of the three incisions to be made in the septum are indicated. The first vertical incision is placed just to the right of the centre of the right coronary valve leaflet. The second vertical incision, is made 8–12 mm (depending upon the diameter of the aortic root) to the left of the first, nearly in the commissure between the right and left coronary leaflets of the valve. The third (transverse) incision is at the base of the right coronary leaflet (which must not be injured) and connects the two vertical ones. The membranous portion of the septum and the region of the atrioventricular (AV) node are well to the right of the first incision.

7

The first vertical myotomy is made. The angle of the knife handle prevents the surgeon's (right) hand from obstructing his view of the septum. (The operation would probably be easier for a left-handed surgeon). Care must be taken to direct the knife parallel to the long axis of the retractor, and not angle it to the right or left.

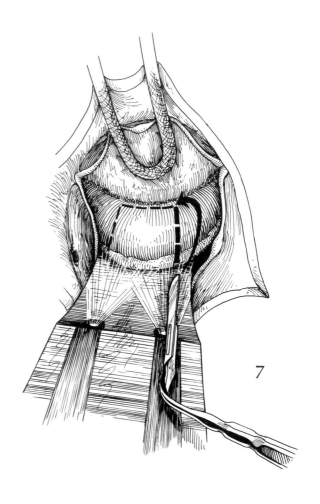

7

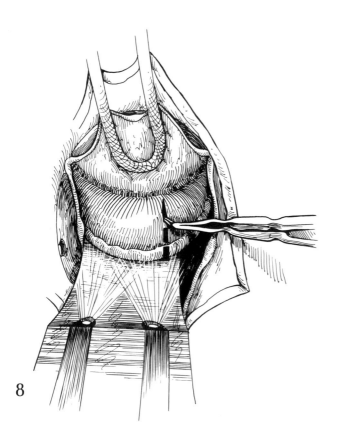

8

8

The vertical incisions must extend sufficiently far toward the apex to ensure that the final resection will be distal (apical) to the free margin of the anterior mitral leaflet. This will be the case if *all* of the No. 10 knife blade and 5–8 mm of the handle are inserted into the septum before the cut toward the retractor and the ventricular cavity is begun.

9a & b

The knife blade and handle are inserted into the hypertrophied septum until the tip of the knife is felt to contact the metal retractor distal (apical) to the most prominent portion of the bulging muscle mass; this must be done blindly. It is important that the knife blade be passed parallel to the plane of the flat of the retractor; the knife and handle must not angle downward toward the lumen or else the apical part of the incision will be shallower than the basal part. After the knife is through the bulging septum (b) it is withdrawn and the handle is raised simultaneously to direct the cutting edge through the muscle and against the retractor blade. The valve leaflets must not be injured as the knife is withdrawn from the aorta.

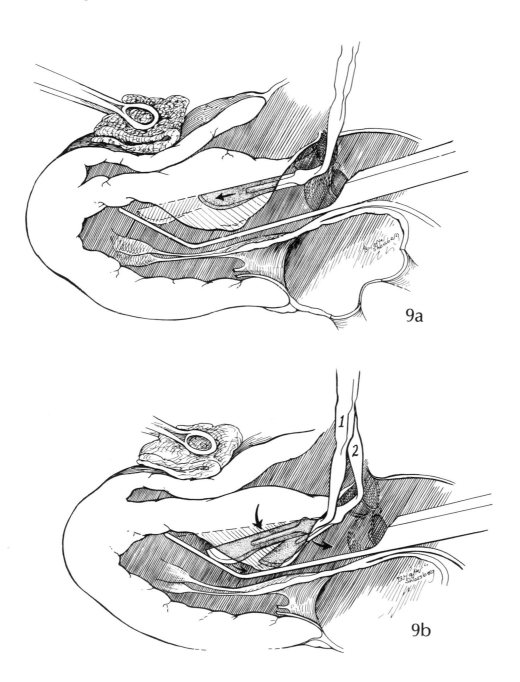

9a

9b

10

The second vertical myotomy is made in the same fashion as the first. As shown, this second incision will usually be quite close to the left edge of the retractor, and the knife blade must not slip off to the left and injure the adjacent mitral leaflet. Another knife (No. 10 blade) angled on the flat is used for the transverse incision which connects the vertical ones. The flat of the blade must be kept parallel to the flat of the retractor; the length of the incision is similar to that of the vertical ones and as previously the knife blade and 5–8 mm of the handle should be inserted into the septum before the cut is begun.

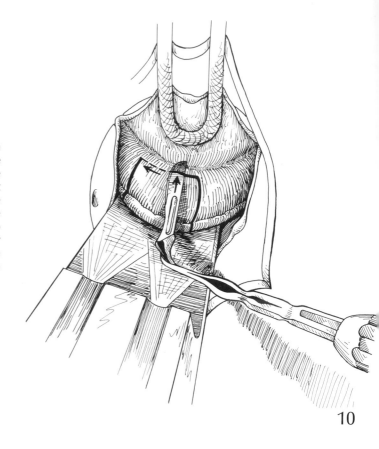

10

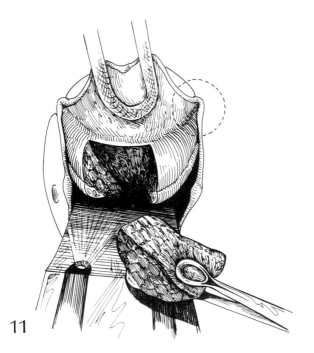

11

11

The crescent-shaped bar of muscle resected from the septum can usually be withdrawn intact from the ventricle (with a sponge forceps, to avoid fragmentation). Sometimes apical attachments remain. In this case the cloth-covered retractor is advanced into the ventricle and the attachments are divided with scissors under direct vision.

12

The endocardial scar on the right edge of the channel is grasped with a small pituitary rongeur, and the muscle is pulled downward and to the left. An additional slice or two of myocardium and scar is then excised from the margin of the resected area. Less frequently the same procedure is carried out on the left.

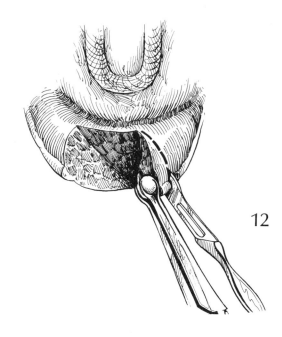

12

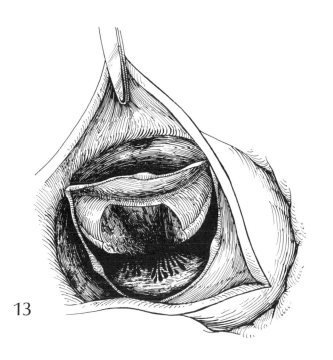

13

13

The final appearance of the new and non-obstructive left ventricular outflow tract created by myotomy and myectomy is shown. The rectangular channel in the septum is easily visualized postoperatively in the short axis view of a two-dimensional echocardiogram.

Both coronary arteries are cannulated and coronary perfusion with arterial blood is begun. The total period of myocardial ischaemia is about 15 min. The clamp on the left ventricular drainage cannula is moved from position A to position B (see *Illustration 1*) to discard the fluid. The left ventricle and aortic root are then irrigated with a large amount of saline solution to remove any particulate matter. Occasionally the heart resumes contractions with the institution of coronary perfusion. When this occurs it is of note that the edges of the channel in the septum *separate* during systole, making the channel largest during the ejection period.

14

The aortotomy is closed with a continuous everting mattress suture as the patient is warmed. Often the aorta is calcified in the aortic sinus, in which case it may be advisable to employ two or three interrupted mattress sutures (reinforced with Teflon pledgets) in the lowermost part of the incision. After the continuous suture is completed the aortic clamp is removed. As this is done the suture line is separated with fine forceps and air is evacuated from the aortic root.

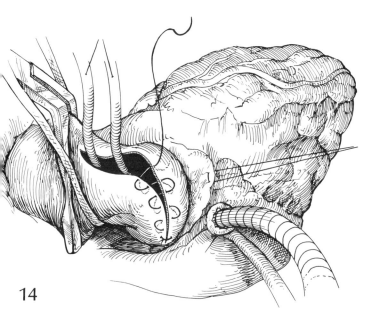

14

15

The everted edges of the aortic incision are approximated with an over-and-over suture.

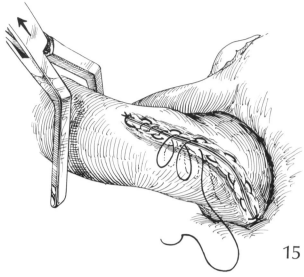

15

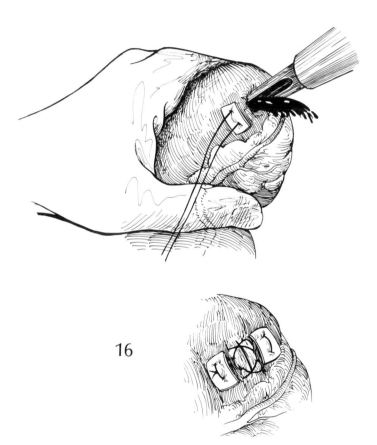

16

16

During closure of the aorta the heart is usually in ventricular fibrillation. When the patient's temperature is normal, the apex is elevated, the drain is removed and a grooved sound is passed in turn into the left atrium, left ventricle and aorta. The lungs are ventilated to expel air trapped in pulmonary veins. The apical stab wound is then repaired, the heart defibrillated and bypass is discontinued. A temporary pacing electrode is attached to the right ventricle. If a conduction abnormality was present before operation (e.g. right or left bundle-branch-block) or if complete heart block is evident at any time during the operation, a pair of permanent pacing electrodes is attached to the left ventricle with the ends placed in a subcutaneous pocket in the upper abdomen. One of the electrodes is used for temporary pacing with a lead extender. If permanent pacing later becomes necessary the pulse generator can be inserted into the pocket under local anaesthesia.

Postoperative care

Postoperative care is similar to that given to any patient operated upon for aortic stenosis. If pressor support is necessary in the early postoperative period dopamine is the agent most often employed. Transient atrial fibrillation occurs in half or more of patients, usually in the first day or two after operation. The compliance of the ventricle is reduced and the loss of atrial contraction may be poorly tolerated in which case, prompt electrical cardioversion is usually indicated. Digoxin and quinidine are administered to patients who have had atrial fibrillation and are continued for 6 weeks after the patient returns home.

Results

Two relatively recent publications have presented in some detail the results of operations for IHSS at the National Heart Institute[1, 2] and these data will only be summarized here. Immediate (perioperative) mortality in the total group of 342 patients is 9 per cent. In the first 198 patients (1960–1977) operative mortality was 9 per cent, while in the last 144 patients (1978 through 1981) it has been 8 per cent. I had assumed that with increasing numbers of operations mortality would decrease but this has not been the case. Deaths in the perioperative period have resulted from a variety of causes: technical misadventure, left ventricular failure, intractable arrhythmia and myocardial infarction have all occurred. Complete heart block can be avoided in most patients by confining the septal resection to that shown. However, complete left bundle-branch-block will be produced in about 85 per cent of all patients, and if right bundle-branch-block is present before operation it is likely that complete AV dissociation cannot be avoided. In several patients a ventricular septal defect was created at operation and recognized immediately when a systolic thrill was palpated over the right ventricle when bypass was terminated. In these patients the defect was closed immediately. In other patients ventricular septal defects apparently occurred several weeks after operation. In these the resection may have interrupted large intramyocardial coronary arteries, and the defect developed as a result of infarction and rupture of the septum. Several of these late-occurring defects were small, were associated with trivial left-to-right shunting and required no treatment. Three others were larger and were closed at second operations.

Almost all patients describe quite gratifying symptomatic improvement after operation and 6–12 months postoperatively are in functional classes I and II. Dizziness and syncope almost never occur after operation and an important increase in exercise tolerance is the rule. The most common residual symptom is precordial pain with exertion, most often described by patients more than 60 years of age.

Clinical improvement is paralleled by haemodynamic improvement, and in virtually all patients the intraventricular pressure gradient is shown to be absent or greatly reduced at the time of postoperative left heart catheterization. We have not recorded systematic changes in left ventricular end-diastolic pressure after operation.

A few final thoughts

It seems appropriate here to recall to the reader the surgical aphorism: 'It is generally undesirable to carry out a local operation in the treatment of a generalized disease.' IHSS is a primary disease of cardiac muscle, principally affecting the left ventricle and the interventricular septum. As a result, left ventricular compliance is more or less reduced, which may be the cause of symptoms. There is no evidence that any operation can increase ventricular compliance in a patient with IHSS. Also, symptoms may result from a discrepancy between the oxygen supply and the oxygen demand of the increased ventricular muscle mass, even when the coronary arteries are normal. But, operation can and does relieve obstruction to left ventricular outflow, and will abolish or ameliorate symptoms caused by obstruction. Operation cannot be expected to arrest progression of the basic cardiomyopathic process, and some patients may have excellent symptomatic improvement after operation only to develop symptoms again in later years as cardiomyopathy progresses. Nevertheless, nearly three-quarters of all patients operated upon, are now alive and have maintained symptomatic improvement during follow-up periods of more than 20 years. Continued application of the operation seems well warranted.

References

1. Morrow, A. G., Reitz, B. A., Epstein, S. E., *et al*. Operative treatment in hypertrophic subaortic stenosis: techniques, and the results of pre and postoperative assessment in 83 patients. Circulation 1975; 52: 88–102

2. Maron, B. J., Merrill, W. H., Freier, A. P., Kent, K. M., Epstein, S. E., Morrow, A. G. Long-term clinical course and symptomatic status of patients after operation for hypertrophic subaortic stenosis. Circulation 1978; 57: 1205–1213

Surgical treatment of aortic valve disease

Denton A. Cooley MD
Surgeon-in-Chief, Texas Heart Institute, Houston, Texas, USA

Introduction

Pathological lesions of the aortic valve may produce different physiological changes from either stenosis, regurgitation or a combination of the two. Aetiological factors are usually rheumatic valvular disease, congenital anomalies, cystic medial necrosis with annuloaortic ectasia and the occasional traumatic lesion. The surgeon's responsibility is to select the proper means of repair for the individual case[1, 2].

Valvuloplasty is seldom possible except in congenital aortic valve disease producing stenosis. Most patients undergoing valvular surgery for congenital stenosis are operated upon during the first 10 years of life, and often a desperately ill infant will require emergency surgery within the first or second week of life. For the most part, operation during these early years is confined to valvotomy (see Chapter on Congenital aortic stenosis, pp. 000–000).

For the vast majority of patients undergoing surgery for aortic valve disease, however, the aetiological factors are acquired and valve replacement indicated. In general, there are three situations which require replacement of the aortic valve.

Aortic regurgitation

The dilated annulus, often referred to as annuloaortic ectasia, is a common cause of 'pure' aortic regurgitation. Such patients often have other stigmata of Marfan's syndrome. The valve replacement usually involves the use of a composite valve fabric conduit placed in the aortic annulus. Direct anastomoses between the coronary orifices and the fabric graft are necessary.

Bacterial endocarditis may cause gross disruption of the valve with perforations or fragmentation. Rheumatic fibrosis and foreshortening of leaflets may also cause regurgitation, and when calcification is superimposed valve replacement is inevitable.

Aortic stenosis

Aortic stenosis may be due to a congenitally bicuspid valve with superimposed fibrosis and calcification. Rheumatic heart disease with valvulitis may also result in stenosis. Often this valve is small and volcano-shaped, with dense fibrosis and calcification. When calcification is present in acquired stenotic lesions valve replacement must be performed.

Combined aortic stenosis and regurgitation

These findings are usually a result of late fibrosis and calcification, predominantly following rheumatic valvular disease. The valve must be replaced in these cases.

The operation

Operation is performed through a median sternotomy approach to the heart. Temporary cardiopulmonary bypass is routine. Although a single large venous cannula may be used for isolated aortic valve replacement, when mitral valve lesions are present or coronary arteries are to be grafted both the superior and inferior venae cavae should be intubated for venous outflow. Arterial return of oxygenated blood from the oxygenator is usually made through a cannula placed through purse-string sutures in the distal ascending aorta. When a dissecting aneurysm is present cannulation of the iliac artery through a common femoral artery is preferred. A vent is necessary, and the preferred method is to vent with a sump catheter placed in the left atrium through an atriotomy placed close to the right superior pulmonary vein.

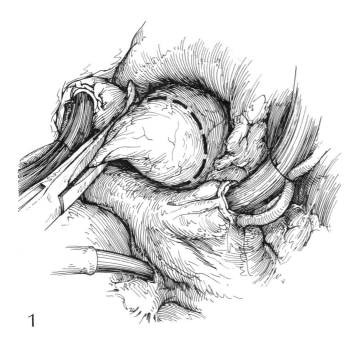

1

1

The aortotomy incision is made in an oblique transverse direction staying clear of the right coronary orifice.

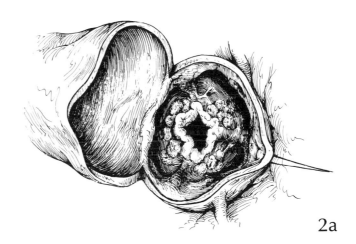

2a

2a & b

The valve is then exposed. This may reveal the typical calcified appearance of a tricuspid aortic valve (a) or the pattern of calcification on a congenitally bicuspid valve (b).

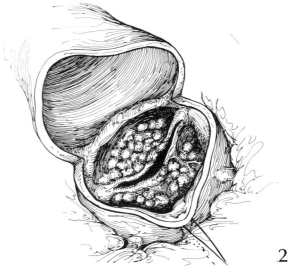

2b

3

The valve is excised, care being taken not to remove an excessive amount of annular tissue, which would prevent secure placement of the valve prosthesis.

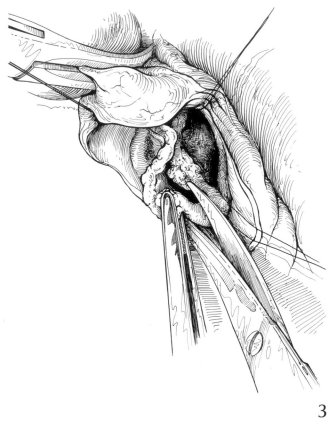

3

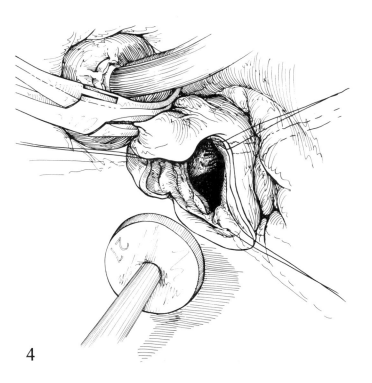

4

4

The appropriate prosthesis is then selected and the annulus sized. Both mechanical and bioprosthetic replacements may be used, the mechanical type being preferred for younger patients and bioprostheses for older ones. This preference is based primarily upon the known favourable durability of the currently available mechanical prostheses.

5

The prosthesis is sutured in place with 2/0 mattress sutures and polyester or Teflon felt pledgets. The pledgets should be placed above the aortic annulus rather than below. The Björk-Shiley prosthesis is illustrated.

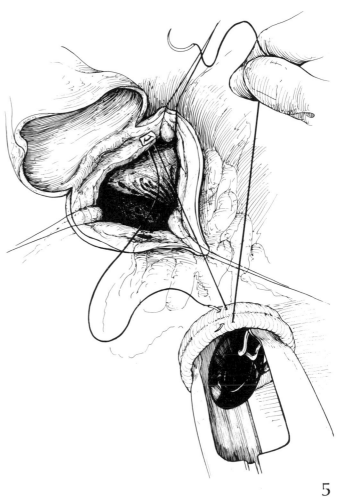

5

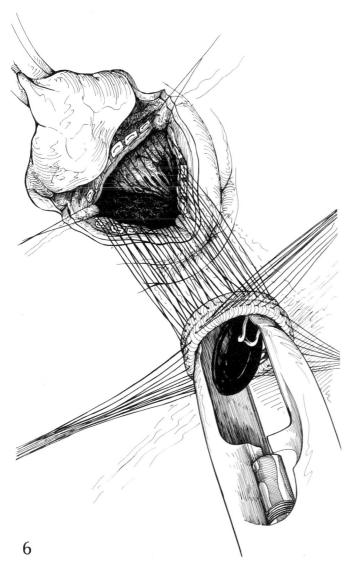

6

6

When all the sutures have been inserted, the valve is slid into place.

7

When the valve has been seated, the sutures are tied and cut.

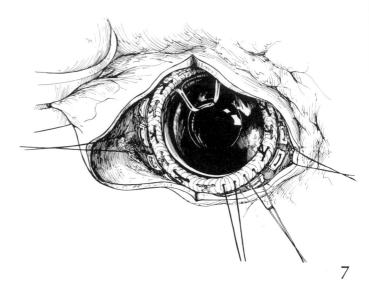

7

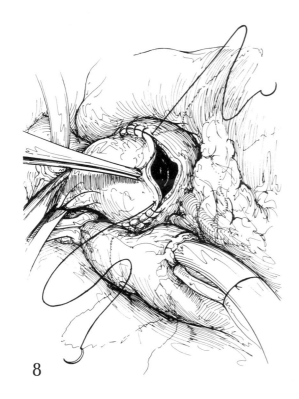

8

8

The aortotomy is closed with a continuous polypropylene monofilament suture.

9

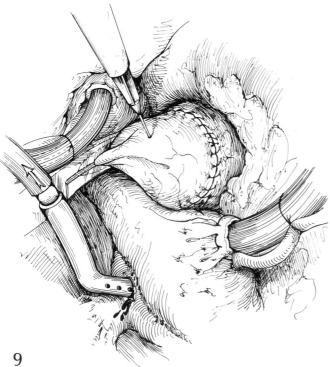

9

Air is aspirated from the ascending aorta and apex of the left ventricle. The sump in the left atrium is removed at the same time. At this point the clamp is removed from the ascending aorta and coronary circulation is restored. When cardiac action resumes the patient is weaned from cardiopulmonary bypass. Catheters and cannulae are then removed from the heart and aorta. The aortotomy is closed with a double purse-string suture and the atriotomy is closed in a similar manner.

Most patients are operated upon at normothermic temperature levels. However, when the entire ascending aorta and proximal aortic arch is involved, with aneurysmal change or dissection, systemic hypothermia is used. Once the patient's body temperature is reduced to 22–24°C the cardiopulmonary circuit is discontinued by occluding the venous outlet cannula and stopping the return pump, and blood is aspirated from the heart and aortic arch. For the aortic replacement a tightly woven Dacron fabric graft of appropriate size is soaked with autologous plasma prepared in the operating theatre[3]. The graft is then placed in the steam autoclave for 3–5 minutes. This technique produces a graft which is impervious to bleeding through interstices between the threads. During circulatory arrest the distal anastomosis can be accomplished in less than 15 minutes. Cardiopulmonary bypass is resumed after cross-clamping the tightly woven Dacron felt fabric graft. The aortic valve replacement may be performed during the period of cooling or after the period of circulatory arrest, depending upon the circumstances.

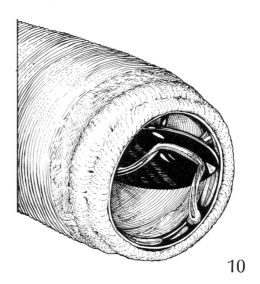

10

10

In patients with true annuloaortic ectasia in which the sinuses of Valsalva are dilated and the coronary orifices have moved cephalad a composite valved tube graft is used.

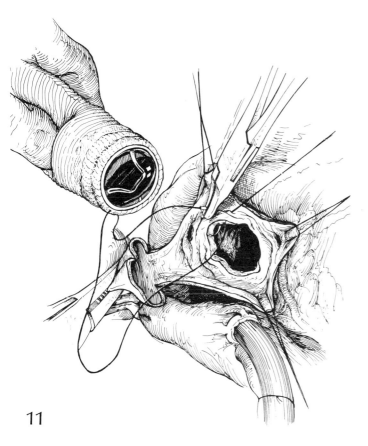

11

11

The composite valve tube graft is sewn directly to the aortic anulus. This may be performed with a continuous running suture of polypropylene as illustrated.

12

A hole is made in the tube graft above the valve, using a hot cautery element. The hole is placed to be opposite the left coronary ostium, and the left coronary artery is now anastomosed to this hole using a continuous running suture of polypropylene.

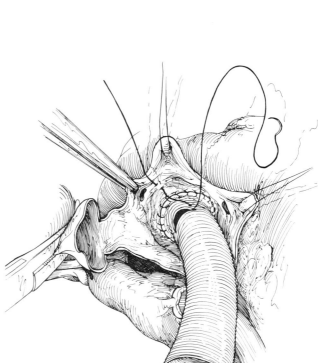

12

13

The anastomosis is begun inferiorly and continued along the inferior rim of the hole that has been made sewing this from the inside.

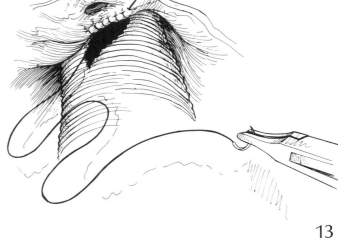

13

14

The anastomosis is completed from above.

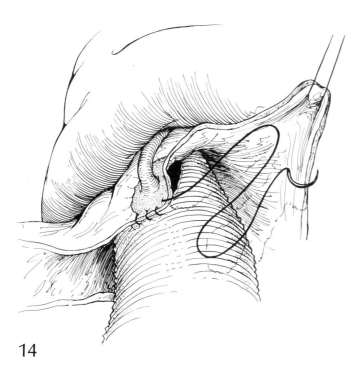

14

15

A similar technique is made for the insertion of the right coronary artery. A suitable hole is made opposite the right coronary orifice, and this is anastomosed in place beginning on the inside inferiorly with completion of the anastomosis above. Finally, the distal graft is anastomosed and continuity of the aorta restored.

Air is removed from the graft in the heart as previously described, and cardiopulmonary bypass discontinued after the heart has taken over circulation.

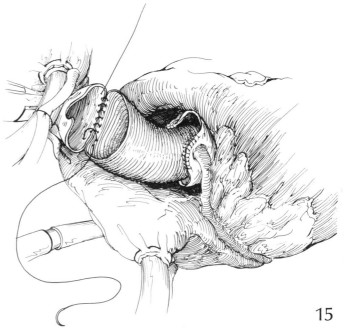

15

Results

Surgical treatment of aortic valve disease has reached a level of safety not enjoyed by replacement of the mitral or tricuspid valve. In the majority of patients with aortic regurgitation, aortic stenosis or a combination of the two, surgical repair and replacement can be accomplished with a surgical mortality of less than 3–5 per cent. In patients with hypertrophied or dilated left ventricles particular attention must be paid to myocardial preservation during the period of mycardial ischaemia. Hypothermia and potassium arrest have greatly improved the results of aortic valve surgery.

References

1. Cooley, D. A. Techniques in cardiac surgery. 2nd edn. Philadelphia: W. B. Saunders, 1984

2. Lefrak, E. A. Database and methology. In Cardiac valve prostheses. Lefrak, E. A., Starr, A. (Eds.) New York: Appleton-Century-Crofts, 1979, 38–63

3. Cooley, D. A., Romagnoli, A., Milam, J. D., Bossart, M. I. A method of preparing woven Dacron grafts to prevent interstitial hemorrhage. Cardiovascular Diseases, Bulletin of the Texas Heart Institute 1981; 8(1): 48–52

Aortocoronary saphenous vein bypass grafting

Stuart W. Jamieson MB, FRCS, FACS
Professor and Head, Cardiothoracic Surgery, University of Minnesota, Minneapolis, Minnesota, USA

Introduction

Coronary artery surgery has evolved over the past decade to be the most commonly performed cardiac procedure in the world, and in the United States alone over 150 000 of these procedures are performed annually. Though there are many ways to perform this operation, the principles remain the same. They are to provide improved blood supply to the myocardium using a venous conduit to bypass fixed lesions in the coronary arteries. A thorough understanding of cardiac anatomy and the interpretation of coronary angiograms is essential.

It used to be thought that coronary artery bypass grafting was only indicated in those patients with good distal vessels and discrete lesions with good or moderate ventricular function. However, with increased expertise a wider application of this operation is warranted. Further, coronary bypass procedures are increasingly being performed in combination with other cardiac procedures such as valve replacement. At the present time most believe that lesions greater than 40 per cent on angiography should be bypassed. The judicious use of sequential anastomoses will allow small vessels to be bypassed, with increased patency rates.

The preoperative angiogram can often be misleading. Although some judgment of the size of vessels may be made by comparing them to that of the catheter, which is generally 2 mm in diameter, vessels will often appear smalller than is found at operation. No decision as to operability should be made entirely on the size of coronary arteries on angiography. Even if these vessels are found to be truly severely compromised at operation, with diffuse and distal disease, endarterectomy, even on the left side, may provide good results. Another common misconception is that total occlusion of a coronary artery is not an indication for surgery since no further muscle could be in jeopardy. This is incorrect thinking. Myocardium supplied by totally occluded vessels is often a source of angina and of course is supplied by collateral flow, causing a 'steal' from other areas. Furthermore, loss of these collateral vessels will result in a further major infarction. Myocardial areas supplied by a totally occluded vessel will either still contain muscle, in which case the vessel is worth grafting, or will be entirely fibrotic, in which case aneurysmectomy is in order.

Other primary conduits have been advocated, including the internal mammary arteries (*see* chapter on 'Internal mammary artery bypass grafting, pp. 471–480). These vessels are not always of sufficient size, however, and cannot be grafted to the most distal vessels of the heart. Furthermore, there are only two internal mammary arteries and even with the use of sequential mammary artery grafting vein grafts will still be needed. Since reoperation is more difficult in the presence of a patent internal mammary graft we prefer to retain elective use of the internal mammary vessels for failed primary operations or younger patients with high grade LAD lesions.

The operations

PREPARATION OF THE VEIN

This is one of the most important parts of the operation.

1

The patient is laid with the leg slightly flexed and externally rotated. It is often convenient to remove the vein through three or four separate incisions in the leg, which slightly reduces postoperative morbidity. However, this is not essential and if the vein is thin and has multiple small branches it is generally preferable to make one continuous vertical incision. The vein should be handled gently at all times to reduce spasm and it should not be allowed to dry.

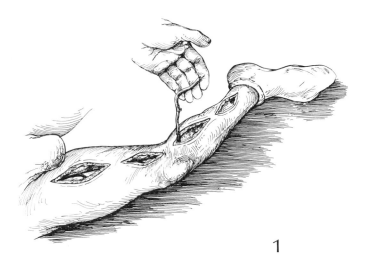

1

2

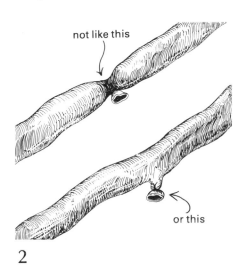

not like this

or this

2

The vein branches are generally tied, though clips may be used. It is important not to place the ties either too close to the vessel wall, producing a constricting band of adventitia, or too far from the lumen, possibly promoting intraluminal thrombosis.

3

Should a small branch be accidentally avulsed a simple mattress suture of 6/0 polypropylene will repair the defect without narrowing the lumen. Loose fatty and connective tissue should be removed from the vein, largely because this may hide small branches. It is generally most convenient to do this final trimming after the vein has been removed from the leg.

The vein is gently perfused with fluid to be sure that the size is adequate and to look for leaks. It is most important to avoid high distension pressures and the constitution of the distending fluid is also important. Though many centres use blood, it is probable that lactated Ringer's solution is satisfactory, but saline, which has a pH below 6, should be avoided; this is a source of direct endothelial injury. The vein should be inspected and ready for use before the institution of bypass.

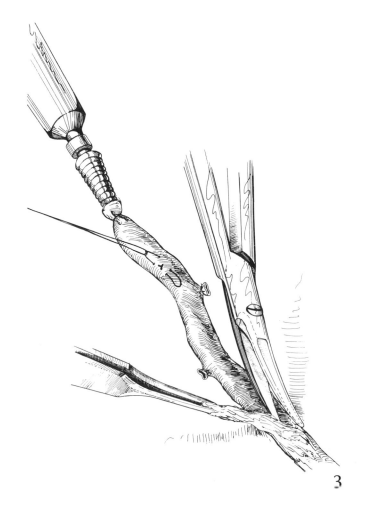

3

DISTAL ANASTOMOSES

The distal anastomoses are performed first and all distal anastomoses are performed during one cross-clamp interval. After the heart has been arrested the coronary arteries are inspected. The heart is elevated on sponges and the operative plan formulated.

4

Anastomosis generally begins with the left anterior descending artery. The use of Silastic retention tapes will allow the area which is to be operated upon to be kept out of the pool of cold saline although the rest of the heart is immersed. These tapes also have the effect of removing any non-coronary collateral flow from the field. The use of a pulmonary artery vent is important; this reduces non-coronary collateral flow and keeps the heart collapsed and cool.

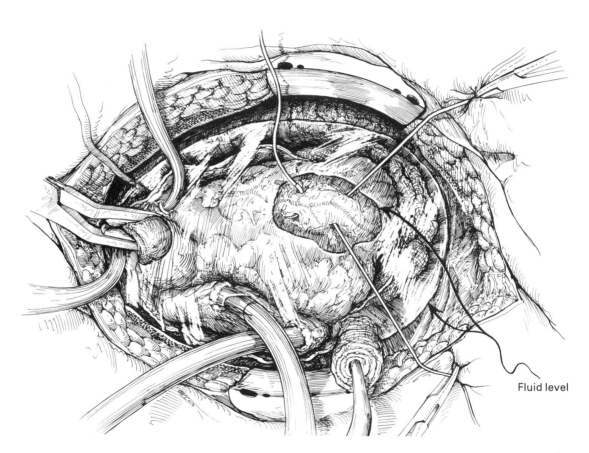

Fluid level

4

5 & 6

A small incision (1–2 mm) is made in the anterior aspect of the vessel. This is enlarged with Pott's scissors to about 4 mm in size but corresponding to the oblique cut previously made in the vein. The vein segment should of course be reversed.

There are numerous methods for anastomosis of the vein to the artery. The general principles are that 6/0 or 7/0 polypropylene should be used, that in general the sutures should be placed from within the artery to the outside so as to avoid raising an intimal flap, and that good exposure is vital.

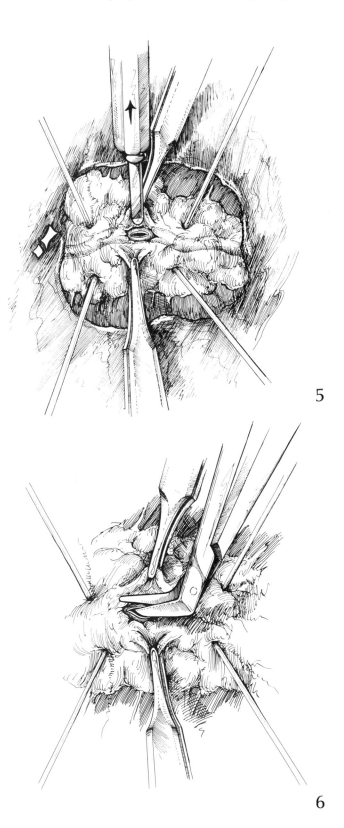

5

6

7, 8 & 9

We generally prefer to anchor the vein at the toe and heel and then sew each of the four quadrants, starting at the anchored portions so that the two knots are tied at the midpoint of the vein.

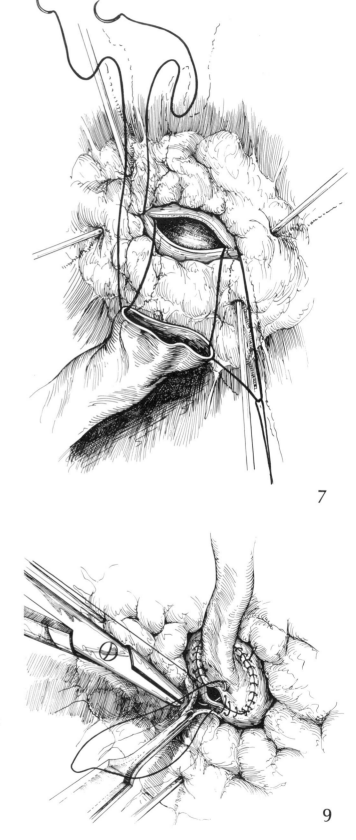

7

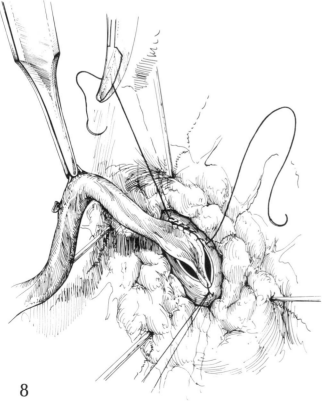

8

9

10 & 11

When the vessels are large and the veins of good quality, and if there is no atheroma within the artery, a continuous technique may safely be used. This generally uses a stitch at the heel followed by a continuous stitch up either side to tie the knot slightly away from the toe.

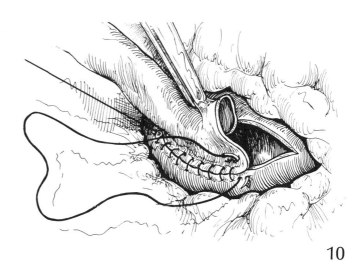

10

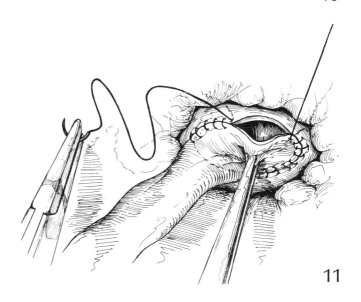

11

12

When the right coronary artery is sewn with a continuous technique the toe is anchored first. The first few sutures are inserted before the suture line is tightened, then the medial side of the anastomosis is fashioned. The other side of the suture is then brought up to complete the suture line.

The order of performance of the distal anastomoses may vary, but generally the left anterior descending artery anastomosis is performed first, followed by anastomosis of other anterior vessels such as the diagonal or intermediate. Attention is then turned to the right coronary artery or posterior descending arteries and lastly to vessels on the lateral wall of the left ventricle, the obtuse marginal coronary arteries. This order of anastomosis means that initially the myocardium is cooled maximally by leaving it immersed in the cold saline while the surgeon is working on the anterior aspect. The left and right ventricles are immersed by elevation of the operative field with Silastic tapes while he is working on the right and inferior vessels and the heart is maximally cooled when finally the obtuse marginal vessels are grafted and the heart lifted out of the cooling solution.

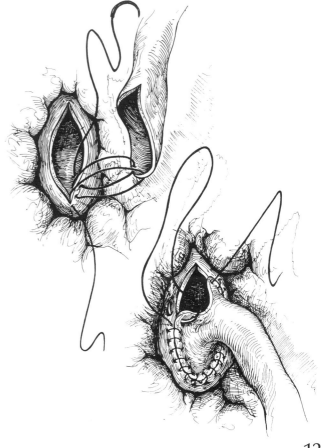

12

13

The right coronary artery is usually exposed below the angle of the heart. The use of silastic tapes and a pulmonary artery vent has the result of immersing the heart, with the exception of the area being worked on, in cold saline.

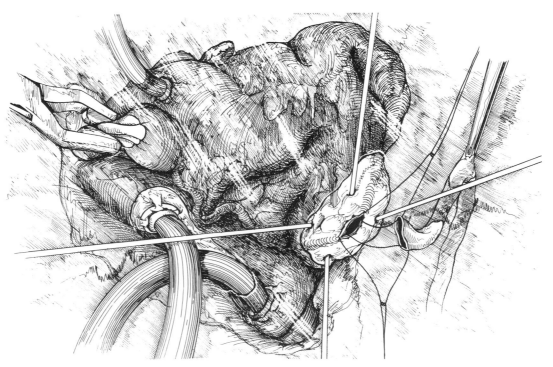

13

Endarterectomy

If the vessel lumen is grossly involved with atheromatous plaque an endarterectomy may be necessary.

14

To do this a slightly longer incision is made in the artery and the plane between the atheromatous plaque and adventitia is found with an elevator.

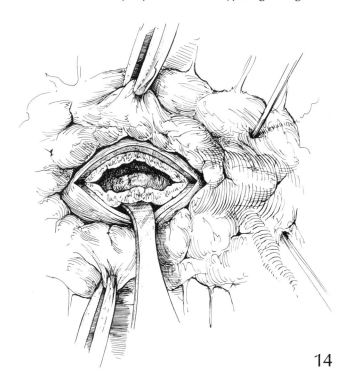

14

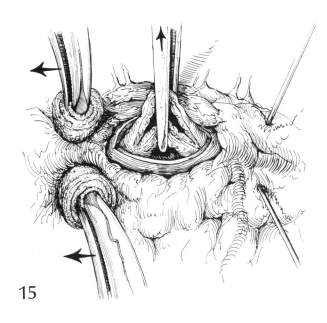

15

15

The plaque is then grasped firmly with a pair of forceps and by gentle traction on either side of the vessel above the incision with two peanut dissectors the atheromatous plaque is withdrawn from the adventitial layer.

16

The plaque is cut short after about 1 cm has been withdrawn proximally. Further withdrawal of the atheromatous plaque here may shear off side branches and lead to infarction. However, complete withdrawal is achieved distally.

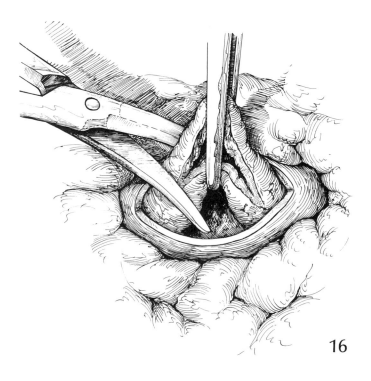

16

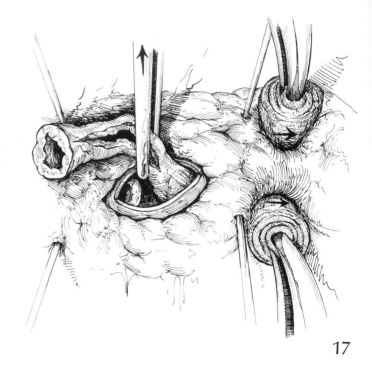

17

For distal withdrawal a similar method is used. The plaque is grasped fully, while again traction is exerted, in a downward direction.

17

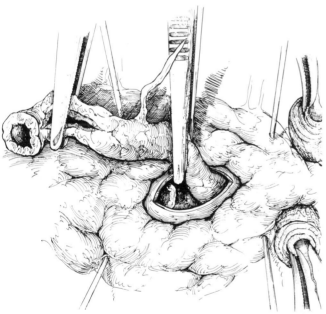

18

18

A second pair of forceps is then used to grasp the atheromatous plaque as it becomes free, followed by the first pair of forceps once more. In this way the vessel is sequentially grasped until all atheromatous cast is removed. It is important to ensure that adequate feathering is obtained distally, confirming complete removal. If the endarterectomy specimen does not include the most distal portion it may be necessary to perform a further distal anastomosis to achieve good runoff.

Endarterectomy is most commonly performed on the right coronary artery. When, however, good runoff cannot be achieved on the left side endarterectomy may be performed here too. With the left anterior descending artery it is especially important not to attempt to withdraw significant portions of atheroma in a proximal direction as important septal arteries may be placed in jeopardy.

Sequential technique

Though most commonly a single vein graft is placed to a single distal vessel, the judicious use of the sequential technique improves long-term patency rates. This technique allows more than one outlet for each vein. Its advantage is that smaller vessels may be bypassed along the route of travel of the vein, thus increasing their chance of long-term patency. Optimally, the most distal vessel should be large, with good run-off. The sequential technique is also useful when the length of vein available is insufficient or when the performance of several proximal anastomoses on the aorta may be difficult or dangerous, as in the presence of severe ascending aortic atherosclerosis or plaquing. The obvious disadvantage of this technique is that the loss of the proximal portion of the conduit will jeopardize all outlets.

The technique of a sequential anastomosis requires the most distal anastomosis to be performed first, in the routine way. The next vessel to be bypassed is then isolated and an incision made. The vein is distended and the point of the sequential anastomosis measured. An incision is made in the vein at a suitable point. It is important that the anastomosis be incorporated in the vein in such a way that it is neither distorted nor its normal route of travel halted, which can lead to kinking. Anastomosis is now made in the routine way.

The most commonly performed sequential anastomosis is carried out from the left anterior descending coronary artery to the diagonal to the aorta. The left anterior descending artery is almost always a vessel of good calibre and runoff and the diagonal artery is generally smaller. The diagonal artery can be bypassed by using the vein as it lies in a gentle curve towards the aorta.

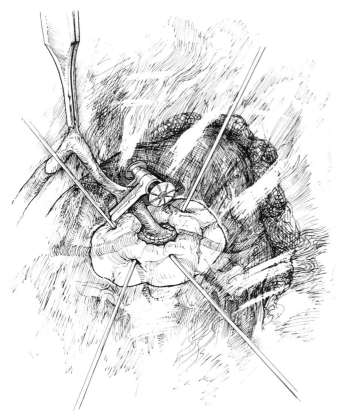

19

Once the left anterior descending anastomosis has been performed a non-traumatic clamp is placed on the distal portion of the vein.

19

20

The diagonal coronary artery is exposed and a longitudinal incision made in this vessel. The vein is distended and the point of anastomosis measured. A longitudinal incision is made in the vein with a No. 11 blade.

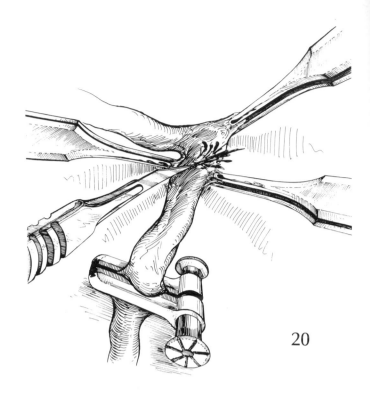

20

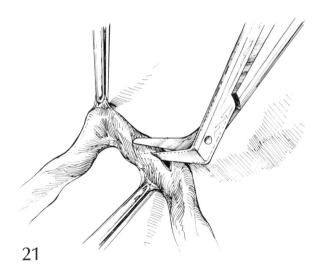

21

21

The incision in the vein is then enlarged with scissors to a slightly bigger size than the incision in the artery.

22, 23, 24 & 25

The vein is anchored heel and toe as before and the anastomosis performed in routine fashion. Again, with suitable positioning of the heart and elevation of the working area with Silastic tapes the heart is kept immersed in cold saline while the anastomosis is performed. After completion of the sequential anastomosis the clamp is placed proximal to the diagonal anastomosis so that the vein can be measured to the aorta and cut to size.

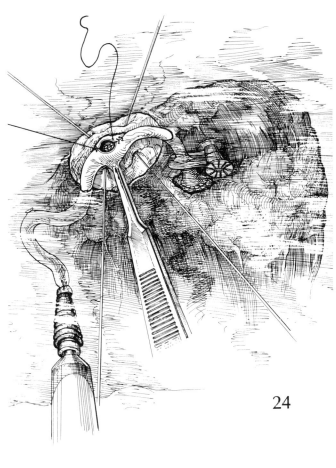

24

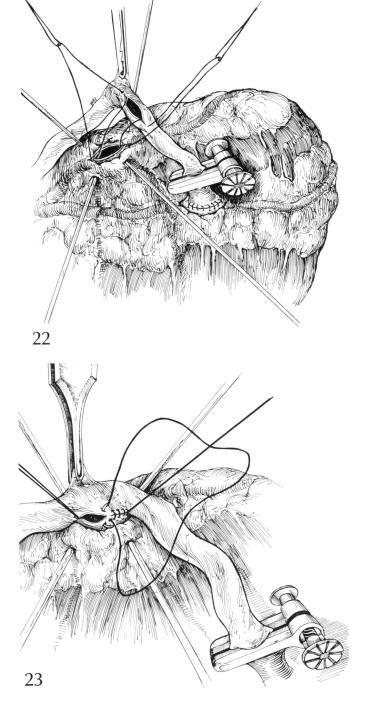

22

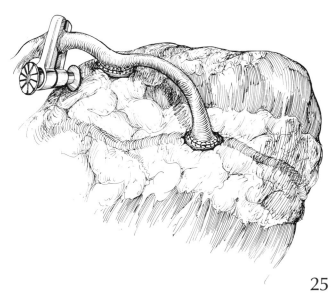

25

23

Other favourable sites for a sequential graft are from the posterior descending to the right coronary artery (if the posterior descending artery contains a discrete lesion and the right coronary artery provides a significant continuation branch supplying posterolateral arteries) (*see Illustration 32*), or where two or three obtuse marginal arteries lie together, where they can be grafted in sequence. A further option is to graft from obtuse marginal artery to posterior descending or main right artery. Again the principle of the biggest outlet being the most distal anastomosis should be maintained.

A longitudinal incision is always made in both the vein conduit and the artery. For the left anterior descending to diagonal (*see Illustration 33*) and the obtuse marginal to right coronary sequential anastomoses the anastomosis is made with the longitudinal cut of the vein overlying the longitudinal cut in the artery. However, for obtuse marginal to obtuse marginal or obtuse marginal posterior descending grafts a smaller incision is made ... both the vein and the artery and they are anastomosed in X fashion. It is easiest to make this latter anastomosis with a continuous suture.

After completion of the distal anastomoses, whether single or sequential, each conduit is measured to the aorta so that it lies in a gentle curve without tension or kinks. The vein is gently distended wih irrigant fluid in order to do this and then cut to size. An oblique cut is made; this enlarges the vein opening maximally, both for the proximal anastomosis on the aorta and for the next distal anastomosis to be performed.

After all distal anastomoses have been completed the aortic cross-clamp is removed.

PROXIMAL ANASTOMOSES

26

In order to perform the proximal anastomosis a side-biting clamp is placed on the aorta on the left side for the left-sided grafts and the right side for right-sided grafts. The aorta should be checked for atheromatous plaquing before the clamp is placed and the aorta grasped in a pair of large forceps while this clamp is put into position.

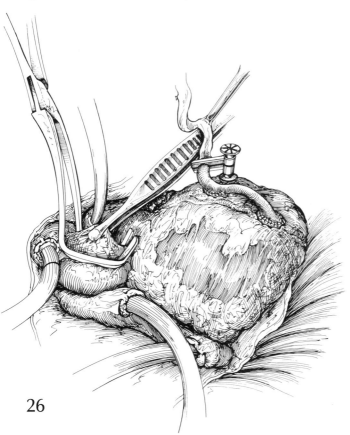

26

27

An incision is made in the aorta with a No. 11 blade and the resultant hole enlarged and made into a circle with a punch. The proximal anastomosis is made with 5/0 polypropylene.

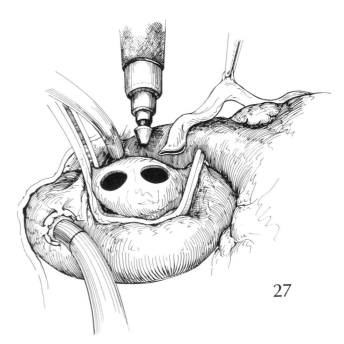

27

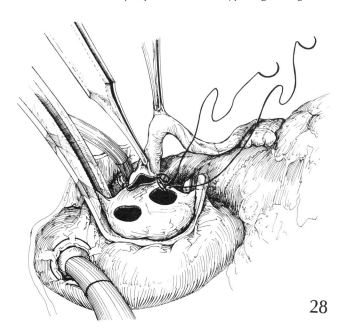

28

28, 29 & 30

Again the principle of anastomosis is that the aorta is sewn from within out to avoid dislodging atheromatous plaques. We prefer to sew the inferior margin first, completing the anastomosis by then bringing the other suture around to tie at the toe of the vein. When the left-sided grafts have been performed the side-biting clamp is removed, air removed from the grafts and the distal anastomoses checked for haemostasis.

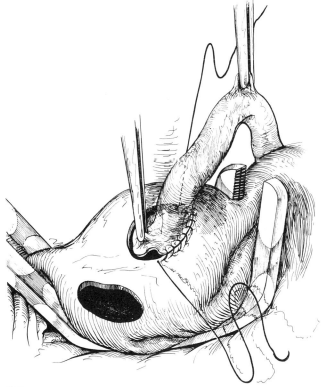

29

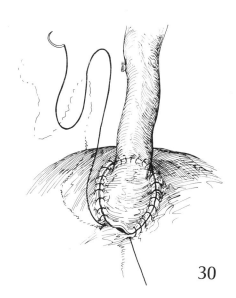

30

31

The right-sided anastomoses are then performed, though for these grafts the suture, which begins at the heel, is placed inferiorally rather than laterally.

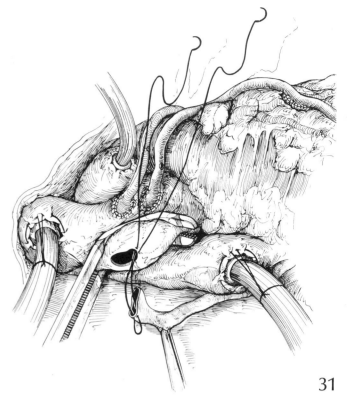

31

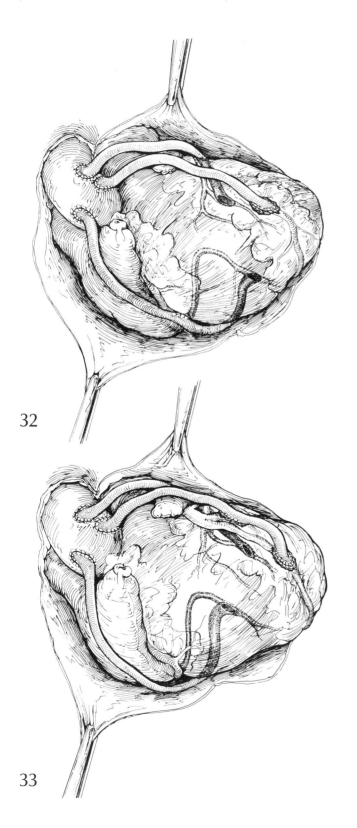

32

32 & 33

After completion of the anastomoses the grafts should lie without tension or kinking and contain gentle curves. Sequential anastomoses, if performed, should not appreciably interrupt the normal course of the vein.

33

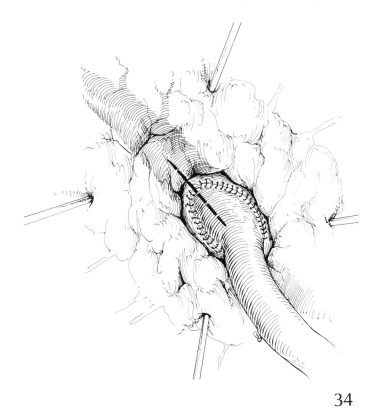

34

REOPERATION

Reoperation in coronary artery surgery is becoming increasingly common. The principle of surgery in this case is to achieve complete mobilization of the heart so as to provide uniform cooling and adequate exposure of posterior vessels. Where previous vein grafts are still patent great caution should be taken to avoid dislodging the loose and friable material that is generally contained within these vessels. It is wise to institute cardiopulmonary bypass and venting before final mobilization of the left ventricle.

34 & 35

The distal anastomoses are generally performed through the toe of the old graft provided no new disease has occurred distally. Anastomosis may now be made using both the native artery distally and the old graft proximally.

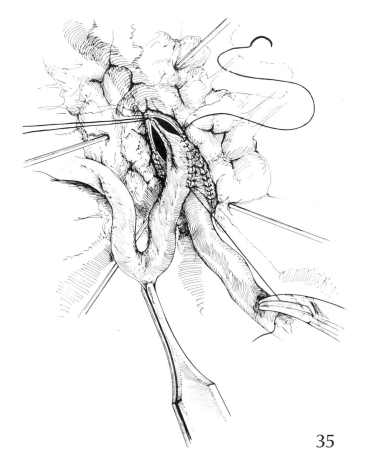

35

36

The proximal anastomoses are most conveniently performed at the site of the old anastomoses. A rim of previously placed vein may be left in situ.

Sequential grafting is more common in reoperation in order to improve revascularization and the long-term patency rate. Where anterior vessels are excessively small or where insufficient vein exists the internal mammary vessels may be used.

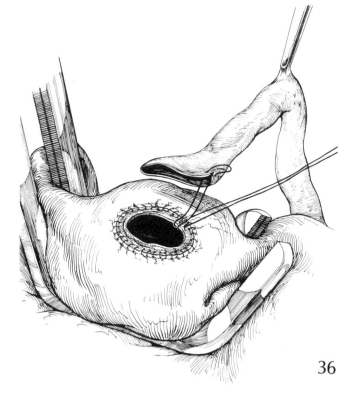

36

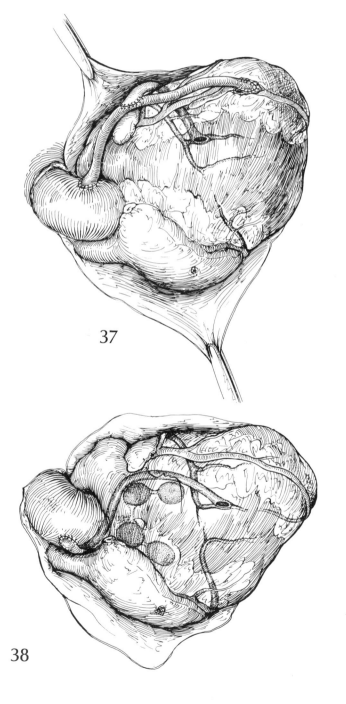

37

38

37 & 38

Other methods that conserve venous material where this is restricted are the anastomosis of a vein to another conduit and, in the case of an obtuse marginal vessel, to pass the vein through the transverse sinus rather than going over the pulmonary artery. If a venovenous anastomosis isused a relatively large ostium should be made in the recipient vessel.

Internal mammary artery to coronary artery bypass grafting

Bruce W. Lytle MD
Staff Surgeon, Department of Thoracic and Cardiovascular Surgery, The Cleveland Clinic Foundation, Cleveland, Ohio, USA

Floyd D. Loop MD
Chairman, Department of Thoracic and Cardiovascular Surgery, The Cleveland Clinic Foundation, Cleveland, Ohio, USA

Introduction

The internal mammary artery (IMA) is an excellent conduit for coronary artery bypass grafting. Studies of IMA grafts up to 5 years after surgery have demonstrated the rate of postoperative patency of IMA grafts to be more than 90 per cent. Since early patency of saphenous vein grafts is also good, particularly when large coronary vessels are grafted, overall early differences between the patency rates of IMA and vein grafts have not been dramatic. However, with thousands of restudied grafts now available for review, early patency of IMA grafts has been shown to exceed that documented for vein bypass grafts to coronary arteries. The superiority of the early patency of the IMA graft is particularly apparent when subgroups of patients tending to have small vessels and diffuse disease, such as women and young adults, are examined.

Atherosclerosis within vein grafts occurs with increasing frequency between 5 and 10 years after operation and provides an additional reason for the use of the IMA arterial graft. Autopsy studies have shown atherosclerosis of the mammary arteries to be rare, and graft atherosclerosis developing in the IMA after bypass grafting has not yet been demonstrated. Although large numbers of IMA grafts have not yet been studied at 10 years after surgery, existing data indicate that IMA graft longevity, in addition to early patency, may be superior to that of vein grafts.

However, use of the IMA for bypass grafting has not become widespread. A survey conducted in 1980 found that only 13 per cent of United States surgeons used this graft, possibly because of several practical and theoretical disadvantages. Preparation of the IMA graft is more time-consuming than is vein preparation and IMA-to-coronary distal anastomoses are technically more difficult to perform than are vein grafts. However, improved anaesthetic techniques, increased surgical experience and modern methods of myocardial protection minimize these problems. Comparative study has demonstrated no increase in morbidity with IMA use, and among 1295 patients for primary myocardial revascularization receiving IMA grafts at the Cleveland Clinic Foundation in 1981, 5 operative deaths occurred (0.4 per cent).

A legitimate matter of concern is that the IMA, a vessel usually 1.5–2.5 mm in diameter at the point of grafting, might not deliver sufficient flow for large coronary vessels. The surgeon must exercise judgement regarding the adequacy of IMA flow and which coronary artery is best suited for an IMA graft. Left ventricular hypertrophy, a heavily dominant anterior descending coronary artery or a small IMA represent relative contraindications to the grafting of the IMA to the anterior descending artery, although for such patients the IMA may function perfectly adequately as a diagonal or circumflex graft. Data concerning patients undergoing exercise testing after IMA grafting as well as the low rate of clinical angina and myocardial infarction experienced by such patients indicate that when proper selection is used the IMA provides more than adequate flow.

The left IMA is used preferentially when grafting the anterior descending coronary artery. The anterior descending is often the patient's most important coronary artery and the IMA will reach this vessel easily in most patients. Specific indications for IMA use include grafts to diffusely diseased vessels of limited outflow, grafts to small coronary vessels, coronary revascularization in young adults, reoperations for vein graft failure and absent or unsuitable leg veins.

471

MAMMARY ARTERY ANATOMY

1

The internal mammary artery is a branch of the subclavian artery, usually arising opposite the thyrocervical trunk. It enters the thorax deep to the sternal end of the clavicle and subclavian vein.

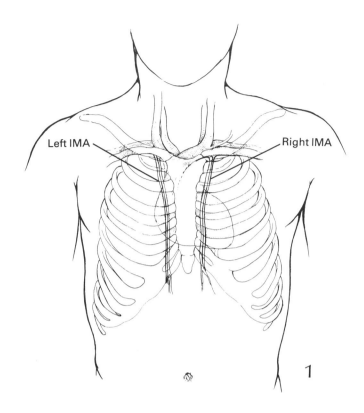

1

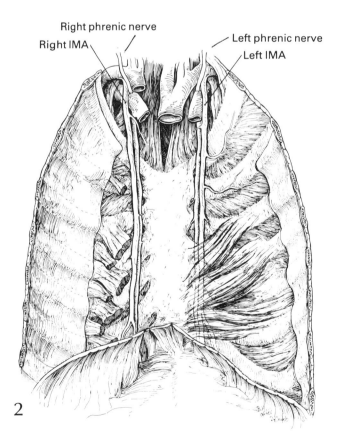

2

2

The phrenic nerve crosses from the lateral to the medial aspect of the IMA near the IMA origin, at which point the pericardiophrenic branch of the IMA joins the nerve. As the IMA descends parallel to the sternum it is related ventrally to the costal cartilages and fascia of the internal intercostal muscles. Dorsally it is covered by pleura in its most cranial portion, but caudal to the third rib it is also covered by fibres of the internal thoracic muscle. Major branches include perforating vessels that extend anteriorly through the intercostal muscle layers of the chest wall and anterior intercostal branches arising in the first five or six intercostal spaces that run laterally to anastomose with aortic intercostal vessels. A major bifurcation occurs between the fifth and seventh intercostal spaces, where the vessel divides into the musculophrenic and superior epigastric arteries.

The operation

Graft preparation

Median sternotomy is used in all cases for IMA-to-coronary bypass grafting.

3

Before heparinization the side of the sternum where the artery is to be dissected is evaluated with the use of a self-retaining retractor which is stabilized by fixation to the operating table. The fingers of the retractor are placed on the sternum. The pleural reflection can be dissected laterally to expose the IMA while maintaining pleural continuity or the pleura may be incised, exposing the left hemithorax. The anaesthetist decreases the patient's tidal volume slightly to allow the lung to fall away from the operative field. The mammary artery and its vein, which runs medial to the artery, are identified and an incision with electrocautery is made in the tissue overlying the fourth or fifth intercostal space at the lateral edge of the sternum. Blunt dissection is then carried out with the tip of the electrocautery instrument. The correct dissection plane lies on the dorsal aspect of the internal intercostal muscle layer, and except for the arterial and venous branches the IMA pedicle can be isolated with only rare use of the electrocautery current. Over costochondral junctions the dissection is dorsal to the perichondrium.

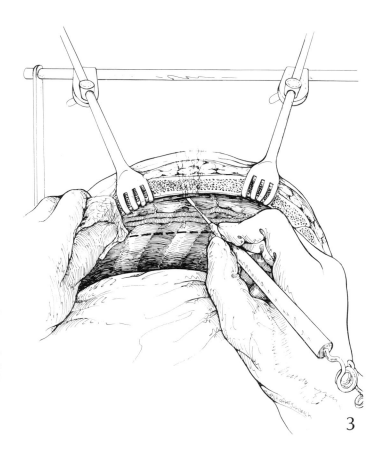

3

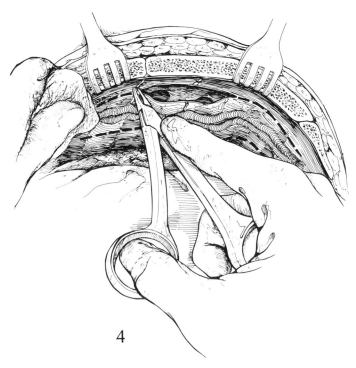

4

4

Perforating vessels and intercostal branches are occluded with a Hemoclip on the IMA side and either a Hemoclip or cautery is used on the chest wall side of the vessels. Any blood shed on to the field is collected with a regionally heparinized blood salvage system and processed into washed, packed erythrocytes which are then available for later transfusion.

Once the correct plane is identified dissection is carried both proximally and distally, exposure being maintained by gentle traction on the pedicle. Traction must be gentle in order to avoid avulsion of IMA branches and intimal damage, which can lead to localized dissection and occlusion of the vessel. The vein is mobilized with the artery. Forceps should never be used to handle the IMA itself. During the caudal part of the dissection it is necessary to take some fibres of the transverse thoracic muscle layer with the pedicle. Proximally the dissection is carried to the superior border of the first rib, avoiding injury to the subclavian vein and phrenic nerve. Caudally, dissection is carried beyond the bifurcation into the superior epigastric and musculophrenic arteries. These vessels, however, are left intact so that flow is maintained throughout the length of the IMA.

5a & b

When the dissection is completed papaverine solution is sprayed on to the vessel to maintain vasodilatation (*a*) and a papaverine-soaked sponge wrapped around the pedicle (*b*). If the pleura has been entered a thoracic catheter is inserted posterolaterally. The mammary artery self-retaining retractor is removed and a sternal spreading retractor inserted.

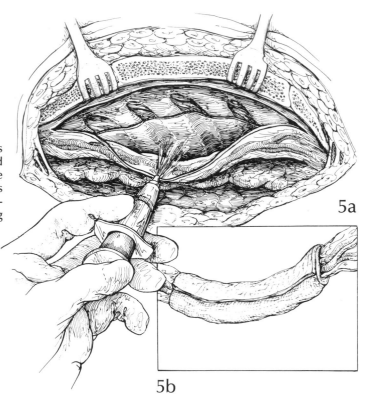

5a

5b

Preparation for cardiopulmonary bypass

6

Before cardiopulmonary bypass is established the IMA is divided distal to its major bifurcation and the distal vessel tied and suture ligated on the chest wall side. An assessment of the length of IMA needed to reach the point where the recipient artery is to be grafted is then made while the lungs are inflated.

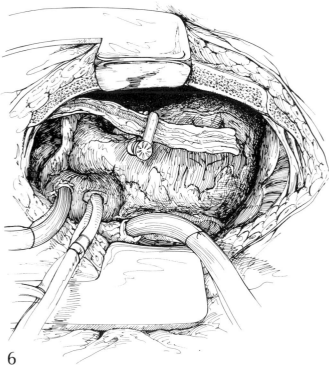

6

7a, b & c

When the site for the ideal anastomosis on the IMA is identified the tissue of the pedicle on either side of the artery itself is divided (a). The IMA is then cut, leaving 1.5 cm beyond the end of the pedicle (b). Small iris scissors are used to make a 5–6 mm ventral slit in the distal end of the IMA (c).

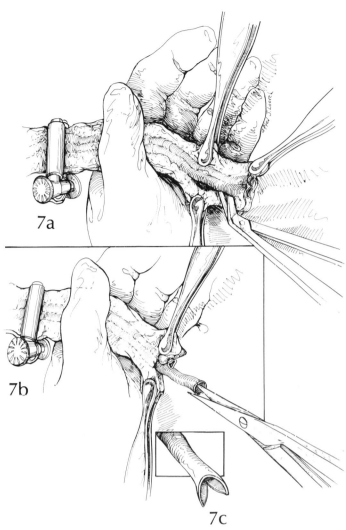

7a

7b

7c

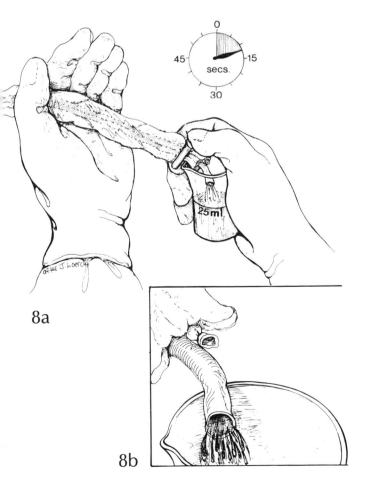

8a

8b

8

Assessment of flow through the IMA is then made at a normal systemic blood pressure. If the flow through the IMA appears low, timed flow is measured into a beaker. At a normal blood pressure IMA flow should be at least 80 ml/minute. Once adequacy of flow is established an atraumatic clamp is placed on the IMA pedicle and a haemostat is used to fix the pedicle to the towel surrounding the operating field, in order to prevent twisting of the IMA.

Distal anastomosis

Cardiopulmonary bypass is then established. Distal anastomoses are performed with the aid of aortic cross-clamping and cold cardioplegia for myocardial protection. A Y-tube allows venting of the aortic root by the catheter used to inject the cardioplegic solution. When multiple grafts are scheduled the vein graft distal anastomoses are performed before the IMA anastomosis. Packs in the pericardium are used to elevate the heart, making the anterior wall more accessible when the IMA is to be grafted to anterior descending or diagonal branches. For anastomoses to circumflex vessels the surgeon stands on the patient's left side and the assistant elevates and retracts the heart to the right.

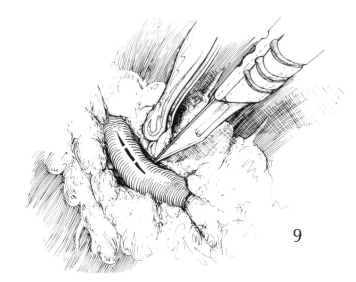

9

9

Epicardial fat and myocardium overlying the host vessel are dissected away with a scalpel. Cardioplegic solution is infused to distend the vessel and the coronary arteriotomy is initiated with the tip of a razor. The arteriotomy is then extended 4–5 mm with iris scissors. The IMA must not be damaged with forceps. However, as the IMA arteriotomy is longer than the coronary arteriotomy it is possible to manipulate the IMA by holding the tip with forceps and excluding it from the anastomosis.

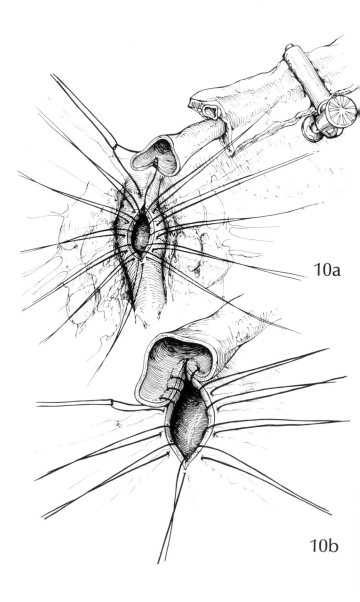

10a

10a & b

An interrupted suture technique using siliconized 7/0 silk suture is preferred for the IMA-to-coronary anastomosis. The IMA diameter is usually 1.5–2.5 mm at the point of anastomosis and care must be exercised not to narrow the conduit itself. The interrupted suture technique has the advantage that all sutures are placed in both the host vessel and the graft under direct vision. Initially all the sutures, 10–12 in number, are placed in the IMA and the IMA tied down. The heel stitch (a) and the sutures on each side of it are the most critical of the anastomosis and are placed carefully in the IMA and tied gently. Sutures on one side of the anastomosis are then individually placed and tied (b).

10b

11a & b

On the other side of the anastomosis, in order to allow adequate visualization, no sutures are tied until all have been placed (a). Once all sutures have been tied the atraumatic clamp is moved from the vessel to allow inspection of the anastomosis under pressure and also evaluation of the area supplied by the IMA. Any adventitial bands on the hood of the graft are divided with iris scissors.

Four sutures are placed in the pedicle to secure it to the epicardium (b). This prevents twisting or adherence of the pedicle to the chest wall. The aorta is then unclamped. Vein grafts to the left-sided coronary vessels are placed beneath the IMA and vein graft proximal anastomoses to the aorta completed.

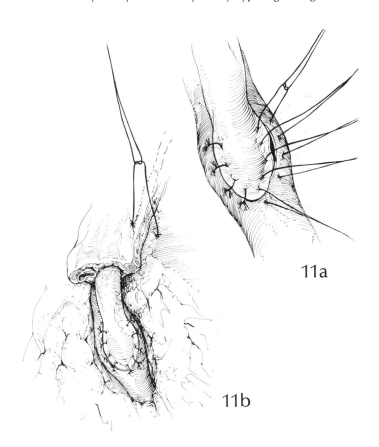

11a

11b

Grafting options with the IMA

In most cases the left IMA is used to bypass obstructing lesions in the proximal left anterior descending coronary artery. However, when the need arises almost any coronary artery can be grafted with either an *in situ* or a free IMA graft. The left IMA will reach the anterior descending, diagonal and many circumflex arteries as an *in situ* graft.

12

To facilitate grafting of circumflex vessels the pericardium is incised posteriorly just to the left of its reflection over the pulmonary artery. This incision is stopped just anterior to the phrenic nerve and allows the left IMA to pass directly to any left-sided vessel without bowing anteriorly around the pericardium. This manoeuvre is particularly useful in reaching posterior circumflex vessels.

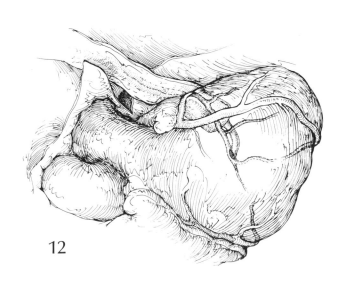

12

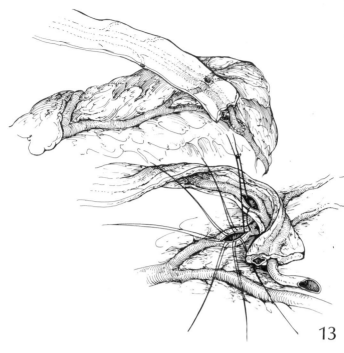

13

Sequential left IMA grafts can be useful. A side-to-side anastomosis is made to the proximal anterior descending artery or a distal diagonal branch with a subsequent end-to-side anastomosis of the more distal left anterior descending artery. The sequential grafts are fashioned in a diamond-shaped manner, placing the IMA arteriotomy at right angles to the coronary arteriotomy.

13

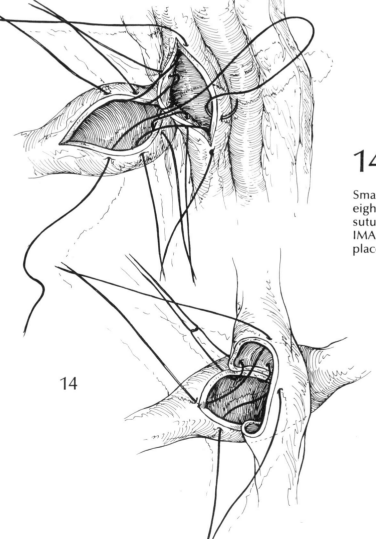

14

14

Small arteriotomies, 3–4 mm in length, are used and six to eight sutures are placed in the coronary vessel. The heel suture of the coronary vessel is placed in the side of the IMA arteriotomy and tied. The remaining sutures are all placed before any are tied.

15

The distal anastomosis is performed in routine fashion. The use of proximal diagonal branches as the initial vessel grafted with a sequential IMA graft is not recommended as angulation at the side-to-side anastomosis tends to occur.

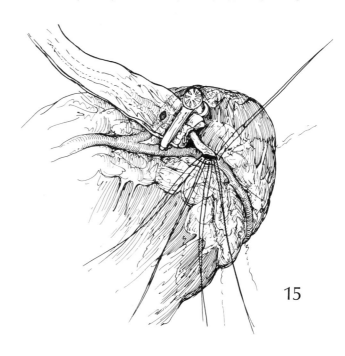

15

16

Right IMA *in situ* grafts may reach the anterior descending (at the junction of the mid and upper one-third), first septal perforating, diagonal, lateral circumflex and proximal right coronary arteries. When bilateral mammary artery grafting is performed the right IMA will often reach the proximal diagonal or circumflex branches if brought anterior to the aorta and posterior to the left IMA, which can be used to graft the left anterior descending artery.

The main disadvantage of the use of right IMA grafts is the difficulty in any subsequent reoperation through a median sternotomy. Therefore, bilateral IMA grafting is not a standard procedure. Specific indications for bilateral IMA grafting include absent or unsuitable veins, operations in the presence of diffuse coronary atherosclerosis and occasionally primary operations in young adults with diffuse atherosclerosis.

16a

16b

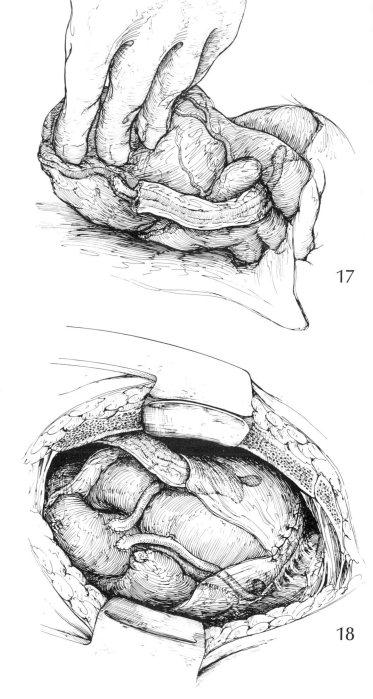

17

18

17 & 18

When *in situ* pedicles will not reach the coronary vessels to be grafted an alternative is to divide the IMA at its origin from the subclavian artery and use the IMA as a free graft. The proximal anastomosis is made to the aorta with interrupted 6/0 siliconized silk suture material after a small button of aorta has been removed with a 4 mm punch. Free grafts may reach extremely distal posterior circumflex and right coronary branches. An additional 1–2 cm of length may be conserved if the proximal anastomosis is made to the posterior aorta and the graft brought through the transverse sinus to the coronary vessel. When the right IMA is used a free graft presents less difficulty if subsequent reoperation is needed than does an *in situ* right IMA graft.

Further reading

Green, G. E. Internal mammary artery-to-coronary artery anastomosis. Three year experience with 165 patients. Annals of Thoracic Surgery 1972; 14: 260–271

Loop, F. D., Irarrazaval, M. J., Bredee, J. J., Siegel, W., Taylor, P. C., Sheldon, W. C. Internal mammary artery graft for ischemic heart disease; effect of revascularization on clinical status and survival. American Journal of Cardiology 1977; 39: 516–522

Lytle, B. W., Loop, F. D. Elective coronary surgery. Cardiovascular Clinics 1982; 12: 31–47

Surgery for the complications of myocardial infarction

Wayne M. Derkac MD
Instructor in Surgery, Harvard Medical School;
Assistant in Surgery, Massachusetts General Hospital, Boston Massachusetts, USA

Willard M. Daggett MD
Professor of Surgery, Harvard Medical School;
Visiting Surgeon, Massachusetts General Hospital, Boston, Masachusetts, USA

Introduction

Mechanical complications resulting from myocardial infarction usually have profound acute or chronic haemodynamic effects. Ruptured mitral valve papillary muscle, left ventricle aneurysm, and ruptured interventricular septum represent the most commonly seen and most often devastating problems. An understanding of the haemodynamic consequences of these problems enables appropriate resuscitative manoeuvres to be instituted and ensures appropriate operative timing. Furthermore, an understanding of the underlying pathophysiology of these problems has proved essential in the successful development of operative techniques to restore good haemodynamic function.

PAPILLARY MUSCLE RUPTURE

Mitral valve papillary muscle rupture is a rare complication of acute myocardial infarction, occurring in 1 or 2 per cent of patients admitted to hospital for treatment of infarction. The clinical course is usually one of fulminant pulmonary oedema and cardiogenic shock. More than 50 per cent of patients die in the first 24 hours[1]. Since the anterolateral papillary muscle is better vascularized (supplied by branches of the left anterior descending and circumflex marginal coronary arteries) than the posteromedial papillary muscle (supplied from either right coronary artery branches or circumflex branches) rupture of the post-eromedial muscle occurs the more frequently. Therefore this complication is most often seen following inferior or posterior myocardial infarction[2].

Preoperative

With the acute development of cardiogenic shock in association with a new holosystolic murmur following acute myocardial infarction pressor support is instituted and, if adequate systemic perfusion pressure can be maintained, vasodilator therapy is also begun. The placement of a Swan-Ganz catheter is useful in both diagnosis and management. During the placement of the Swan-Ganz catheter it is possible to exclude postinfarction ventricular septal rupture by obtaining measurements of oxygen saturation in the right atrium and pulmonary artery, thereby detecting an oxygen step-up at the right ventricular level. In addition the Swan-Ganz catheter can assess V waves in the pulmonary capillary wedge tracing and is useful in monitoring left heart filling pressures. Radionuclide ventriculography is often a useful bedside technique to help differentiate the patient with mitral regurgitation as a result of papillary muscle rupture with relatively well preserved left ventricular ejection from the patient with functional mitral regurgitation from annular dilatation and left ventricular failure as a consequence of massive infarction, which will be associated with a very low ejection fraction.

The placement of an intra-aortic balloon pump before catheterization can often stabilize the patient temporarily and has been shown to improve postoperative survival. After emergency catheterization, including left ventriculography and coronary angiography, emergency operation is indicated to correct the mitral regurgitation and prevent concomitant end-organ failure.

The operation

Extrocorporeal circulation

Operation is undertaken through a standard median sternotomy incision. An ascending aortic perfusion cannula is placed and venous return to the pump is effected with two caval cannulae. After the aorta has been cross-clamped myocardial protection is carried out in routine fashion.

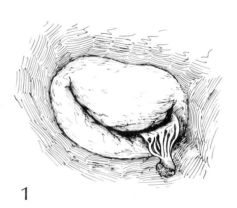

1

If bypassable coronary artery stenoses are present the proximal aortosaphenous vein graft anastomoses may be performed before the initiation of cardiopulmonary bypass or, in the case of unstable patients, during cooling. Distal anastomoses are then performed after placement of a right superior pulmonary vein-left ventricular vent and after the administration of cardioplegia.

1

Inspection of mitral valve

Attention is then turned to the mitral valve. The operating table is rotated away from the operator during cardioplegic infusion. Care is taken not to retract the heart at this point as this may render the aortic valve incompetent and make effective infusion of cardioplegic solution difficult. The left atrium is then widely opened in the atrial groove with an incision which begins anterior to the right superior pulmonary vein and extends superiorly to just behind the superior cavo-atrial junction. This incision is then carried down to the inferior margin of the left atrium. Since the left atrium is often quite small it has been found convenient to extend the atrial incision beneath the inferior vena cava and to mobilize both venae cavae by sharp dissection. A retractor is then placed in the left atrium and the mitral valve is inspected. A ruptured papillary muscle head is easily visible. Mitral valve repair is regarded as inadvisable in this group of patients.

2

Excision of mitral valve

The chordae of the anterior leaflet are snared with a large nerve hook. Retraction on the nerve hook posteriorly serves to demonstrate the anterior leaflet. The valve is then excised entirely, beginning with the anterior leaflet and leaving a rim of approximately 3 mm of valve tissue. Subsequently the heads of the remaining papillary muscles are divided in order to free the chordal attachments of the valve. The mural or posterior leaflet is excised with angled oesophageal scissors. Care is taken to avoid injury to the atrial wall during excision of the posterior leaflet.

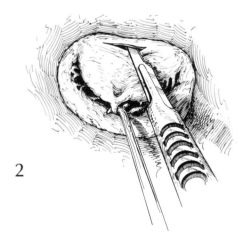

2

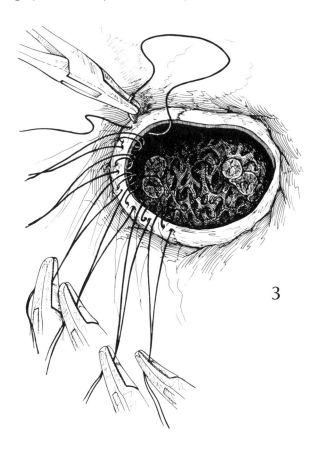

3

3

Insertion of mitral prosthesis

The annulus is then sized. Since the left ventricular cavity is invariably small, employment of a low-profile (Björk-Shiley tilting disc) prosthesis is preferred. In the rare case of thickened annular tissue interrupted figure-of-eight 2/0 Tycron sutures are placed in the annulus.

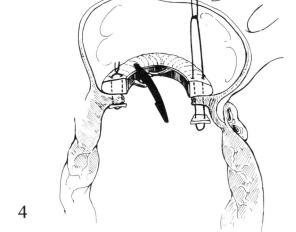

4

4

Usually, however, in these cases the annulus is very thin and interrupted horizontal mattress sutures of 2/0 Tycron reinforced with Teflon felt pledgets are placed. In order to avoid stress on the annulus during tying of the sutures the pledgets are placed on the ventricular side of the annulus. The first suture is placed at 8 o'clock and the remainder in clockwise fashion. Care is taken to avoid deep placement of sutures in the region of the aortic valve anterosuperiorly, in the region of the conduction system inferiorly and in the region of the circumflex coronary artery posteriorly. During placement of the sutures care should be taken to avoid passing the needles or sutures through the left ventricular musculature. Passage of sutures should be only through the annulus in order to avoid a site for potential dissection of blood and later ventricular rupture.

These sutures are then passed through the prosthetic valve annulus, care being taken to ensure that they emerge from the valve ring at its very edge. The valve is then seated in place and the sutures are tied. Rewarming is begun during the later stages of tying the valve sutures. It is important that the knots are on the outside of the valve ring so that after they are cut they will not interfere with disc motion. The disc is orientated so that the larger orifice is anterior.

5

Free mobility of the disc is then tested, a cotton-tipped swab being used to prevent injury to the surface. The disc should open and close freely and if any restriction is noted its orientation should be changed by means of the valve holder until full excursion of the disc is obtained. A small (size 8) Foley catheter is placed across the minor orifice of the valve and the Foley catheter balloon inflated to render the valve incompetent and thus prevent ejection of air during the atrial closure.

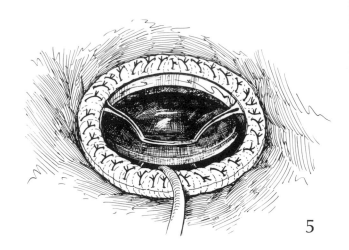

5

Closure of atriotomy

The left atriotomy is then closed with two running sutures of 3/0 polypropylene, one from below and one from above. The ascending aortic cross clamp is removed after the cardioplegic infusion has been finished and the aortic root monitoring catheters removed in order to vent air from the ascending aorta. The heart is immediately defibrillated if necessary, although it is usual for cardiac rhythm and contraction to resume spontaneously after removal of the cross clamp.

Extreme care should be exercised during elevation of the heart during removal of residual air in order to avoid avulsion of the valve and consequent initiation of left ventricular posterior wall rupture. As air is removed from the left ventricular apex the Foley catheter is deflated and withdrawn from the heart and the running 3/0 polypropylene suture is held taut. The vent holes in the ascending aorta are continuously bleeding as the Foley balloon is deflated and the catheter removed as the patient begins to eject blood into the ascending aorta. The left atriotomy is closed by tying after a polypropylene catheter has been placed across the left atriotomy into the left atrium for measurement of left atrial pressure.

Intra-aortic balloon pumping at full balloon volume is resumed as soon as the patient regains rhythm. Right atrial and right ventricular epicardial pacing electrodes are placed. Caval tourniquets are subsequently released and the patient is then weaned from cardiopulmonary bypass.

Postoperative management

Postoperative management consists of pressor support, maximal vasodilator therapy and intra-aortic balloon pumping.

Since the first successful replacement of a ruptured mitral valve papillary muscle by Austen et al. in 1965[3], operative mortality has steadily improved, rates as low as 19 per cent being reported. Actuarial 5-year survival has been reported as high as 75 per cent, justifying an early aggressive approach to this problem[4].

LEFT VENTRICULAR ANEURYSM

Left ventricular aneurysm formation occurs in 10–20 per cent of patients after an acute myocardial infarction[5]. Natural history studies have documented a 5-year mortality as high as 90 per cent in patients with left ventricular aneurysms following acute myocardial infarction[6]. Aneurysms involving the anterior, lateral and apical portions of the left ventricle are more common than posterior or inferior aneurysms because of the higher incidence of anterior myocardial infarctions and the position of the diaphragm.

With large segments of dyskinesis extending over 20 per cent of the left ventricular free wall, a higher end-diastolic volume must be maintained in order to secure adequate stroke volume. By the law of LaPlace, with increasing end-diastolic volume left ventricular systolic wall tension must increase, causing further left ventricular dilatation with concomitant increased myocardial oxygen consumption.

Preoperative

While congestive heart failure, angina, recurrent ventricular tachyarrhythmias and systemic emboli are the major indications for left ventricular aneurysmectomy, congestive heart failure and angina are by far the most common indications. Recurrent ventricular tachycardia has been reported in 8 per cent of patients with left ventricular aneurysms[7, 8]. Although the presence of left ventricular thrombus is very common in left ventricular aneurysms, systemic emboli are not[8]. In recent years early surgery has been increasingly recommended for sizeable ventricular aneurysms as it has been observed that a number of initially asymptomatic patients treated medically develop progressive non-aneurysmal impairment of left ventricular muscle function in a manner similar to that which occurs in patients with chronic mitral regurgitation.

The operation

Extracorporeal circulation

The patient is placed on total cardiopulmonary bypass as previously described. Epicardial adhesions to the pericardium are invariably present over the aneurysm. These are divded by sharp dissection after the initiation of cardiopulmonary bypass with the heart decompressed and only after ventricular fibrillation has occurred or been induced in order to prevent embolization of intramural thrombus.

6

A laparotomy pack is then placed behind the heart and, with the ventricular vent on suction, the outlines of the ventricular aneurysm are seen. The ascending aorta is now cross-clamped and cold cardioplegia is induced. If coexistent bypassable coronary artery disease exists proximal aortosaphenous vein anastomoses are performed either before the initiation of cardiopulmonary bypass or during cooling. The distal coronary arteries are identified after induction of ventricular fibrillation and before aortic cross-clamping. The distal anastomoses are then constructed.

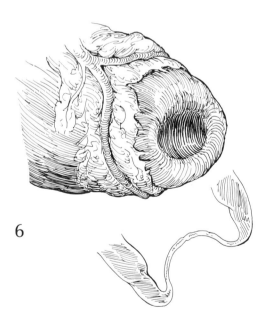

6

Repair of aneurysm

7

Attention is then turned towards repair of the left ventricular aneurysm. An incision is made longitudinally through the aneurysm.

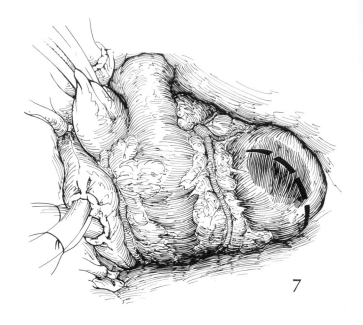

8

Laminated clot is carefully removed, the Penfield No. 4 elevator being used to remove the scarred endocardial layer to which the thrombus is adherent.

9

The walls of the aneurysm are then resected to within 2 cm of normal left ventricular muscle.

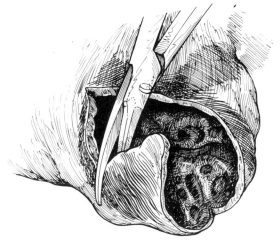

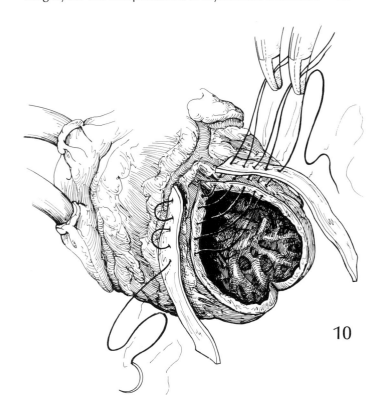

10

10

Two strips of Teflon felt are cut, and interrupted No. 0 Tevdek (No. 7–7052, C–3 needle, Deknatel) sutures are placed in horizontal mattress fashion in order to close the defect. Alternatively, a two-layer (running horizontal mattress followed by over-and-over) running 3/0 polypropylene suture technique may be used to close the ventriculotomy. This is a more expeditious technique and gives an excellent result.

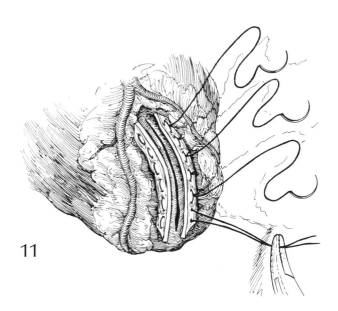

11

11

The sutures are then tied, beginning with those towards the base of the heart and finishing with the apical sutures. Before the apical sutures are tied the left ventricular vent is turned off and the aortic cross clamp removed.

12

The cardioplegic infusion catheter site in the ascending aorta is allowed to bleed freely and any air is subsequently vented from the apex of the left ventricle during vigorous ventilation and manual inversion of the left atrial appendage.

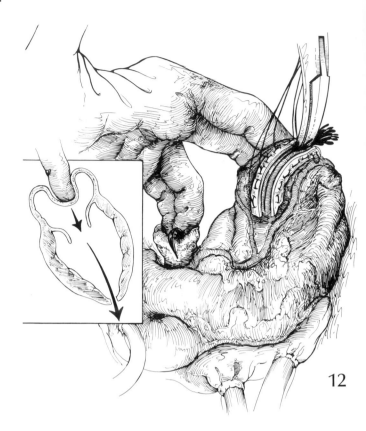

12

13

The patient is rewarmed as the remaining horizontal mattress sutures are tied and cut. Again starting from the base of the heart, a second layer of running over-and-over No. 0 Tevdek suture is carried out. The suture line is constructed so that it lies superficial to the horizontal mattress suture line already in place (b). Care should be taken to extend the suture line approximately 1–2 cm beyond the ends of the ventriculotomy.

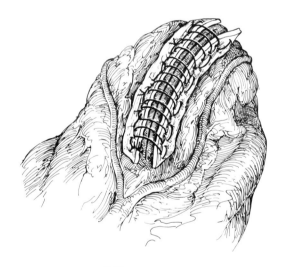

13

Termination of bypass

The heart is defibrillated if necessary and a polypropylene catheter is placed into the left atrium from the right superior pulmonary vein for pressure monitoring. Right atrial and right ventricular epicardial pacing electrodes are also placed. Normal sinus rhythm, atrial pacing or atrioventricular sequential pacing is maintained as indicated and the patient weaned from cardiopulmonary bypass.

If concomitant mitral valve replacement is necessary the transatrial approach already discussed is preferred. Mitral valve replacement is performed after construction of any distal coronary anastomoses and after closure of the left ventricular aneurysm site.

Postoperative management

The degree of contractile performance of the non-aneurysmal left ventricle has been correlated with operative mortality and postoperative functional results, and patients with an ejection fraction of the non-involved left ventricle greater than 30 per cent achieve better operative results[9, 10]. Current mortality rates for left ventricular aneurysmectomy range from 7 to 20 per cent, depending on the presence of preoperative congestive failure, extent of coexistent coronary artery disease and the degree of left ventricular dysfunction present in the non-aneurysmal segment. Long-term survival rates of 51 to 69 per cent 7–9 years after operation have been reported, depending on the degree of associated coronary artery disease and the degree of revascularization of the remaining myocardium[7, 11, 12].

The technique of left ventricular aneurysmectomy and electrophysiological studies for recurrent ventricular tachycardia are discussed in the chapter on 'Surgical treatment of cardiac arrhythmias', pp. 564–583.

VENTRICULAR SEPTAL DEFECT

Postinfarction ventricular septal defect (VSD) is an uncommon but usually devastating mechanical complication of acute myocardial infarction. Experience has demonstrated that patients in cardiogenic shock and those with posterior or inferior infarction are at highest risk[13–15].

Preoperative

The timing of operation is critical. At present all patients with postinfarction ventricular septal defect and cardiogenic shock undergo intra-aortic balloon pump placement, emergency catheterization, coronary arteriography and emergency operation. Delay of operation in these patients results in end-organ failure which is associated with a significantly lower postoperative salvage rate. Patients who are completely stable are operated upon more than 4 weeks after infarction. Those patients who are not in cardiogenic shock but not completely stable require operation within 3 weeks and need immediate intervention whenever early signs of haemodynamic or end-organ deterioration occur. Ventricular septal rupture should generally be regarded as a surgical emergency. To operate early is far less dangerous than to operate too late.

Surgical techniques have gradually evolved since the first successful operation for postinfarction VSD was perfomed by Cooley et al. in 1956[16]. Since postoperative right ventricular dysfunction is significant in this group of patients the VSD is no longer approached through the right ventricle but rather through the left ventricular infarct site. Differences in the geometry of the left ventricular anterior and posterior walls resulted in a high rate of postoperative left ventricular rupture following primary left ventricular closure with inferior or posterior defects. Prosthetic patch replacement of the left ventricular free wall defect remaining after inferior infarctectomy has significantly reduced this complication and generally improved the survival of patients undergoing operations for posterior VSD following inferior or inferoposterior myocardial infarction.

The operation

A median sternotomy incision and the institution of cardiopulmonary bypass with two caval drainage cannulae are perfomed as previously described. The patient is cooled to 25°C and when ventricular fibrillation occurs a left ventricular vent is placed via the right superior pulmonary vein.

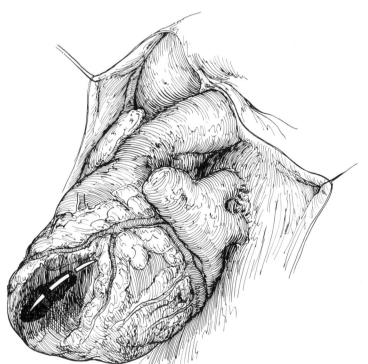

DEFECTS OF THE ANTERIOR SEPTUM

14

The limits of the anterior infarct are noted. The ascending aorta is cross-clamped and cold cardioplegic solution is infused into the aortic root as previously described. If bypassable coronary artery lesions are present proximal anastomoses are constructed either before the initiation of cardiopulmonary bypass or during cooling. Similarly, distal anastomoses are now constructed so that cardioplegic infusions can be given sequentially through newly constructed bypasses to diminish overall myocardial ischaemia.

14

15

The left ventricle is elevated by means of packs in the posterior pericardium. The anterior left ventricular infarct is then opened and the ventricular septum inspected for a ventricular septal defect. Once the defect is located and the margins debrided a piece of Teflon felt is placed posterior to its rim.

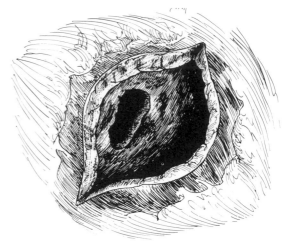

15

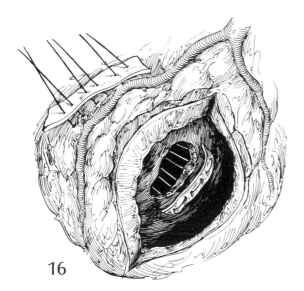

16

16

Interrupted No. 0 Tevdek sutures are then placed through this Teflon felt strip, through the posterior surface of the lower margin of the ventricular septal defect and out through the anterior wall of the right ventricle, and another Teflon felt strip is placed just to the right of the left anterior descending coronary artery. Multiple interrupted horizontal mattress sutures are placed in this fashion and tied down with subsequent obliteration of the septal communication.

17

The left ventriculotomy is then closed between two additional layers of Teflon felt using the two-layered No. 0 Tevdek approach previously described for aneurysm closure. During closure of the left ventriculotomy the ascending aortic cross clamp is removed and air is vented from the apex of the left ventricle and from the ascending aorta and the patient is rewarmed to 37°C.

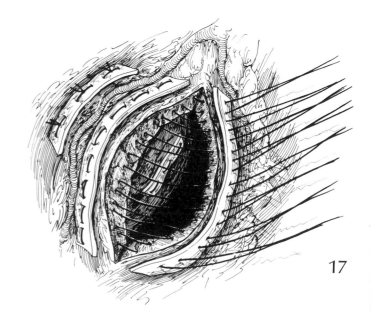

17

18

If on close inspection of the ventricular septum the loss of septal tissue is significant an elasticized knitted Dacron patch must be used in order to prevent dehiscence of the septal repair. 2/0 Teflon-pledgeted sutures are placed in horizontal mattress fashion through and through the interventricular septum, with the pledgets on the right ventricular side across the inferior rim of the defect. The anterior row of sutures is placed through a Teflon felt strip on the right ventricular free wall to the right of the septum and left anterior descending coronary artery, emerging at the anterior margin of the ventricular septal defect. A Dacron patch (DeBakey Dacron elastic fabric, USCI), is cut to size and the Tevdek stutures are passed through it.

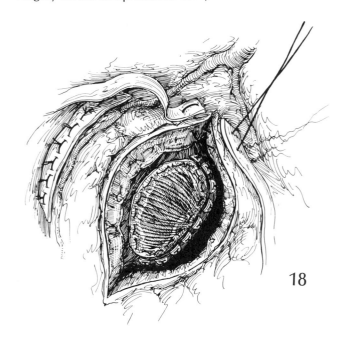

18

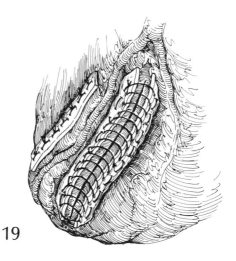

19

19

The patch is then seated on the left side of the septum and tied in place. After debridement of non-viable left ventricular tissue the left ventriculotomy is closed as previously described.

DEFECTS OF THE APICAL SEPTUM

20

Defects of the apical septum are approached through the
left ventricular apex.

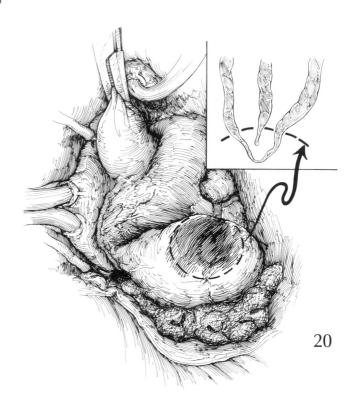

20

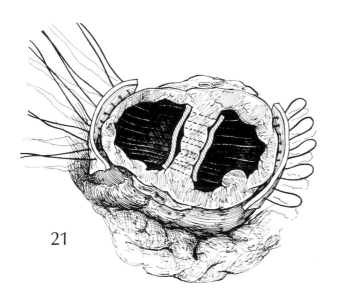

21

21

After debridement of left ventricular and right ventricular
apical non-viable tissue four strips of Teflon felt are placed
as follows: on the right ventricular free wall, right
ventricular septum, left ventricular septum and left
ventricular free wall.

22

Closure is accomplished with No. 0 Tevdek horizontal
mattress sutures through and through all layers of Teflon
felt.

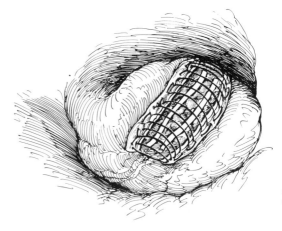

22

DEFECTS OF THE POSTERIOR SEPTUM

Median sternotomy, cardiopulmonary bypass with right heart exclusion and systemic hypothermia to 25°C are instituted as previously described. Topical cooling is employed and a vent is placed.

Minor septal loss

23

The heart is lifted out of the pericardial well and the inferior wall inspected. The margins of the inferior left ventricular infarct are noted. If concomitant coronary artery bypass grafting is to be performed proximal anastomoses are performed either before initiation of cardiopulmonary bypass or during cooling. The aorta is then cross-clamped and cold cardioplegic solution is infused into the aortic root. Subsequently, after aortic cross-clamping, the distal anastomoses are carried out. The heart is then elevated out of the pericardial well and retracted superiorly. It is helpful if the operator now moves to the patient's left side.

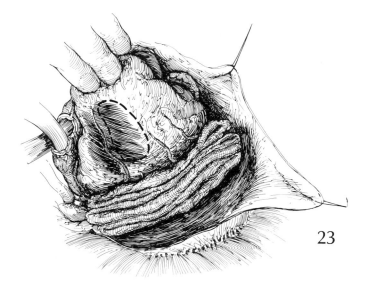

23

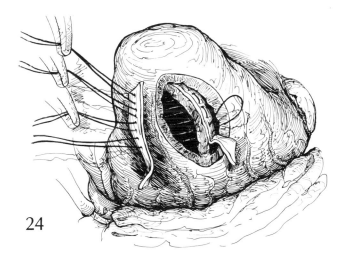

24

24

The left ventricular inferior infarct is opened and the margins of the infarct are debrided back to healthy tissue. Care is taken to avoid injury to the papillary muscles. Mitral valve replacement is not performed unless concomitant papillary muscle rupture is present. Close inspection of the inferior interventricular septum is carried out. If the posterior septum is only cracked or split off from the posterior left ventricular wall without significant loss of septal tissue the defect may be closed by plicating the septum to the free wall of the diaphragmatic right ventricle.

25

This is carried out with No. 0 Tevdek interrupted horizontal mattress sutures through a strip of Teflon felt on the left ventricular surface of the septum and through a second strip of Teflon felt on the inferior right ventricular wall to the right of the septum as in primary closure of a small anterior ventricular septal defect.

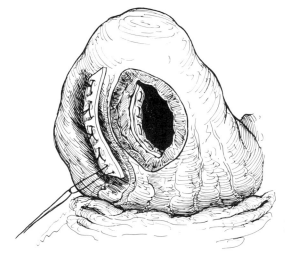

25

Major inferior septal loss

26

If, however, significant inferior septal muscle loss is noted
a patch must be placed. Mattress sutures of interrupted
2/0 Tevdek sutures buttressed by Teflon felt pledgets are
brought through from the right ventricular side of the
septum to its left ventricular side. Those sutures that are
placed on the diaphragmatic right ventricular surface are
placed with the pledgets on the epicardial surface of the
right ventricle.

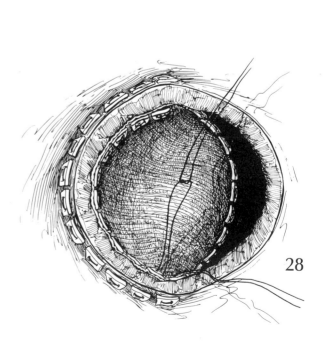

26

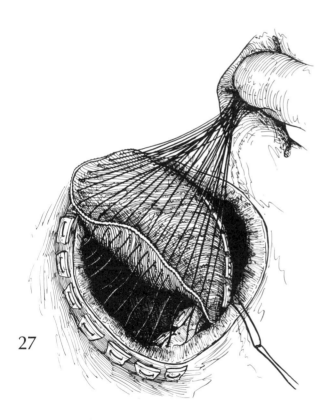

27

27

An elasticized patch of DeBakey Dacron elastic fabric is
then cut and the sutures are placed through the patch.

28

The patch is tied in place after additional Teflon felt
pledgets have been placed (*b*).

28

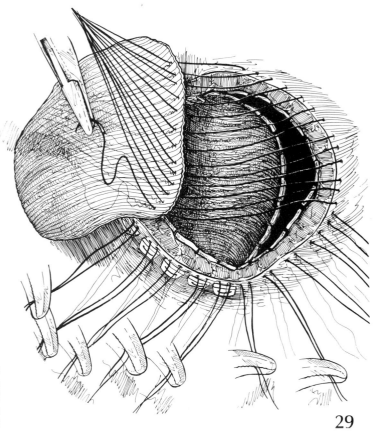

29

29 & 30

Subsequently, interrupted No. 0 Tevdek sutures are placed mattress-fashion circumferentially around the margins of the left ventricular surface. A segment of Cooley low-porosity woven Dacron patch (Meadox Medicals) is cut oversized. The sutures are then passed through this patch and tied after additonal Teflon pledgets have been placed beneath the ties.

The ascending aortic cross clamp is subsequently removed and the patient is rewarmed. The heart is defibrillated if indicated. Two polypropylene catheters are inserted into the left atrium through the right superior pulmonary vein. Two right atrial and two right ventricular epicardial pacing electrodes are placed. Once the patient has been rewarmed the left ventricular vent is clamped and the repair is inspected for leaks. It is important to place additional haemostatic sutures while the patient is on cardiopulmonary bypass so that these may be tied down under no tension with the brief discontinuation of extracorporeal circulation.

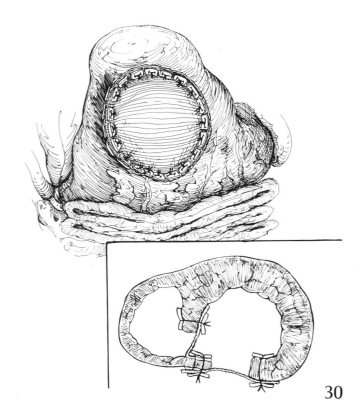

30

Postoperative management

After the repair has been completed right ventricular dysfunction is frequently seen. This is managed by continuing cardiopulmonary bypass and the institution of increased left ventricular perfusion pressure with inotropic support administered through a left atrial line. This has been shown to improve right ventricular function by increasing right ventricular myocardial perfusion without causing pulmonary vasoconstriction. Intra-aortic balloon pumping is continued for 3–4 days.

Results

Our recent results indicate 85 per cent survival after posterior septal rupture with recent progressive improvement in results. It is suggested that the reasons for improved surgical management of postinfarction VSD are: (1) an early aggressive operative approach, particularly in those patients with haemodynamic instability (which gives the best chance for the prevention of kidney, liver and brain dysfunction): (2) perioperative intra-aortic balloon; (3) a transinfarct approach to repair of the VSD; (4) closure of the left ventricular free wall defect with a prosthetic patch in cases of posterior septal rupture; and (5) improved intraoperative myocardial protection with cardioplegia.

References

1. Sanders, R. J., Neuberger, K. T., Ravin, A. Ruptures of papillary muscles: occurrence of rupture of the posterior muscle in posterior myocardial infarction. Diseases of the Chest 1957; 31: 316–323

2. Vlodaver, Z., Edwards, J. E. Rupture of the ventricular septum for papillary muscle complicating myocardial infarction. Circulation 1977; 55: 815–822

3. Austen, W. G., Sanders, C. A., Averill, J. H., Friedlich, A. L. Ruptured papillary muscle: report of a case with successful mitral valve replacement. Circulation 1965; 32: 597–601

4. Killen, D. A., Reed, W. A., Wathanacharoen, S., Beauchamp, G., Rutherford, B. Surgical treatment of papillary muscle rupture. Annals of Thoracic Surgery 1983; 35: 243–248

5. Schliechter, J., Hellerstein, H. K., Katz, L. N. Aneurysm of the heart: a correlative study of 102 proved cases. Medicine 1954; 33: 43–86

6. Nagle, R. E., Williams, D. O. Natural history of ventricular aneurysm without surgical treatment. British Heart Journal 1974; 36: 1037

7. Cosgrove, D. M., Loop, F. D. Long-term results and life expectancy after ventricular aneurysmectomy. In: Moran, J. M., Michaelis, L. L., eds. Surgery for the Complications of Myocardial Infarction. New York: Grune and Stratton, 1980: 289–302

8. Simpson, M. T., Oberman, A., Kouchoukos, N. T., Rogers, W. J. Prevalence of mural thrombi and systemic embolization with left ventricular aneurysm: effect of anticoagulation therapy. Chest 1980; 77: 463–469

9. Watson, L. E., Dickhaus, D. W., Martin, R. H. Left ventricular aneurysm. Preoperative hemodynamics, chamber volume and results of aneurysmectomy. Circulation 1975; 52: 868–873

10. Shaw, R. C., Connors, J. P., Hieb, B. R. et al. Postoperative investigation of left ventricular aneurysm resection. Circulation 1977; 56 (Suppl. II): 7–11

11. Cooperman, M., Stinson, E. B., Griepp, R. B., Shumway, N. E. Survival and function after left ventricular aneurysmectomy. Journal of Thoracic and Cardiovascular Surgery 1975; 69: 321–328

12. Cooley, D. A., Walker, W. E. Surgical treatment of postinfarction ventricular aneurysm: evolution of technique and results in fifteen hundred and thirty-three patients. In: Moran, J. M., Michaelis, L. L., eds. Surgery for the Complications of Myocardial Infarction. New York: Grune and Stratton, 1980: 273–287

13. Gaudiani, V. A., Miller, D. C., Stinson, E. B. et al. Postinfarction ventricular septal defect: argument for early operation. Surgery 1981; 89: 48–55

14. Radford, M. J., Johnson, R. A., Daggett, W. M. et al. Ventricular septal rupture: a review of clinical and physiologic features and an analysis of survival. Circulation 1981; 64: 545–553

15. Daggett, W. M., Buckley, M. J., Akins, C. W. et al. Improved results of surgical management of postinfarction ventricular septal rupture. Annals of Surgery 1982; 196: 269–277

16. Cooley, D. A., Belmonte, B. A., Zeis, L. B., Schnur, S. Surgical repair of ruptured interventricular septum following acute myocardial infarction. Surgery 1957; 41: 930–937

Trauma to the heart and great vessels

Panagiotis N. Symbas MD
Professor of Surgery, Emory University School of Medicine, Atlanta, Georgia, USA

Introduction

Injury to the heart may be due to penetrating or non-penetrating trauma and is a major cause of death in injured patients. Trauma to the heart of sufficient severity to be the sole cause of death is found in a significant number of the victims of blunt trauma. Over 50 per cent of patients who sustain penetrating trauma to the heart die shortly after their injury. Prompt and proper management of these accident victims will improve their survival.

Penetrating wounds of the heart

A penetrating wound of the heart is one of the most dramatic and urgent problems confronting the surgeon. It is most often due to a knife or bullet wound and is usually associated with a precordial wound of the chest wall, although it is seen with wounds in other areas of the chest, upper abdomen and neck. The clinical manifestations of penetrating cardiac wounds usually depend upon the site and size of both the pericardial and cardiac wounds and are those of blood loss, haemothorax and/or cardiac tamponade. Cardiac wounds which manifest with bleeding are treated initially by repletion of the decreased intravascular blood volume, drainage of the thoracic cavity with tube thoracostomy and other appropriate resuscitative measures. Expansion of the circulating blood volume may be readily accomplished by autotransfusion of blood drained from the thoracic cavity.

Patients with cardiac tamponade are immediately treated by expansion of the intravascular blood volume and pericardiocentesis. All patients with suspected or proved cardiac wounds are definitively managed by exploration and surgical repair as soon as feasible.

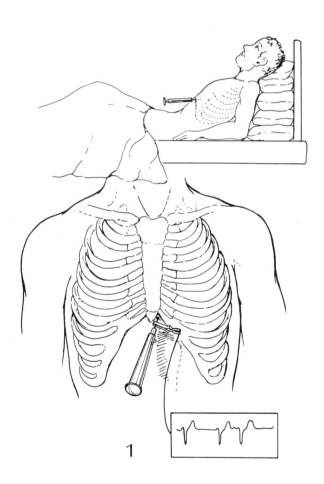

1

1

Pericardiocentesis

With the patient in a supine position with the chest raised to 40–50° the lower sternal and upper abdominal area is appropriately prepared and draped. The skin to the left of the xiphoid process is infiltrated with local anaesthetic and a thin-walled 18-gauge needle, or preferably a plastic needle, is inserted into the skin slightly below the tip of the angle formed by the xiphoid process and left costal margin. The needle is then advanced upward towards the left shoulder and backwards at about 30° from the skin surface. Approximately 6 cm under the skin a tough structure, the membranous portion of the diaphragm and pericardium, can be felt. This structure is carefully pierced, at which point the needle is in the pericardial sac and the beating heart may be felt tapping against it. As much blood as possible is aspirated and, if a plastic needle was used, it is left in place for constant decompression of the pericardial space until thoracotomy can be performed.

Repair of cardiac wound

2

With the patient still in the supine position but with the left chest elevated to 30° the entire chest from the lateral margin of the left latissimus dorsi muscle to the right anterior axillary line is rapidly prepared and draped while the operating team is ready or preparing to perform a rapid thoracotomy if needed. An anterolateral submammary incision is made extending from the left lateral sternal border to the midaxillary line. The fourth intercostal space is identified by first identifying the sternomanubrial junction, which corresponds to the second rib. If necessary the left breast is elevated and the pectoralis muscle incised as well as the fourth intercostal muscles.

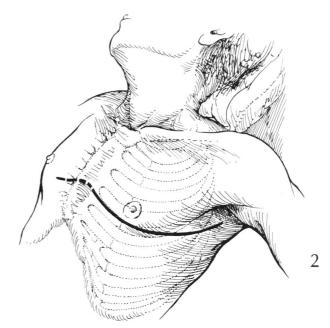

2

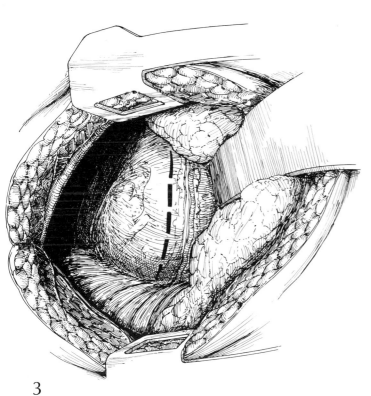

3

Once the incision is completed a standard chest wall retractor is inserted with the handle towards the left axilla, the left lung is retracted laterally and the phrenic nerve is identified. The bluish and tense pericardium is lifted either with tissue forceps or with clamps and is incised anteriorly and parallel to the phrenic nerve. Non-clotted blood is aspirated and pericardiotomy is completed by incising the pericardium anteriorly and parallel to the phrenic nerve, extending from the diaphragm inferiorly to the great vessels superiorly. If necessary the pericardial incision is converted to a T incision, the vertical limb of the T passing anteriorly from the first incision.

3

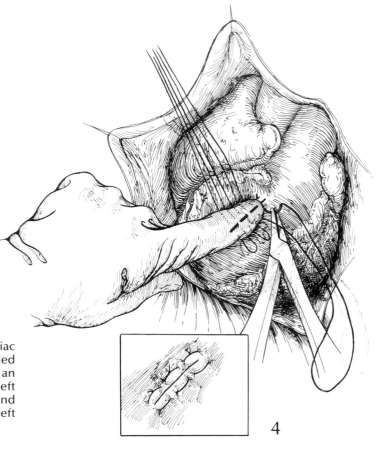

4, 5 & 6

The clotted blood is then evacuated manually, the cardiac wound is identified and bleeding, if present, is controlled digitally, with crossing sutures or, if the wound is in an atrium, with a vascular clamp. The heart is then left undisturbed for a period of time to regain function and restore tissue perfusion. Similarly the heart is left undisturbed if no evidence of bleeding is present.

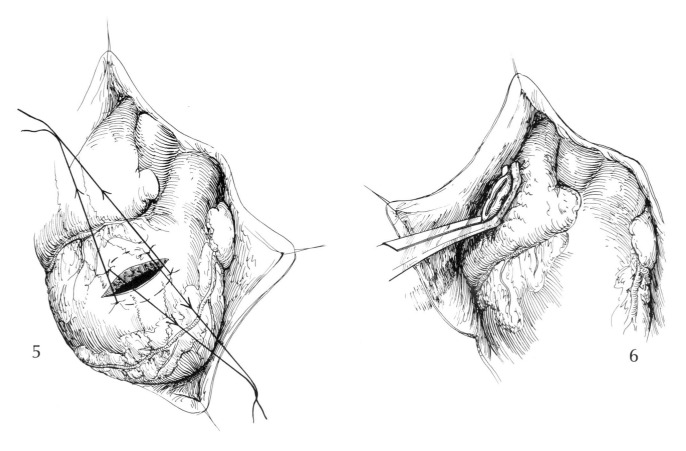

7

The wound is then repaired with over-and-over or horizontal pledgetted mattress sutures. When the cardiac wound is close to a coronary artery care is taken not to incorporate the artery into the sutures. If the wound is into the opposite pleural space or for any reason cannot be visualized the thoracotomy incision is extended by a submammary incision into the opposite chest. The sternum is transversely transected with a Gigli's saw passed behind the sternum, thereby creating a bilateral thoracotomy.

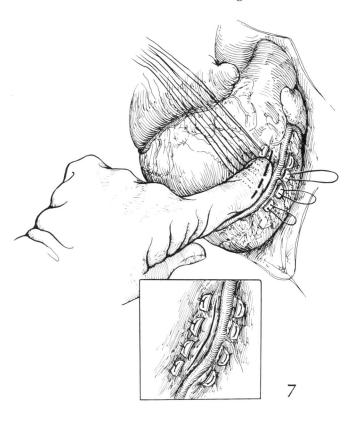

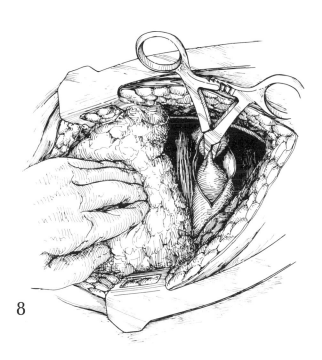

8

If cardiac arrest occurs when the pericardium is opened the left lung is quickly retracted anteriorly and the descending aorta exposed. The aorta is then grasped with one of the operator's hands and is cross-clamped at the midthoracic level, special care being taken to avoid the adjacent oesophagus.

9

The heart is then massaged bimanually to control the bleeding through the wound as much as possible and to avoid extension of the cardiac wound. The cardiac wound is then rapidly repaired and cardiac massage is continued until a normal heartbeat resumes. Once the heart resumes vigorous beating the vascular clamp of the descending aorta is slowly released as the patient's blood volume is restored. The surgical wound is closed without closing the pericardium and the pleural space is drained through a thoracostomy tube.

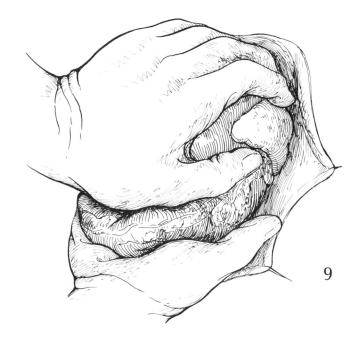

Non-penetrating wounds of the heart

Blunt trauma to the heart may result in rupture of the free cardiac wall, the ventricular septum or the aortic or atrioventricular valves. Few patients survive such an injury and the management of these patients is a challenging problem.

RUPTURE OF THE FREE CARDIAC WALL

Rupture of the free cardiac wall may occur at the time of injury or be delayed for up to 2 weeks as a result of the softening of the contused myocardial segment, whereas rupture of the ventricular septum or cardiac valves usually occurs at the time of injury.

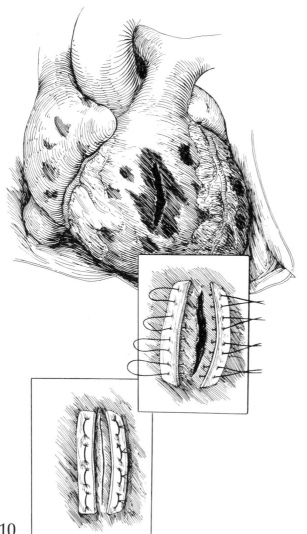

10

Patients with acute rupture of the free cardiac wall usually die immediately or within hours of the injury. The clinical manifestations are cardiac tamponade, haemothorax and shock. Delayed rupture of the heart manifests itself similarly to rupture following a myocardial infarction, the patient presenting with chest pain, cardiac tamponade or decreased cardiac output.

Patients with rupture of the free cardiac wall should undergo immediate exploration if operating facilities are available, otherwise pericardiocentesis should be performed immediately to relieve the cardiac tamponade. This should be followed as soon as possible by thoracotomy.

The incision

Thoracotomy is performed through a left anterolateral submammary incision through the fourth intercostal space or through a vertical sternum-splitting incision, the operative management being similar to that for the patient with a penetrating wound of the heart.

Repair of the wound

The method of repair of the cardiac wound is dependent upon the site, size and extent of the coexisting cardiac contusion. Atrial wounds amenable to tangential clamping are repaired by first controlling the bleeding with an appropriate vascular clamp. When the myocardium adjacent to the wound is not significantly injured the wound is repaired with running over-and-over sutures or with interrupted horizontal pledgetted sutures.

10

The bleeding from atrial wounds not amenable to occlusion with a vascular clamp or through ventricular wounds is controlled digitally and the repair is performed with interrupted horizontal pledgetted sutures or continuous horizontal mattress sutures buttressed with Teflon felt strips. Inaccessible or large wounds usually necessitate the use of cardiopulmonary bypass for their repair. After cardiopulmonary bypass has been instituted the wound is repaired with the use of Teflon pledgets or strips to buttress the interrupted horizontal sutures since the myocardium is often softened and contused at the site of the injury.

11

When the defect is too large to be closed primarily a Dacron prosthetic patch graft may be used for the repair.

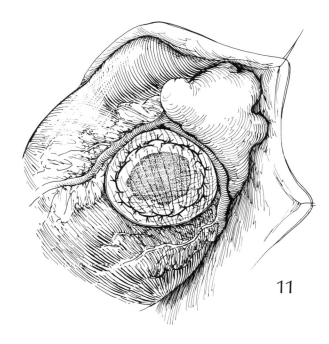

11

VALVULAR RUPTURE

The clinical manifestations of valvular rupture depend upon which valve is injured, the extent of the injury, the time lapse between the injury and examination and the other coexisting injuries to the heart and other organs. Symptoms and signs of congestive heart failure, cardiac tamponade or intrathoracic bleeding may be present if rupture of the free cardiac wall is also present. The diagnosis can usually be made by auscultation or by echocardiographic, phonocardiographic, haemodynamic and angiocardiographic studies. Cardiac valve injuries are best initially managed medically; however, if the injury is haemodynamically significant, then valve replacement will be necessary.

RUPTURE OF VENTRICULAR SEPTUM

The ventricular septum is particularly vulnerable to rupture by blunt trauma during late diastole or early systole since the compression-type force is applied while the ventricular chambers are filled and the valves are closed.

The clinical manifestations during the acute period depend upon the size of the defect, the absence or presence of cardiac tamponade and/or the presence of coexisting cardiac or other organ injuries. The symptoms and signs are similar to those of a ventricular septal defect following myocardial infarction. Symptoms and signs of cardiac tamponade and haemothorax may also be present if rupture of the free cardiac wall has also occurred. A systolic thrill and murmur are usually noted, but their appearance may be delayed for several hours or days after the injury. The definitive diagnosis of this injury is made by cardiac catheterization.

The prognosis of patients with traumatic septal defect depends upon the size of the defect and the existence of other cardiac or non-cardiac injuries. If possible, surgery should be performed electively at 4–8 weeks after injury. If there is extensive myocardial contusion in addition to the ventricular septal defect, then circulatory support with the intra-aortic balloon pump can be used for a few days to help stabilize the patient's condition.

Repair of the defect

12

The repair of the ventricular septal defect is performed through a median sternotomy incision. Since the vast majority of the defects require closure during the acute post-injury period and since in most of the patients contusion of the ventricular wall is present and the defect is located in the muscular septum near the apex its closure must include contused ventricular tissue.

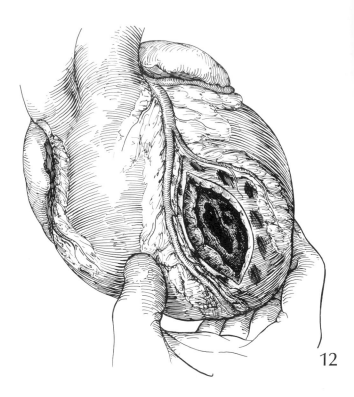

12

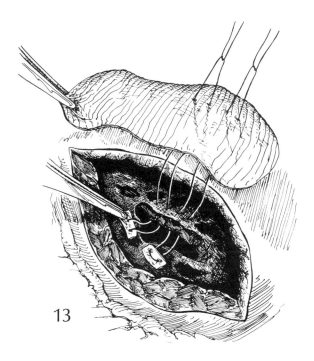

13

13

The defect is therefore closed with the use of a patch sutured with horizontal pledgetted sutures placed through the non-contused ventricular septum.

14

The ventriculotomy is then closed with interrupted horizontal pledgetted mattress sutures or with Teflon strips similar to the closure of rupture of the free cardiac wall by placing the sutures through the right ventricular wall next to the anterior descending coronary artery, through the patch and then through the left ventricular wall.

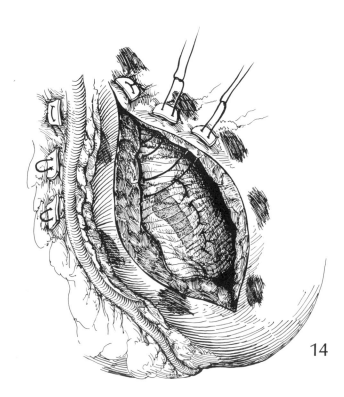

14

Penetrating wounds of the great vessels

Penetrating injury to the great vessels is frequently associated with massive bleeding, which makes the treatment of this injury challenging. Clinical manifestations of great vessel injuries include massive haemothorax with or without symptoms and signs of haemorrhagic shock, cardiac tamponade, haematoma of the lower neck, absent or weak carotid or radial pulses and/or symptoms and signs of arteriovenous, aortocardiac or aortopulmonary fistula. The management of these patients depends on the clincial presentation of the injuries but usually includes maintenance of an adequate airway, relief of cardiac tamponade and restoration of the circulating blood volume until the patient can be transferred to the operating theatre for the repair of the wound.

The incision

The patient is placed in the supine position with the thorax and neck prepared over a wide area and draped so that the median sternotomy or thoracotomy incision can be extended if necessary.

Lower cervical or thoracic injuries manifesting themselves with bleeding are usually approached through a left anterolateral thoracotomy through the fourth intercostal space. This incision can be extended if necessary to the right pleural space after transection of the sternum, to the neck by transection of the upper sternum and to the supraclavicular area parallel to the clavicle.

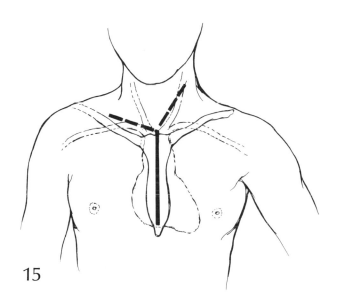

15

15

All aortic injuries other than those in the descending aorta and injuries of the great vessels diagnosed by arteriography are repaired through a median sternotomy with or without extension of the incision into the neck or supraclavicular region. Injuries of the descending aorta are approached through a posterolateral thoracotomy.

Repair of wound

Most of the aortic wounds can be repaired after tangential clamping of the aorta. Stab wounds are then repaired with a running over-and-over 3/0 non-absorbable synthetic suture whereas bullet wounds are preferably repaired with interrupted horizontal 3/0 pledgetted sutures. Aorto-pulmonary and aortocardiac communications or ascending aortic wounds requiring cross-clamping of the aorta are repaired under cardiopulmonary bypass in a similar manner to those of congenital origin.

16

Wounds of the descending aorta which necessitate cross-clamping of the aorta when the required aortic occlusion time is less than 25 minutes may be repaired without any distal aortic perfusion. When the required occlusion time would be greater than 25 minutes the repair is performed either with the use of an external shunt (as illustrated) or under femoral vein to femoral artery bypass. Innominate or left common carotid wounds are preferably repaired with the use of an internal shunt, though repair may be possible without a shunt. When bypass or a shunt is used for the repair during the aortic cross-clamping period the arterial pressure of the right arm and lower extremities is constantly monitored and balanced perfusion of both vascular compartments is maintained.

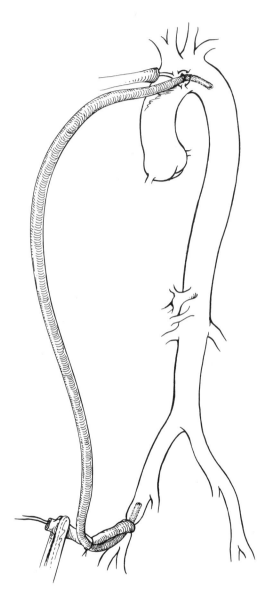

16

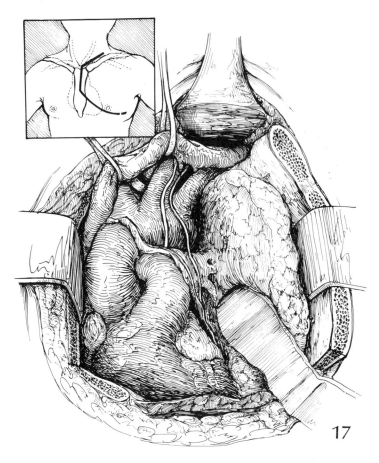

17

In penetrating trauma to the arch or great vessels exposure can be readily obtained by a combined thoracotomy-sternotomy with extension into the neck. The innominate vein is shown here protected by encircling tapes, but it may be sacrificed if necessary.

17

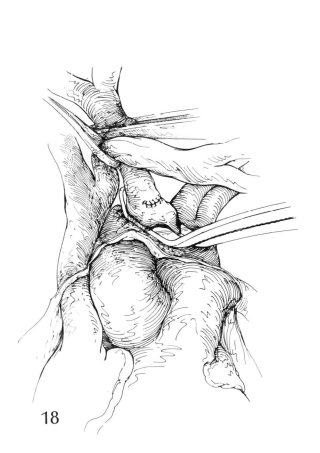

18

Repair of penetrating wounds to the vessels to the brain may be carried out with the use of a small shunt from the ascending aorta.

18

Traumatic rupture of the aorta

Rupture of the aorta and great vessels may result from blunt trauma. The aortic isthmus and ascending aorta are the most frequent sites of injury, although rarely an injury may occur in the aortic arch or the descending or abdominal aorta. The majority of patients who survive the injury and reach hospital alive have rupture at the aortic isthmus. The stresses applied to the aorta which cause rupture are torsion, shearing and bending stresses.

Rupture of the aorta manifests itself with bleeding or increased pulse amplitude and blood pressure in the upper extremities, decreased pulse amplitudes and blood pressure in the lower extremities and radiographic evidence of widening of the mediastinum. The diagnosis can only be established by aortography, which should be performed on all patients with blunt trauma and one or more of the above findings.

Repair of aortic rupture should be carried out as an emergency. If for any reason this cannot be done immediately after the injury the patient should be treated as any patient with aortic dissection to protect him from complete aortic rupture and exsanguination and the repair should be performed as soon as possible thereafter.

Repair of rupture

Repair of isthmic rupture of the aorta is performed through a posterolateral thoracotomy in the fourth intercostal space. The correction of the lesion may be attempted without provision for perfusion of organs distal to aortic cross-clamping only if the repair can be completed in less than 25 minutes. When the repair cannot be performed within that period some form of bypass, left atrial to femoral artery or femoral vein to femoral artery, or external shunt from proximal to distal aorta or femoral artery should be used. When systemic anticoagulation is contraindicated an external shunt should be employed.

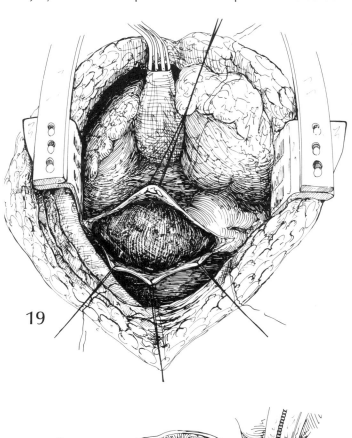

19

19

While the thoracotomy is being performed the left common femoral vessels are exposed for cannulation. The left lung is collapsed and retracted medially and ventilation is maintained with the right lung. The aorta distal to the mediastinal haematoma is dissected out and encircled with a tape. The femoral vein and artery are then cannulated and the venous cannula is advanced into the inferior vena cava for partial femoral vein to femoral artery bypass if this is decided upon.

When aorta to femoral artery shunt is chosen as a bypass procedure (see illustration 16) the ascending aorta and femoral artery are cannulated with a heparin-bound Gott shunt. After bypass has been initiated the ligamentum arteriosum is divided if this has not been done previously and the aorta is cross-clamped between the left common carotid and left subclavian artery and distal to the rupture; the left subclavian is also clamped.

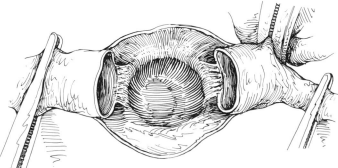

20

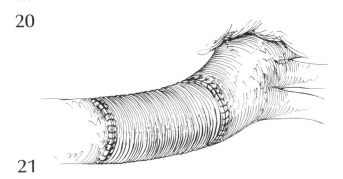

21

20 & 21

The false aneurysm is then opened along the axis of the aorta and the continuity of the aorta is restored with a woven graft interposition.

Surgical treatment of thoracic aortic aneurysms

D. Craig Miller MD
Associate Professor of Cardiovascular Surgery, Stanford University School of Medicine, Stanford, California, USA

Introduction

Discussion of aneurysms of the thoracic aorta and aortic dissections involving the thoracic aorta has been divided into three chapters since the aetiology, indications for operation and many technical details differ markedly in these conditions. The aim of these chapters is to describe and illustrate the important technical features of the operative procedures.

Extracorporeal circulation

Although this is discussed in the chapter on 'Cardio-pulmonary bypass and circulatory support', pp. 51–64, certain of its features are unique in the operative treatment of thoracic aortic aneurysms (both ascending and descending), aortic dissections and aortic arch aneurysms. Therefore these features are briefly summarized here for operative procedures involving the ascending and descending aorta and interspersed at later points in this and the following two chapters where necessary.

1

Total cardiopulmonary bypass with femoral artery arterial cannulation is used for all procedures for the treatment of aneurysms or dissections of the ascending aorta. This entails bicaval cannulation using two multifenestrated 28 Fr cannulae without snaring the superior and inferior vena cavae. The use of separate catheters results in better right heart decompression and facilitates the operative procedure because the venous return line (to the oxygenator) can be placed out of the operative field, this not being easily achieved with the use of a single large (52 Fr) two-stage cavoatrial cannula. In patients who have extremely large aneurysms peripheral venous cannulation can be used, a long 28 Fr caval catheter being inserted via the right femoral vein into the right atrium; a second 'Y-ed' caval catheter can be inserted in the usual manner once the sternum is opened. The right femoral vein is preferred to the left because the anatomy of the abdominal aorta and inferior vena cava junctions favours successful passage of a catheter from the right. This is due to the fact that the left iliac vein passes under the right iliac artery and the angulation is more severe at the caval junction on the left. As will be discussed below, this also applies to cases in which partial femoral-femoral cardiopulmonary bypass is used, even though exposure in the right (or 'down') groin is not as easy as the left.

For arterial cannulation the right common femoral artery is used. If severe peripheral atherosclerotic disease is present, or in patients with aortic dissection, the femoral artery containing the best pulse or found by angiography to be perfused by the true lumen should be used. In complicated cases extension of the incision into the retroperitoneum may be necessary in order to cannulate the external or common iliac artery. This may also be the case in children.

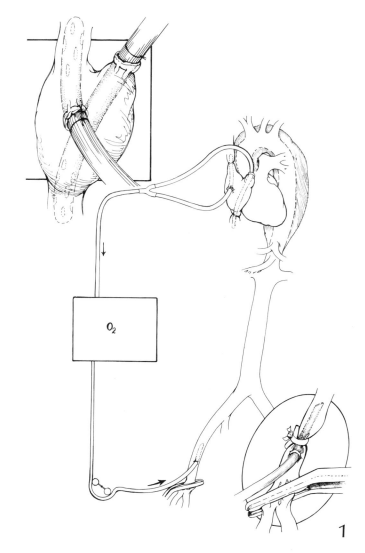

1

2

Partial femoro-femoral cardiopulmonary bypass is used for all procedures involving the descending thoracic aorta. While this method and all other methods of spinal cord protection do not provide complete immunity from paraplegia, experience indicates that this is the safest of all options in terms of protecting both the spinal cord and the kidneys. Serious disadvantages associated with systemic heparinization, which is necessary with this technique, have not been encountered. This is due in part to the advent of low-porosity soft woven Dacron grafts, better suture materials (polypropylene) and single-lung ventilation with endobronchial intubation.

Venous cannulation is accomplished via the femoral vein, a long (28 Fr or 24 Fr) multifenestrated catheter being threaded up into the right atrium. If the venous cannula can only be inserted as far as the iliac vein bifurcation inadequate venous return may result. In such circumstances the opposite common femoral vein should be dissected out and cannulation attempted. If the long venous cannula again cannot be advanced into the right atrium, then the catheter can be left in the common iliac vein, but supplemental venous return must be provided; this can be done by simply 'Y-ing' a second venous cannula into the venous return line. The second cannula is a 22 or 24 Fr Bardic catheter inserted through a purse-string suture into the main pulmonary artery. While it is rarely necessary to have to resort to pulmonary artery supplemental venous cannulation, this is preferable to attempting to use partial cardiopulmonary bypass with only a common iliac vein cannula.

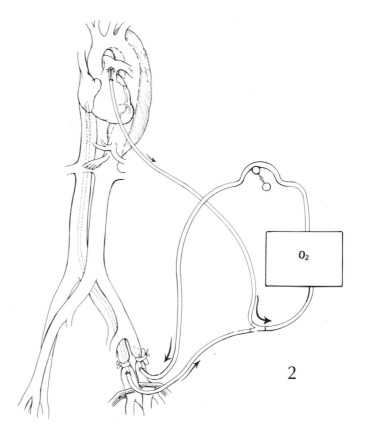

2

The operations

ASCENDING THORACIC ANEURYSMS

Aneurysms of the ascending aorta are approached through a standard median sternotomy incision. If the aneurysm is entered on opening the sternum or difficulties arise in patients who have been operated upon previously, cardiopulmonary bypass with peripheral cannulation can be instituted at that time. In very rare cases, e.g. a false aneurysm which is intimately adherent to the entire posterior sternum, entry into the chest may be most safely accomplished with profound hypothermia and circulatory arrest.

3

The pericardium is opened and preparation for bicaval cannulation performed. Dissection continues to expose fully the distal extent of the aneurysm, but only to the degree that this is safe. If previous rupture or presence of a huge aneurysm has resulted in the tissue planes between the aneurysm and other contiguous structures (such as the superior vena cava, innominate vein, pulmonary artery and lung) becoming obliterated, then these tissues are not dissected free at this time. For the purposes of this chapter it is assumed that the aneurysm terminates proximal to the origin of the innominate artery; if the aneurysm involves the proximal portion of the transverse aortic arch then special cannulation with cross-clamping of the transverse arch may be necessary (*see* chapter on 'Aortic arch aneurysms').

Cardiopulmonary bypass is started and the patient is cooled to 30°C. During this time more dissection of the aneurysm can be accomplished safely, including circumferential control of the distal aorta if the aneurysm is not densely adherent to surrounding structures. Mobilization of the innominate vein allows complete exposure of the proximal arch. Care must be taken not to avulse large branches of the innominate vein, including the left and the right internal mammary veins. In patients who have undergone previous surgery the innominate vein should be mobilized before the sternal retractor is opened too widely, which might result in avulsion of the vein from the superior vena cava.

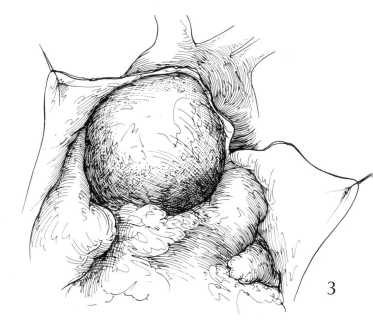

3

4

After the heart has either fibrillated spontaneously owing to the systemic hypothermia or is fibrillated deliberately with either topical hypothermia or transient electrical stimulation, the distal ascending aorta is cross-clamped at the level of the innominate artery with a large angled clamp. The aneurysm is then opened obliquely. A single dose of cardioplegia (500 ml of cold hyperkalaemic crystalloid solution into each coronary ostium) is then used to arrest the heart. Since many of these patients have aortic regurgitation, injection of cardioplegic solution into the aortic root is contraindicated. In addition, attention is paid to keeping the heart submerged under a continuous (100–200 ml/minute) bath of cold lactated Ringer's or saline solution during the entire period of aortic cross-clamping. This supplemental profound topical hypothermia obviates the need for repeated doses of cardioplegic solution and/or resorting to very low (20°–24°C) systemic temperatures on cardiopulmonary bypass. The use of a pulmonary artery vent (as illustrated) is optional. This 14 Fr sump vent effectively reduces the amount of bronchial circulation returning to the left ventricle. This has been found to obviate the use of a left ventricular vent in almost all cases, though in cases of long-standing aortic regurgitation with resultant massive left ventricular hypertrophy and dilatation the use of an apical left ventricular vent (20 Fr sump vent) may allow more effective resuscitation of the heart after the cross clamp has been removed.

If annular dilatation or the aneurysmal process itself has resulted in important aortic regurgitation or if severe valvular pathology is present the aortic valve is excised as illustrated. It is important to emphasize here that this is generally not necessary in patients with *acute* aortic dissections (*see* next chapter) in most of whom the native aortic valve can be preserved by means of reconstructive techniques.

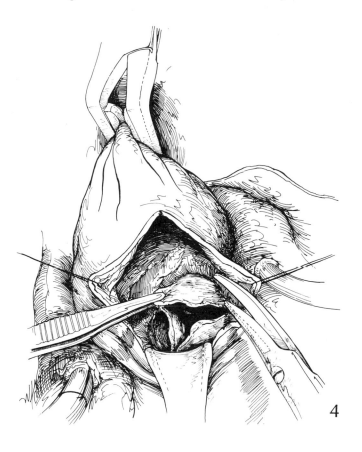

4

5

The majority of patients with ascending thoracic aortic aneurysms today have either annuloaortic ectasia (with or without Marfan's syndrome) or coexistent aortic regurgitation, so that usually aortic valve replacement is performed concomitantly with resection of the aneurysm. (If concomitant aortic valve replacement is not necessary, then the techniques of graft insertion are the same except that the aorta below the sinotubular ridge must be retained so as not to disrupt the commissural support of the aortic valve; portions of the sinus can be resected and replaced with graft material if the proximal end of the graft is tailored appropriately.) The aortic valve is replaced with a bioprosthesis or a mechanical prosthesis of the surgeon's choice. The preferred technique is to take interrupted horizontal mattress sutures from the aortic to the ventricular aspect of the annulus, using braided Dacron on a sharp half-circle needle. After the prosthesis has been carefully seated into place and the sutures tied and cut attention is directed to the aneurysm.

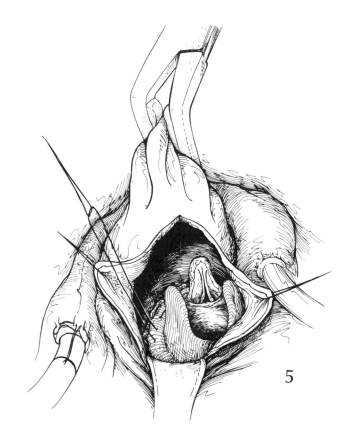

5

6

With the aneurysm open more dissection can be carried out, which was impossible previously with the heart beating on cardiopulmonary bypass and the aneurysm closed. It is still important, however, not to attempt to dissect the entire aneurysm free from adjacent structures when it is densely adherent. In such cases portions of the aneurysm wall can be left in continuity with these structures; important details include careful and meticulous dissection of the aortic root just above the level of the annulus. This must be done in an assiduous fashion, sweeping all aortic adventitia off the right ventricular infundibulum, main and right pulmonary arteries, superior vena cava and left and right atria. Small tongues of aorta are dissected free above the left and right main coronary ostia. If the coronary ostia are displaced markedly (>3 cm) cephalad (as is sometimes the case in patients with Marfan's syndrome and/or annuloaortic ectasia), then such a technique is not applicable and the coronary arteries must be reimplanted (*see Illustrations 12–14*). A small (8 Fr) rubber catheter can be inserted into the main coronary arteries to facilitate dissection of these full-thickness tongues of aortic cuff around the ostia.

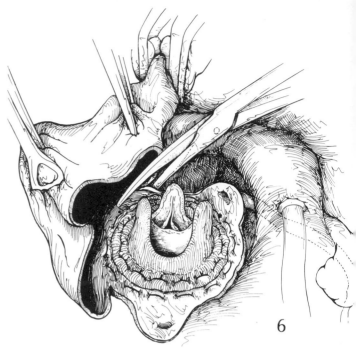

6

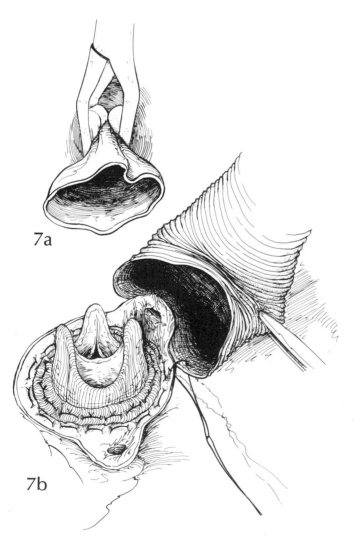

7a

7b

7a & b

When the proximal aortic cuff has been suitably prepared (*a*) a long 3/0 polypropylene suture (140 cm (54 inches)) is used for the proximal graft anastomosis. The suture is started on the left posterolateral aspect of the aorta, taking a generous needle bite of the remaining aortic cuff (*b*). The other needle is passed through the graft, which has been tailored appropriately to conform to the configuration of the proximal aortic root. Currently the low-porosity very soft woven Dacron grafts mentioned above (*see* p. 511) are preferred. These grafts are so impervious to blood that they can be used without preclotting, though it is probably safest to preclot them with non-heparinized autologous blood. Preclotting techniques applicable to other grafts also include autoclaving the graft with either blood, fresh frozen plasma, albumin or platelet concentrates. One advantage of not having to preclot the low-porosity grafts is that graft size selection can be deferred until the aorta is open and the aortic cuff prepared. This advantage is even more apparent in patients with aortic dissections, as discussed in the next chapter.

The distal aortic cuff can be prepared at this time or after the proximal anastomosis is completed. Again a circumferential, full-thickness aortic cuff is prepared, leaving 5 mm or more of aorta to be used for the distal anastomosis. As was emphasized in describing dissection of the proximal aortic cuff, meticulous attention must be paid to sweeping all aortic adventitia towards the aorta so that this tissue can be incorporated into the distal anastomosis. This point is important because the adventitial layer contains the greatest amount of tensile strength and incorporation of this layer into the suture line produces the soundest and most haemostatic anastomosis.

8

The proximal suture line is first constructed in a continuous fashion along the posterior rim of the aortic cuff. The graft is displaced caudad and is held on gentle traction. Deep bites of aorta are taken and constant traction is applied to the continuous suture line as it is constructed. In many cases the tissue is quite friable and great care is necessary in passing the needle through the aortic cuff, pulling it through on the curve of the needle and maintaining the proper amount of following traction on the suture by the assistant. The suture bites are taken down close to the prosthetic valve sewing ring except in the areas of the coronary ostia, where the needle point is passed right into the ostium of the coronary artery. This effectively obliterates the bulk of the aortic root without resorting to 'composite' techniques. A second polypropylene suture can be placed opposite the initial suture to aid alignment of the graft circumference; this is not mandatory, but is occasionally helpful. The proximal end of the graft has been tailored to conform to the tongues of aortic root left around the coronary arteries. If the graft is still relatively small compared with the aortic root circumference, then the effective circumference of the graft can be enlarged by excising a scalloped 'half moon' portion of the graft with shallow angles in the bias cut. Similar techniques can be used distally, but usually the distal aorta is much smaller than the graft and other modification techniques are necessary.

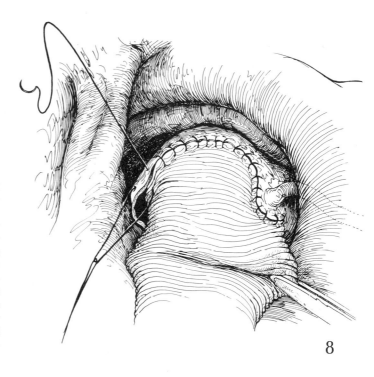

8

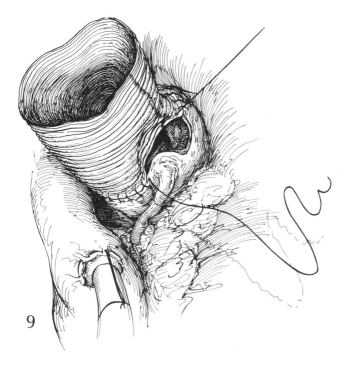

9

9

The same 140 cm 3/0 polypropylene suture is continued around anteriorly; the anterior portion of the anastomosis is most easily performed forehand by the assistant. To ensure that the right coronary artery is not compromised it is preferable to terminate this arm of the suture to the right of the right coronary artery; the other arm of the initial suture is then run anteriorly up and over the ostium of the right coronary. Again the suture bites are taken right down close to the prosthetic sewing ring except in the region of the right coronary ostium, where the needle is passed into the coronary ostium. In the right antero-lateral and anterior portions of the aorta it is important to ensure that the sutures do not inadvertently compromise the portion of the right coronary artery that lies superficially in the atrioventricular groove. A helpful manoeuvre is to insert a small (8 Fr) blunt-tipped rubber catheter into the coronary artery to prevent injury to this vessel.

10

After completion of the proximal suture line the graft is trimmed to the appropriate length, which is usually surprisingly short. The graft is transected on a bias to produce longer graft length along the greater curvature of the ascending aorta and a shorter length along the lesser curvature (frequently measuring only 2–5 cm). Too long a graft will result in buckling and anterolateral displacement of the reconstructed aorta. The distal anastomosis is constructed between the graft and this circumferential full-thickness cuff of aorta with another long (140 cm) 3/0 polypropylene suture. If there is no atherosclerosis involving the aorta the suture line can be taken from graft to aorta on the inside; this may be preferable in certain patients since the needle is first passed through the stiffer graft and then through the soft and fragile aorta; passing the needle in the opposite direction must be done with care since the force necessary to pass the needle through the graft may result in small tears around the needle holes in the aorta. As was true for the proximal suture line, extreme gentleness is necessary both in passing the needle through the aorta and also in maintaining a constant amount of 'following' traction on the suture. After the posterior wall is completed the suture is passed to the outside and the remainder of the anastomosis performed in the usual fashion.

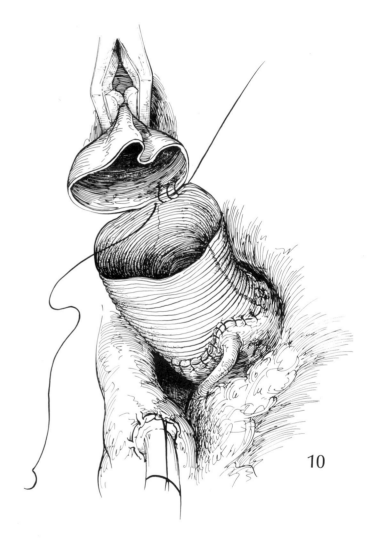

10

11

Before the aorta is unclamped it is important to turn off any left-sided vents in use and fill the heart with blood from the oxygenator. While the heart is filling with blood and the distal anastomosis is nearing completion the anaesthetist is asked to inflate the lungs with increasing amplitude and frequency. Before the last suture bite is placed the left atrial appendage is invaginated, the pulmonary veins massaged, and the entire heart gently agitated with the assistant's left hand to ensure that most of the air is evacuated through the anastomosis. The suture line is then completed and the cross clamp removed while any retained air is continuously evacuated from the highest portion of the graft with a syringe and needle.

Attention should then be directed to ensure that both the right and left ventricles and other portions of the heart are warming equally (disparities in the rate of warming can be the first sign of compromise of a coronary artery). During gentle saline irrigation both suture lines are inspected, but it is exceedingly important not to twist or pull the graft to any extreme as this can cause suture line disruption and bleeding from needle holes. If major bleeding from the posterior aspect of either suture line is seen at this time it is prudent to reclamp the aorta and control the bleeding with additional sutures; to attempt to do this with pump perfusion pressure in the graft can easily result in additional trauma to the suture lines and major haemorrhage. Bleeding points in the lateral or anterior portions of the suture line can be controlled without reclamping the aorta.

If coexistent severe coronary artery disease makes concomitant myocardial revascularization necessary the distal anastomoses are constructed before the aorta is opened. The proximal ends of the vein grafts are anastomosed to the ascending aortic graft before unclamping, after 5–6 mm diameter holes have been cut out of the graft in appropriate locations with a sterile disposable ophthalmic cautery unit. Attempting to construct the proximal vein graft anastomoses to the Dacron

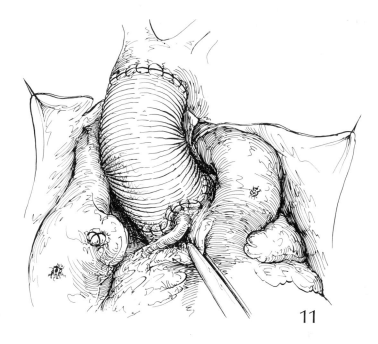

11

graft after releasing the cross clamp can be treacherous. It is difficult to achieve a bloodless field for this with a partial occlusion or side-biting vascular clamp. An alternative (which is rarely necessary) is to anastomose the proximal vein graft to the distal aortic arch or the innominate artery using a small partial occluding clamp.

When the heart has been satisfactorily resuscitated cardiopulmonary bypass is gradually and slowly discontinued. It is extremely important in these patients not to allow episodes of hypertension to occur as this may result in haemorrhage or even suture line disruption. Liberal use of an intravenous sodium nitroprusside drip reduces this threat and lowers myocardial oxygen consumption. The patient's mean arterial pressure is kept in the range of 60 to 75 mmHg, depending on the patient's age and any coexistent atherosclerotic occlusive arterial disease.

Special situations

12

In younger patients with degenerative ascending aneurysms the coronary ostia may be displaced far cephalad as part of the disease process. This is most common in patients with Marfan's syndrome and to a lesser extent in patients with annuloaortic ectasia. Most frequently the right coronary artery is displaced farther than is the left. In such circumstances it is impracticable to dissect out a tongue of aorta surrounding the ostium of the coronary artery; reimplantation of the coronary ostium as a full-thickness button is the preferred technique. The coronary arteries are excised from the aneurysm, leaving a 4–5 mm rim of aorta surrounding the coronary ostium.

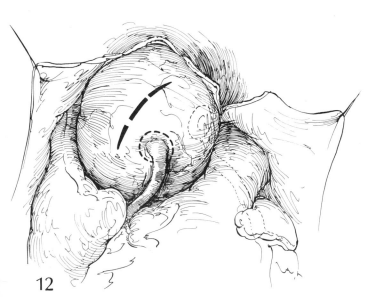

12

13

Since the right coronary artery is more frequently displaced cephalad than the left it is commonly only necessary to reimplant the right coronary artery, using the conventional aortic tongue technique for the left coronary. If the left coronary artery must be reimplanted this is done after completion of the proximal anastomosis to facilitate exposure in this area. The end-to-side anastomosis of the full-thickness button is carried out with running 4/0 or 5/0 polypropylene. Care must be taken to ensure that the coronary artery is not kinked or otherwise compromised. The distal anastomosis is then completed as described above. Finally, the appropriate location for reimplantation of the right coronary artery button is determined and a generous defect made in the graft with a disposable cautery. The right coronary artery is then reimplanted, a similar running suture of fine polypropylene being used. The anastomoses must be performed with care since bleeding from the left coronary anastomosis may be almost inaccessible after completion of the procedure.

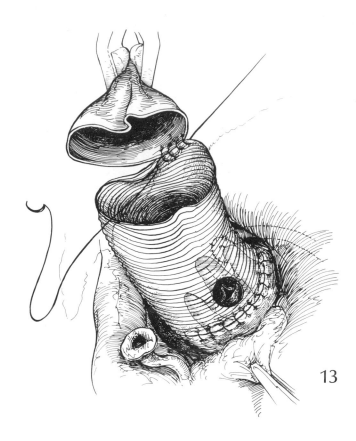

13

14

14

The completed reconstruction when both coronary arteries require reimplantation is shown here. As the heart is filled with blood to evacuate air before the aorta is unclamped haemostasis at the coronary anastomoses should be checked. Adjuncts which can help control diffuse haemorrhage include correcting the patient's coagulation profile immediately using specific factors as indicated (including fresh frozen plasma, cryoprecipitate and platelet concentrates in addition to protamine sulphate). In extreme circumstances, especially in patients with severe preoperative hepatic failure, factor IX concentrates (Proplex or Koyne) can be administered, but their use carries a high risk of hepatitis. Local adjunctive manoeuvres include packing large areas of diffuse oozing with Gelfoam soaked in topical bovine thrombin. Microcrystalline collagen (Avitene) can also be used, but is expensive. If available, fibrin glue works well in these situations. However, the key to the prevention of major bleeding complications remains strict attention to meticulous surgical technique.

DESCENDING THORACIC ANEURYSMS

Descending thoracic aortic aneurysms are approached through a left posterolateral thoracotomy with the patient in the right lateral decubitus position. Selective endo-bronchial intubation greatly facilitates these procedures and prevents damage to the left lung. Serial blood gas concentrations or transcutaneous oxygen saturation values must be monitored with the left lung deflated, however, as arterial desaturation can occur. Partial cardiopulmonary bypass is used for all cases (see *Illustration 2*). The right common femoral vein is preferred for venous cannulation. This can be facilitated if the patient's hips are rotated from the table to 45–60° and the shoulders are fully perpendicular to the table.

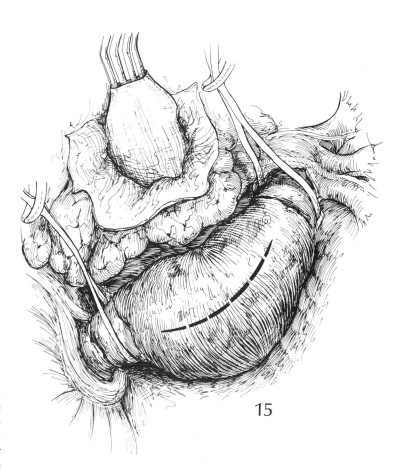

15

15

While the right femoral vessels are being dissected free in preparation for cannulation the aorta proximal and distal to the aneurysm is dissected free and encircled with large Silastic tapes. Most descending thoracic aortic aneurysms are atherosclerotic in aetiology (excluding aortic dissections – see next chapter) and very few are degenerative. These aneurysms may be either saccular or fusiform in configuration. Diffuse dilatation or ectasia involving the entire thoracic aorta is a different disease and may well not be best managed by surgical treatment unless a localized saccular component exists. In general it is always best to limit the amount of aorta resected in order to minimize the chance of paraplegia. This implies that segments of modestly dilated aorta can probably be safely left *in situ* when a large saccular aneurysm is being resected. When a rather extensive fusiform aneurysm involves the greater part of the descending thoracic aorta, there is no option but to resect the aneurysm in its entirety.

Proximal control is obtained just proximal or distal to the left subclavian artery, depending on the extent of the aneurysm. If the aneurysm involves the distal transverse arch, then proximal control can be obtained between the innominate and left carotid arteries. The operative approach to this area can be facilitated by opening the pericardium far anteriorly and working distally from the ascending aorta to the arch. Care must be taken not to damage the phrenic, vagus and recurrent laryngeal nerves. If a segment of the aneurysm is densely adherent to a portion of the lung it is prudent not to continue dissection of the lung off the aneurysm as rupture of the aneurysm into the lung parenchyma may have occurred previously. In these cases dissection of this region of the aneurysm is deferred until the aorta has been clamped and opened, and the relevant segment of aortic wall can be left attached to the lung. Care must also be taken to avoid injury to the oesophagus, which can become densely adherent to some of these aneurysms.

Partial femoral-femoral cardiopulmonary bypass is insti-tuted slowly, with adjustment of the venous return to the oxygenator to maintain the patient's preload (pulmonary artery diastolic (PAD) pressure measured by a Swan-Ganz catheter) in a targeted range (as determined before going on bypass). Perfusion rates range from 1000 to 2000 ml/minute; no hypothermia is employed. The conduct of

partial cardiopulmonary bypass is markedly simplified and made safer by tracking the filling (PAD) pressure instead of the mean arterial pressure. Frequently a supplemental sodium nitroprusside drip is also required to prevent excessive proximal hypertension.

Once the patient's haemodynamics are stable and the targeted flow rate has been reached the distal descending aorta is cross-clamped. Adjustments in the rate of venous return to the oxygenator and/or nitroprusside infusion rate may be necessary at this point, after which the proximal aortic clamp is applied at the appropriate location. The subclavian (and when necessary the left common carotid) arteries are then clamped separately. The preferred location for placement of the proximal cross clamp is between the left carotid and left subclavian arteries (or in some cases even distal to the left subclavian). When necessary, however, it can be placed proximal to the left common carotid without greatly increasing the risk of stroke. If one desires to know with certainty beforehand whether or not the patient can safely tolerate temporary clamping of the left common carotid artery a 'non-invasive' carotid stump pressure can be measured with a balloon catheter during the time of cerebral arteriography. Alternatively, an intraoperative stump pressure can be measured in the left common carotid artery before cardiopulmonary bypass is started.

16a & b

The aneurysm is then opened longitudinally; the aorto-tomy is extended with scissors proximally and distally (*a*). Laminated clot is evacuated manually; lost blood is returned to the pump oxygenator by the coronary suckers. After the debris within the aneurysm has been evacuated and the aorta irrigated copiously with saline, bleeding from intercostal branches can be controlled from within by suture ligation (*b*). It has been stated that reimplantation of large intercostal vessels may reduce the incidence of paraplegia, but this remains unproved. In patients with atherosclerotic aneurysms the technique described only infrequently entails reimplantation of a large left-sided intercostal artery between the levels of T7 and T12; this is not the case in patients with extensive aortic dissections (*see next chapter*), but again it remains conjecture whether or not reimplantation of these vessels will reduce the risk of paraplegia. Perhaps the most worrying situation is when there is a large left-sided intercostal artery in the region of T8–T10 which is obviously patent but not copiously back-bleeding; reim-plantation of such an intercostal into the graft is preferred, though no method of spinal cord protection or operative technique provides complete immunity from the threat of paraplegia.

Proximal and distal circumferential full-thickness aortic cuffs are dissected free (*a*) after the bleeding from intercostal arteries has been controlled. The Silastic tubing which had encircled the aorta before clamping falls freely out of the field when the aortic cuff has been dissected free in the proper plane. This guarantees that all of the aortic adventitia is retained with the aortic cuff, ensuring a stronger and more haemostatic anastomosis. Care is necessary to avoid injury to the oesophagus, and any bleeding deep in the mediastinum should be controlled at this time with metallic clips, suture or electrocautery.

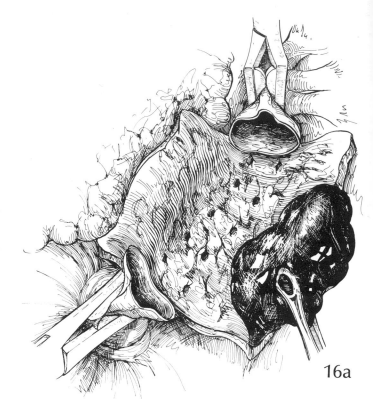

16a

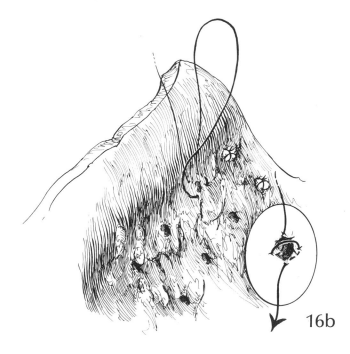

16b

17

The proximal graft anastomosis is constructed first, usually starting on the posterior wall at its most medial aspect and performing the posterior portion of the anastomosis from the inside with a 140 cm 3/0 polypropylene suture, taking the needle from the aorta to the graft. Very soft low-porosity woven Dacron grafts are again used for these cases. Large, deep, full-thickness suture bites are taken of the aortic cuff; gentle yet constant 'following' traction is necessary on this continuous suture line.

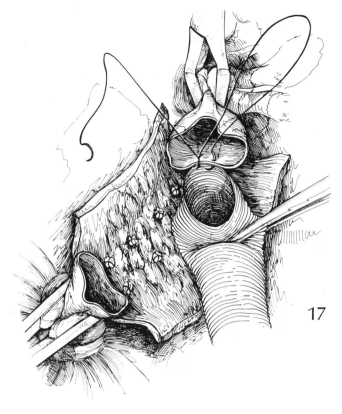

17

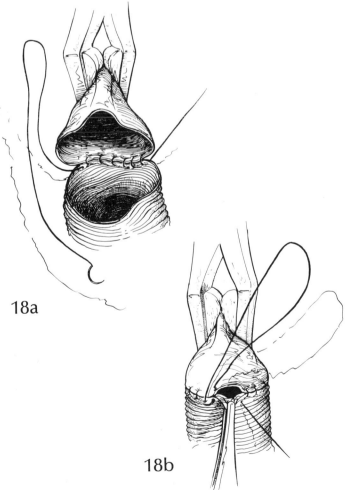

18a

18b

18a & b

After the back wall of the proximal anastomosis has been constructed (a) the anterior portion of the anastomosis is completed (b).

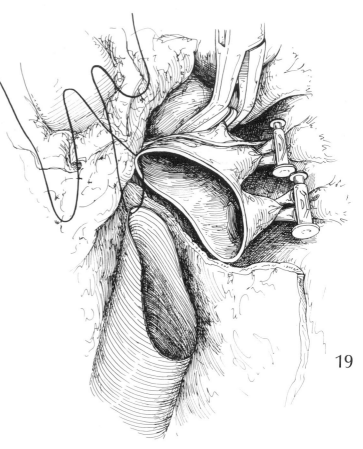

19

19 & 20

Saccular atherosclerotic aneurysms frequently involve the distal aortic arch. In such cases it may be necessary to clamp the aorta proximal to the left common carotid artery. In these circumstances the proximal anastomosis is constructed along a long bevel with the proximal end of the graft tailored appropriately along the bias. A 'reversed bias' approach is favoured, the toe of the graft being attached to the lesser curvature of the arch and the 'heel' of the graft to the point of the arch just beyond the origin of the left subclavian artery along the greater curvature. This results in a more gentle arc of the graft which lies nicely in the mediastinum.

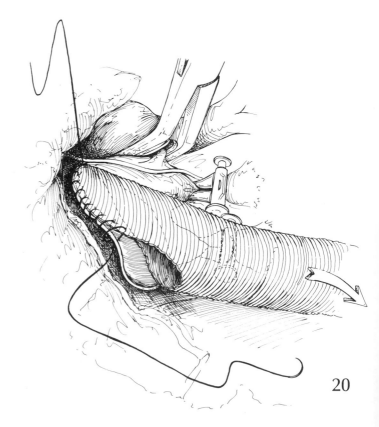

20

21

In patients in whom a portion of the distal arch is also being resected in continuity with the descending thoracic aortic aneurysm it may be easier to use an alternative suture technique for construction of the proximal anastomosis. A 140 cm 3/0 polypropylene suture is started at the toe of the graft far up under the aortic arch along the lesser curvature. The graft is held anteriorly and the posterior suture line is constructed from the outside, going from graft to aorta and working towards the origin of the subclavian artery. The anterior portion of the suture line is then completed.

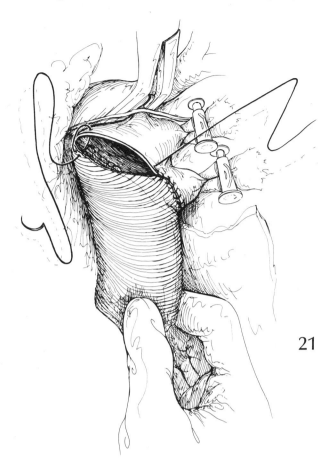

21

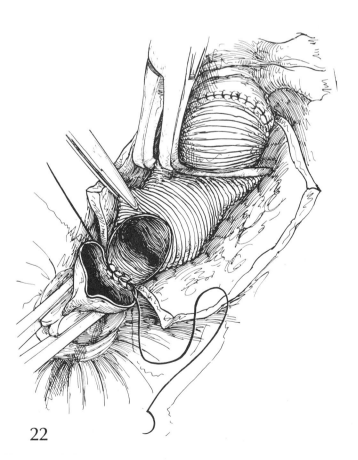

22

22

Attention is then directed to the distal anastomosis. A full-thickness aortic cuff is anastomosed to the graft (after the graft has been trimmed to the appropriate length) with a 140 cm continuous 3/0 polypropylene suture. Many suture techniques can be used satisfactorily, depending on the location of the distal anastomosis in the thorax and the extent of the pathological changes in the aorta. In one method (illustrated) the back wall of the anastomosis is constructed from the inside, taking the needle bites from graft to aorta. This technique is applicable when extensive (calcified) atherosclerotic changes are not present. If such are encountered the back wall of the anastomosis can also be constructed from the inside, but the suture line is started on the most posterior aspect and is carried anteriorly, taking aorta to graft. Deep, large and generous full-thickness bites of distal aortic cuff are mandatory. If the aneurysm is degenerative in aetiology great care is necessary in passing the needle through the fragile aorta.

23

The front wall of the anastomosis is then completed in a conventional running fashion. Before completion of the anastomosis the aorta and graft are flushed in both antegrade and retrograde directions to remove any retained particulate debris as well as to evacuate air from the graft. Inspection of the distal anastomosis for haemostasis is then carried out. If necessary, additional horizontal mattress sutures (with or without Teflon pledgets on the aortic aspects) are placed.

If no significant bleeding from either anastomosis is present partial cardiopulmonary bypass can be rapidly discontinued, taking care to maintain the patient's filling pressure at the predetermined level. Adjustments during this transition phase in the rate of nitroprusside infusion may also be necessary. As was true for patients with ascending aortic aneurysms, it is important to avoid hypertension so as to minimize stresses on the suture lines during the early postoperative period. The mean arterial pressure is kept in the range of 65–80 mmHg, the higher levels being reserved for older patients with associated atherosclerotic occlusive arterial disease elsewhere.

Shortly after cessation of cardiopulmonary bypass the venous cannula is removed and the femoral venotomy is repaired with running 6/0 polypropylene. This is performed before or during the administration of protamine sulphate to reduce the chance of venous thrombosis. After an appropriate amount of blood volume has been returned to the patient from the pump oxygenator the arterial cannula can be removed and the arteriotomy closed with continuous 5/0 or 6/0 polypropylene. Care must be taken to avoid the formation or embolization of any thrombus during arterial cannula removal and arteriotomy repair.

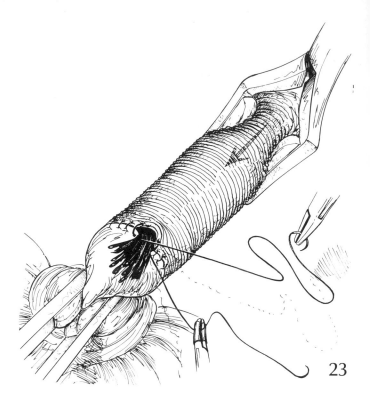

23

24

It should be noted that after resection of an extensive fusiform atherosclerotic aneurysm involving most of the descending thoracic aorta the residual aneurysm sac is left *in situ*; if the sac is very large and redundant, then portions can be excised and the remainder closed loosely over the graft. Without distorting the graft excessively, previous ligated intercostal arteries and the back wall of the aneurysm sac should be inspected because occasionally intercostal arteries which were not bleeding previously may now require suture ligation. Haemostasis is achieved with standard methods and the left lung reinflated by the anaesthetist. A few moments or prolonged periods of high airway pressure to expand the left lung fully and eliminate any residual atelectasis are well worth while. Large (36–40 Fr) chest tubes are inserted and the chest wall closed in standard fashion.

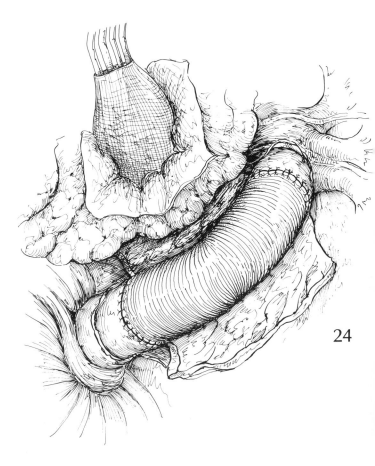

24

Special problems

The vast majority of patients with descending thoracic aortic aneurysms have either atherosclerotic aneurysms as shown above or aortic dissections (see next chapter). Rarely, young patients with or without Marfan's syndrome present with degenerative aneurysms of the descending aorta. Other less common forms of aneurysm involving the descending aorta include acute traumatic tears, chronic post-traumatic false aneurysms, aneurysms of the ductus diverticulum, mycotic aneurysms and luetic aneurysms. The operative techniques for dealing with these patients are not illustrated separately because their details differ little from those described above. All patients with descending thoracic aortic aneurysms, including those with acute traumatic tears, are preferably treated under partial femoral-femoral cardiopulmonary bypass. The only exception to this is in victims of multiple trauma with acute tears of the aortic isthmus who also have severe closed head injuries. In these circumstances systemic heparinization may exacerbate the cerebral injury; therefore a heparinized Gott shunt is used from either the left ventricular apex or the ascending aorta to the distal descending thoracic aorta. Most patients with acute traumatic tears of the thoracic aorta have been found to require graft replacement; however, those with limited tears not involving the entire circumference of the thoracic aorta and those with small false aneurysms may be amenable to primary repair without graft interposition.

Patients with mycotic aneurysms present a unique collection of very challenging problems. In the face of gross contamination or in the presence of an aorto-bronchial or aorto-oesophageal fistula it is imperative to avoid the use of synthetic material. This usually implies exclusion of the descending aorta and reconstitution of aortic flow via an extra-anatomical graft (e.g. ascending aorta to infrarenal abdominal aorta). An alternative technique might be the use of autologous tissue to effect orthotopic reconstruction. This entails the use of the patient's infrarenal abdominal aorta as an arterial autograft to replace a segment of descending thoracic aorta. Another option might include construction of a spiral aortic graft from the patient's common and external iliac arteries. A high-porosity knitted double velour Dacron graft (Microvel) can be used in the abdomen to reconstitute aortic and/or iliac continuity after the donor arterial autograft has been harvested. The clinical results of such innovative techniques are not yet known, in part because such problems are exceedingly rare, though medium-term success has been reported even when a new synthetic graft has been implanted in a contaminated field.

Surgical treatment of aortic dissections

D. Craig Miller MD
Associate Professor of Cardiovascular Surgery, Stanford University School of Medicine, Stanford, California, USA

Introduction

The surgical management of patients with acute and chronic aortic dissections has been assigned a separate chapter by the editors for good reason. Not only do these entities differ in aetiology but the technical features and strategies of treatment also differ markedly from some described for patients with atherosclerotic or other non-dissecting thoracic aortic aneurysms.

While enthusiasm for emergency surgical intervention in patients with acute dissections involving the aorta has waxed and waned over the past two decades, this has emerged as the optimal treatment for patients with acute dissections involving the ascending aorta and has also been advocated for those with acute dissections involving the descending aorta. Patients who have survived acute dissections and later present in the chronic phase of the disease are also candidates for surgical treatment in selected cases. The indications recommended here for operative intervention include all patients with acute aortic dissections (irrespective of whether they involve the ascending or the descending aorta) unless the false lumen of the aortic dissection cannot be opacified at the time of aortography. Other contraindications include the presence of persistent systemic illness or neoplasm that is judged to make a surgical procedure ill advised. The situation differs markedly for patients with chronic aortic dissections, it being recommended that only those who have symptoms referable to the dissection *per se*, those with documented expansion of the chronic dissection and those with a localized false aneurysm segment of the dissection which is greater than 10 cm in diameter should be operated upon.

Terminology

Many systems of nomenclature have been advocated for aortic dissections. This relatively confusing situation has been clarified recently since it has been agreed that the most important factor is whether or not the ascending aorta is involved in the dissection, irrespective of the location of the primary intimal tear and regardless of the extent of distal propagation of the dissection. Such an understanding conforms to the concepts of the original Stanford Type A or B terminology.

1a, b & c

This simplified classification is determined by the expected outcome of the pathological process. If the ascending aorta is involved, then the patient has a Stanford Type A, Massachusetts General Hospital 'proximal' type, University of Alabama 'ascending' type, or DeBakey Type I dissection: This classification is independent of the site of the primary intimal tear; in a patient with a Type A aortic dissection the intimal tear may be located either in the ascending aorta (*position 1*) which ecompasses the vast majority of cases, the transverse aortic arch (*position 2*), the proximal descending thoracic aorta (*position 3*) or all three. Thus even if the tear is located distal to the left subclavian artery an acute retrograde dissection should be treated as Type A with resection and replacement of the ascending aorta.

2

The other category of aortic dissection consists of those in which the ascending aorta is not involved and is termed Type B. In the majority of these patients the primary intimal tear is located in the proximal descending thoracic aorta (*position 3*), but it may also be located in the aortic arch (*position 2*). The key angiographic feature is that the ascending aorta is not involved, a fact that is more easily discovered than the exact position of the primary intimal tear. If the tear occurs in the arch the dissection usually propagates either backwards to involve the ascending aorta (thereby becoming Type A) or extends distally to involve the descending aorta (Type B).

3

A small minority of patients have dissections confined to the transverse aortic arch (*b*); fortunately such cases are exceedingly rare. The optimal treatment for these patients remains unclear.

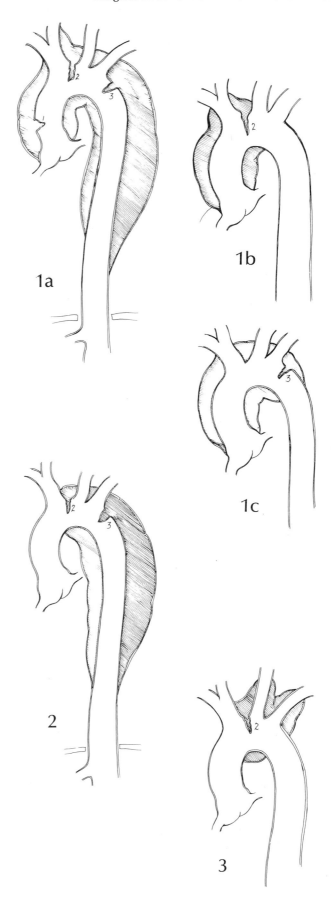

4

The clinical manifestations of acute aortic dissection may mimic those of many other diseases and are truly protean in nature. This is because of the unpredictable consequences as the dissecting haematoma advances down the aorta.

In a large majority of cases blood flow from the false lumen simply re-enters into the true lumen through a fenestration or more usually multiple fenestrations. If this occurs proximal to an important aortic tributary (a) there is no compromise of the circulation to the end organ. This is also the case if the false lumen should re-enter at the origin of its aortic tributary (b).

Distal end-organ ischaemia and/or infarction occurs when the false lumen extrinsically compresses and/or obliterates an important aortic tributary (c, d). Infarction may also be caused by thrombosis of the aortic branch after its lumen has been extrinsically compromised by the false lumen (e). Finally, the false lumen may re-enter directly into the branch artery (f), which results in no important threat to the end organ supplied by this vessel.

These examples explain the varied and manifold presentations of patients with aortic dissections; moreover, each possible pathoanatomical situation can be extremely important in determining the surgical treatment. For example, if a patient with an aortic dissection has a false lumen which has re-entered both the coeliac axis and superior mesenteric artery (f) the intimal flap adherent to the opposite wall of the vessel may heal with time. If surgical intervention is then undertaken in the chronic phase of the disease and perfusion of the aortic false lumen is obliterated it is easy to understand why life-threatening visceral ischaemia may result. Although the surgical maxim has traditionally been to obliterate all flow in the false lumen, numerous studies have shown that this goal is rarely achieved; indeed, such 'failures' may be fortunate for patients in the chronic phase of their disease who are undergoing surgical treatment.

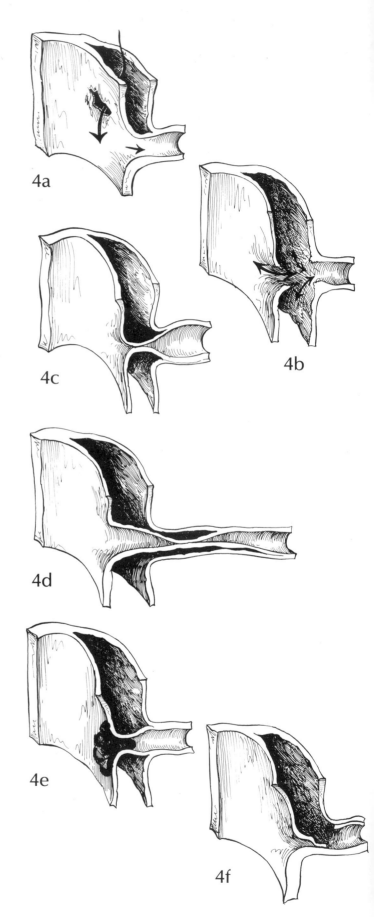

4a

4c

4b

4d

4e

4f

The operations

Type A aortic dissections

5

The surgical goal in patients with Type A aortic dissections is to resect a limited segment of ascending aorta and replace it with a tubular Dacron graft. As discussed in the chapter on 'Thoracic aortic aneurysms', pp. 509–525 peripheral aterial cannulation is used, with central bicaval venous cannulation.

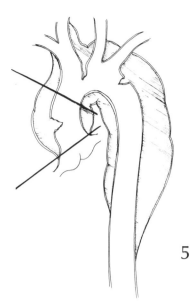

5

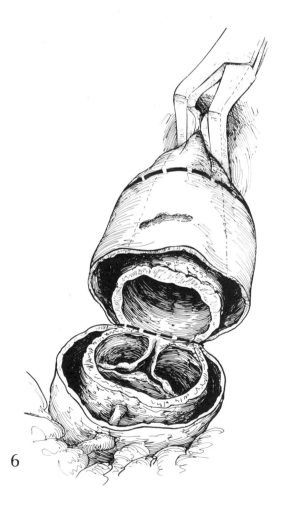

6

6

The ascending aorta is clamped just proximal to the innominate artery. Continuous profound topical hypothermia is used for myocardial protection throughout the period of aortic cross-clamping, supplemented by arresting the heart initially by instilling hyperkalaemic cold crystalloid cardioplegic solution directly into the coronary ostia. The most common position of the primary intimal tear in patients with Type A aortic dissections is illustrated. It is usually transverse in orientation and involves the right anterolateral aspect of the true lumen; in some cases, however, the primary intimal tear is not located in the ascending aorta (see above). The aorta is opened obliquely and the false lumen entered, revealing the septum between the true and the false lumen. This septum is then opened and the true lumen exposed. The right coronary artery may be involved in the dissecting process in some cases, resulting in myocardial ischaemia and/or infarction. The left coronary artery is involved only rarely.

7

In cases of acute Type A dissection aortic regurgitation is frequently caused solely by lack of commissural support of the valve with subsequent prolapse of the aortic valve leaflets. The leaflets themselves are normal and commonly there is no annular dilatation. Since the perfect prosthetic or bioprosthetic valve substitute does not yet exist it is preferable to salvage the native aortic valve whenever possible. Indeed, this is feasible in the large majority (approaching 85 per cent) of patients with acute Type A dissections. However, patients with Marfan's syndrome or annuloaortic ectasia should invariably undergo aortic valve replacement instead of attempted reconstruction because the durability of valvular reconstruction appears to be limited in these cases. Moreover, patients with a chronic Type A dissection frequently have irreparable aortic valve damage and concomitant aortic valve replacement is necessary in a large proportion (50 per cent).

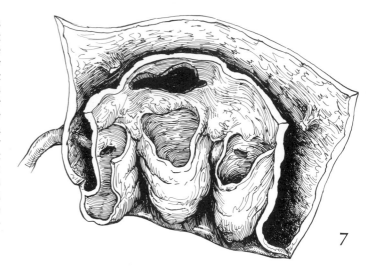

7

8

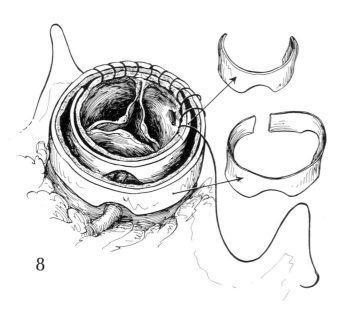

8

Extensive reconstruction of the aortic root is necessary not only to preserve the native valve in cases of acute Type A dissection but also to ensure long-term durability of the valve reconstruction and to minimize the chances of late acute redissection in the remaining aortic root. The key features of the reconstruction include obliteration of the false lumen at the level of the aortic root and preservation of coronary blood flow while still maintaining or creating satisfactory commissural support for the aortic valve. Most commonly a two-layer Teflon felt 'sandwich' technique is satisfactory; this may be extended to include a third layer of Teflon felt inside the endothelium of the true lumen. The collar of Teflon felt inserted into the false lumen is custom-tailored to conform to the topography of the false lumen. It curves over the origin of a dissected coronary artery and extends down into the proximal depths of the false lumen. Frequently this layer of Teflon felt is non-circumferential since the false lumen does not include the entire aortic root at this level. The external layer is circumferential, but its width is not as great as the layer inserted into the false lumen since its only purpose is to reinforce the tensile strength of the adventitia. If a third layer of Teflon felt is added the running polypropylene suture line which reconstructs the aorta and obliterates the false lumen cannot cut or tear through the inner layer, which is formed by the aortic endothelium. Whether two or three layers of Teflon felt are used is immaterial as long as the key objective of obliterating the entire proximal extent of the false lumen is achieved.

9

In a patient with excellent tissue integrity or with a chronic dissection in which the aortic valve is not irreparably damaged, if there is not a tremendous disparity in circumference between the true and the false lumens all layers can be reapproximated with a single running 4/0 polypropylene suture and only one layer of external Teflon felt used. However, such a reconstructive procedure is not possible in many patients with chronic Type A dissections and the more extensive and elaborate reconstructive procedure described above (see *illustration 7*) is preferable.

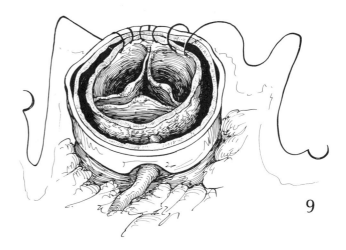

9

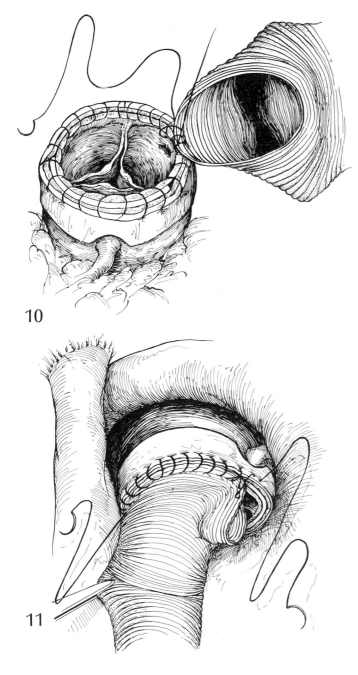

10

11

10 & 11

If the native aortic valve can be preserved the proximal graft anastomosis is started at the left posterolateral aspect of the aortic root with a long (140 cm (54 inch)) 3/0 polypropylene suture. Low-porosity very soft woven Dacron grafts (*see* chapter on 'Thoracic aortic aneurysms', pp. 509–525) are preferred in these circumstances. One advantage of these grafts in patients with acute dissections is that the graft does not necessarily have to be preclotted; therefore the exact size of graft to be selected can be determined after the patient has been heparinized and the aortic root reconstructed. The posterior suture line is constructed from the outside, taking the needle bites from graft to aorta. The graft is held downwards so that it does not interfere with exact apposition. Meticulous care is necessary in carrying the needle through the friable diseased aorta (along the curve of the needle) and guaranteeing that gentle yet constant 'following' traction is always placed on the suture line by the assistant. These important points cannot be over-emphasized when it comes to acute dissections; the tissue integrity is extremely poor and every needle hole tends to tear and bleed unless these precautions are taken. The Teflon felt collars reduce the risk of major technical complications, but use of such buttressing material should not detract from the meticulous attention to detail and gentleness that is mandatory in these cases.

12

A similar but less extensive reconstruction of the distal aorta is necessary in patients with chronic Type A aortic dissections. A single external layer of Teflon felt is used to buttress a running suture of 4/0 polypropylene which obliterates the false lumen and reapposes the aortic intima with the adventitia. A second layer on the intimal surface may rarely be necessary if the tissues are extremely friable. It should also be noted that the aorta has been dissected out as a full-thickness circumferential cuff before anastomosis. The distal graft anastomosis is constructed using techniques similar to those illustrated and described in the chapter on 'Thoracic aortic aneurysms'.

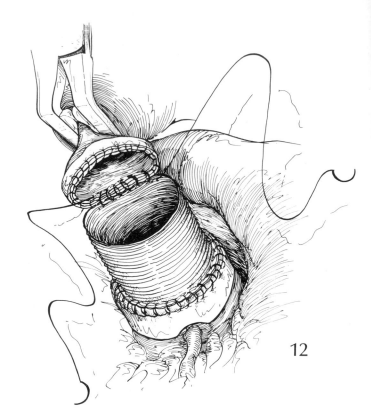

12

13

The anterior aspect of the distal anastomosis is constructed by running both arms of the polypropylene suture towards the middle. The last suture bite is not secured until the patient has been placed in a steep Trendelenberg position, any left-sided vent being used has been turned off, the heart has been filled with blood from the oxygenator and the anaesthetist has fully inflated the lungs. When all air in the left atrium and left ventricle has been expelled the suture is pulled up and tied down. The most superior portion of the graft is then aspirated with a syringe and needle and the aortic cross clamp is slowly removed. Immediate attention is directed to both suture lines to inspect haemostasis. If a major site of bleeding is discovered the cross clamp should be replaced so that this can be repaired before the heart is rewarmed and with no pressure in the ascending aortic graft. Some bleeding from needle holes under the Teflon felt is commonplace and generally does not require additional repair sutures, which may exacerbate the problem. There is probably no other cardiac surgical procedure in which such great care is necessary in handling the diseased tissue and the suture lines; assiduous and meticulous attention to technical details will be rewarded with less bleeding.

If the presence of severe coexisting coronary artery disease or unreconstructable coronary compromise due to the dissection *per se* has made necessary concomitant coronary artery bypass grafting, the vein grafts should be anastomosed to the ascending aortic Dacron graft before the release of the cross clamp. When the heart has been adequately resuscitated cardiopulmonary bypass is slowly discontinued. During this transition period attention must be paid to controlling the mean arterial pressure in the range of 60–70 mmHg. This is most easily accomplished with a continuous infusion of nitroprusside. It is important to avoid episodes of hypertension since the fragile nature of the aortic tissues may lead to anastomotic disruption. Assuming that the cardiopulmonary bypass time is not excessively long and appropriate attention has been paid to the technical details, significant haemorrhage is infrequent.

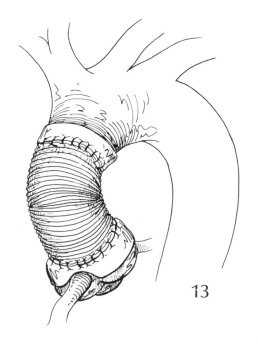

13

14

When concomitant aortic valve replacement is necessary in patients with Type A aortic dissections the above technique is combined with those illustrated in the chapter on 'Thoracic aortic aneurysms'. (A case in which the irreparably damaged aortic valve has been replaced with a porcine bioprosthetic valve is illustrated here.) The false lumen proximally and distally is obliterated and the aortic cuffs reinforced with a single layer of external felt. These layers are approximated with a running 4/0 polypropylene suture. The short ascending aortic graft is then anastomosed proximally, using the technique described above. The proximal end of the graft can be tailored appropriately to conform with the tongues of the aortic root left surrounding the coronary ostia.

One (or rarely both) coronary ostia can be reimplanted into the graft if they should be displaced far cephalad from the aortic annulus (*see Illustration 15*).

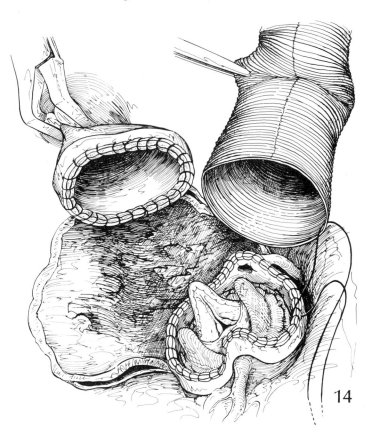

14

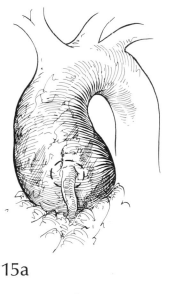

15a

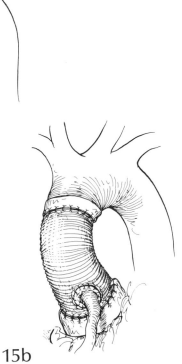

15b

Special features in chronic Type A dissections

As stated above, the indications for surgical intervention are relatively conservative for patients with chronic Type A dissections. Nevertheless, such surgical procedures require slightly different technical manoeuvres in many cases.

15a & b

There is usually a marked disparity in circumference between the true and the false lumens in the chronic phase of the disease (a). For many years the policy was to attempt to obliterate the false lumen and reapproximate the aortic intima with the adventitia in these cases, but life-threatening infarction of an important end organ (brain, kidney, small and large bowel) may result. This is due to the healing that occurs with time in the aortic tributaries. Therefore it is now recommended that distal perfusion should be deliberately directed into both the true and the false lumen in chronic dissections. The critical reader will note that this is a marked departure from the strategy to be adopted when dealing with patients with acute aortic dissections.

16a & b

In a chronic dissection a portion of the septum between the true and the false lumen is excised (a, b) and the distal graft anastomosis is constructed to the false lumen or aortic adventitia. In the chronic phase of the disease the external layers of the aorta are densely fibrotic and hold sutures well. For similar reasons the distal true lumen is densely adherent to the false lumen in most cases. Thus resection of the exposed portion of the septum dividing the two lumens does not predispose to intussusception of the false lumen or other problems and it is probable that surgical resection of chronic aortic dissections ameliorates symptoms and extends life expectancy by virtue of the resection of the large saccular false aneurysmal component and not by the elimination of all flow in the distal false lumen.

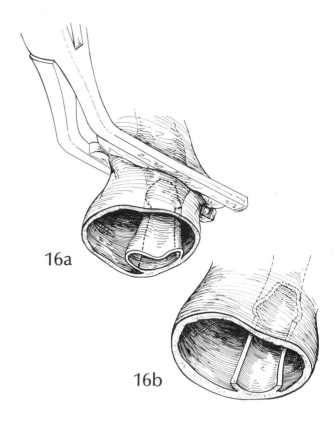

16a

16b

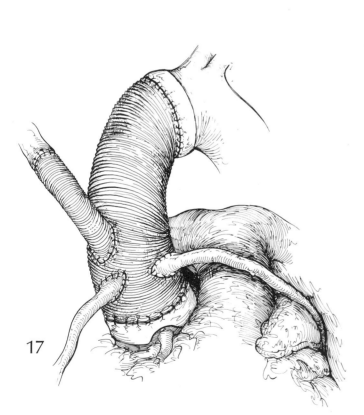

17

17

In certain circumstances ancillary concomitant procedures may be extensive, as illustrated here. This patient with a chronic Type A dissection, severe coronary disease and right cerebral hemispheric transient ischaemic attacks required replacement of the entire ascending aorta as well as the proximal half of the transverse aortic arch. Aortic valve replacement was performed for irreparable valvular incompetence and coronary artery bypass grafts were established to the left anterior descending and right coronary arteries. Occlusion of the innominate artery also required concomitant replacement of the proximal innominate artery with a separate Dacron tube graft.

TYPE B AORTIC DISSECTIONS

18

The surgical goal in a patient with an acute Type B aortic dissection is to resect only a short segment of descending aorta containing the most severe degree of injury and replace it with a tubular Dacron graft. In the case of a patient with a chronic aortic dissection the extent of graft replacement is tailored to the area of saccular aneurysm enlargement that has either produced symptoms or has been documented to be expanding. Preservation of as many intercostal vessels as possible is advised, particularly in cases of acute Type B dissections.

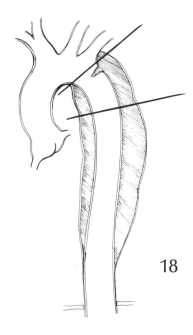

18

19

The descending aorta is approached through a left posterolateral thoracotomy. In these cases proximal control can usually be obtained either just proximal or distal to the left subclavian artery. A limited length of aorta containing the area with the most severe damage (as visualized externally) is excluded by clamps. In cases of acute aortic dissection this segment should be limited to minimize the risk of paraplegia.

With acute dissections the false lumen proximally and distally is obliterated (with or without external layers of Teflon felt) with a running 4/0 polypropylene suture. Bleeding from intercostals is controlled by suture ligation. The incidence of paraplegia is higher in patients with aortic dissections than in those with non-dissecting descending thoracic aortic aneurysms, and perhaps this is due to the fact that with the natural evolution of atherosclerotic aneurysmal disease many intermediate vessels have already been occluded. Intercostal vessels are not reimplanted.

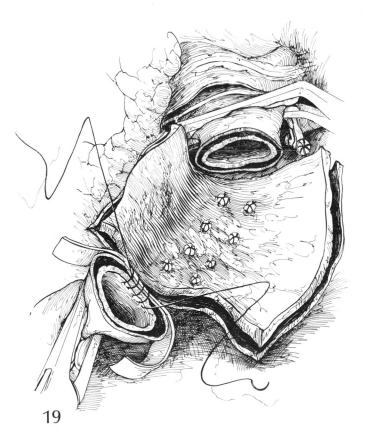

19

20

After dissection and preparation of the full-thickness aortic cuff as described above, the proximal graft anastomosis is performed with a long (140 cm) continuous 3/0 polypropylene suture. If the site of the anastomosis is just beyond the subclavian artery this anastomosis can be started from the inside. Since the aorta in these patients does not contain extensive atherosclerotic disease it is relatively safe to take the needle bites from the graft to the aorta, at least in constructing the posterior wall of the anastomosis. Otherwise the suture can be started at the right posteromedial aspect of the aorta and the posterior wall sewn from inside, taking the suture from aorta to graft. The external layer of Teflon felt does not guarantee that troublesome bleeding will not result; great care is necessary in passing the needle through the aorta and carrying it through along the curve of the needle.

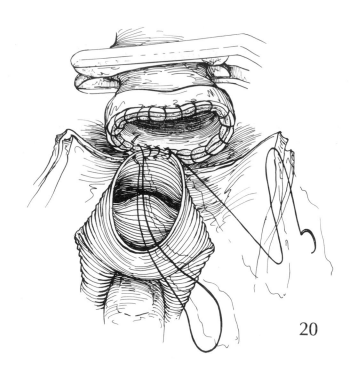

20

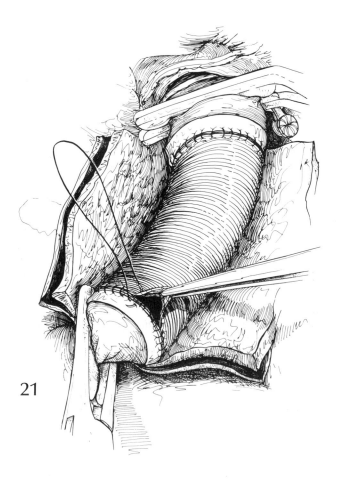

21

21

The front portion of the anastomosis is constructed in standard fashion, the left subclavian artery being occluded with a clip. The distal anastomosis (after preparation of the distal aortic cuff with or without Teflon felt) is then performed using standard techniques. If a disparity exists between the circumference of the graft and the aorta the graft can be made smaller by excising a triangular portion and closing this defect with a running (longitudinal) suture. This is analogous to constructing a dart in a dress, but the 'pleated' segment is excised.

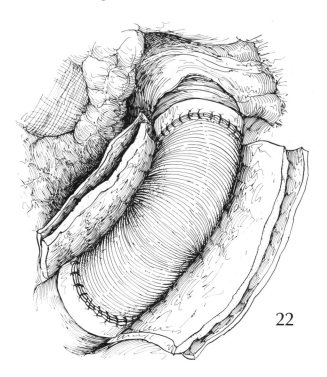

22

Before release of the clamps any retained particulate debris and air is exhausted through the suture line before the suture is tied and cut. Haemostasis should be adequate at this point before the clamps are fully released as subsequent bleeding may be relatively inaccessible.

22

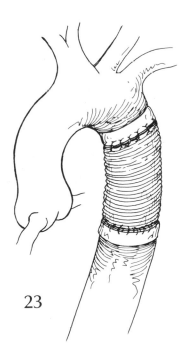

23

23

When the procedure has been completed (as shown) cardiopulmonary bypass can be discontinued quickly, adequate left ventricular filling pressure being maintained by adjusting the volume of blood transfused from the oxygenator.

Although this type of operation for patients with acute Type B dissection does not result in resection of all the diseased aorta it is probably the most appropriate course of action in such cases. The primary intent during operation for acute aortic dissection is to eliminate the leading causes of death, which is accomplished by the procedures outlined above. Subsequent postoperative follow-up of the residual false lumen with serial CT scanning or angiography is indicated and should detect any late problems that may arise. It must be mentioned in this context that surgical treatment of patients with aortic dissection essentially implies combined surgical and medical therapy, since indefinite control of hypertension, administration of beta-blocking agents and assiduous general medical care is necessary to prolong the life expectancy of these patients.

Surgical treatment of aneurysms and dissections involving the transverse aortic arch

D. Craig Miller MD
Associate Professor of Cardiovascular Surgery, Stanford University School of Medicine, Stanford, California, USA

Introduction

While they are uncommon, aneurysms of the aortic arch are not rare and are most frequently the result either of atherosclerosis or of chronic dissections. Two fundamental surgical techniques are used for resection of aortic arch aneurysms. These methods are complementary and not mutually exclusive and both will be illustrated and described in this chapter. For patients undergoing elective operation who have atherosclerotic or degenerative arch aneurysms a simplified cardiopulmonary bypass perfusion technique is favoured for protection of the brain, myocardium and lower body. On the other hand patients with aortic arch aneurysms due to acute or chronic aortic dissection, infection, trauma or syphilis are probably best treated with cardiopulmonary bypass, profound systemic hypothermia and circulatory arrest. Circulatory arrest is probably also the best technique for patients with ruptured aneurysms and those undergoing emergency procedures.

Irrespective of which method is chosen for perfusion and end-organ protection, an important issue is graft haemostasis. Recent improvements in textile manufacturing have produced grafts which are extremely safe (very low-porosity; Meadox Medicals Inc.) soft woven Dacron grafts. However, even these grafts, whether or not they are autoclaved with various protein solutions (autologous blood, autologous platelet-rich plasma, fresh frozen plasma, platelets or albumin), may be associated with massive haemorrhage through the graft interstices if fibrinolysis occurs, as occasionally happens when cardiopulmonary bypass time is unduly prolonged or the patient has severe preoperative hepatic failure. Assiduous surgical haemostasis at the suture lines is important since, after reconstruction of the aortic arch, bleeding from the distal suture line may be inaccessible.

SIMPLIFIED CARDIOPULMONARY BYPASS PERFUSION TECHNIQUES

1

The initial incision is a standard median sternotomy which can be extended into the left neck, dividing the sternocleidomastoid and strap muscles, if necessary.

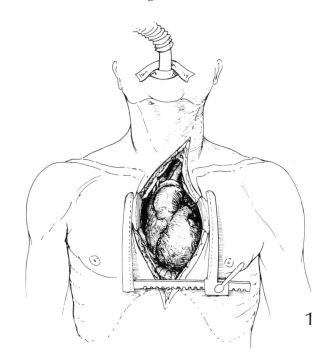

2

The innominate vein can be divided and ligated if necessary to enhance exposure. If the vein is not reconstructed the left arm should be elevated at the end of the procedure and wrapped with an external elastic compression dressing to minimize oedema formation. Since it is not known until the sternum is opened whether or not the innominate vein must be divided it is prudent to insert all major intravenous lines, including Swan-Ganz catheters, via the right internal jugular or subclavian vein. Similarly, large peripheral intravenous lines should be inserted into the right arm.

Certain arch aneurysms which are eccentric in nature or aneurysms of the ductus diverticulum can be repaired with simple aneurysmorrhaphy or Dacron patch techniques. In these cases selected perfusion of the cerebral circulation and total cardiopulmonary bypass may not be necessary; the procedure can be carried out with a modified form of partial cardiopulmonary bypass, the proximal aortic cross clamp being placed proximal to the left carotid or subclavian artery or a large partially occluding vascular clamp being used to exclude the saccular aneurysm. When partial bypass is thus used the heart continues to perfuse the coronary arteries and the innominate artery. Ventilation must therefore be continued during cardiopulmonary bypass, but exposure of the distal arch and proximal descending thoracic aorta can be enhanced if the left lung is deflated with selective endobronchial intubation and single-lung ventilation. On the other hand if total cardiopulmonary bypass, with or without circulatory arrest, is necessary a large endotracheal tube is favoured. This facilitates suctioning and, of course, both lungs can be completely deflated. An example of an atherosclerotic aneurysm involving the distal ascending aorta and the entire transverse aortic arch is illustrated. The great vessels may be ectatic and have modest amounts of mural atherosclerosis, but it is extremely rare to encounter true saccular aneurysms of these vessels.

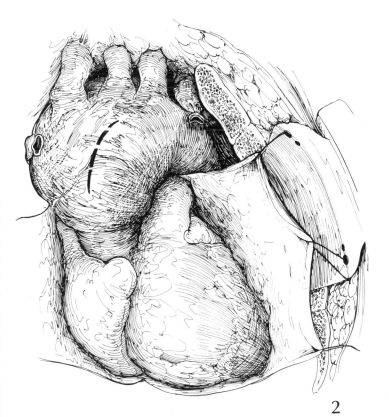

The innominate artery is dissected free up to its bifurcation into the subclavian and carotid arteries, the left common carotid for a distance of 6–7 cm and the left subclavian for a distance of 3–4 cm. All vessels are encircled with small Silastic tapes. The lymphatic tissue in the anterior and posterior mediastinum is carefully dissected and all lymphatics are controlled with tantalum clips to avoid chylothorax. The bulk of the aneurysm itself is deliberately avoided during these preliminary steps to reduce the chance of inadvertent injury to adjacent structures or entry into the aneurysm. This is especially important in the region of the ligamentum arteriosum and under the lesser curvature of the aortic arch between the pulmonary artery and the aorta at the level of the pericardial reflection. Before bypass is started selective endobronchial intubation allows the left lung to be deflated to facilitate distal dissection of the proximal descending thoracic aorta just beyond the level of the left subclavian artery. This can be helpful even if the tube must then be changed to a standard endotracheal tube if total cardiopulmonary bypass, with or without circulatory arrest, is to be employed. Careful attention must be paid to avoid injury to the phrenic nerve; similarly the left vagus and recurrent laryngeal nerves may be invoved with the aneurysmal process or even fused with the aneurysm wall.

In preparation for cardiopulmonary bypass standard bicaval cannulation is then performed through the right atrium, two 28 Fr multifenestrated caval cannulae being used and secured on short purse-string sutures. As will be shown subsequently a pulmonary artery vent can also be used to decompress the left-sided chambers if total cardiopulmonary bypass is to be employed, obviating the need for a left ventricular or left atrial vent. Of course, if the procedure can be accomplished with partial cardiopulmonary bypass careful attention must be paid to the volume of venous return to the oxygenator so that left ventricular preload remains adequate to support the cerebral and the coronary circulation.

If the simplified cardiopulmonary bypass method can be used a single arterial roller pump is connected to a Y connector. Two custom-measured lengths of tubing are then connected to the Y connector in anticipation that one will perfuse one of the common femoral arteries and the other the innominate artery. Appropriately sized Bardic catheters are coupled to this 'Y-ed' arterial line. In most adults a 20, 22 or 24 Fr Bardic catheter can be inserted into the femoral artery; the size of the innominate Bardic catheter varies between 14 and 16 Fr. Cardiopulmonary bypass is then started and the pulmonary artery sump vent (14 Fr) is inserted through a small stab wound in the pulmonary artery.

3

The patient is cooled by means of the heat exchanger in the oxygenator to the range of 24–28°C (nasopharyngeal). Cardiopulmonary bypass flows are kept in the usual range, which varies between 30 and 50 ml/kg/minute. Subsequently, after clamping of the innominate artery and occlusion of the descending thoracic aorta, the flow rate can be reduced slightly. The absolute volume of flow delivered to the cerebral circulation is then dependent on the vascular resistance of the regional bed and is not controlled by the perfusionist using a separate pump head. The ascending aorta is clamped (temporarily) and the heart arrested with crystalloid cardioplegia.

An appropriately sized low-porosity very soft woven Dacron graft and a large aortic occlusion balloon catheter are then brought on to the field. The balloon catheter is placed through the graft. The innominate artery is occluded with a clamp; the left common carotid and left subclavian arteries are then also occluded. Cardiopulmonary bypass flow is reduced to the range of 400–500 ml/minute and the aneurysm is opened. Any laminated clot is quickly evacuated with gauze sponges and the aortic occlusion balloon is threaded down into the proximal descending thoracic aorta and inflated. Pump flow is then increased back to baseline level.

Many methods of myocardial protection can be used, but the technique preferred consists of an initial 500–1000 ml infusion of cold hyperkalaemic crystalloid cardioplegic solution followed by continuous profound topical hypothermia, care being taken to keep the entire heart submerged under the cold saline. The cardioplegic solution can be injected into the aortic root or directly into the coronary ostia after the aorta has been opened. Supplemental doses of cardioplegic solution injected into the coronary ostia may be necessary later if the clamp time is prolonged, since the level of topical cold saline must necessarily be kept low during dissection of the distal aorta and completion of this anastomosis. The aortotomy is extended both proximally and distally to expose the extent of the aneurysm.

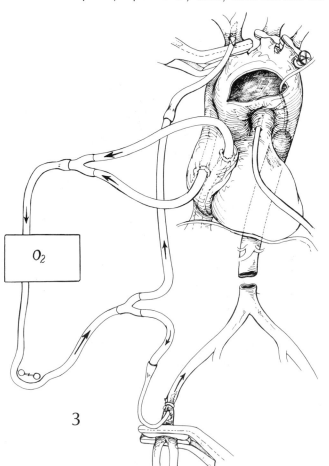

3

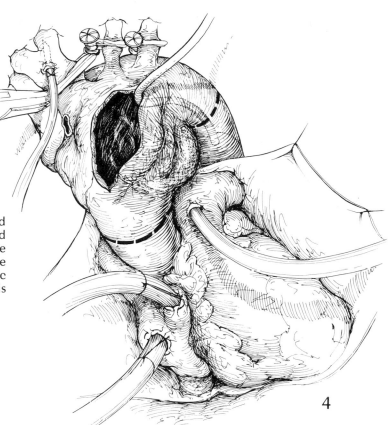

4

4

Any remaining thrombus and debris are irrigated free and appropriate lines of aortic transection are determined both proximally and distally. The entire interior of the aneurysm is then irrigated several times, including the ostia of the great vessels, to ensure that no particulate debris remains or has been trapped. The distal aorta is then transected at the appropriate level.

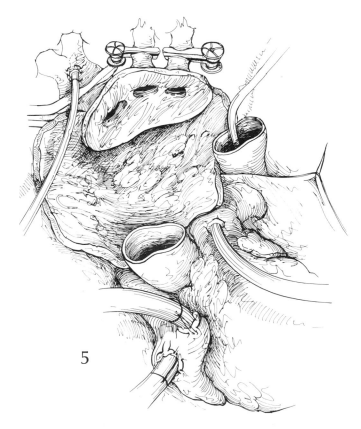

5

5

A full-thickness cuff of distal aorta is dissected completely free. Any major intercostal vessels or other bleeding points are controlled with clips and/or cautery. If desired the proximal ascending aortic cuff can also be dissected free (again in a full-thickness fashion) at this time, but this is usually done later after reinstitution of flow to all the great vessels. A button or island surrounding the ostia of the arch vessels is dissected free, care again being taken to ensure that this is of full thickness and that all aortic adventitia is retained. Since the tissue integrity of these aortic arch aneurysms may be extremely poor, this dissection of the aortic button (especially distally, surrounding the origin of the left subclavian artery) must be done delicately and meticulously.

6

The graft is then slid over the catheter to the region of the distal aorta. The distal suture line is constructed with a long (140 cm (54 inch)) 3/0 polypropylene suture, the back wall being started from the inside. The catheter leading to the balloon can be manipulated out of the way as the suture line is continued. An extreme degree of technical care and detail is necessary in constructing this particular suture line. Deep, large bites of descending aorta must be taken and care must be taken in placing the needle through the aortic tissue, pulling it through the aorta along the curve of the needle and maintaining gentle but constant traction on the suture. One or other limb of the suture is then carried around anteriorly as deemed most convenient for each individual case.

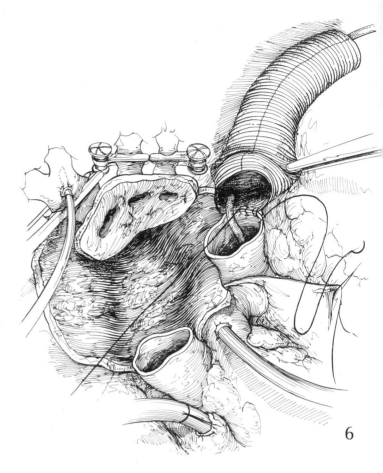

6

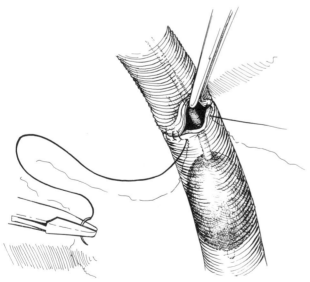

7

7

The distal anastomosis is then completed and the aortic occlusion balloon partially deflated, allowing blood from the femoral perfusion cannula to fill the graft so that the suture line can be inspected for haemostasis. Aortic tears or other serious bleeding problems in the distal anastomosis should be corrected with 3/0 or 4/0 horizontal mattress sutures and Teflon felt pledgets on the aortic aspect because this area becomes inaccessible later on. This manoeuvre also allows particulate debris to be flushed retrograde up into the graft, where it can be irrigated free and aspirated from the field.

8

The end-to-side anastomosis of the three great vessels is then accomplished. This is most easily done by constructing the back wall from inside the aorta, taking the needle from aorta to graft. Both limbs of the suture are then continued around the oval-shaped defect in the graft, which is made with a disposable ophthalmic cautery or scissors.

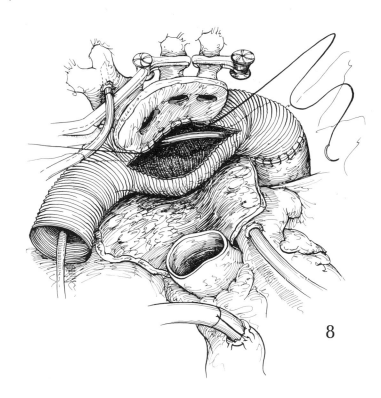

9

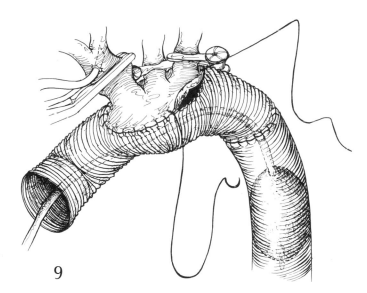

The anterior portion of this end-to-side anastomosis is then completed from the outside. A single long (140 cm) 3/0 suture can be used for the entire perimeter. Rewarming should be started when one half of the anastomosis is completed.

10

The patient is then placed in a steep Trendelenburg position and the ostia of the great vessels are again irrigated and inspected to make sure that no particulate debris has become lodged or hidden in these locations. With the great vessels still clamped the balloon is partially deflated, the anterior aspect of the graft being held upwards; the entire graft and great vessels are then allowed to fill with blood from the femoral cannula. All three great vessels are 'milked' retrograde back to the graft and/or needle-aspirated to ensure that all air has been evacuated, care being taken not to injure the vessels or dislodge any atherosclerotic debris. The left subclavian and left common carotid arteries are then unclamped; frequently perfusion of the innominate artery is sufficient to result in profuse back bleeding down these vessels, helping further to eliminate any possibly retained air or debris, which is flushed up and out of the graft. Finally, the innominate artery clamp is released. Pump flow can be reduced to minimize haemorrhage during these steps if necessary. The aortic occlusion balloon catheter is extracted. The graft is cross-clamped just proximal to the button of aorta, pump flow restored to normal and rewarming accelerated. As mentioned before, the nature of these very soft low-porosity woven Dacron grafts makes it difficult to accomplish complete occlusion with ordinary vascular clamps. Therefore long Kocher clamps applied obliquely should be used (see *illustration 11*).

11

Once reperfusion of the cerebral vessels from both arterial cannulae has been accomplished attention is directed to haemostasis of the end-to-end suture line containing the origins of the great vessels. Significant problems should be corrected at this time. The innominate arterial cannula can be removed either now or later, after completion of the proximal anastomosis. The defect is secured with a full-thickness diamond-shaped purse-string suture.

12

The proximal anastomosis is then constructed, care again being taken to incorporate full-thickness bites of the proximal aortic cuff. The back wall is completed from the inside; as before, a long (140 cm) 3/0 polypropylene suture is used to expedite the construction of this anastomosis since one or other limb can be used sequentially to complete the anastomosis. As always, care is necessary in the construction of this anastomosis to ensure that the aorta is not torn as the needle passes through it and that a proper constant degree of traction is maintained on the 'following' end of the suture.

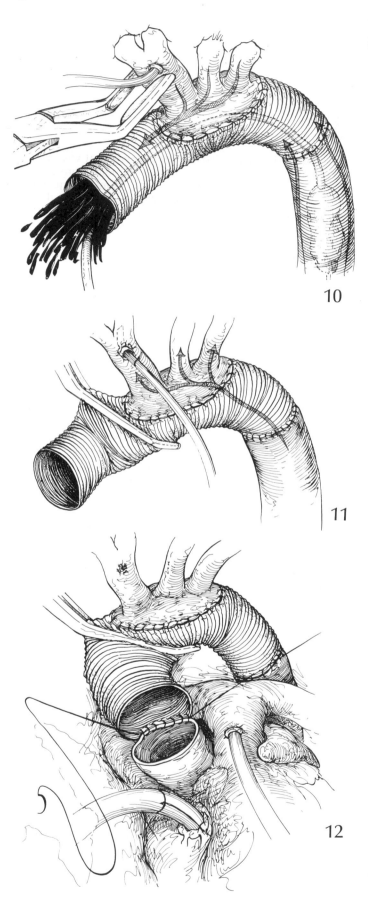

10

11

12

13

The front wall of the proximal suture line is then completed with the other limb of the 3/0 polypropylene suture. The patient has remained in a steep Trendelenburg position since the restoration of flow to the cerebral vessels; any vents in use are then turned off and blood returned to the patient from the oxygenator. The anaesthetist then ventilates the patient, using progressively more amplitude and frequency. The heart is elevated (or needle-aspirated if necessary) and all air evacuated from the left-sided chambers of the heart before completion of this proximal suture line.

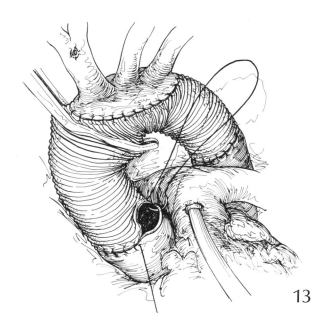

13

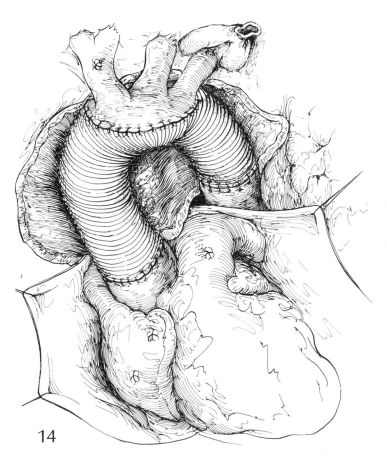

14

14

The procedure has now been completed, the heart resuscitated and cardiopulmonary bypass discontinued. If any concomitant procedures are necessary, such as aortic valve replacement, coronary artery bypass grafting or replacement of the entire ascending aorta, these can be performed after restitutuion of flow to the great vessels.

CARDIOPULMONARY BYPASS WITH PROFOUND HYPOTHERMIA AND CIRCULATORY ARREST

This technique is preferred for patients with acute or chronic aortic dissections resulting in false aneurysms of the aortic arch, emergency cases or patients with ruptured arch aneurysms. A standard median sternotomy incision is used (see illustration 1), with or without extension into the neck. Preparation for total cardiopulmonary bypass is carried out as previously described, though of course the arterial pump line does not have to be 'Y-ed'. Surface cooling before the institution of core cooling on bypass may be used to ensure that the peripheral adipose and muscular tissues are adequately cooled, thereby eliminating heat shifts during the period of circulatory arrest, though this preliminary step is not essential. During the cooling phase (the rate of which should be limited to 1°C/minute) haemodilution is carried out; fresh autologous blood is withdrawn for later use and replaced on a ml-per-ml basis with crystalloid or colloid solutions, or both. Associated concomitant procedures may be performed during this cooling phase (e.g. aortic valve replacement or coronary artery bypass grafting), although most prefer to delay these until the rewarming phase in order to make more efficient use of the total time on cardiopulmonary bypass.

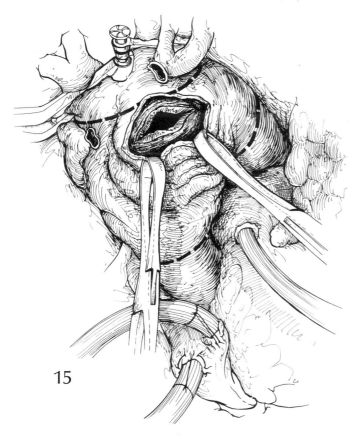

15

15

When the patient's rectal temperature is about 15°C the great vessels are clamped as described above. The pump flow is reduced to the range of 100–200 ml/minute and the venous lines are clamped without exsanguinating the patient into the cardiopulmonary bypass circuit. The heart is arrested with cardioplegic solution and continuous profound supplemental topical hypothermia is started. The aneurysm is then opened longitudinally. The almost complete cessation of bronchial blood flow and the use of the pulmonary vent usually completely eliminate any blood return to the left heart, thereby avoiding the need to clamp the ascending aorta.

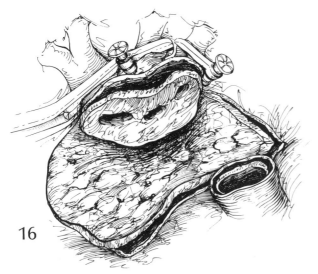

16

16

The use of circulatory arrest for resection of an aortic dissection involving the aortic arch is illustrated here. The basic surgical techniques are similar to those outlined earlier for patients with aortic dissections involving other segments of the thoracic aorta. The points of aortic transection both distally and proximally are determined and full-thickness aortic cuffs are dissected free. A full-thickness button of the convex surface of the aortic arch incorporating the origins of all three great vessels is dissected free. Portions of the posterior aneurysm sac need not be completely resected.

17

The aortic cuffs proximally and distally and the button for the great vessels are then prepared by obliterating the false lumen (with or without the use of external layers of Teflon felt) with a running 4/0 or 3/0 polypropylene suture. The back wall of the button surrounding the great vessels can be reapproximated from the inside, but care is necessary to avoid tearing the fragile aortic intima when the needle traverses this layer. Back bleeding from the distal aorta can be intermittently aspirated with the pump suckers if necessary.

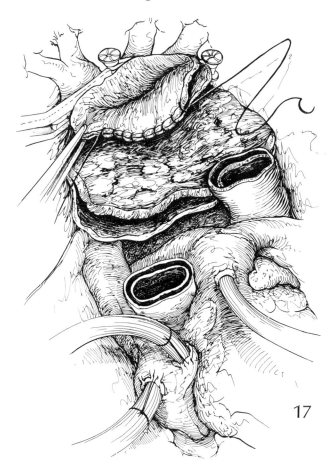

17

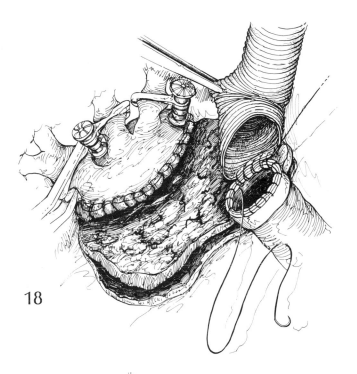

18

18

After preparation of the aortic cuffs the distal anastomosis is constructed end to end using a 140 cm 3/0 polypropylene suture. If the tissue integrity of the aorta is poor a single external layer of Teflon felt (secured circumferentially with a running 4/0 polypropylene suture) can be helpful. Construction of the back wall of the anastomosis is performed from the inside; the distal anastomosis is then completed in standard fashion from the outside.

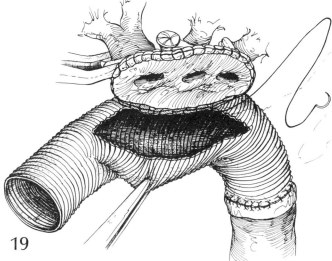

19

19

An appropriately sized oval-shaped defect is cut into the greater curvature of the graft with a disposable ophthalmic cautery. The end-to-side anastomosis of this island containing the great vessels is then constructed, again starting at the middle of the back wall from the inside and using both limbs of a 140 cm polypropylene suture.

20

The patient is then placed in a steep Trendelenburg position and the ostia of the great vessels as well as the proximal portion of the descending thoracic aorta are all irrigated copiously and suctioned clean to ensure that no particulate debris is retained. Pump flow is then gradually increased, the proximal end of the graft being held straight up in the air before release of the clamps on the great vessels. These vessels are then carefully 'milked' back towards the graft to drive any possibly retained air up into the graft and out of the cerebral circulation. The clamps on the arch vessels are then briefly removed to guarantee again that no air has become lodged in their proximal portions. When this has been accomplished pump flow is brought back up to the normal range, the great vessels are unclamped and rewarming started. The graft is clamped just proximal to the end-to-side anastomosis. Rewarming should be limited to a rate of 1°C every 3 minutes. After perfusion has been restarted it is important to inspect the distal and great vessel anastomoses critically for haemostasis. Serious bleeding must be repaired at this time, and if necessary the pump can again be turned off to facilitate placement of repair sutures, avoiding undue twisting or tension of the graft. Exposure and control of such major bleeding points later in the procedure will be difficult and may lead to even more troublesome bleeding. During rewarming the proximal anastomosis and any necessary concomitant procedures (aortic valve replacement, coronary artery bypass grafting etc.) are performed.

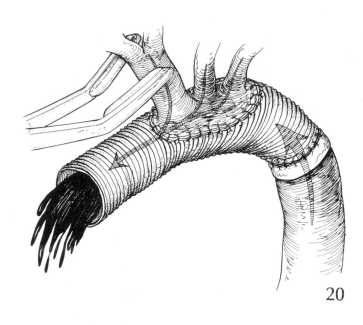

20

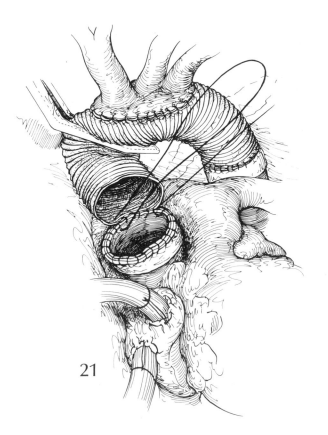

21

21

The proximal anastomosis in a patient with a dissection in which the distal ascending aorta was involved but concomitant aortic valve replacement was not necessary is illustrated. This anastomosis is constructed with a 140 cm 3/0 polypropylene suture, starting on the back wall and running both limbs round anteriorly.

22

When the patient's temperature has reached 37°C, the heart has been adequately resuscitated on bypass and all other concomitant procedures have been completed bypass is gradually and slowly discontinued. Decannulation is routine.

When haemostasis is complete the heparin effect is neutralized with protamine sulphate and the coagulation profile corrected with appropriate components. Rapid and serial assessment of the entire coagulation pattern is necessary to guide such component therapy. Platelets and fresh frozen plasma are used frequently and cryoprecipitate occasionally, but Factor IX concentrates (Proplex or Koyne) only rarely and only when absolutely necessary, owing to the high risk of hepatitis. Retransfusion of the patient's fresh (autologous) warm whole blood also helps to normalize coagulation.

The completed procedure whereby the proximal descending thoracic aorta, the entire arch and the majority of the ascending thoracic aorta have been replaced is illustrated. It should be noted that the technique described does not include wrapping the graft with the aneurysm sac. This is usually not necessary and, since the preferred technique involves dissection of, and, anastomosis to full-thickness aortic cuffs, wrapping the prosthesis with the aneurysm sac would not result in effective tamponade as blood could escape from these areas. There are cases, however, in which the 'inclusion' anastomotic method may be preferred, but it is recommended only for the distal descending aortic anastomosis. This technique can be helpful in cases of large degenerative aneurysms when exposure of the distal aorta is difficult. If one is to use such a technique, then it is extremely important to use a large needle and very large bites of aorta to guarantee that the suture bites are of full thickness. On the other hand care must be taken not to injure adjacent structures or possibly incorporate the oesophagus into the anastomosis with large 'blind' bites taken from the inside when the 'graft inclusion' technique is used.

Even in the best of hands, it is probably realistic to expect that the operative mortality rate for aortic arch aneurysm resection will be in the region of 10 per cent, with a slightly lower incidence of stroke, regardless of what type of perfusion technique is used. Thus while this risk is acceptable (and markedly superior to earlier surgical attempts), it is still relatively high. Operation

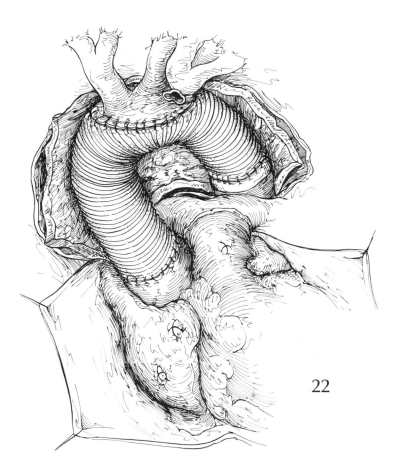

22

should be reserved for patients with symptomatic arch aneurysms, those with arch aneurysm expansion documented by CT scanning or aortography, those with aneurysms 10 cm or larger in diameter and, possibly, those with acute aortic arch dissections. Fortunately the vast majority of patients with acute dissections who have involvement of the arch present either as acute Type A or as acute Type B (see Chapter on 'Surgical treatment of aortic dissections', pp. 526–537) and can be handled safely by just resecting the ascending or descending aorta as appropriate. In the rare patient who has an acute dissection that is confined to the transverse arch, then replacement may be the only viable option.

Cardiac tumours

W. R. Eric Jamieson MD, FACC, FACS, FRCS(C)
Clinical Associate Professor, Division of Cardiovascular and Thoracic Surgery, Department of Surgery, Vancouver General Hospital, University of British Columbia, Vancouver, Canada

Bonnie G. Massing MD, FRCP(C)
Clinical Assistant Professor, Department of Pathology, University of British Columbia, Vancouver; Associate Pathologist, British Columbia Children's Hospital, Vancouver, Canada

Noel F. Quenville MD, FRCP(C)
Clinical Professor, Department of Pathology, University of British Columbia, Vancouver; Head, Division of Anatomical Pathology, Vancouver General Hospital, Vancouver, Canada

Introduction

Primary cardiac tumours are extremely rare in all age groups and probably have an annual incidence of less than 1 per cent. They are of special interest to both the cardiologist and the surgeon. The majority of tumours primary to the heart are benign and the cardiac myxoma represents approximately 25 per cent of primary tumours of the heart. A high index of clinical suspicion is necessary to diagnose a cardiac tumour; protean manifestations can mimic a variety of other cardiac and non-cardiac diseases. Because of the uncommon occurrence of these lesions no surgeon has a broad experience with any cardiac tumour.

Of the variety of cardiac tumours the surgeon is most likely to encounter the myxoma in adults and the rhabdomyoma in children. Surgery for rhabdomyoma should be aggressive when the child does not have tuberous sclerosis. The surgery for cardiac myxoma must be designed to prevent recurrence, minimize the dangers of intraoperative embolization and permit exploration of all cardiac chambers. The approach of choice for surgical management of left atrial tumours is via the right atrium and the interatrial septum. This technique allows exposure for wide excision of the septal stalk and helps avoid fragmentation and embolization. The combined right and left atriotomies are advisable for large left atrial tumours. Surgery for benign cardiac tumours can be successful with minimal morbidity and mortality.

Pathology

The cardiac myxoma arises from embryonic mesenchymal remnants with multipotential capabilities for cellular differentiation[1-4]. The accompanying tables document the relative incidence, common sites, gross appearance and pathological features important for the surgeon to consider in the management of cardiac tumours.

Consultation with the pathologist may be useful before attempting excision or biopsy of a cardiac neoplasm in order to ensure an accurate diagnosis. The possibility of frozen section examination should be discussed as well as the appropriate handling of the specimen for electron microscopic or other special studies. Malignancy is difficult to determine from frozen sections, and radical resection is suggested whenever possible, including radical resection of the septum or posterior wall of the left atrium for attached myxoma. Embolic tissue removed from a peripheral vessel should always be examined for myxomatous tissue, especially in a patient without a cardiac history and in sinus rhythm.

Table I Benign cardiac tumours – adults[1-6]

Tumour	Relative incidence*	Common sites	Gross appearance	Additional comments
Myxoma	25 per cent	75 per cent lt atrium 20 per cent rt atrium 7 per cent ventricular 5 per cent multiple	Polypoid mass, 5–6 cm., soft, gelatinous with mucoid appearance arising from endocardium. Pedunculated narrow stalk. Myxoma right atrium tends to be solitary with wider attachment. Tumour may be bilateral and multicentric.	Majority of atrial myxomas arise from septum and require resection of atrial portion. There is a tendency to embolize during surgery.
Papillary elastofibroma	10 per cent	Endocardium, usually valvular surface	Multiple papillary fronds attached to endocardium by a short pedicle, resembles sea anemone.	Most commonly an incidental finding on surgically removed valves.
Lipomas 1. Lipomatous hypertrophy atrial septum	10 per cent	Atrial septum	Circumscribed but unencapsulated mass of firm brown fat which distorts atrial septum.	Rhythm disturbances usually present.
2. True lipoma		Myocardium, pericardium	Encapsulated mass of mature fat.	Asymptomatic

*Relative incidence refers to per cent of all heart and pericardial tumours in the large AFIP series of 533 cases[4].

Table II Benign cardiac tumours – children[4, 7, 8]

Tumour	Relative incidence*	Common sites	Gross appearance	Additional comments
Rhabdomyoma	60 per cent neonates 40 per cent children	Intramyocardial tumour which occurs in all chambers. Left and right ventricle most common, 50 per cent have intracavity portion.	Vary in size from millimetres to several centimetres. White to yellow mass.	Approximately ⅓ cases associated with tuberous sclerosis. Hamartomas primarily result from arrested cardiocyte maturation. Usually multiple.
Fibroma	13 per cent	Ventricular free wall. Frequently involve septum. Occasionally atria.	Single tumour, may be as large as 10 cm. White, firm, appears circumscribed.	Often calcified on X-ray. May occur in association with generalized fibromatosis. Though circumscribed, tumour usually infiltrates muscle on microscopy; therefore wider excision may be necessary.
Haemangioma	3 per cent	Occurs any site in heart including epicardium. May have intracavity portion.	Vascular appearance (red, haemmorrhagic) grossly appear circumscribed but extensive spread into myocardium is the rule.	Must be distinguished from varix of the heart, which usually occurs on subendocardium.
Teratoma	20 per cent neonates 12 per cent children	Majority are intrapericardial and arise at base of the heart.	May reach very large size (>15 cm) Smooth and lobulated surface. Cut surface reveals multiple cysts.	Have definite malignant potential. Usually attached to root of pulmonary artery and effective removal includes dissection of root of great vessels.

Table III Cardiac tumours – malignant[4, 9–12]

Tumour	Relative incidence	Common sites	Gross appearance	Additional comments
Angiosarcoma	7 per cent	80 per cent right heart	Vascular tumour which may extensively involve heart and pericardium.	Cardiomegaly present. Electron microscopy recommended.
Rhabdomyo-sarcoma	5 per cent	Occurs in all chambers.	Multiple nodules of soft tumour, may invade cardiac valves. Usually myocardial and intracavitary portions.	Electron microscopy recommended.
Fibrosarcoma	3 per cent	Occurs in all chambers.	May have nodular or infiltrative appearance. Firm tumours, white. May have intracavitary portion with valvular invasion.	Electron microscopy recommended.
Secondary	Most common cardiac tumours.	All sites in heart.	Multiple, small, nodules are typical.	Metastases to the heart have been reported with most kinds of malignancy. Most common are: 1. Melanoma 2. Lung 3. Leukaemia 4. Thyroid The majority are asymptomatic.

Presentation of cardiac myxomas

The classic triad of presentation of cardiac myxomas is atrioventricular valvular obstruction, embolism and constitutional manifestations. The protean manifestations may mimic many disease processes with chronic systemic involvement such as rheumatic fever, bacterial endocarditis or collagen diseases. The presentation of myxomas is embolic in 40 per cent of cases, intracardiac obstruction in 94 per cent and manifestations of systemic illness in 82 per cent[13]. Embolization may be systemic, pulmonary or coronary depending on the site of the primary lesion and the presence of intracardiac shunts.

The intracardiac obstruction is usually either intermittent subvalvular obstruction of the left ventricle, partial obstruction of the mitral valve during diastole by a left atrial myxoma or obstruction of the tricuspid orifice by a right atrial myxoma, which may cause a large right-to-left shunt through a patent foramen ovale. A left atrial myxoma may interfere with the mitral valve apparatus, causing regurgitation.

The presentation of obstruction may be progressive and rapid, sometimes with syncope, palpitations, dyspnoea and unusual variation of symptoms with posture. Cardiac murmurs may be atypical and vary with posture. The constitutional manifestations of cardiac tumours are weight loss, fatigue, fever, urticaria, clubbing, Raynaud's phenomena, anaemia, elevated exythrocyte sedimentation rate, thrombocytopenia and alteration of serum immunoglobulin levels[14].

Abnormalities of cardiac rhythm and conduction may be the presenting features. Left atrial tumours may mimic mitral stenosis, often with pulmonary hypertension, while right atrial tumours may mimic tricuspid stenosis or insufficiency, cor pulmonale, Ebstein's anomaly, carcinoid heart disease, pulmonary embolism, constrictive pericarditis, acute rheumatic pericarditis and caval syndromes. Right ventricular tumours may cause outflow obstruction and simulate pulmonary valve stenosis, and left ventricular tumours may mimic aortic stenosis. Embolic material may cause systemic, cerebral or pulmonary infarction and, if infected, lead to aneurysms and abscess formation.

Diagnosis

Echocardiography is the most important procedure available today for the imaging of cardiac tumours. M-mode echocardiography is dependent on tumour movement for visualization. The classic imaging of the left atrial myxoma is reflected echos behind but separate from the anterior mitral leaflet as the tumour prolapses into the ventricle during diastole[15]. The findings are independent of the size of the tumour, though small tumours may not be identified. Right artial myxomas may present similar findings, with a mass of echos behind the tricuspid leaflets holding the valve open during diastole and causing abnormal valve motion. The mass usually disappears into the atrium during systole; persistence of the mass throughout the cardiac cycle indicates fixation of the tumour to the mitral or tricuspid valve.

Real-time two-dimensional (2D) echocardiography provides quantitative information regarding size, shape and mobility of the tumour, as well as the effects on cardiac function. The 2D study can evaluate simultaneously both the left and right atrial, identifying bilateral tumours if present. 2D evaluation will detect smaller space-occupying lesions than M-mode imaging because of better resolution. Besides determining the presence, size and mobility of the tumour, the 2D assessment can determine the site of the stalk attachment and determine more accurately the extent of tumour obstruction. Isolated right atrial or ventricular tumours that would be missed otherwise can be identified by real-time studies.

Echocardiography should obviate the need for contrast studies, which could be detrimental to the patient. If angiography is deemed necessary the right atrial myxoma should be visualized by an inferior vena caval contrast injection and the left atrial myxoma by pulmonary artery injection with laevophase visualization so as to avoid fragmentation of the tumour in both instances. Transseptal catheterization can be hazardous owing to the risk of fragmentation and embolization.

The operations

Surgery following early diagnosis may be lifesaving, and once the diagnosis of an endocardial tumour, most commonly a left atrial myxoma, has been established prompt surgical intervention is mandatory. The surgical management must be designed to permit exploration of all cardiac chambers, minimize the dangers of intra-operative embolization and prevent recurrence.

ENDOCARDIAL MYXOMAS

Left atrial myxoma

Total cardiopulmonary bypass and myocardial protection with hypothermic cardioplegia is used. The right atriotomy and interatrial septal approach affords better exposure of the left atrium than the left atriotomy approach. The stalk of the tumour should be excised with an oval-shaped full-thickness segment of the atrial septum. The site of attachment of the tumour stalk may be other than the fossa ovalis, and sites along the atrial wall are not uncommon. This approach affords full examination for residual tumour fragments and multicentric tumours. The left ventricle and right ventricle are examined through their respective atrioventricular valves for tumour fragments or multicentric myxomas.

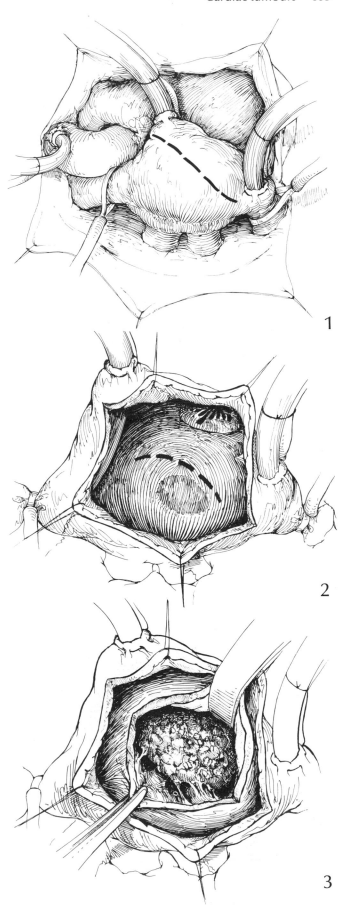

1

1

The patient is placed on cardiopulmonary bypass with two caval cannulae and the use of caval tapes so that the right atrium may be explored.

2

2 & 3

Right atriotomy is performed and the right atrium, tricuspid valve and right ventricle examined for tumour involvement. The atrial septum, including the fossa ovalis, is exposed and an incision made in the position illustrated. The tumour can now be seen through the interatrial incision. It is usually attached to the left atrial side of the fossa ovalis.

3

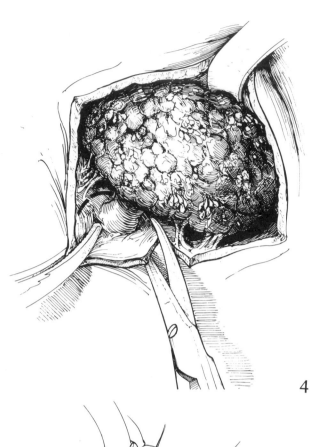

4

4 & 5

A portion of the septum containing the stalk and incorporating a satisfactory margin around the tumour is excised, the septum and stalk are firmly grasped and the entire tumour removed. A spoon is sometimes helpful to deliver excessively large and fragile tumours.

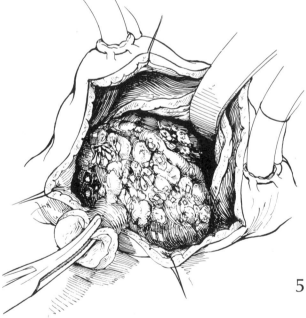

5

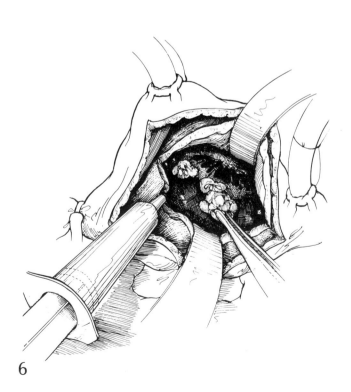

6

6

Careful examination for tumour remnants is carried out and irrigation performed of the atria and left ventricle to ensure that no residual fragments exist. The mitral valve is examined for abnormalities that may require repair or replacement.

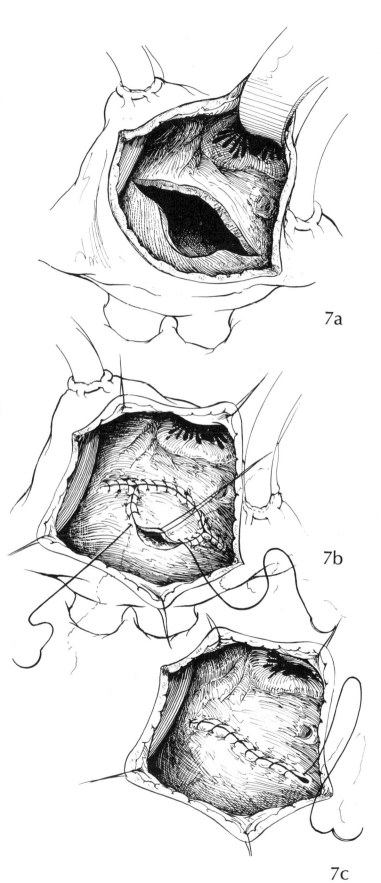

7a

7b

7c

7a, b & c

The residual defect in the atrium (*a*) is repaired with a pericardial patch if large (*b*) or may be repaired primarily (*c*).

8

The right atriotomy is now closed. The release of the superior caval tape allows the evacuation of air. Residual air should be aspirated from the ascending aorta and left heart with manual ventilation of the lungs by the anaesthetist before release of the aortic cross clamp.

The right atriotomy approach, besides providing better exposure of the left atrium, affords less traction on the septum and lessens the risk of fragmentation. The atrioventricular valves must alway be assessed for concomitant valvular disease or valve destruction by tumour. The tumour can cause fibrous thickening of the endocardium and especially the atrial surface of the leaflets. Damage to the tricuspid valve from a right atrial myxoma is more common than damage of the mitral valve from a left atrial myxoma.

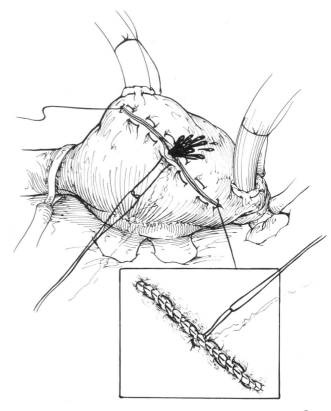

8

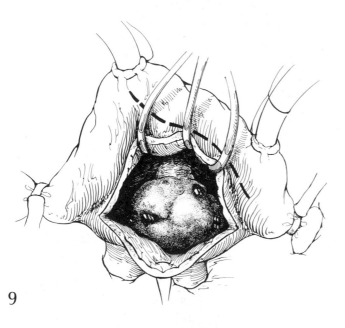

9

9

The combined right and left atriotomy approach is probably only necessary for very large tumours. The left atrial incision is made in the usual place, revealing the tumour, and the right atrial incision planned in the position shown.

10a & b

Excision of the base of the tumour, together with the surrounding septum, is performed from the right atrial side (a) and the tumour can then be removed from the left side (b).

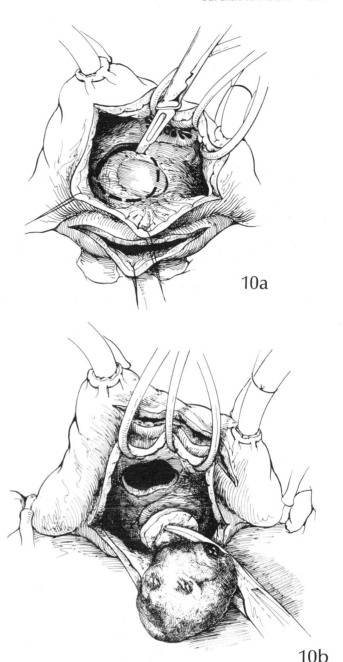

10a

10b

Right atrial myxoma

The surgical management of the right atrial myxoma requires special attention. To minimize the risk of embolization the superior vena cava should be cannulated from the high right atrial wall or superior vena cava and the inferior vena cava indirectly from a common femoral vein. Excision of the atrial myxoma with a full thickness of septum affords better protection against recurrence. Right atrial tumours often require extensive resection and reconstruction. The repair should consist of reconstruction of the tricuspid valve annulus, if indicated, and right atrial reconstruction with autologous pericardium[16].

Ventricular myxomas

Cardiac myxomas may also occur within the right and left ventricles. Right ventricular tumours are approached by ventriculotomy. These tumours usually involve the anterior wall of the right ventricle in close association with the papillary muscles and anterior leaflet of the tricuspid valve, within the tricuspid valve or pulmonary outflow tract. Left ventricular tumours can be approached by three routes – through the aorta, through the left atrium with detachment of the anterior leaflet of the mitral valve or by left ventriculotomy. The septal excision site of the left ventricular myxoma can be repaired with a patch.

Recurrent myxomas

Cardiac myxomas can be recurrent in all cardiac chambers. The excision of the interatrial septum is not universally accepted, but a radical approach at the primary operation affords the best opportunity for cure. Extraseptal sessile tumours are more likely to recur because of implantation and the removal of an inadequate amount of atrial wall. Recurrences at extraseptal sites are often multiple and sessile. Extraseptal resections tend to be less radical for it is not as easy to resect and replace external atrial walls as septum. Malignant tumours or malignant recurrences of myxomas are very difficult to manage successfully.

The metastatic eventuality of the local recurrence of a myxoma cannot be predicted from the microscopic assessment of the primary tumour. Metastatic lesions often have a more malignant appearance than the original tumour. Recurrent lesions must be totally excised along with their attachment to the cardiac or vessel wall. Surgery for recurrent malignant tumours is usually only palliative.

11a & b

PAPILLARY FIBROELASTOMA

A papillary fibroelastoma on the anterior leaflet of the mitral valve is shown here (a). This tumour resembles a sea anemone with multiple papillary fronds attached to valve endocardium by a relatively short pedicle. After resection of the tumour with a portion of the leaflet patch repair is carried out (b).

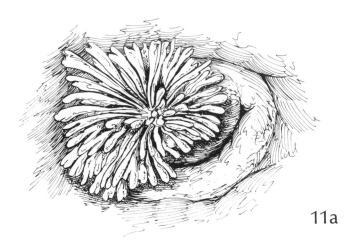

11a

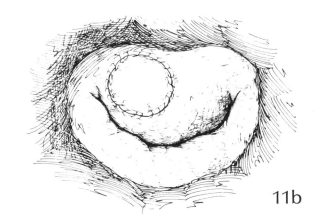

11b

Complications

The morbidity and mortality of excision of atrial myxoma is minimal. Strict attention must be paid by the surgical team to avoid perioperative tumour embolization. Supraventricular arrhythmias occur after extensive atrial surgery but reflect injury to the sinoatrial node rather than to internodal conduction pathways. One study showed an incidence of supraventricular arrhythmias in 28 per cent of patients, all of whom were discharged in sinus rhythm[17].

Follow-up

After removal of atrial tumours the echocardiographic pattern becomes normal. Echocardiographic assessment is necessary for follow-up evaluation for recurrence.

MYOCARDIAL TUMOURS

Myocardial tumours, in contrast to endocardial myxomas, are usually fibromas and hamartomas. The principles of surgical management of these tumours include preservation of major coronary arteries, papillary muscles and valves and reconstruction of the ventricle to allow satisfactory myocardial filling. Cardiac transplantation is an alternative for a left ventricular tumour, such as a fibrous histiocytoma, when the tumour is otherwise inoperable[18].

The benign tumours in children are usually rhabdomyomas. The hamartomas are usually multiple and occur in both atria and ventricles. Children who do not have tuberous sclerosis should be managed aggressively.

12

Ventricular hamartoma

The unusual tumour illustrated here by courtesy of Dr A. Ian Munro, Clinical Associate Professor, Vancouver General Hospital, University of British Columbia[19], is a large hamartoma of the anterior right ventricular wall adjacent to the atrioventricular groove. (The insert is a drawing of a computerized tomography showing the relationship of the tumour).

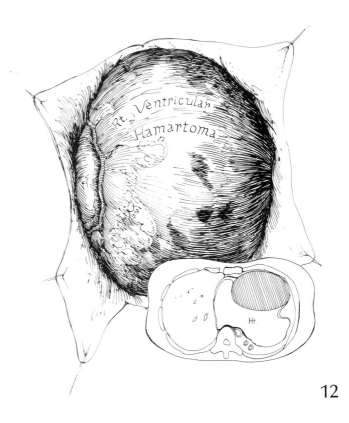

12

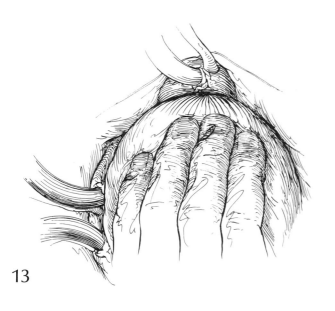

13

13

Cannulation of the ascending aorta and superior and inferior vena cavae has been carried out and a hand placed over the tumour to demonstrate its size (18 × 12 × 10 cm).

14

The operative site after resection of the tumour is demonstrated here. The tumour extended from the infundibulum superiorly to the posterior descending artery inferiorally, and medially from the right atrium to midway towards the anterior descending artery. The right coronary artery was involved in the tumour.

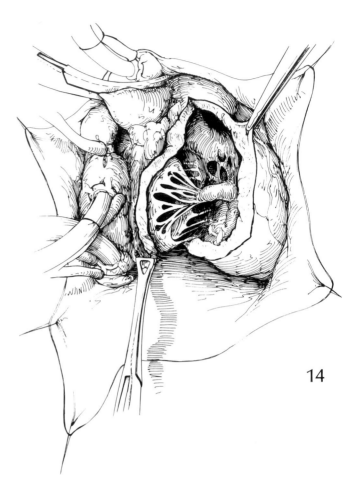

14

15

The repair consisted of primary closure superiorly and inferiorly, while the remainder of the defect was closed with Teflon cloth as shown.

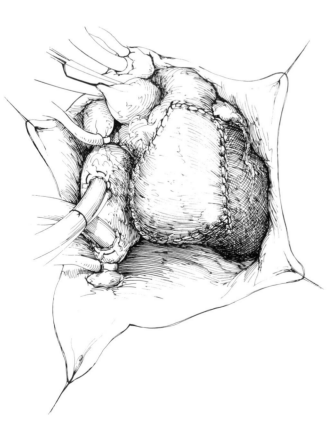

15

16 & 17

Ventricular septal fibroma

These illustrations demonstrate resection of a ventricular septal fibroma. A right transverse ventriculotomy is performed and the portion of interventricular septum encompassing the tumour excised. The tricuspid and mitral valves remain intact. The ventricular septum is reconstituted with a synthetic patch.

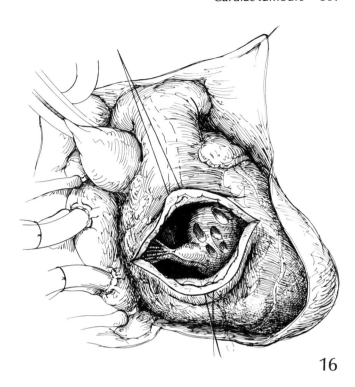

16

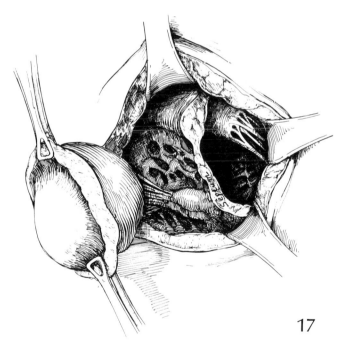

17

RENAL CELL CARCINOMA

Renal cell carcinoma frequently extends into the inferior vena cava and the tumour thrombus occasionally extends into the right atrium. The presentation usually includes inferior veva caval obstruction and right-sided congestive heart failure. The renal carcinoma thrombus may be confused with a right atrial myxoma. The abdominal procedures without the support of cardiopulmonary bypass include finger dissection and Foley catheter removal of the cardiac tumour extension. Cardiopulmonary bypass increases the likelihood of safe and complete removal of the tumour thrombus. Extension of tumour thrombus into the right heart must not be considered a sign of inoperability.

18

The illustration shows a hypernephroma with tumour thrombosis to the right atrium. The recommended management is with total cardiopulmonary bypass, using cannulation of the ascending aorta, superior vena cava and femoral vein with a long cannula to the infrarenal inferior vena cava. Nephrectomy and tumour thrombosis removal can now be performed.

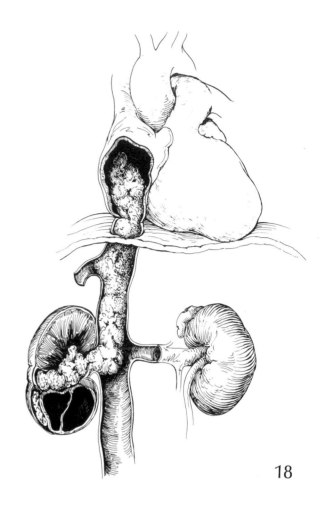

18

References

1. Feldman, P. S., Horvater, E., Kalman, K. An ultrastructral study of seven cardiac myxomas. Cancer 1977; 40: 2216–2232

2. Ferrans, V. J., Roberts, W. C. Structural features of cardiac myxomas. Human Pathology 1973; 4: 111–146

3. Morales, A. R., Fine, G., Castro, A., *et al.* Cardiac myxoma (endocardioma): an immunocytochemical assessment of histogenesis. Human Pathology 1981; 12: 896–899

4. McAllister, H. A., Fenoglio, J. J. Tumours of the cardiovascular system. Atlas of Tumor Pathology, 2nd series, Fascide 15, Washington, D.C. Armed Forces Institute of Pathology, 1978

5. Fishbein, M. C., Ferrans, V. J., Roberts, W. C. Endocardial papillary elastofibromas. Histologic, histochemical and electron microscopic findings. Archives of Pathology 1975; 99: 335

6. Page, D. L. Lipomatous hypertrophy of cardiac interatrial septum: Its development and probable clinical significance. Human Pathology 1970; 1: 151–163

7. Fenoglio, J. J., MacAllister, H. A., Ferrans, V. J. Cardiac rhabdomyoma: A clinicopathologic and electron microscopic study. American Journal of Cardiology 1976; 38: 241–251

8. Feldman, P. S., Meyer, M. W. Fibroelastic hamartoma (fibroma) of the heart. Cancer 1976; 38: 314–323

9. Rossi, N. P., Kiosdros, J. M., Aschinbrener, C. A., Threnhaft, J. L., *et al.* Primary angiosarcoma of the heart. Cancer 1976; 37: 891–894

10. Yang, H. Y., Wasiebuski, J. F., Lee, W., *et al.* Angiosarcoma of the heart: ultrastructural study. Cancer 1981; 47: 72–80

11. Ramu, M. Rhabdomyosarcoma of the heart. Postgraduate Medical Journal 1976; 52: 310–312

12. Lockwood, Wm. B., Broghamener, W. L. The changing prevalence of secondary cardiac neoplasms as related to cancer therapy. Cancer 1980; 45: 2659–2662

13. Trimakas, A. P., Maxwell, K. D., Berkay, S., Gardner, T. J., Achuff, S. C. Fetal monitoring during cardiopulmonary bypass for removal of a left atrial myxoma during pregnancy. Johns Hopkins Medical Journal 1979; 144: 156–160

14. Attar, S., Lee, Y. C., Singleton, R., Scherlis, L., David, R., McLaughlin, J. S. Cardiac myxoma. Annals of Thoracic Surgery 1980; 29: 397–405

15. Wolfe, S. B., Popp, R. L., Feigenbaum, H. Diagnosis of atrial tumours by ultrasound. Circulation 1969; 39: 615–622

16. Culliford, A. T., Isom, O. W., Trehan, N. K., Doyle, E., Gorstein, F., Spencer, F. C. Benign tumour of right atrium necessitating extensive resection and reconstruction. Journal of Thoracic and Cardiovascular Surgery 1978; 76: 178

17. Silverman, N. A. Primary cardiac tumours. Annals of Surgery 1980; 191: 127–138

18. Jamieson, S. W., Gaudiani, V. A., Reitz, B. A., Oyer, P. E., Stinson, E. B., Shumway, N. E. Operative treatment of an unresectable tumour of the left ventricle. Journal of Thoracic and Cardiovascular Surgery 1981; 81: 797–799

19. Larrieu, A. J., Jamieson, W. R. E., Tyers, G. F. O., Burr, L. H., Munro, A. I., Miyagishima, R. T., Gevein, A. N., Allen, P. Primary cardiac tumours. Journal of Thoracic and Cardiovascular Surgery 1982; 83: 339–348

Surgical treatment of cardiac arrhythmias

Richard Cory-Pearce MB, BS, FRCS, FACC
Senior Research Fellow, British Heart Foundation;
Consultant Cardiothoracic Surgeon, University of Cambridge and Papworth Hospital, Cambridge, UK

Introduction

The direct and indirect operative treatment of cardiac arrhythmia, begun in the late 1960s with the surgical induction of complete heart block, has expanded to cover a large field of supraventricular and ventricular arrhythmias and has been associated with the development of more and more specific techniques with improvement of success rates and an increase in the indications. All of the advances in this field have been based on the rapidly enlarging sphere of electrophysiology, culminating most recently in the achievement of interruption of some tachycardias by transvenous techniques.

Active treatment of cardiac arrhythmias can be based on three principal forms of therapy, used separately or in combination. These are pharmacological, stimulatory and surgical. Pharmacological treatment is essentially the sphere of the cardiologist in association with the specialist electrophysiologist. Stimulatory treatment is based on a variety of implantable devices ranging from conventional pacemaker systems to specialized scanning antitachycardia devices. This chapter is not concerned with either of these options but only with a direct surgical approach to the disorder of rhythm. It should be noted, however, that following such a direct approach post-operative permanent cardiac pacing may well be required.

SCOPE OF SURGERY

There are many different types of cardiac arrhythmia amenable to surgery, each with its appropriate operative technique or techniques. It is convenient to divide the arrhythmias into four principal groups:

1. supraventricular tachycardia with a distinct accessory pathway;
2. supraventricular tachycardia in which the accessory pathway, if present, is not distinguishable from the normal conduction system;
3. ventricular tachycardia in the absence of coronary artery disease; and
4. ventricular tachycardia associated with coronary artery disease.

Surgical options are divisible into two broad categories – namely, the interruption of a specific conduction pathway (albeit pathological or physiological) and the excision of the site of origin of tachycardia. The former implies interruption of one limb of a cyclical re-entrant mechanism and is limited to the region where atria and ventricles meet; it also applies to that group of arrhythmias in which an atrial tachyarrhythmia is associated with a rapid ventricular rate mediated by the junctional conduction tissue responding at a pathologically fast rate. The latter is applicable to local re-entrant circuits or areas of unstable automaticity and regional excision of the entire focus.

Preoperative investigation

Thorough investigation in the catheterization and electro-physiological laboratories is mandatory in all cases. This can be time-consuming and demanding of both patient and physician. In patients selected for surgery the principal objectives are the elucidation or confirmation of the specific type of arrhythmia, the localization of an ectopic focus of activity or an accessory pathway, the diagnosis of an associated condition (such as coronary artery disease or a hypertrophic cardiomyopathy) and the identification of the most potent techniques for inducing and terminating tachycardia.

Intraoperative mapping

Localization of an accessory pathway or the origin of ventricular tachycardia before operation is not sufficiently precise to allow the surgeon to proceed directly to ablation. A more accurate identification must be carried out as a preliminary to surgical treatment. For this reason, it is important to be able to induce tachyarrhythmia during operation. To render conditions optimal it is mandatory to cease active medication at an appropriate time before surgery to ensure that there is no significant residual drug effect and to conduct the mapping during surgery at normothermia.

Direct mapping of the sequence of activation of the heart during tachycardia is the best way of localizing an abnormal focus of origin or conduction pathway. In the event of failure of induction of tachycardia there are several indirect methods for localizing the appropriate site, such as mapping during sinus rhythm, atrial or ventricular pacing, 'pace mapping' and 'cryothermal mapping'.

The principle of intraoperative mapping is to plot abnormal activation sequences, so identifying their origin or abnormal conduction. In the special instance of localizing the atrioventricular (AV) nodal-His bundle junction local mapping based on knowledge of anatomical postition allows accurate identification of the operative site by observation of the characteristics of the His-bundle electrogram (see below). In all other instances the activation of the epicardial surface is plotted by derivation of surface electrograms from multiple sites. Comparison of the time of activation of each site by reference to a fixed bipolar electrode allows the construction of isochrone maps depicting the spread of activation. Where appropriate this is also applied to the endocardial surface.

The multiple epicardial sites can be sampled sequentially with a roving hand-held probe or synchronously with a sock-like net which fits over the ventricle to the AV groove and on which are multiple electrodes. The first alternative has the advantages of simplicity and flexibility. Direct measurements can be made so that there is no reliance on complex software. It is the only method that can be used for endocardial or atrial mapping. It does not, however, allow the mapping of a single beat and in mapping the posterior surface of the heart it is usually associated with very unstable rhythms not typical of the symptomatic tachycardia. It is a little slower, but in the hands of experienced operators this is not a significant disadvantage. Synchronous one-beat analysis by the sock technique has the advantage of being somewhat faster and is more effective in mapping the posterior ventricular walls. It is, however, necessarily more complex and therefore more expensive. Reliance on software also exposes it to the vulnerability of sampling error or system failure. The sock electrode is essentially restricted to epicardial mapping of the ventricles.

1

Mapping system

The layout of a typical mapping system is depicted diagrammatically here. The three principal components are a programmable stimulator as used in electrophysiological laboratories, a large-screen display for simultaneous monitoring of the procedure and a recording device to facilitate detailed study and measurement. The control box allows the selection of the electrodes in current use as pacing or sensing channels and directs the sensing channels to the appropriate areas of the display and recorder. The patient is connected to the control box with the interposition of an isolation interface on both sensing and pacing channels. The roving probe or bipolar electrodes in the sock are exclusively used for sensing. The other electrodes are in the form of bipolar hooks which are attached to specific parts of the atrium or ventricles for pacing or sensing as appropriate.

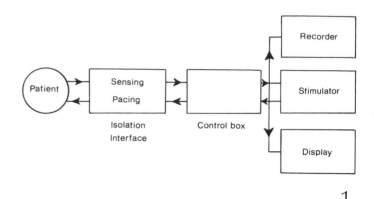

1

SPECIAL CONSIDERATIONS IN LEFT ATRIAL ENDOCARDIAL MAPPING

When it is necessary to map part of the left atrial endocardium, as in localization of a left atrial free wall accessory pathway, then open access to the mitral annulus is required during a period when the heart is beating at normothermia. Special precautions need to be taken, therefore, to prevent the possibility of embolization of air to the cerebral or coronary circulations. A suitable technique involves the provision of a coronary perfusion line fixed into the ascending aorta with a purse-string suture combined with aortic cross-clamping and maintenance of mitral valve incompetence by a retractor passing through the valve from the left atrium into the left ventricular cavity. Should the aortic valve be regurgitant or rendered so by mitral valve retraction, separate coronary cannulations would be indicated.

Intraoperational testing

Assessment of the success of the technique is of the utmost importance at two junctures – during the postprocedural intraoperative period and at the end of in-hospital convalescence before the patient's discharge. The intraoperative procedures are specifically designed to establish whether the procedure is effective in preventing tachyarrhythmia. After AV node – His bundle ablation permanent heart block should be observed. Successful removal of an accessory pathway is demonstrated by examination of the electrocardiogram (ECG) for evidence of pre-excitation and by repeat mapping during appropriate rhythms. In all cases repetition of the techniques found before ablation to be the most reliable in inducing tachycardia is required; it is at this stage that the presence of alternative tachyarrhythmias may be discovered. These are likely to be caused by either a second accessory pathway or a secondary focus of ventricular tachycardia.

The operations

Ablation techniques

According to the procedure planned a variety of techniques are available. They include dissection with transection, excision or exclusion, ligation, diathermy and cryothermy. The cryothermy technique has advanced the surgery of appropriate disorders principally by reducing the amount of dissection required and thereby reducing morbidity and speeding up the procedure. A cryothermy probe of tip diameter 5 mm is used and must be able to attain temperatures of between −60 and −70°C. Excision and exclusion techniques are principally restricted to ectopic foci in the ventricles.

ABLATION OF THE AV NODAL-HIS JUNCTION

Preparation of the patient for cardiopulmonary bypass is undertaken according to normally established techniques with some special considerations. Venous cannulation requires two cannulae placed well into the venae cavae and the additional use of caval snares. Introduction of the caval cannulae posteriorly in the right atrium near the cavoatrial junctions facilitates good exposure of the atrial endocardium for mapping purposes. This cannulation technique should be used in all instances as it cannot be known with certainty that a procedure involving opening the right atrium or ventricle will not be required. It is important to induce tachycardia for mapping during normothermia and so the pump prime should be kept at body temperature. After induction of cardiopulmonary bypass normothermic perfusion should be maintained.

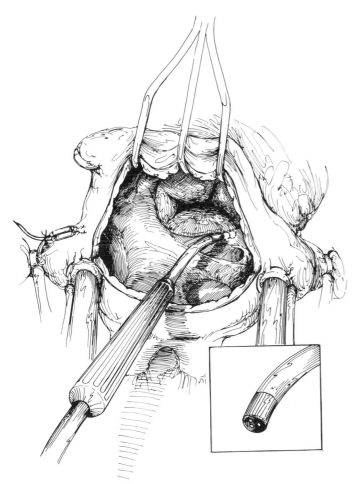

2

A vertical right atriotomy is made and retraction applied to expose the posterior tricuspid annulus. With the hand-held probe the right atrial border of the tricuspid annulus is mapped from the coronary sinus orifice to the right fibrous trigone by taking recordings of the endocardial electrogram from adjacent sites along the whole area.

2

3

The anatomical landmarks for mapping the position of the AV node-His bundle are the tricuspid annulus, the coronary sinus orifice, the tendon of Todaro and the right fibrous trigone marked by the supraventricular portion of the membranous interventricular septum. It is essential to adopt a reliable code for identifying the sites by consecutive numbering as shown here.

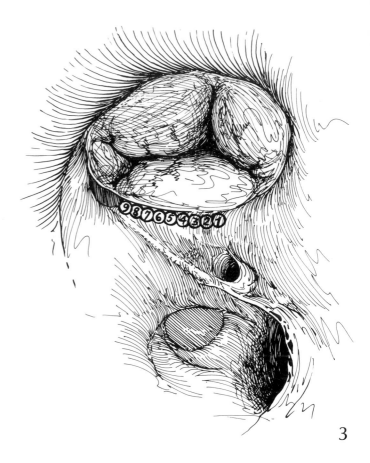

3

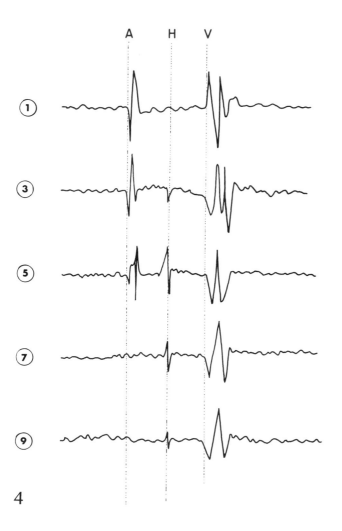

4

4

Serial recordings identify a progression from sites showing only atrial and ventricular activity through those demonstrating atrial (A), His (H) and ventricular (V) activity, from which first the atrial and then the His spike are lost. The ablation technique is centred on the site showing maximal amplitude of the His signal (trace 5).

5

The cryoprobe is applied to the site of maximal activity for one minute at 0°C during sinus rhythm. If appropriately selected this will result in complete AV block. The ventricular escape rhythm is usually of a narrow complex variety indicating origin in the lower His bundle. This is an acceptable, indeed desirable, variety of escape rhythm. Efficacy having thus been confirmed, the cryoprobe is then applied for 2 minutes at −60°C in the selected site and in at least two immediately adjacent sites.

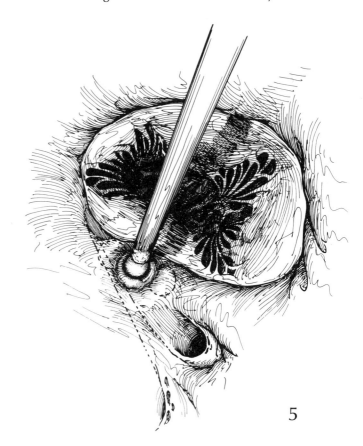

5

6

The intracardiac operative procedure is now complete and the right atriotomy is sutured in a single layer of 4/0 polypropylene, following which intraoperative post-procedural testing is performed and, a successful outcome having been achieved (the demonstration of complete heart block), the operation is completed by established techniques.

As indicated previously, permanent pacing is indicated after His bundle ablation. The type of system selected will depend on the careful cardiological assessment of the individual case, but temporary epicardial atrial and ventricular bipole electrodes are usually applied before chest closure and a permanent transvenous pacing system is implanted after electrophysiological reassessment and before discharge from hospital.

6

ABLATION OF ACCESSORY PATHWAYS

The surgical approach and technique employed for the ablation of accessory AV pathways is determined by the anatomical location of the pathological connection. It is convenient to deal with them in four regions. These are the right atrial free wall, the left atrial free wall and the anterior and posterior septal pathways. Although pre-operative mapping in the electrophysiological laboratory is unable to define the precise location of abnormal conduction tissue, it is invaluable in indicating in which of these regions it lies, so directing the surgeon's approach.

7

Right atrial free wall pathways

The region concerned is shown in this diagrammatic illustration. It extends around the right atrial border of the tricuspid annulus from the base of the aorta to the orifice of the coronary sinus.

Cardiopulmonary bypass is established and reference electrodes positioned as described in the preceding section.

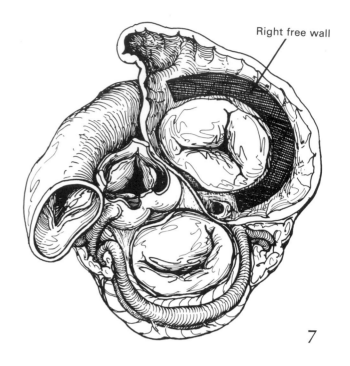

Right free wall

7

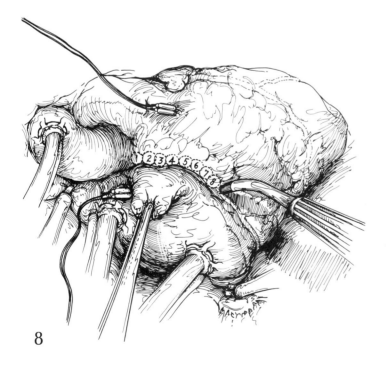

8

8

During normothermic perfusion re-entrant techycardia is induced and the AV groove mapped externally. Preoperative localization in the electrophysiological laboratory would usually indicate a short section of the AV groove for mapping. Should it prove impossible to induce tachycardia, mapping may be performed in sinus rhythm or atrial or ventricular pacing. An early site of activation during sinus rhythm or atrial pacing will be shown in overt pre-excitation (Wolff-Parkinson-White syndrome), but in the case of a concealed pathway it will only be apparent during retrograde conduction (tachycardia or ventricular pacing).

9

The crossing point of the accessory pathway having been localized, an epicardial incision is made in the AV groove and extended generously to either side of the crossing point. The dissection is deepened in the epicardial fat, the right coronary artery being kept to the ventricular side. Removing much of the fat exposes the AV junction.

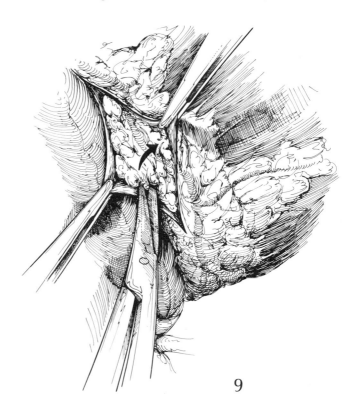

9

10

10

The crossing point is then ablated by cryothermy, a similar technique being used to that described for His bundle ablation. First a test freeze to 0°C is carried out to confirm that interruption of the pathway is achieved. Should this not prove successful adjacent points are tested to 0°C until a successful point is found. This is then treated to −60°C for 2 minutes, along with adjacent sites as before. With this approach the procedure can be accomplished without cardiopulmonary bypass. However, the patient should be cannulated and the benefit of avoiding perfusion is debatable.

11

The alternative technique of transection of the accessory pathway is performed by exposing a generous length of the AV junction in the appropriate area indicated by mapping.

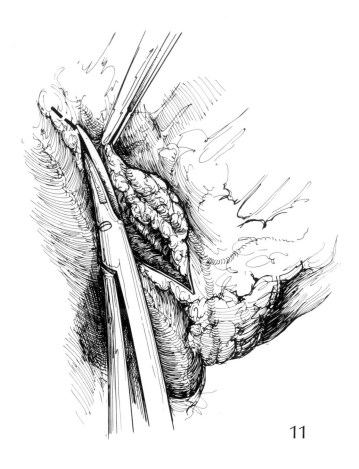

11

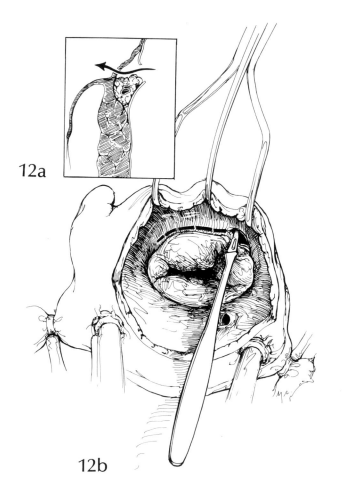

12a

12b

12

The groove having been carefully displayed, thereby protecting the right coronary artery, the transection is completed by an endocardial incision immediately to the atrial side of the tricuspid annulus. The plane of disconnection of the right atrium and its epicardium from the right ventricle is shown diagrammatically in the inset.

13

The endocardial incision is then extended to cover the entire region exposed externally, keeping as close to the tricuspid annulus as possible.

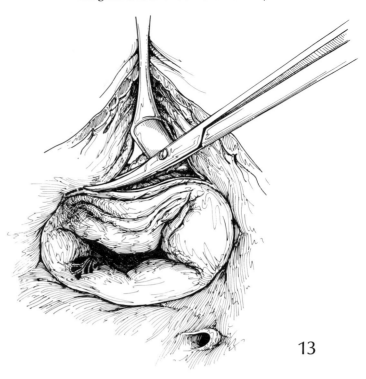

13

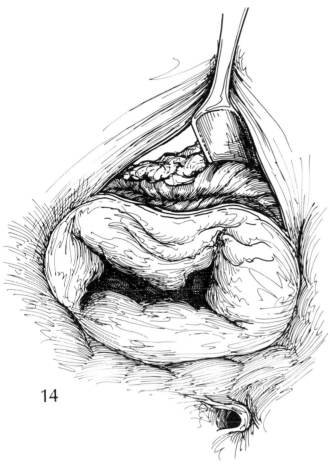

14

14

It is important to be sure that the right atrium is totally disconnected over the entire site chosen.

15

The endocardial incision is then closed with a continuous 4/0 polypropylene suture in one layer.

If cardioplegia has been used coronary perfusion is now restored. If spontaneous defibrillation does not occur the heart is electrically defibrillated. The tricuspid valve is kept regurgitant by retraction of one of the leaflets. When an overt accessory pathway has been ablated the abolition of pre-excitation on the surface ECG will immediately be apparent. Repeat of the local mapping of the AV groove should, however, be performed in all cases, followed by attempts to initiate tachycardia. It is possible for pre-excitation to remain and yet tachycardia prove impossible to initiate, presumably owing to alteration of the conduction characteristics of the accessory pathway. In this circumstance it is, however, advisable to relocate the crossing point of the pathway and make a further attempt at ablation or interruption to prevent the possibility of further recovery in the early postoperative period, allowing the recurrence of tachycardia.

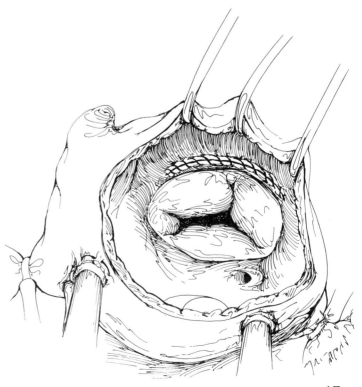

15

16

The epicardial incision is closed with a single continuous 4/0 polypropylene suture followed by routine closure of the right atriotomy and withdrawal of cardiopulmonary bypass by the usual techniques.

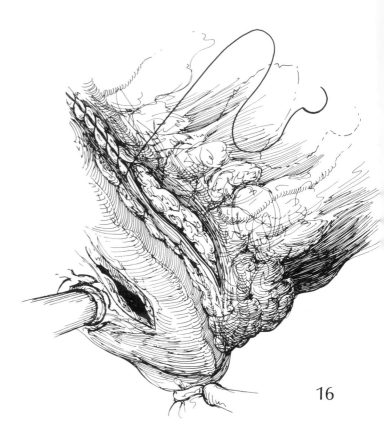

16

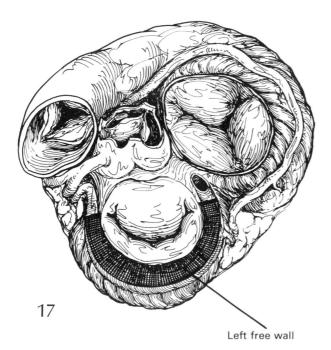

17

Left free wall

17

Left atrial free wall pathways

The left atrial free wall pathways are those that cross from atrium to ventricle over the portion of the annulus fibrosus of the mitral valve corresponding to the attachment of the posterior mitral leaflet. It can easily be seen that the right-hand portion of this overlaps with the posterior septal area (see below) and this exposes one of the limitations of preoperative localization whereby it is difficult to distinguish between free wall pathways occurring in this area and those truly placed in the posterior septal region. Preoperative localization, however, is extremely helpful in another direction. If the pathway is shown to be in the right half of the left free wall sector, then dissection epicardially in the AV groove is likely to lead to interruption of the pathway without opening the left atrium. This is performed in the same way as for right free wall pathways. If it is present in the left (lateral) part, however, dissection is difficult and potentially hazardous to the circumflex coronary artery. In these circumstances it is preferable to perform a left atriotomy, map the activation of the left atrium around the mitral valve annulus and ablate with cryothermy application. The presence of a dominant right coronary artery is particularly favourable to epicardial treatment of pathways in the right part of the left atrial free wall.

18

Many of these patients will have a left atrium of normal size, and to facilitate the exposure of the mitral annulus mobilization of the pericardium around the venae cavae and the right-sided pulmonary veins is followed by dissection of the interatrial groove (see inset). Access may be further facilitated by reducing the amount of blood in the right atrium with caval snares; this would need to be accompanied by pulmonary artery venting to remove the coronary sinus return.

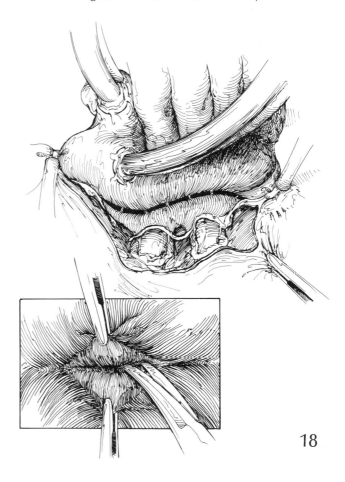

18

19

19

The vertical left atriotomy exposes the mitral valve in the usual way and the free wall pathways are mapped by sampling from the atrial side of the mitral annulus along the course of attachment of the posterior leaflet as described for localization of the AV node-His bundle. Mapping is performed during re-entrant tachycardia and during ventricular pacing when retrograde conduction in the accessory pathway will be revealed as an early point of activation on the left free wall. During this part of the operation it is essential to prevent air embolism by the techniques previously described under 'Special considerations in left atrial endocardial mapping' (p. 566). Mapping should be carried out well on to the septal portion as preoperative localization is not always sufficiently sensitive to differentiate clearly between the posterior septal and the left free wall pathways. The result of mapping may therefore indicate a different approach as for posterior septal pathways (see below).

The pathway having been localized, a test freeze and definitive ablation by cryothermy are performed as for AV node-His bundle ablation. When the procedure has been shown to be effective the left atrium is closed with a continuous suture of 3/0 polypropylene, air is removed and the heart is taken from bypass in the manner usual to the operator's practice.

20

Anterior septal pathways

Atrioventricular communication in the anterior septal region is almost exclusively on the right side because of the anatomical relationship of the root of the aorta to the right fibrous trigone. The supravalvar portion of the membranous interventricular septum is an invaluable landmark in procedures in both the anterior and posterior septal regions. The approach to the anterior septal portion of the tricuspid annulus is as for the localization of the AV node-His bundle.

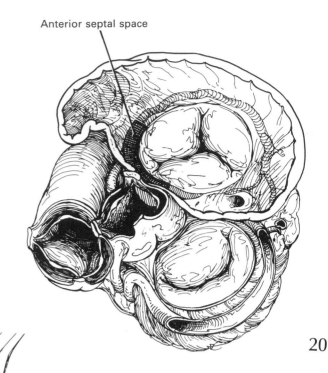

Anterior septal space

20

21

The endocardial incision to approach the anterior septal space is immediately adjacent to the fibrous annulus of the tricuspid valve, beginning at the supravalvar membranous septum and proceeding anteriorly on to the free wall, where the right atrium loses its relationship to the aortic root and comes into relation with the right coronary artery. Caution is required in the mid-region of this incision to avoid entering the adjacent non-coronary sinus of Valsalva.

21

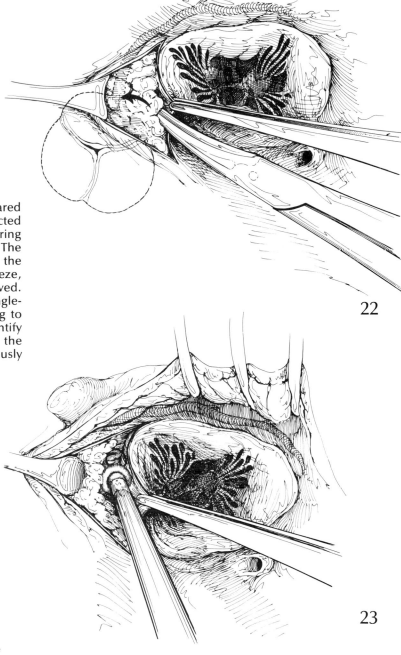

22 & 23

The contents of the space, primarily fat, are cleared carefully, the right coronary artery being deflected anteriorly towards the aortic root to protect it during dissection and to expose the ventricular muscle. The cryoprobe is applied at the site of crossing of the accessory pathway and, after confirmation by test freeze, the usual cluster of freezing points at −60°C is achieved. The endocardial closure is again with continuous single-layer 4/0 polypropylene, and after complete retesting to confirm the effectiveness of the procedure and to identify any previously concealed additional pathways the atriotomy is closed and bypass withdrawn as previously described.

22

23

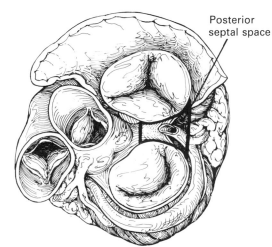

24

24

Posterior septal pathways

The posterior septal space is the most difficult in which to work and to produce successful ablation of accessory pathways. It meets the anterior septal space at the right fibrous trigone adjacent to the supravalvar membranous septum and broadens out to its epicardial marking deep to the coronary sinus at the point where it turns to enter the right and left atrium. Between these limits it is related to the right and left atria and also to the portion of the left ventricle which lies between the mitral annulus and the interventricular septum.

25

The posterior septal space can be entered from the epicardial surface of the heart between the origin of the posterior descending coronary artery and the coronary sinus. This approach is more favourable in the presence of a dominant right coronary artery than a dominant left coronary artery. However, a more complete exposure of the entire contents of the space is obtained by an endocardial approach from the right atrium, which is preferred.

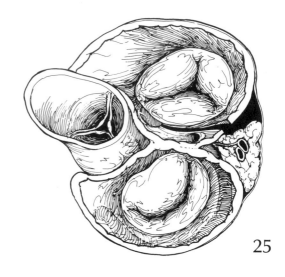

25

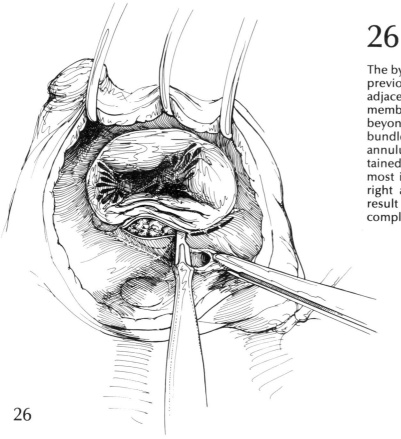

26

26

The bypass technique and right atriotomy are as described previously. The endocardial incision is immediately adjacent to the tricuspid annulus and extends from the membranous interventricular septum to a point well beyond the coronary sinus orifice. The AV node-His bundle is protected by keeping the incision close to the annulus fibrosus when the conduction tissue is maintained in the right atrial tissues retracted proximally. It is most important for the same reason not to separate the right atrium from the right fibrous trigone as this will result in division of the His bundle and permanent complete heart block.

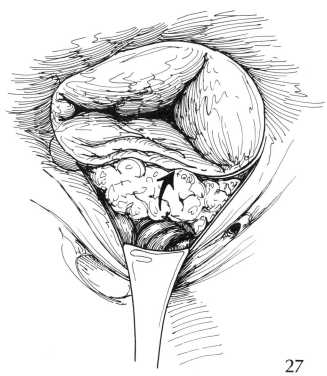

27

Blunt dissection is used to clear the fat from the space, retracting the coronary sinus with the conduction tissue to the atrial and leftward side and exposing the AV nodal artery in the floor.

27

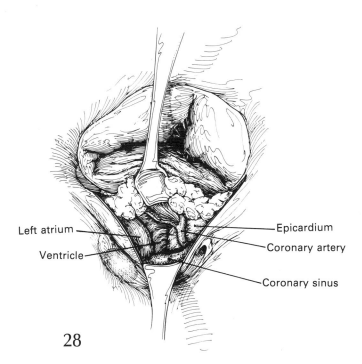

Left atrium

Ventricle

Epicardium

Coronary artery

Coronary sinus

28

28

The space is cleared of its contents protecting the artery, coronary sinus and conduction tissue and the limit of the space is reached when the left atrial wall is encountered by dissecting beneath the coronary sinus. The left atrial wall is followed up to the right fibrous trigone and the right side of the space is cleared to the extent of the incision beyond the coronary sinus. Should this fail to interrupt the accessory pathway the left atrium can be entered from this space and resutured. If pre-excitation still exists the pathway is likely to be running with the His bundle and cryothermal ablation of the bundle may be indicated, producing complete heart block. The endocardial incision is closed with continuous single-layer 4/0 polypropylene as usual, followed by closure of the right atriotomy and withdrawal of bypass in the operator's customary manner.

ABLATION OF ECTOPIC VENTRICULAR FOCI

Ectopic foci of tachycardia situated in the ventricular muscle or specialized fibres are usually associated with a primary cardiomyopathy or coronary artery disease, usually involving infarction. Where neither coronary artery disease nor evidence of a myopathy is readily apparent the latter should always be suspected. Evidence from detailed electrophysiological studies of these disorders indicates that the former has an underlying mechanism of pathological automaticity and the latter is based on a re-entrant mechanism. The re-entrant circuit substrate arises as a result of changes in conduction properties secondary to ischaemic damage and is of a microscopic nature so that in both types complete excision of the area is the principle on which treatment is based. In the presence of coronary artery disease coronary grafting or resection of aneurysmal tissue is performed according to conventional indications. With the greater specificity of electrophysiologically directed procedures has come an improved efficacy in the abolition of ventricular tachycardia which has rendered the alternative procedures of coronary grafting with or without aneurysmectomy inadequate as the definitive procedure.

The site of the ectopic focus is localized by construction of a complete map of ventricular epicardial activation by reference to the electrogram recorded from a bipole hook electrode fixed in the ventricular epicardium in a region indicated by preoperative study to be distant from the tachycardia focus. The principal techniques of epicardial ventricular mapping are described in the section on 'Intraoperative mapping' (pp. 565–566).

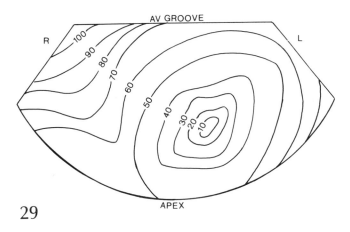

29

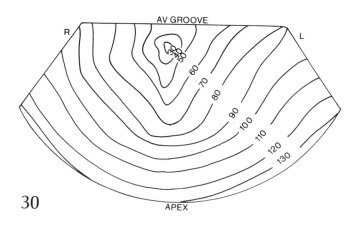

30

29 & 30

The samples are taken according to a previously agreed grid reference system, each sample point being identified by a unique number so that the point on the epicardium from which any individual electrogram was obtained can be reliably identified. It is of immense help to use a standard diagrammatic two-dimensional depiction of the ventricular surface. In this example the septum is 'removed' and the ventricles opened along the course of the posterior descending coronary artery. A vertical line dividing the map into two equal portions would mark the course of the anterior descending branch of the left coronary artery. Points activated at the same time with reference to the fixed bipole electrode are joined to form isochrone contours in the construction of an isochrone map of the ventricular surface. Mapping is undertaken during sinus rhythm and ventricular tachycardia, thereby identifying the site at which tachycardia first appears on the epicardium. In almost all cases endocardial activation precedes epicardial activation, indicating the endocardial location of the focus. The epicardial breakthrough point is at the shortest electrical distance from the endocardial origin and is most commonly the epicardium directly overlying the focus. In a small number of cases, however, it may be geographically distant as, for example, when the endocardial origin is septal or in an area of diffuse fibrosis.

Ventricular tachycardia with normal coronary arteries

As has been stated, ventricular tachycardia in the absence of significant coronary arterial disease is usually associated with a primary cardiomyopathy. This may add considerably to the morbidity and mortality of the procedure and emphasizes the importance of detailed preliminary investigation not restricted to the electrophysiological laboratory. Cryoablation of the focus has been shown to be effective in this condition and is, in our opinion, the technique of choice.

31

The epicardial breakthrough point is frequently found on the right ventricle, often in the region of the outflow tract. After surface mapping the cryoprobe is applied to the epicardial breakthrough point and a test freeze to 0°C performed. If this proves effective in preventing induction of tachycardia the temperature is reduced to −60°C for 2 minutes and repeated at a cluster of points surrounding the first. Should the test freeze prove ineffective it is repeated in immediately adjacent sites, but in the event of continued tachycardia a distant endocardial focus must be suspected and ventriculotomy is indicated. This is performed over the epicardial breakthrough point, due consideration being given to the coronary artery anatomy.

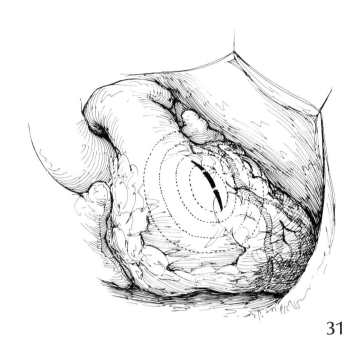

31

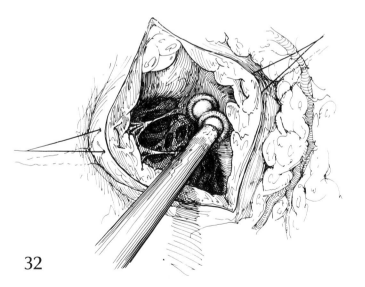

32

32

Endocardial mapping is then performed; this requires the use of a hand-held probe. The septum may well be the site of the ectopic focus and its identification is followed by the usual procedure of test freeze followed by −60°C application at a cluster of adjacent points. Induction of tachycardia should now prove impossible; should tachycardia occur, it is due either to a failure to ablate the identified focus or to the unmasking of a secondary focus. The latter may be indicated by an altered electrocardiographic morphology. It is mandatory to perform careful remapping and ablate the secondary focus if shown.

The ventriculotomy is closed with a continuous 3/0 polypropylene suture in one full-thickness layer. Buttresses may be used if deemed appropriate.

Ventricular tachycardia associated with coronary artery disease

In cases in which ventricular tachycardia is associated with coronary artery disease previous infarction is usual, and in almost all other cases diffuse fibrosis is found. The substrate for postulated micro re-entrant circuits is in the border zone of relative ischaemia, and hence resection of an infarcted area which by accepted surgical techniques involves the border zone remaining, is associated with an unacceptably high recurrence rate. Thus the approach to the resolution of tachycardia is based on accurate localization and extirpation of the region of origin, but of course aneurysm resection and coronary grafting to other areas are undertaken on the commonly accepted criteria.

33

Mapping of the surface of the ventricles will usually indicate an epicardial breakthrough point at the margin of an infarcted or aneurysmal area. The approach to an aneurysm is therefore biased in favour of the region of origin of tachycardia, as illustrated.

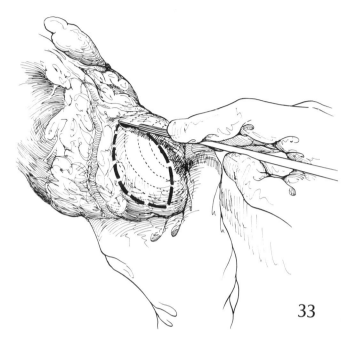

33

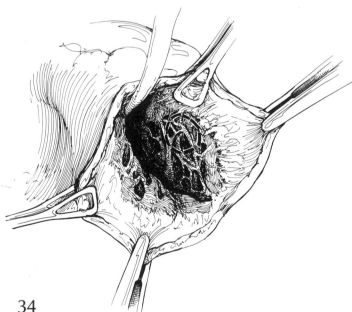

34

34

Once the aneurysmal area is opened endocardial mapping is performed, concentrated on the region indicated by epicardial mapping. This requires the use of a hand-held probe as previously described.

35

The area of origin of ventricular tachycardia having been identified, the subendocardium is removed as illustrated; it is most important to carry this stripping beyond the fibrous margin of the aneurysm, recognizing that the focus of origin of tachycardia is likely to be in the borderline zone. The subendocardial extent of infarction is usually more extensive than the epicardial demarcation and, as electrophysiological study has shown the vast majority of ventricular tachycardias in ischaemic heart disease to arise in the border zone, the strip must be carried to the region of normal muscle as is commonly indicated by the endocardial mapping.

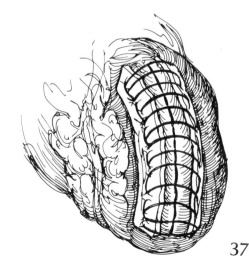

35

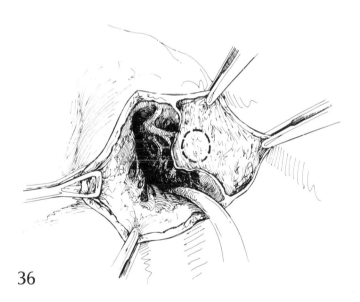

36

36

The strip being completed, the flap of endocardial tissue is excised and excision of any aneurysmal or scar tissue is performed according to conventional techniques. At this stage of the operation induction of tachycardia should prove impossible and remapping is therefore not applicable. However, should tachycardia be induced at this stage endocardial remapping is indicated, with further resection according to the result. It is possible that the primary area of origin of tachycardia having been ablated, a secondary unstable focus may be revealed by reinduction techniques. This should be treated in the same way as the primary origin.

37

Closure of the ventriculotomy is carried out according to the operator's usual practice, with the use of Teflon buttresses where indicated. Removal of air from the heart and withdrawal of cardiopulmonary bypass are also performed according to the surgeon's customary technique.

37

Transplantation

Stuart W. Jamieson MB, FRCS, FACS
Professor and Head, Cardiothoracic Surgery, University of Minnesota, Minneapolis, Minnesota, USA

Introduction

Cardiac transplantation was first performed in man in 1964[1] and achieved international attention in 1967[2]. In the early years clinical cardiac transplantation was unsuccessful at most centres and the number of hospitals performing transplantation fell from 64 in 1968 to 3 or 4 throughout the world in the 1970s. During this period well over half of all cardiac transplants reported were performed at Stanford University by Shumway's group, who indeed had achieved the first consistent success in the laboratory[3]. Cardiac transplantation at Stanford has been performed with increasing frequency since its first clinical application in January 1968, and about 50 transplants are performed yearly at the present time (1984). The survival after one year has improved from 22 per cent in 1968 to 88 per cent for 1984. There is an attrition rate of approximately 5 per cent per year thereafter. The procedure therefore provides superior survival compared with many other operations in cardiac surgery, and indeed in so far as it provides satisfactory palliation for lethal conditions followed by complete rehabilitation it compares most favourably with most other operations in surgery, especially those for cancer.

The clinical institution of heart-and-lung transplantation at Stanford has also shown early success, with 75 per cent one-year survival. However, the limitation of donor availability and the still substantial expertise required to achieve postoperative rehabilitation both for heart and heart-lung transplantation require that these procedures should be carried out only in specialized centres for the foreseeable future.

HEART TRANSPLANTATION

The donor

Selection of donor

Potential donors for cardiac transplantation require the diagnosis of brain death and confirmation of the absence of cardiac impairment by history or physical examination. It is important that cardiac donors should be free of excessive inotropic support, systemic infection or malignancy. At the present time it is recommended only to use donors under the age of 35 since over this age there is an increased incidence of immune-mediated coronary atherosclerosis in the transplanted heart.

Harvesting of other organs

If a donor is deemed to be satisfactory, arrangements are usually made for the simultaneous harvesting of other organs. These may include the kidneys, liver, pancreas, bone, skin and cornea. Dissection and mobilization of the kidneys and/or liver is usually carried out after a median sternotomy incision has confirmed that the heart is morphologically normal.

Harvesting of donor heart

1

Cardiopulmonary bypass is not necessary for procurement of either the heart or the heart-lung block. The aorta, main pulmonary artery and superior vena cava are mobilized. When the dissection of abdominal organs has been completed systemic heparinization of the donor is carried out.

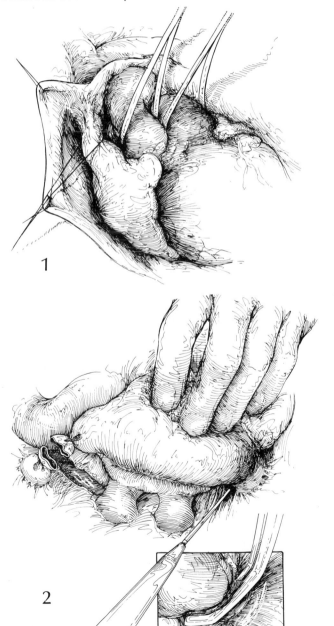

2

The superior vena cava is doubly tied and cut between ligatures. This should be done well away from the right atrium so as to preserve sinus node function. The inferior vena cava is mobilized and clamped at the diaphragm, then divided above the clamp. This prevents the excessive spillage of inferior vena caval blood into the chest cavity during the remainder of the dissection.

3

The heart is now decompressed and a line for the insertion of cardioplegic solution is inserted into the aortic root. The aorta is clamped. Cardioplegic infusion is begun.

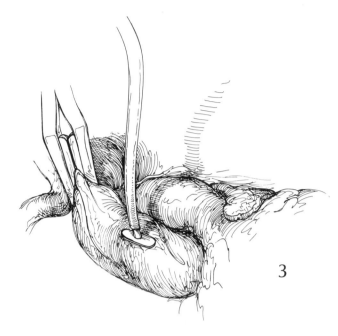

3

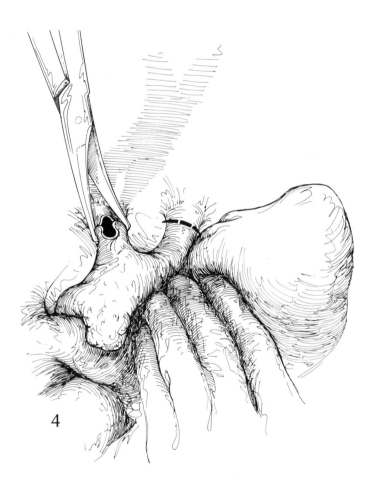

4

4

The left superior pulmonary vein is divided to allow egress of cardioplegic solution and thorough decompression of the heart. The heart is kept immersed in cold (4°C) saline during the remainder of the cardioplegic infusion and then the left inferior pulmonary vein is divided.

5

The aorta is divided aş high as possible. The right pulmonary veins are then divided, followed by division of the right and left pulmonary arteries. The heart may now be lifted out of the chest and transferred to a bowl containing cold saline solution. This may then be carried into the recipient operating theatre, but if the heart is to be transported to another hospital it is placed in a plastic bag containg cold saline which is sealed in a similar sterile plastic bag, the whole being then transferred to a sealed container containing cold saline which is packed in ice. With this method a total ischaemic time of 4 hours is readily tolerated.

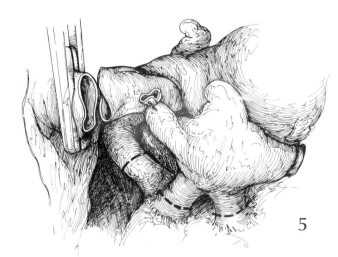

5

Preparation of donor heart

When the donor heart is brought to the recipient operating theatre it is trimmed for subsequent implantation. During this time it is kept largely immersed in a bowl of cold saline.

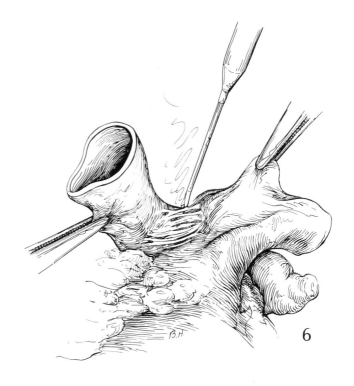

6

6

The aorta and pulmonary artery are separated by electrocautery, care being taken to stay above the coronary arteries.

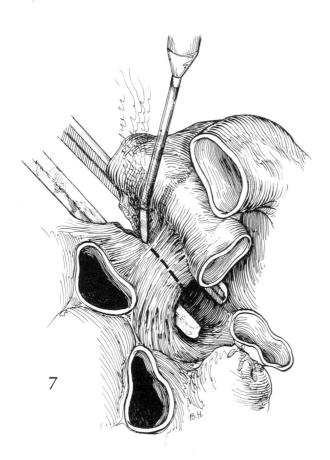

7

7

The pulmonary artery is then separated from the pulmonary veins along the line of the transverse sinus.

8

The right and left pulmonary arteries are now joined, leaving a large ostium for subsequent implantation. This may be further trimmed, but a larger pulmonary artery orifice than usual is generally required because of the large diameter of the recipient's pulmonary artery as a result of moderate pulmonary hypertension.

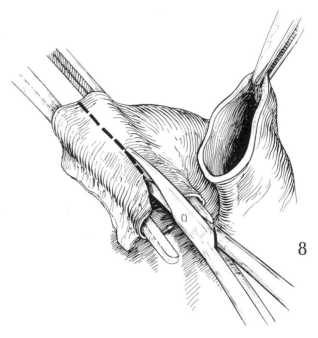

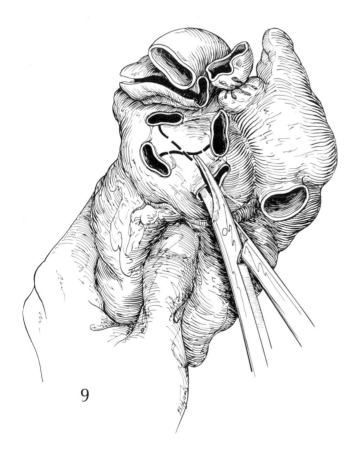

9

Finally the atrial veins are connected, leaving the left atrium opened out ready for subsequent reimplantation.

The recipient

Selection for transplantation

At the present time suitable recipients for cardiac transplantation are less than 55 years of age and suffer from end-stage heart disease that will not respond to any other therapy. There clearly should not be other factors that may limit the patient's survival, such as malignancy, and existing renal and hepatic failure must be judged to be the result of cardiac failure and potentially reversible. Because of the indefinite necessity for immunosuppression any active infection provides a contraindication, and the patient must be aware of, and likely to adhere to, the strict necessity for regular medication.

Excision of recipient's heart

10

Bypass in the recipient is established in the routine way, though the aortic cannula is placed as high in the ascending aorta as convenient and the two caval cannulae are placed low in the atrium passing into the venae cavae. After institution of bypass the venae cavae are snared, the aorta cross-clamped and the heart excised as shown.

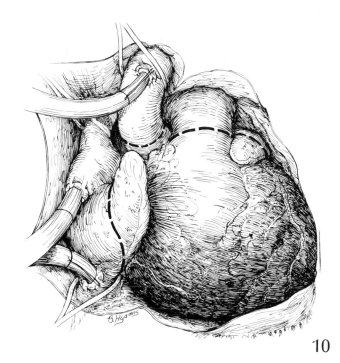

10

11

The excision starts at the right atrium, which is cut at the atrioventricular junction except that the appendage is removed. The atrial septum is now divided at its junction with the ventricle and the left atrium incised at the atrioventricular junction, though again the appendage is excluded.

11

12

The aorta is then cut as low as possible, care being taken not to undercut this vessel. The pulmonary artery is similarly cut. A sucker should be placed down both right and left pulmonary arteries in order to eliminate the possibility of fresh thrombus. It is often convenient to place a clamp on the pulmonary artery in addition to the aorta as this probably helps to prevent the presence of excessive air in the pulmonary circuit.

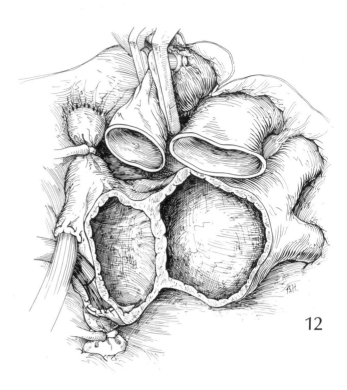

12

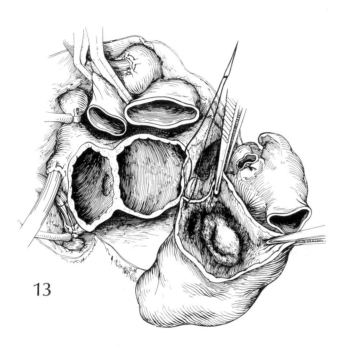

13

Implantation of donor heart

13

Implantation begins at the level of the left superior pulmonary vein in the recipient. This site corresponds to the left atrial appendage of the donor. The suture line is then continued in a clockwise direction along the lateral edge of the left atrium until the septum is reached.

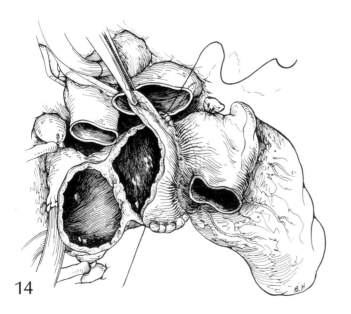

14

14

The other end of the suture is now brought anticlockwise across the top of the atrium to reach the septum and finally to join the other end of the suture. Once the left atrium is closed the suture is tied and cut.

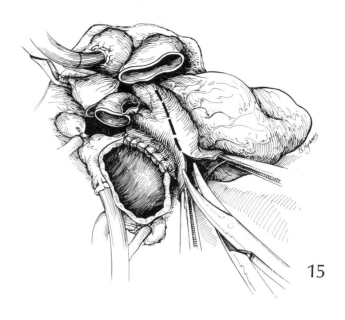

15

15

The donor right atrium is now opened, starting at the inferior vena cava. A curvilinear incision is made up towards the appendage. This has the effect of avoiding the sinus node during subsequent implantation.

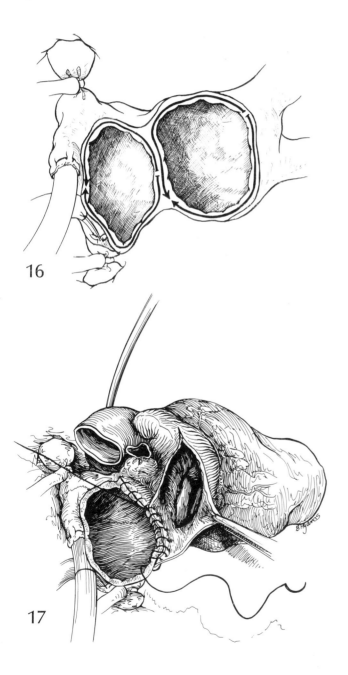

16

17

16 & 17

The right atria are now anastomosed, beginning at the midpoint of the septum and proceeding clockwise until the midline atrial point laterally is reached.

18

The other end of the suture is now brought in an anticlockwise fashion to meet the first, to which it is tied.

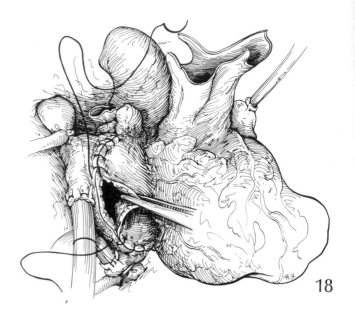

18

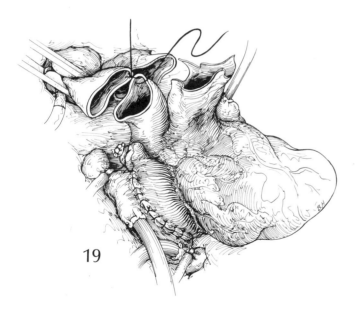

19

19

The aortic anastomosis is now performed with a continuous suture, starting posterolaterally and sewing the posterior wall from inside, proceeding clockwise. At the completion of this anastomosis air is removed from the heart and the aortic cross clamp is removed.

20

The caval snares are now removed and the pulmonary artery anastomosis is completed in the same fashion as the aorta.

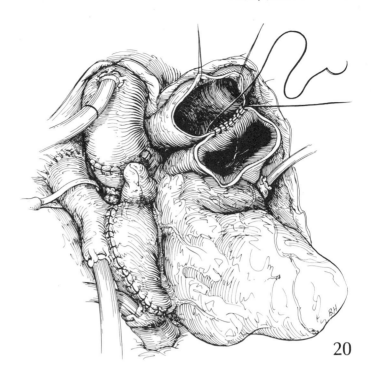

20

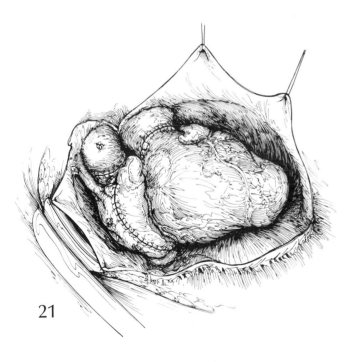

21

21

A suture ligature should be placed on the superior vena cava. Once the heart resumes satisfactory activity bypass is discontinued and protamine administered. Postoperative care is routine save for the institution of immunosuppression and reversed isolation techniques.

HEART-LUNG TRANSPLANTATION

Heart-and-lung transplantation provides successful therapy for end-stage heart and lung disease. Many patients with cardiac disease are not treatable by heart transplantation because of pulmonary hypertension, the normal donor right ventricle being unable to adapt to this workload acutely. Further, many patients with isolated end-stage pulmonary disease, with or without cor pulmonale, are more satisfactorily treated by heart and lung transplantation for the following reasons: all diseased pulmonary tissue is removed; a single tracheal anastomosis is perfomed; the coronary-bronchial anastomoses are left intact; and assessment of rejection by cardiac biopsy guides immunosuppression for both organs.

The results for combined heart-lung transplantation have thus been immensely superior to those for single lung transplantation, which is a suboptimal therapeutic procedure with little to recommend it, especially since retention of a diseased lung is likely to result in a continual source of ventilation-perfusion disparity and infection.

The donor

Selection of donor

Donors for heart-lung transplantation are very much more scarce than for heart transplantation alone. Normal lungs are required of course, in addition to a normal heart, and in the brain-dead population this is rare. Many factors make this so. A prospective donor having sustained a lethal cerebral injury may well have aspirated gastric contents, is generally intubated as an emergency and thus with less than optimally sterile procedure and tends rapidly to develop pneumonic changes. Fluid balance is often difficult to achieve because of diabetes insipidus and, of course, pulmonary oedema tends to develop rapidly in patients who are brain-dead.

A prospective donor must have a totally normal chest X-ray appearance, absence of grossly contaminated pulmonary secretions, an arterial oxygen partial pressure of at least 100 mmHg on a forced inspired oxygen content of 40 per cent and peak inspiratory pressures of less than 30 mmHg. The donor is matched for a given recipient on size criteria as well as ABO blood group compatibility. If time permits the donor's lymphocytes are matched against recipient serum, though this is probably not necessary if the recipient has neither been pregnant nor had blood transfusions and has a negative match against a panel of random lymphocytes.

Size matching is important, and the most convenient way of achieving this is simply to compare the chest X-rays of both donor and recipient. It is probably optimal to have the donor lungs slightly smaller than those of the recipient; certainly it would be unwise from the point of view of subsequent ventilation to allow them to be larger.

Harvesting of donor heart and lungs

The donor heart and lungs are removed without bypass after systemic heparinization. The heart is exposed and both pleura incised above the hila of the lungs. The phrenic nerves may be sacrificed. The superior vena cava is doubly ligated and then cut as for cardiac transplantation. An infusion line is placed in the main pulmonary artery; a No. 14 pulmonary artery vent catheter is convenient for this purpose. A cardioplegic infusion catheter is placed in the ascending aorta and after division of the inferior vena cava the aorta is clamped and cardioplegic infusion begun. Simultaneously an infusion is begun into the pulmonary artery, consisting of Collins' solution with the addition of 8 mEq magnesium and 65 ml 50 per cent dextrose per litre. A total of 500 ml of cardioplegic solution is infused into the aortic root and 1500 ml of modified Collins' solution into the main pulmonary artery. As soon as infusion of these solutions has been established the tip of the left atrial appendage is excised to allow egress of fluid from the heart.

Ventilation is continued with unheated room air only. High levels of inspired oxygen are assiduously avoided in the donor and later in the recipient after implantation of the lungs. After completion of the infusions the aorta is divided as high as is convenient. The trachea is identified to the right and posterior to the divided aorta and is clamped as high as possible, with the lungs approximately two-thirds inflated. With the clamp used as a retractor the trachea is pulled forward out of the wound and the lungs progressively freed on both sides, electrocautery being used to divide the posterior reflections of the pleura. Care must be taken not to enter the oesophagus here, though of course integrity of the vagus nerves may be ignored. It is essential to handle the lungs with care and gentleness at all times.

The heart and lung block can now be lifted out of the chest and is placed in a large bowl containing cold saline solution.

The recipient

Selection for transplantation

Recipients for the combined operation must have the general characteristics outlined for recipients for cardiac transplantation. In addition, of course, there must be inoperable pulmonary disease. All patients in the Stanford series have suffered from pulmonary hypertension, whether this be due to Eisenmenger's syndrome or primary pulmonary hypertension. Though palliation of many other conditions may be possible by this operation, it seemed most sensible to initiate a clinical series with patients with pulmonary hypertension because of the established poor prognosis of the condition and the lack of any other available therapy. In addition, these patients are relatively young and generally have a sterile tracheo-bronchial tree, and there is little likelihood of recurrence of disease in the transplanted organs.

Excision of recipient's heart and lungs

The most difficult and important aspects of the recipient operation are to remove the heart and lungs without injury to the phrenic or vagus nerves and to ensure haemostasis. A standard median sternotomy is performed.

22

The left pleura is now divided anteriorly with electro-cautery. Should the presence of adhesions be anticipated before operation it is wise to attempt to divide these with electrocautery before heparinization and the insertion of the cannulae, though this is often impossible owing to cardiomegaly.

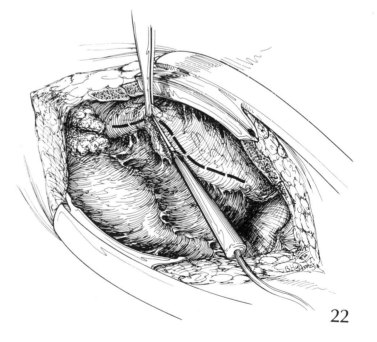

22

23a & b

The pericardium is opened. The cannulae for bypass are inserted as for cardiac transplantation. Bypass is instituted and, after the aortic cross clamp has been placed, the venae cavae are snared and the heart is removed as previously described.

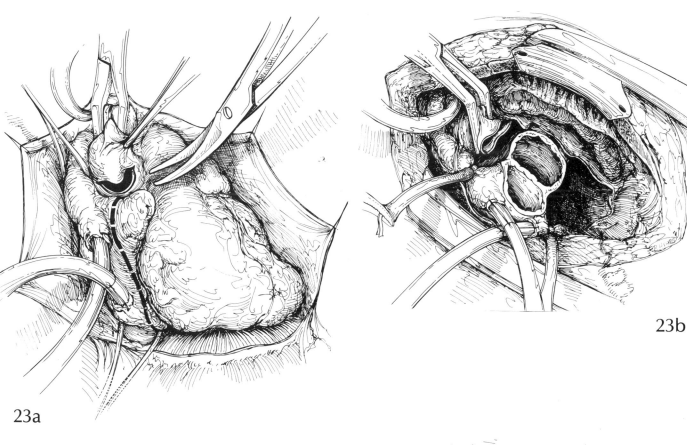

23b

23a

24

Two clamps are now placed on the pericardium on the left side and retracted anteriorly and to the left. The pericardium is now incised 3 cm posterior to the left phrenic nerve. This incision is carried down to the diaphragm, care being taken to stay well clear of the nerve. Superiorly it is carried as far as the pulmonary artery. This incision should not be continued further cephalad, where it would get too close to the vagus and phrenic nerves, which begin to come together after this point.

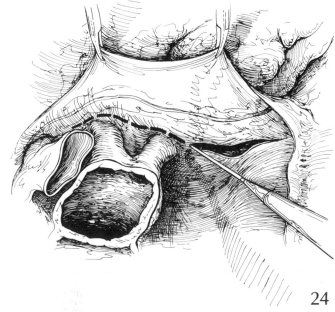

24

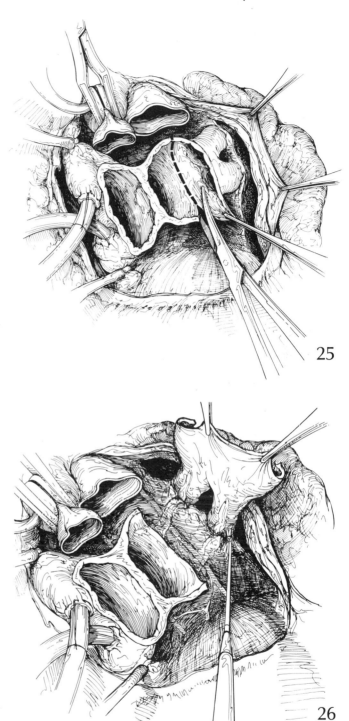

25 & 26

The left atrium is now incised posteriorly between the pulmonary veins. This incision is carried through the oblique sinus and electrocautery used to free the remnants of the left atrium and pulmonary veins from the posterior pericardium. The left atrium and left pulmonary veins are retracted anteriorly. The dissection should stay right on the pulmonary veins since the vagus nerve lying on the oesophagus is immediately posterior.

25

26

27

The pulmonary ligament on the left side is now ligated and cut. The whole left lung is now retracted up out of the wound anteriorly and towards the right side and electrocautery used to separate the remaining pleura posteriorly so that the whole hilum comes free.

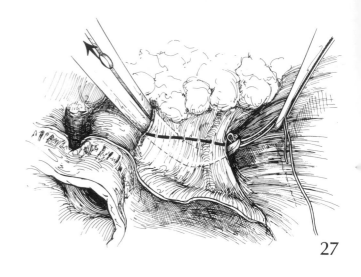

27

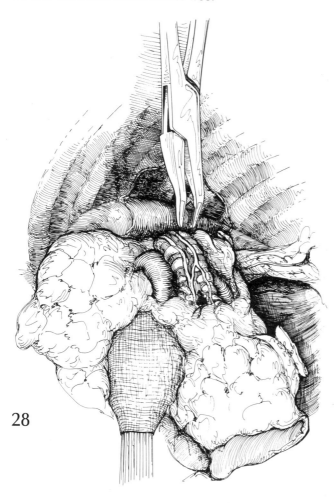

28

28

Several large bronchial arteries will be found, especially in patients with Eisenmenger's syndrome. These are individually secured with clips. The bronchus is now exposed. This is retracted well out towards the surgeon and freed from the surrounding tissue and bronchial arteries.

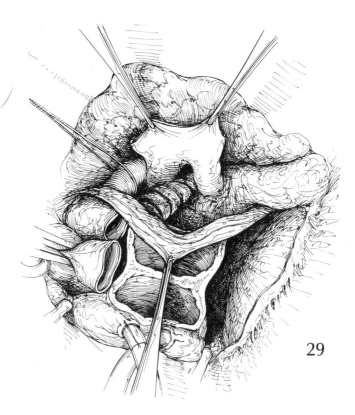

29

29

The left main bronchus has now been freed. The pulmonary veins, still attached to the atrial remnant, are clear of the posterior chest wall and the left pulmonary artery is now cut. The left lung is attached only by the left main bronchus.

30

A TA 30 stapler with 35 mm staples is used to clamp the left bronchus. The bronchus is now cut distal to the staples and the left lung passed off the table. It should be considered unsterile, together with the instruments used in cutting the bronchus.

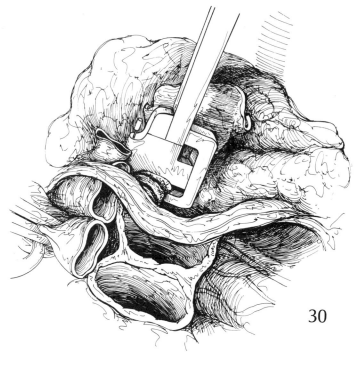

30

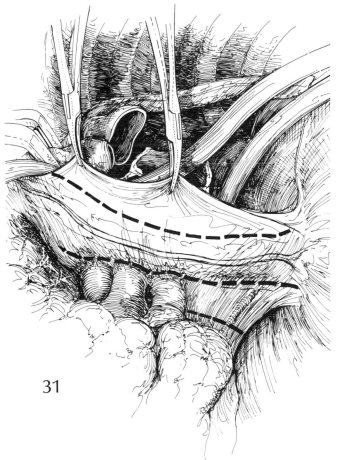

31

31

Attention is now turned to the right side. The right pleura is incised in a similar manner to the left, leaving a ribbon of approximately 3 cm on either side of the right phrenic nerve. It should be noted that as the phrenic nerve proceeds cephalad over the pulmonary artery it lies surprisingly anterior next to the superior vena cava. The ribbon of pericardium is now retracted anteriorly and an incision made on the right side immediately anterior to the pulmonary veins but as far away as possible from the phrenic nerve. The phrenic nerve on the right lies closer to the hilum than on the left. Once the pulmonary veins have been freed from the pericardium the incision proceeds inferiorly, electrocautery being used until the posterior pericardium is entered at the level of the tape encircling the inferior vena cava. The pulmonary ligament may now be ligated and divided.

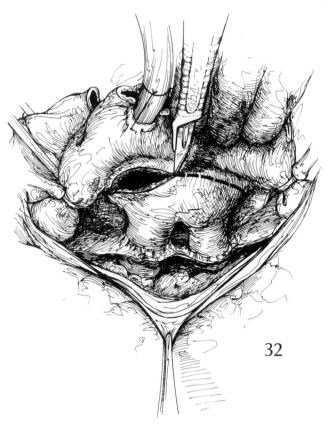

32

32

An incision is now made in the left atrium posterior to the interatrial groove, as if opening the left atrium for a mitral valve replacement. This incision passes superiorly and inferiorly.

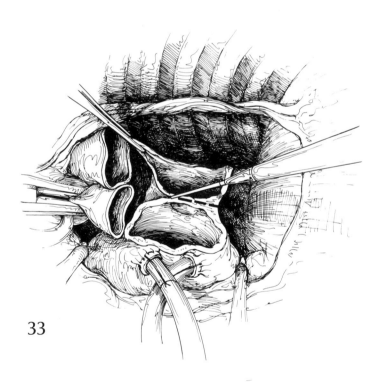

33

33

The right atrium is now separated from the remnants of the pulmonary veins.

34

The pulmonary veins will come free after dissection from the posterior mediastinum with electrocautery, care being taken to preserve the phrenic nerve anteriorly and the vagus nerve immediately posteriorly.

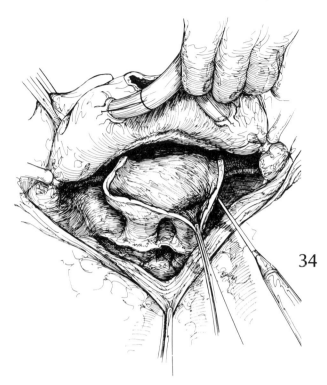

34

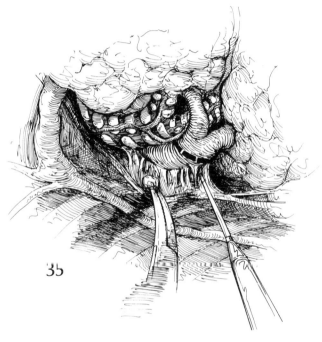

35

35

The whole right lung is now retracted anteriorly and towards the left, and again the pulmonary veins and the bronchus are freed from the posterior pleura with electrocautery. The bronchial arteries should be ligated. The vagus nerve lies immediately posterior to the hilum and care must be taken not to injure this structure. The right pulmonary veins will become free. The right pulmonary artery is now divided at the level of the hilum, and the right bronchus can be freed.

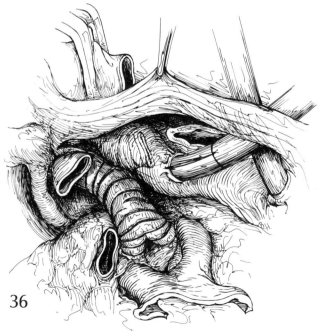

36

36

Again the surrounding structures and bronchial arteries are swept free of the bronchus and the lung is retracted out towards the operator. The bronchus is now secured with a TA 30 stapler and divided and careful inspection for haemostasis is carried out within the thoracic cavity.

37

The remnants of the pulmonary artery are now excised, leaving a small button in the area of the ductus ligament. This preserves the recurrent laryngeal nerve.

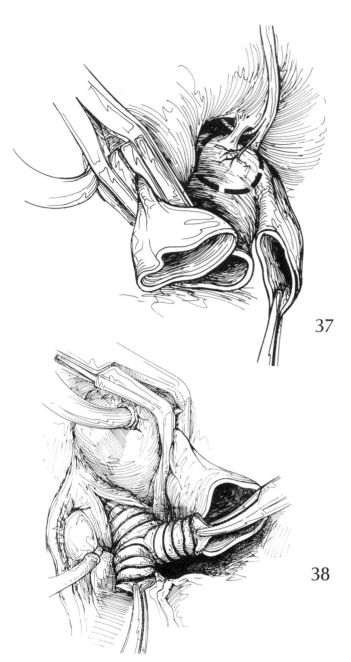

37

38

A posterior incision is now made with electrocautery immediately to the right of the aorta. The trachea can be palpated here and is exposed at the carina. The stumps of the left and right bronchi are found, both stapled. The left is longer than the right, which has generally been stapled at the carina. The distal trachea is freed by grasping the bronchial stumps with clamps, but great care should be taken to leave the surrounding tissue and blood supply intact. A large bronchial artery generally lies posterior to the trachea and should be ligated here.

38

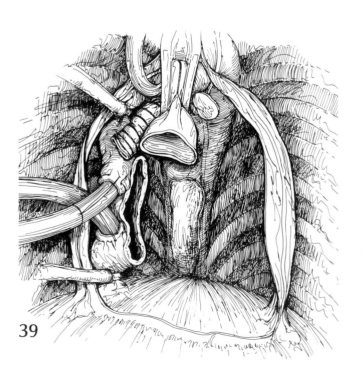

39

The finally empty chest is illustrated. The bronchi have not yet been removed. Meticulous haemostasis is now effected since after implantation of the new heart-lung block the identification of bleeding points in the posterior mediastinum is almost impossible.

39

Implantation of donor heart and lungs

40

When the donor heart and lungs are received two lines for the infusion of topical cold solution are passed off, one to each chest. The donor trachea is trimmed immediately above the carina with a scalpel. Cultures are taken from the donor trachea, which is then sucked out well but gently with a small sucker.

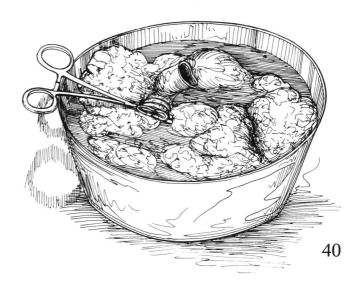

40

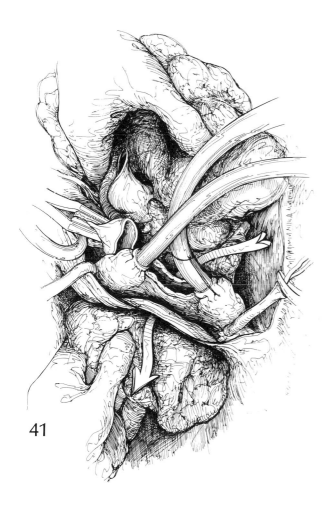

41

41

The right lung is passed beneath the right atrium and vena cava and the left lung beneath the left phrenic nerve.

42

The recipient trachea is cut immediately above the carina. Again this is cultured. The tracheal anastomosis is performed with continuous polypropylene (3/0). The level of cold irrigant solution is adjusted so that it does not rise excessively and run into the trachea. Both lungs tend to float on the fluid and should be covered with wet laparotomy sponges.

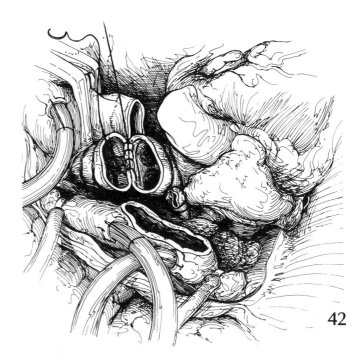

42

43

After the tracheal anastomosis has been completed the atrial anastomosis is performed. The donor right atrium is opened as for cardiac transplantation, the incision avoiding the sinus node. The anastomosis is performed with a continuous suture of polypropylene. On the posterior side all remnants of the left atrium and the intra-atrial groove are included.

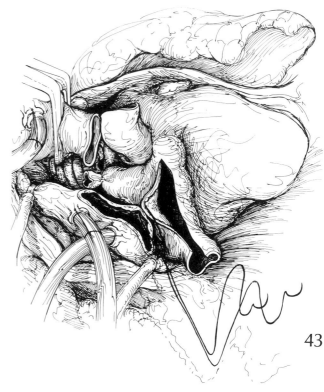

43

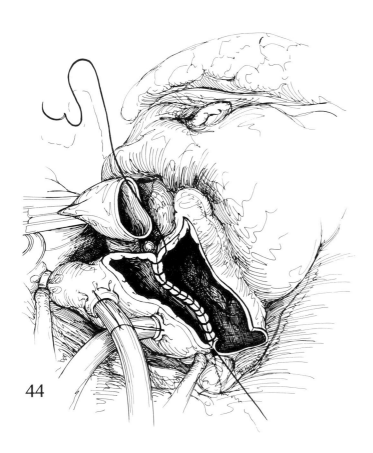

44

44

The suture is now brought anticlockwise to meet the other suture, to which it is tied.

45

Finally the aortic anastomosis is performed with a 4/0 polypropylene suture. Before final closure the aorta is filled with saline.

All anastomoses having been completed, the chest cavity is emptied and the caval snares removed. Air is removed from the heart and the aortic cross clamp removed. Gentle respirations are begun with 5 cm of PEEP and the operation continues as routine.

Postoperative care is similar to that for cardiac transplant surgery save that the chest tubes are generally left in for a further 24 hours and aggressive diuresis is instituted.

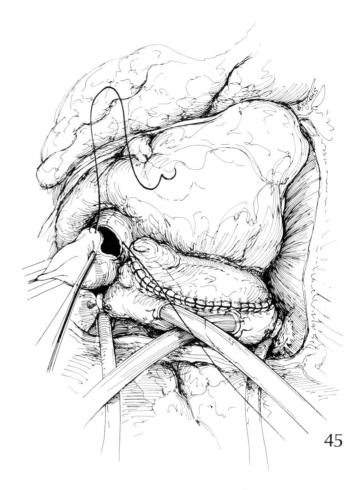

45

References

1. Hardy, J. D., Chavez, C. M., Kurrus, F. D. Heart transplantation in man: developmental studies and report of a case. Journal of the American Medical Association 1964: 188; 1132–1140

2. Barnard, C. N. The operation. A human cardiac transplant: an interium report of a successful operation performed at Groote Schuur Hospital, Cape Town. South African Medical Journal 1967: 41; 1271–1274

3. Lower, R. R., Shumway, N. E. Studies on orthotopic homotransplantation of the canine heart. Surgical Forum 1960: 11; 18–19

Reoperation

William A. Baumgartner MD
Assistant Professor of Surgery, The Johns Hopkins Hospital, Baltimore, Maryland, USA

Introduction

The emergence and expansion of cardiac surgery over the past decade has resulted in an increasing number of patients undergoing cardiac operations. At present coronary artery bypass grafting is the most frequent operation performed in the United States. During this time it has been realized that this and many other kinds of heart surgery are only palliative, resulting in increasing numbers of secondary cardiac procedures. These reoperations are indicated for progressive coronary atherosclerosis occurring in native coronary arteries or in the previously placed bypass grafts, with resultant pre-occlusive or occlusive disease. Other common indications for reoperation include malfunctioning prosthetic valves, prosthetic valve endocarditis or native valve replacement for failure of a previously performed valvuloplastic procedure.

Special consideration should be given to this subgroup of cardiac patients. Previous operative notes provide details of the technique used in the original operation, including the location of bypass grafts. Assessment of the proximity of the right ventricle and aorta to the overlying sternum may be partially determined by a lateral chest radiograph.

The operation

It is firmly believed that a second median sternotomy can be performed safely and with minimum morbidity to the patient[1]. Although it sometimes requires tedious and meticulous dissection, the exposure afforded by this approach is unequalled when dealing with intracardiac procedures.

1

Skin incision

Routine skin incision is carried down to the level of the wires previously inserted. The total number of wires having been identified from the chest radiograph, these are removed with wire cutters and a heavy needle holder or clamp.

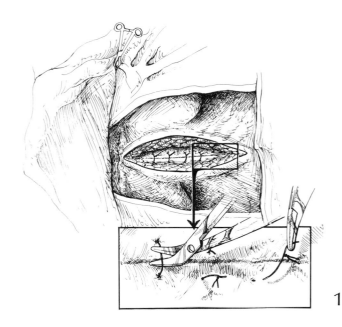

1

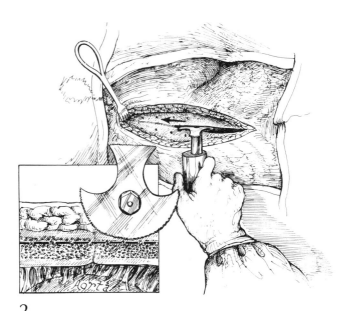

2

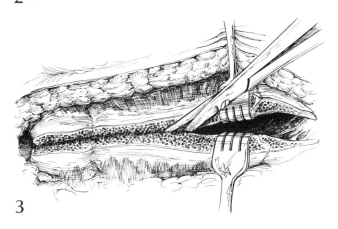

3

2 & 3

Division of sternum

With a rake in the superior portion of the incision for exposure purposes, an oscillating saw is employed to divide the outer table of the sternum only (*inset*). Extension of the saw cut through the inner table could result in aortic, coronary graft or right ventricular perforation. With penetration of the outer table there is usually a palpable yielding of the saw, signifying extension into the marrow portion.

Division of the inner table is performed with heavy scissors starting at the inferior portion of the sternum. In addition to cutting, the scissors act as a wedge to prise the sternum apart.

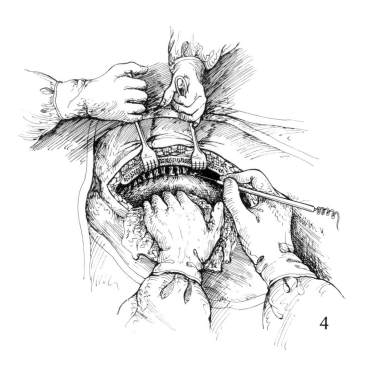

4 & 5

Visualization of heart and great vessels

With the assistant gently lifting the left side of the sternum the surgeon divides adhesions between the sternum and the anterior surface of the heart and great vessels with electrocautery. Gentle counter-traction is used by the operating surgeon to visualise these adhesions adequately so that they may be divided. The electrocautery unit is an effective tool for dissection with maintenance of haemostasis. Both sides of the sternum are dissected laterally for several centimetres to allow safe placement of a retractor. With the retractor in place further dissection can be continued laterally. Before the aorta is dissected out, scar tissue overlying the innominate vein is divided, preventing tearing of this structure when the retractor is opened.

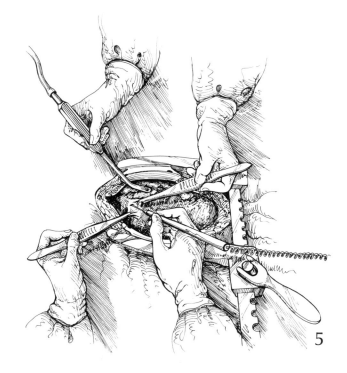

6 & 7

Dissection of the aorta and ventricles

Complete dissection of the aorta is then carried out circumferentially. The aorta having been dissected free, emergency cannulation can proceed if necessary, with arterial inflow via the aorta and venous drainage by the pump suckers. A plane is then developed between the right atrium and the pericardium and/or lung with the electrocautery unit. Gentle traction and counter-traction on the heart and lung respectively facilitate this dissection. Once the pericardium is identified and dissected free from the area of the right atrium it is suspended from the retractor.

Completion of the dissection over the anterior surface of the right and left ventricles can be carried out directly laterally. The remaining dissection of the diaphragmatic, apical, lateral and posterior walls of the left ventricle is performed on cardiopulmonary bypass with the heart decompressed.

In situations (reoperation involving a large ascending aortic aneurysm) in which the aorta lies in close proximity to the sternum, the femoral artery is cannulated simultaneously with the opening of the chest.

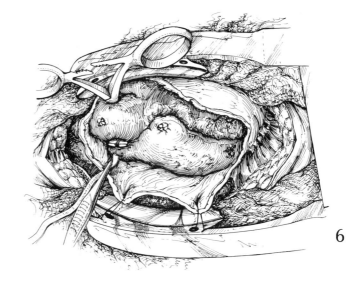

6

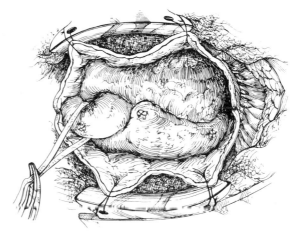

7

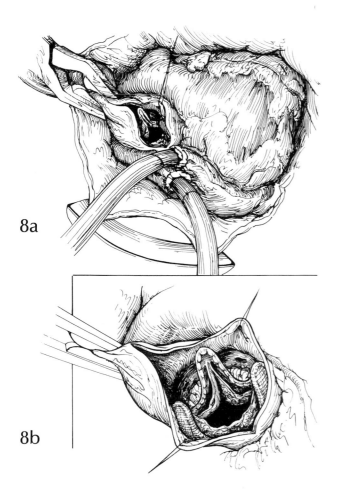

8a

8b

8a & b

Replacement of malfunctioning prosthetic valves, whether in the aortic or mitral positions, requires special consideration. Upon opening the chest, using the techniques previously described, routine cannulation with two caval cannulae and an aortic arterial cannula is carried out. Using the aortic location as an example, an oblique aortotomy is made, starting anteriorly with extension inferiorly in the direction of the non-coronary sinus.

9a & b

The valve is then removed by first grasping individual sutures with a pituitary rongeur. This instrument grasps firmly, suture division being facilitated with a No. 15 blade (a).

The surrounding ingrowth of endothelium that has occurred on the valve sewing ring is then dissected free with a blunt instrument (b). The valve annulus is then trimmed and this is followed by valve replacement in the routine manner. This is generally performed without pledgets, but these may be used if the annulus is friable.

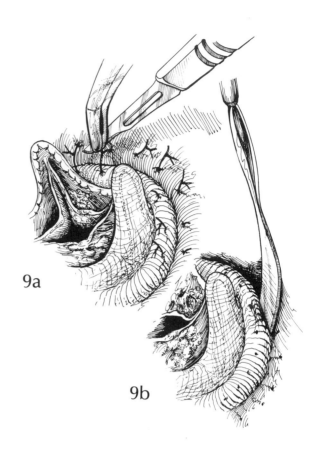

9a

9b

Prosthetic valve endocarditis

Prosthetic valve endocarditis can be present with a variety of anatomical situations requiring special operative techniques. A not infrequent pathological finding in this group of patients is perivalvular necrosis, either as gross abscess or sinus tracts extending below the region of the aortic annulus into the intraventricular septum or left ventricular free wall[2].

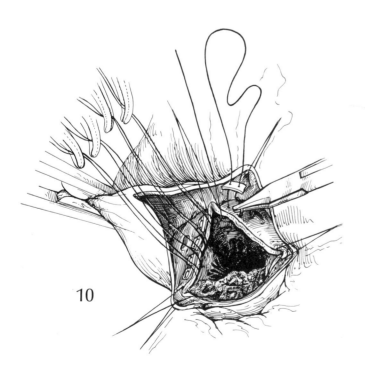

10

10

When an abscess cavity is present beneath the non-coronary sinus, debridement of this area is performed with subsequent closure if anatomically feasible. Pledgeted sutures are used if the annulus has been weakened by the inflammatory process. If the abscess cavity is large debridement alone is performed with replacement of the sutures above the abscess cavity in the native annulus. Occasionally these abscess cavities extend to and include the anterior leaflet of the mitral valve. Small perforations in this leaflet can be repaired primarily, but if there is extensive necrosis or loss of tissue, the valve should be replaced.

11, 12 & 13

A much more serious anatomical defect created by prosthetic valve endocarditis is extensive necrosis of the upper ventricular septum below the region of the right sinus of Valsalva. With this amount of destruction suture placement in the native annulus is not feasible. Translocation of the aortic valve must then be performed, with median sternotomy and standard cardiopulmonary bypass. Arterial cannulation can be accomplished via the ascending aorta or femoral artery, depending on the technical considerations in each case. After establishment of cardiopulmonary bypass and complete dissection of the ascending aorta, the aorta is cross-clamped and the proximal arotic root opened. Myocardial protection is provided by the infusion of cardioplegic solution into each of the coronary artery ostia and supplemented with topical cold saline. The valve is removed and the annulus is debrided of all necrotic tissue. The interior of the heart is lavaged with cold saline to remove any particulate matter and to further cool the heart. The coronary ostia are oversewn and a valved Dacron conduit is interposed in the ascending aorta.

Saphenous vein is then used to perform aortocoronary bypass grafts to the left anterior descending coronary artery and the distal right coronary artery. If coronary artery disease is present a separate anastomosis may be necessary to the obtuse marginal branch of the left circumflex coronary artery. Proximal anastomoses may be performed in a portion of the ascending aorta or, if this has been resected, into the Dacron graft.

Ideally, if it can be ascertained before operation that the translocation procedure will be employed the proximal anastomoses are sewn into the Dacron conduit before the period of ischaemia, thereby reducing this critical time.

This operation was first described by Danielson et al.[3] and should be reserved for those patients in whom the annulus has been destroyed to such an extent that satisfactory placement of a new prosthesis is impossible. It has, however, been successful in curing the infection as well as restoring valvular function in their patients as well as in those reported on by Reitz et al.[4]. The long-term results, however, remain unclear at the present time.

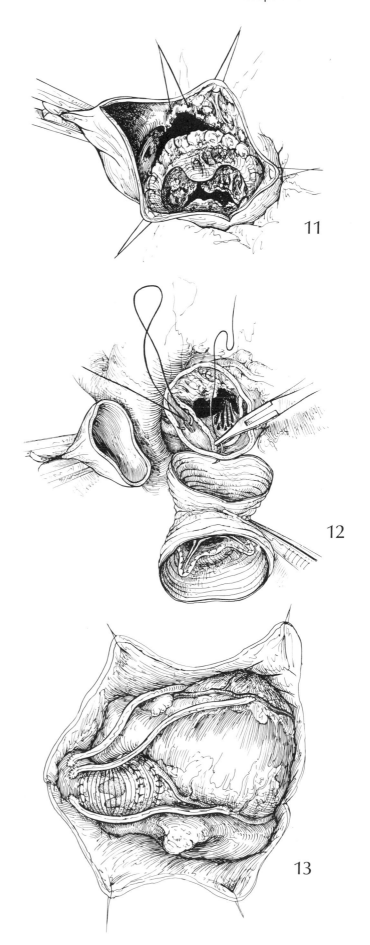

11

12

13

References

1. Oyer, P. E., Shumway, N. E. Again, via the median sternotomy. Archives of Surgery 1974; 109: 604

2. Baumgartner, W. A., Miller, D. C., Reitz, B. A. et al. Surgical treatment of prosthetic valve endocarditis. Annals of Thoracic Surgery 1983; 35: 87–104

3. Danielson, G. E., Titus, J. L., DuShane, J. W. Successful treatment of aortic valve endocarditis and aortic root abscesses by insertion of prosthetic valve in the ascending aorta and placement of bypass grafts to coronary arteries. Journal of Thoracic and Cardiovascular Surgery 1974; 67: 443–449

4. Reitz, B. A., Stinson, E. B., Watson, D. C., Baumgartner, W. A., Jamieson, S. W. Translocation of the aortic valve for prosthetic valve endocarditis. Journal of Thoracic and Cardiovascular Surgery 1981; 81: 212–218

Index

Acid base balance,
  during bypass, 59
  postoperative, 72
Acidosis, 72
Alkalosis, 72
Anaesthesia, 32–50
  cardiopulmonary bypass and, 40
  in children, 43, 44
    drugs used, 44
  classification, 32
  drugs in, 38
    for children, 44
  infusion drugs, dilutions and rate of administration, 38
  intraoperative management, 33
  introduction of, 38
  intubation, 39
  line placement, 33
  monitoring, 33–37
    central venous pressure cannula, 34
    direct arterial blood pressure cannula, 33
    pulmonary artery catheter, 36
    temperature, 37
  in neonate, 43
  postbypass period, 41
  prebypass period, 40
  preoperative evaluation, 32
  preoperative medication, 32
  special considerations, 43
  transfer of patient to ITU, 42
Anatomically corrected malposition, 92
Aneurysm,
  aortic,
    mycotic, 525
    reoperation, 609
  aortic arch, 522, 538–550
  ascending thoracic aorta, 512
  descending thoracic aorta, 519
  left ventricular, postinfarction, 481, 485
  thoracic aortic, 509–525

Angiography, 6–8
  coronary, 6
  pulmonary, 8
Annuloaortic ectasia, 446, 451, 513, 514, 517, 530
Anomalous anterior antrioventricular node, 104
Anomalous pulmonary venous connection,
  partial, 123
  total, 5
    anatomy, 122–128
    diagnosis, 130
    surgical repair, 129–137
Anterolateral thoracotomy, 28
Anticoagulation,
  in bypass, 54
  postoperative, 75
Aorta,
  aneurysm,
    ascending thoracic, 512
    descending thoracic, 519
    mycotic, 525
    reoperation, 609
    thoracic, 23
    surgical treatment of, 509–525
    extracorporeal circulation in, 510
  cannulation, 57
  coarctation of, see Coarctation of aorta
  dissection of, 7, 609
    coronary artery disease with, 532, 534
    surgical treatment of, 526–537
      indications and contraindications, 526
      operations, 529
      reconstruction of aortic root, 530
    surgical repair,
      valve replacement, 533, 534
    symptoms of, 528
    terminology of, 527
    type A, 527, 533
    type B, 527, 535
  penetrating wounds of, 505

Aorta (*cont.*)
  shunt to pulmonary artery, 114
  traumatic rupture of, 508
Aortic arch,
  aneurysms of, 522
    anastomosis in repair, 543
    treatment of, 538
  congenital abnormalities of, 381–392
    investigations, 384
    operations for, 385
    preoperative considerations, 384
    symptoms of, 384
  development of, 381
  dissections,
    anastomosis in repair, 543
    treatment of, 538
  division of vascular ring, 386
  double, 386
  false aneurysms, 546
  incomplete vascular ring, 385
  penetrating wounds of, 507
  right, 388, 391
  ruptured aneurysm, 546
  transverse, aneurysms and dissections, 538–550
Aortic atresia, with double inlet ventricle, 178
Aortic interruption, 368
Aortic regurgitation, 7, 446
  anaesthesia and, 48
  in aortic dissection, 530
  cardiac catheterization, 14
  pathophysiology and, 48
Aortic root,
  narrow, 280
  reconstruction of, 530
Aortic stenosis, 69, 446
  anaesthesia and, 48
  combined with regurgitation, 446
  congenital, 275–280
    incidence of, 275
    indications for operation, 275
    operations for, 276
    preoperative considerations, 275
    subvalvular fibrous, 278
    supravalvular, 279
    valvular, 276
    variations in, 279
  grading of, 13
  pathophysiology of, 48
  valvular stenosis, congenital, 276
Aortic valves,
  anatomy, 100
  annuloaortic ectasia, 446, 451, 513, 514, 517, 530
  homograft, in Fontan operation, 197
  prosthetic, 416, 420
  replacement,
    myocardial protection during, 69
    postoperative anticoagulants, 75
    in treatment of aneurysm, 513
    with aortic dissection, 533, 534
Aortic valve disease,
  congenital, 446
  surgical treatment of, 446–453
    operations, 447
    prostheses, 448
    results of, 453
Aortocoronary saphenous vein bypass grafting, 454–470, 611
  anaesthesia for, 45
  distal anastomosis, 456
  endarterectomy, 461
  operations, 455
  preparation of vein, 455
  proximal anastomoses, 466

Aortocoronary saphenous vein bypass grafting (*cont.*)
  reoperation, 454, 469
  sequential technique, 463, 470
Aortography, 7
Aortoplasty,
  in repair of coarctation, 375
  Vosschulte, 377
Arteries, penetrating wounds of, 505–508
Ascending thoracic aortic aneurysm, repair of, 512
Asplenia, 91
Atherosclerosis, in vein grafts, 471
Atrial appendages,
  anatomy, 91, 101
  juxtaposition of, 90
    in transposition, 293, 313
  thrombosis, 400
Atrial cannulation, 55
Atrial isomerism, 142, 159, 254, 291
Atrial septal defects, 5, 101
  anatomy, 90
  closure of,
    incision for, 28
  coronary sinus defect, 139, 142
  Ebstein's anomaly with, 207
  inferior sinus venous defect, 141
  mitral regurgitation with, 149
  ostium primum, 139, 152
    repair of, 148
  Rashkind procedure for, 284
  repair of, 143–150
    atrial incision, 145
    closure, 146, 147
    contraindications, 143
    incisions, 144
    indications, 143
    myocardial protection, 145
    postoperative care, 150
    preoperative considerations, 143
  secundum defects, 139, 144
    surgical repair, 145
  sinus venosus defects, 140
    repair of, 148
  surgical anatomy, 138–142
  transcatheter closure, 284
  types, 139
  within dual fossa, 145
  within oval fossa, 139
Atrial situs, 101
Atrioventricular canal ventricular septal defects, 220
Atrioventricular concordance, 102, 104, 184, 187, 189
  in coarctation, 368
  in pulmonary atresia, 254
  univentricular, 103
Atrioventricular conduction axis, 215
Atrioventricular conduction tissues, 158
Atrioventricular discordance, 102, 104, 184, 187, 207
  in pulmonary atresia, 253
Atrioventricular junction,
  anatomy of, 94, 97, 98, 102, 154, 155, 156, 157
  in transposition, 294
  sequential analysis, 102
Atrioventricular muscular septum, 96
Atrioventricular node, in transposition, 292, 293
Atrioventricular septal defect,
  anatomy, 151–159
    compared with normal, 152
    valve morphology, 162
  associated malformations, 172
    anatomy, 159
  bileaflet valve, 172
  complete type, 161
    repair of, 162

Atrioventricular septal defect (*cont.*)
  conduction tissues and, 158
  diagnosis, 162
  double orifice, 172
  Ebstein's anomaly with, 207
  intermediate type, 161
    repair of, 170
  mitral cleft, 154, 157, 162
  ostium primum, 161, 167, 170
  ostium secundum, 167
  parachute valve, 172
  partial type, 161
    repair of, 168
  Rastelli type A, anatomy, 157
  Rastelli type C, 162
  Rastelli type I, 162
  repair of, 160–172
    atrial patch, 165, 167
    complications of, 172
    indications and contraindications, 162
    leaflet mobilization, 164, 168
    operations for, 162
    ostium primum closure, 169, 170
    preoperative considerations, 162
    septal patch, 165
    valve reconstruction, 169
  septal morphology, 161
  subcategorization, 156
  types, 161
  with tetralogy of Fallot, 236
Atriventricular spetum,
  membranous, 152, 153
  muscular, 153
Atriventricular valve,
  atresia, 184
  malformations of, 179
Atrium,
  double outlet, 156
  myxomas, 552, 553
  renal cell tumour in, 562
Atrium, left,
  anatomy of, 94
  free wall pathways, ablation of, 574
  myxoma, 553
  pressure, 2
Atrium, right,
  anatomy of, 92
  free wall pathways, ablation of, 570
  isomerism, 101
  myxoma, 557
AV nodal-His junction, ablation of, 567

Bacterial endocarditis, 223, 446
Bilateral conus, 105
Bjork-Shiley valve, 421, 430, 449
Blalock-Taussig anastomosis,
  left, 247
  right, 241
Blalock-Taussig PTFE prosthetic shunt, modification of, 243
Blalock-Taussig shunt, 108
  subclavian arterioplasty for, 112
Blood coagulation,
  during bypass, 63
  postoperative, 74
Blood flow, measurement of, 4
Blood platelets, during bypass, 74
Blood pool scanning, 12
Blood pressure,
  during cardiopulmonary bypass, 40
  measurement by direct arterial cannula, 33
  postbypass, 41
Bubble oxygenators, 52

Calcium levels, during bypass, 59
Cannulation, in bypass, 54
Cardiac arrest, 65
  by cardioplegic solutions, 66
  in hypertrophic subaortic stenosis, 437
  postoperative, 75
Cardiac arrhythmias,
  after Mustard and Senning operations, 312
  after repair of atrial septal defect, 150
  anterior septal pathways, ablation of, 576
  groups, 564
  in Ebstein's anomaly, 214
  intraoperational testing, 566
  in tumours, 552
  left atrium free wall pathways,
    ablation of, 574
  posterior septal pathways,
    ablation of, 577
  postoperative, 74
  right atrium free wall pathways,
    ablation of, 570
  surgical treatment of, 564–583
    ablation of accessory pathways, 570
    ablation techniques, 567
    anterior septal pathways, 576
    AV nodal-His junction, 567
    ectopic ventricular foci, 580
    intraoperational testing, 566
    intraoperative mapping, 565
    left atrium free wall pathways, 574
    operations for, 567
    posterior septal pathways, 577
    preoperative considerations, 565
    right atrium free wall pathways, 570
    scope, 564
    ventricular tachycardia, 581, 582
Cardiac biopsy, 9
  after transplantation, 76
Cardiac catheterization, 2–5
  applications of, 1, 2
  assessment of ventricular function, 5
  basic methods, 2
  in children, 15
  complications of, 7, 8
    in children, 15
  detection of shunts, 5
  interpretation of data, 2
    anaesthesia and, 32
  left heart, 4
  measurement of blood flow, 4
  in newborn, 43
  normal haemodynamic values, 3
  right heart, 2
  during pulmonary artery banding, 121
  measurement, 5
  postoperative, 72, 74
Cardiac reserve, 32
Cardiac resuscitation, after bypass, 59
Cardiac tamponade,
  anaesthesia in, 49
  diagnosis, 16
  from arterial injury, 505
  from trauma, 498, 503
  management of, 49
  pathophysiology of, 49
  postoperative, 74
Cardiac transplantation, 584–605
  anaesthesia in, 49
  contraindications, 49
  donor heart,
    harvesting, 585
    implantation of, 590

Cardiac transplantation (*cont.*)
  donor heart (*cont.*)
    preparation of, 587
  from tumour, 559
  immunosuppression in, 49, 76, 593
  postoperative biopsy, 76
  postoperative care, 76, 593, 605
  recipient, 589
    excision of heart, 589
    implantation of donor heart, 590
    selection of, 589
  rejection, 76
  selection of donor, 585
  survival rates, 584
  with lungs, 594–605
    excision of recipient heart, 595
    harvesting of donor heart and lungs, 594
    implantation of heart and lungs, 603
    recipient, 595
    selection of donor, 594
Cardiomyopathy, *see* Congestive cardiomyopathy and
  Hypertrophic cardiomyopathy
Cardioplegia, 67
Cardioplegic solutions, 66, 67
Cardiopulmonary bypass, 51–64
  acid base balance during, 59
  anaesthesia and, 40
  anticoagulation in, 54
  apparatus, 51
  bubble oxygenators, 52
  cardiac arrest in, 66
  cardiac resuscitation after, 59
  coming off, preparations for, 40
  commencement, 58
  complications, 63
  extracorporeal membrane oxygenation, 63
  for children, 44
  heat exchangers, 53
  humoral factors, 59
  hypothermia during, 40, 54
  intra-aortic balloon assistance, 62
  left ventricular assist devices, 63
  membrane oxygenators, 53
  in neonates, termination of, 44
  platelets during, 74
  preparations for, 21
  pressure and flow, 59
  pump prime, 54
  purposes, 51
  simplified, 539
  special devices, 62
  techniques, 54
  termination, 59
  ventilation during, 59
  venting, 58, 66
Carpenter-Edwards valve, 418
Central venous pressure, measurement by cannula, 34
Children (*see also* Congenital heart disease)
  anaesthesia for, 33, 43, 44
  cardiac catheterization in, 15
  cardiac tumours in, 550, 551, 559
  cardiopulmonary bypass for, 44
  postoperative care, 75
  premedication in, 44
  prosthetic valves for, 416, 423
  pulmonary atresia in, 268
  pulmonary stenosis in, 268, 271
  valve protheses for, 448
Circulatory support, 51–64
Coarctation of aorta, 221
  adult form, 366
  anatomy, 364–370

Coarctation of aorta (*cont.*)
  aortic interruption, 368
  forms of, 364, 365
  isthmic, 366
  pulmonary artery banding in, 117
  relationship to ductal tissue, 367
  repair of, 371–380
    aortoplasty with dacron patch, 375
    choice of operation, 371
    insertion of bypass prosthesis, 378
    incision for, 23
    mortality, 371, 379
    operations for, 372
    postoperative care, 379
    resection with end-to-end anastomosis, 374
    results of, 379
    subclavian angioplasty, 372
    Vosschulte aortoplasty, 377
    with resection and insertion of prosthesis, 375
  shelf like lesion, 366
  ventricular septal defect in, 368
  with persistent truncus, 344
  with transposition, 299, 310
Congenital heart disease,
  anesthesia for, 43
  anatomy of, 88–106
  cardiac catheterization in, 15
  sequential segmental analysis of, 101–105
    philosophy of, 101
    subsequent steps, 105
  shunting in, 5
Congenital malformations (*see also specific lesions*)
Congestive cardiomyopathy,
  cardiac catheterization in, 15
Coronary angioplasty, percutaneous transluminal, 10
Coronary arteries,
  anatomy, 97, 98
  anomalies, in tetralogy of Fallot, 250
  in transposition, 296
Coronary arteriography, 6, 7
Coronary artery,
  anatomy, 91
  atherosclerosis, obstructive, 10
  blood flow, 45
  in correction of transposition, 334, 335, 336
  injury during pericardiectomy, 397
  obstruction, hypertrophic subaortic stenosis and, 436
  in repair of aortic aneurysm, 517, 518
Coronary artery bypass grafting,
  atherosclerosis in, 471
  bypass in, 58
  internal mammary artery, 471–480
    distal anastomoses, 476
    graft preparation, 473
    operation, 473
    options, 477
    preparation for cardiopulmonary bypass, 474
    sequential technique, 478
  postoperative anticoagulants, 75
  reoperation, 606
  saphenous vein, 454–470
    distal anastomosis, 456
    endarterectomy, 461
    operations, 455
    preparation of vein, 455
    proximal anastomoses, 466
    reoperation, 454, 469
    sequential technique, 463, 470
Coronary artery disease,
  anaesthesia and, 38, 45
    induction, 46
  evaluation of, 7

Coronary artery disease (*cont.*)
  ventricular tacycardia in, 582
  with aortic dissection, 532, 534
Coronary sinus, absent, with AVSD, 172
Cor triloculare biatriale, 173
Cricothyroidotomy, postoperative, 72
Criss cross hearts, 103, 192
Crista, 235
Cyanosis, causes of, 43

Descending thoracic aortic aneurysms, repair of, 519
Diagnosis,
  invasive methods, 8
  non-invasive methods, 1
    complementing invasive methods, 11
  nuclear medicine in, 12
Doppler echocardiography, 11
Double inlet ventricle, 173–183
  Fontan operation for, 192, 201
  indeterminate, 182
  left, 175–180
  repair of, 179
  right, 181
  terminology, 173
  valve malformation with, 179
Double outlet atrium, 156
Double outlet right ventricle, 235
  anatomy, 92
  with transposition, 291
Down's syndrome, 162
Ductus arteriosus,
  persistent, *see* Persistent ductus arteriosus
Ductus diverticulum, aneurysms of, 539
Duromedics (Hemex) valve, 422

Ebstein's anomaly, 188, 189, 253
  affecting tricuspid valve, 204
  anatomy of, 204–207
  diagnosis, 208
  features of, 204
  Fontan operation in, 192
  surgical repair, 207, 208–214
    closure of atriotomy and decannulation, 214
    closure of defects, 210
    electrophysiological mapping and cannulation, 209
    plication of atrialized right ventricle, 211
    postoperative care, 214
    technique, 209
    tricuspid valve replacement, 213
  with other lesions, 207
Echocardiography, 11
Eisenmenger complex, 358, 595, 598
Electrocardiography,
  anaesthesia and, 32
  intracardiac, 8
Electrophysiological studies, 8
Endarterectomy, with coronary artery bypass, 461
Endocardial cushion defects, *see* Atrioventricular septal defects
Endocarditis,
  from prosthetic valves, 610
  postoperative, 75
Endocardium,
  biopsy, 9
  myxoma, 553

Fallot's tetralogy, *see* Tetralogy of Fallot
Femoral cannulation, 55
Fluids and electrolytes, postoperative, 72

Fontan operation, 191–203
  anaesthesia and position of patient, 193
  aortic valve homograft in, 197
  for double inlet ventricle, 179
  history of, 192
  indications for, 192
  patch closure of the right atrioventricular valve, 201
  physiology of, 192
  postoperative care, 202
  results of, 202
  right atrial-to-pulmonary arterial anastomosis, 197
  right atrial-to-right ventricular anastomosis, 193
  technique, 193

Glenn shunt, 115
Goretex graft in shunt procedures, 111
Great vessels,
  penetrating wounds of, 505–508
  surgical access to, 17–31
  transposition, *see* Transposition of great vessels

Haemyodynamic values, normal levels, 3
Haemorrhage, postoperative, 74
Hall-Kaster valve, 422
Hancock valve, 417
Heart,
  approach to, 89
  biopsy, 9
  chambers,
    anatomy of, 92
    breaching of, 397
  endocardial myxoma, 553
  exposure of, 21
  myocardial tumours, 559–561
  myxoma, 551
    complications of, 558
    diagnosis, 552
    endocardial, 553
    operation for, 553
    presentation of, 552
    recurrent, 557
  non-penetrating wounds, 502
  papillary fibroelastoma, 558
  penetrating wounds, 498
    repair, 499
    tamponade in, 498
  rhabdomyoma, 550
  surface anatomy of, 90
  surgical access to, 17–31, 89
  transplantation, *see* Cardiac transplantation
  trauma to, 497–504
  tumours of, 550–563
    benign, 551
    classification, 551
    incidence, 550
    malignant, 552
    pathology, 550
  ventricular hamartoma, 559
  ventricular septal fibroma, 561
  wall rupture, 502
Heart disease, assessment of, 1
Heart failure,
  congestive,
    anaesthesia and, 46
    in newborn, 43
  in coarctation, 371
  in pulmonary atresia with VSD, 261
Heat exchangers, 53
Hypernephroma, 562
Hypertension, during bypass, 40

Hypertrophic obstructive cardiomyopathy, 15
    cardiac catheterization in, 15
Hypertrophic subaortic stenosis, 15, 435–445
    anaesthesia in, 49
    cardiac arrest in, 437
    coronary artery obstruction and, 436
    indications for operation, 435, 436
    operation for, 437
        mortality rate, 445
        myotomy and myectomy, 440, 442, 443
        postoperative care, 44
        results of, 445
    preoperative considerations, 435
    symptoms, 435
    valve disease and, 436
Hypotension, postoperative, 75
Hypothermia, 54
    during bypass, 40
    for newborn, 43

Immunosuppression, in cardiac transplantation, 49, 76, 593
Infarction scintigraphy, 12
Innominate artery, anomalous, 392
Intensive care units, 71 (see also Postoperative care)
    monitoring in, 71
    patient information, 42
    transfer of patient to, 42
Interatrial shunting of blood, 138
Intra-aortic balloon pump, postoperative, 73
Intraventricular spetum, postinfarction rupture, 481
Ionescu-Shiley valve, 419

Judkins technique, 6

Kidney,
    during bypass, 63
    postoperative failure, 75

Left atrial pressure, 2
Left atrium, anatomy, 94
Left subclavian artery, aberrant, 391
Left ventricle,
    anatomy, 97, 99–100
    catheterization, 4
    double inlet, 175–180
    hypertrophy, 435 (see also Hypertrophic subaortic stenosis)
        myocardial protection and, 69
        outflow tract obstruction with transposition, 310
    postinfarction aneurysm, 481, 485
Left ventricular assist devices, 63
    postoperative, 73
Left ventricular outflow tract obstruction,
    transposition with, 319–327
        complications, 325
        indications for surgery, 319
        preoperative, 319
        with intact septum, 326
        with VSD, 320
Left ventriculography, 6
Lillehei-Kaster valve, 422
Lungs,
    during bypass, 63
    transplantation, see Cardiac transplantation

Magnesium, levels, during bypass, 59
Mammary artery,
    anatomy of, 472

Mammary artery (cont.)
    coronary artery bypass, 471–480
        distal anastomoses, 476
        graft preparation, 473
        operation, 473
        options, 477
        preparation for cardiopulmonary bypass, 474
        sequential technique, 478
Marfan's syndrome, 446, 513, 514, 517, 525, 530
Medastinitis, postoperative, 75
Median sternotomy, 18, 89
Medtronic Hall valve, 422
Membrane oxygenation, extracorporeal, 63
Mitral cleft, 154, 157, 162
Mitral commissurotomy,
    closed, 399–404
        operation, 399
        reoperation, 404
Mitral regurgitation,
    anaesthesia and, 47
    aortography in, 7
    cardiac catheterization in, 14
    causes of, 405
    diagnosis, 11
    mitral commissurotomy and, 403
    pathophysiology of, 47
    valve replacement in, 425
    with atrial septal defect, 149
Mitral stenosis, 412
    anaesthesia in, 47
    commissurotomy for, 399
    diagnosis, 11
    grading of, 13
    pathophysiology, 47
    reconstructive surgery in, 405
    replacement in, 425
Mitral valve,
    anatomy, 94, 95, 96, 100, 427
    annulus dilatation, repair of, 408
    annulus remodeling, 408
    chordal elongation, 411
    damage from myxoma, 556
    Ebstein's anomaly affecting, 204
    leaflets, 100
        repair of, 410
    papillary fibroelastoma, 558
    postoperative competence, 414
    prosthetic, 420
    reconstructive surgery, 405–414
        assessment of repair, 414
        indications for, 405
        inspection of valve, 407
        operation, 406
        postoperative care, 414
    replacement, 425–434
        excision of valve, 428
        indications for, 425
        myocardial protection during, 70
        operation, 426
        positioning, 431
        preoperative considerations, 425
        reorientation, 430
    restricted leaflet motion, repair, 412
    ruptured chordae, 410
Mitral valve disease,
    hypertrophic subaortic stenosis and, 437
    pathology of, 407
Mitral valve papillary muscle, postinfarction rupture, 481
Mitral valve prostheses, for postinfarction papillary muscle rupture, 483
Mitral valvotomy, closed, incision for, 28
Mitral webs, 279

Monitoring, 33–37
   central venous pressure, 34
   pulmonary artery catheter, 36
   temperature, 37
Muscle relaxants, 38
Mustard's operation for transposition, 301–311
   additional lesions, 310
   complications, 308, 312
   indications, 301
   pericardial patch, 302, 303
   placement of pericardial baffle, 306, 307
   preoperative considerations, 301
   reoperation, 309
   results, 308
   technique, 302
Mycotic aortic aneurysms, 525
Myocardial infarction,
   complications, surgery of, 481–496
   intraventricular septum rupture following, 481
   left ventricular aneurysm following, 481, 485
   papillary muscle rupture following, 481
   ventricular septal defect following, 481, 489
Myocardial protection, 65–70
   during repair of atrial septal defect, 145
   during specific operations, 68
   preferred methods, 66
   techniques, 65
Myocardial tumours, 559–561
Myocardium,
   contractility,
      measurement, 5
      oxygen consumption and, 45
      postoperative, 73
   disease of, cardiac catheterization in, 15
   dysfunction, assessment of, 5
   failure, left ventricular assist systems in, 73
   ischaemia, 40
   oxygen supply and demand, 45
   perfusion imaging, 12
   restrictive disease, 16

Neonatal period,
   anaesthesia in, 43
   cardiac catheterization in, 43
   congestive heart failure in, 43
   cardiopulmonary bypass in, termination, 44
Nuclear cardiography, 12

Omniscience valve, 421
Oxygenators, 52, 53
Oxygen uptake, measurement of, 4

Pacemakers,
   implantation, 77–87
      atrial lead placement, 83
      catheter insertion, 80
      epicardial lead placement, 85
      permanent, 79
      preoperative preparation, 79
      temporary, 78
      testing, 87
      testing catheter, 82
      veins used, 80, 81
      ventricular lead placement, 81
Papillary fibroelastoma, 558
Papillary muscle rupture, postinfarction, 481
Parietal band, 235
Partial anomalous pulmonary venous connection, 123
Patient,
   position on table, 17
   transfer to ITU, 42
Pericardial effusion, diagnosis, 11

Pericardiectomy, 393–397
   approach to, 394
   hazards of, 397
   history of, 393
   indications for, 393
   method, 394
   preoperative considerations, 393
Pericardiocentesis, 16, 498
Pericardiotomy, 398
Pericarditis, postoperative, 75
Pericardium,
   disease of, cardiac catheterization in, 16
   exposure of, 20, 89
   patch, 302, 303
Persistent atrioventricular canal malformations, see
      Atrioventricular septal defects
Persistent ductus arteriosus, 5
   anatomy, 356–357, 359
   aneurysmal, 363
   calcified, 363
   incidence, 358
   incision for, 23
   Rashkind procedure for, 286
      double disc prosthesis, 289
      hooked prosthesis, 286
   spontaneous closure, 358
   surgery of, 358–363
      aims, 358
      division, closure and ligation, 361, 363
      identification of ductus, 360
      postoperative care, 363
      preoperative considerations, 358
      technique, 359
   transcatheter closure, 286
      double disc prosthesis, 289
      hooked prosthesis, 286
   transposition with, 299, 310
Persistent truncus arteriosus,
   anatomy of, 341–345
      in relation to correction, 342
   coarctation with, 344
   correction, 346–355
      conduit replacement, 354
      indications, 347
      infundibular type, 351
      operations, 347
      perimembranous type, 351
      pulmonary artery banding in, 117, 353
      results, 354
      in special circumstances, 353
      steps in, 348
   definition, 341, 346
   incidence of, 346
   natural history, 347
   right aortic arch with, 388
   truncal valve regurgitation and, 354
   types, 343, 347
   with interruption of aortic arch, 354
Phrenic nerve injury, during percardiectomy, 397
Polysplenia, 91
Positive and expiratory pressure, postoperative, 74
Posterior tricuspid annuloplasty, 212
Postlateral thoracotomy, 23
Postoperative care, 71–76
   acid base balance, 72
   anticoagulants, 75
   arrhythmias, 74
   cardiac arrest during, 75
   cardiac output, 72
   cardiac tamponade, 74
   children, 75
   coagulation problems, 74

Postoperative care (*cont.*)
  endocarditis and medastinitis, 75
  fluids and electrolytes, 72
  haemorrhage, 74
  intra-aortic balloon pump, 73
  left ventricular assist systems, 73
  monitoring during, 71
  pericarditis, 75
  renal failure, 75
  respiration, 71
  sepsis, 75
Potassium concentration, during bypass, 59
Pott's anastomosis, in Fallot's tetralogy, 243
Pregnancy, prosthetic valve and, 423
Pressure volume loops, in valvular disease, 47
Prostaglandin infusion, 192, 371
Pulmonary angiography, 8
Pulmonary artery,
  absence of, 237
  banding, 117–121, 312
    coarctation, 373
    in correction of transposition, 331
    complications of, 121
    for double inlet ventricle, 180
    incision for, 28
    indications for, 117
    mortality, 117
    persistent truncus, 353
    removal of, 121
    technique of, 118
  branches, stenosis of, 274
  catheter in, monitoring by, 360
  conduit between right ventricle and, 324
  constriction of, 117
  exposure of, 28
  obstructive lesions, 267
Pulmonary atresia, 104
  anatomy of, 252–257, 258
    Fontan operation in, 192
    in infancy, 268
  types of, 252
  with ventricular septal defect, 236, 254, 258–266
    closure of VSD, 262
    continuity between right ventricle and pulmonary arteries, 264
    corrective procedures, 262
    diagnosis, 258
    heart failure in, 261
    indications for surgery, 251
    management of collateral arteries, 259
    multifocal blood supply, 261
    operations for, 260
    palliative procedures, 260, 266
    preoperative considerations, 258
    relief of peripheral stenosis, 260
    results of treatment, 246
    right ventricular outflow tract enlargement in, 260
    systemic-to-pulmonary artery shunt in, 260
  with double inlet ventricle, 178
  with intact ventricular septum, 253
Pulmonary stenosis,
  in childhood, 271
  in infancy, 268
  spontaneous regression, 272
  with transposition, 310
Pulmonary thromboembolism, 8
Pulmonary valve, absence of, 237

Radionuclides, in diagnosis, 12, 14
Rashkind procedures, 281–290
  equipment, 281
  indications for, 281
  technique, 282

Rastelli operation, 319, 320, 343
Rastelli atrioventricular septal defect,
  type A, 157
  type C, 162
  type I, 162
Renal cell carcinoma, 562
Renal failure, postoperative, 75
Reoperation, 606–611
  dissection of aorta and ventricles, 609
  division of sternum, 607
  operative details, 607
  replacing valves, 609
  visualization of heart and vessels, 608
Respiration, during intensive care, 71
Restrictive cardiomyopathy, cardiac catheterization in, 16
Rheumatic valvular disease, 446
Right aortic arch, 358
Right atrium,
  anatomy of, 92
  isomerism, 101
Right subclavian artery, aberrant, 390
Right ventricle,
  anatomy, 97–99
  catheterization, 2
  conduit to pulmonary artery, 324
  double inlet, 181
  double outlet, 235
Right ventricular outflow tract obstruction, with intact ventricular
    septum, 267–274

Scimitar syndrome, 123
Senning operation for transposition, 312–318
  indications for, 313
  principles of, 313
  technique, 314
Sepsis, postoperative, 75
Septal band, 235
Septal myectomy, 15
Septoparietal trabeculae, 236
Shunts,
  detection and quantification of, 5
  left-to-right, 5
  right-to-left, 5
Shunt procedures, 107–116
  Blalock-Taussig, 108
    subclavian arterioplasty for, 112
  central aorta to pulmonary artery, 114
  Glenn, 115
  subclavian artery to pulmonary artery, Goretex graft, 111
  subclavian to pulmonary, 108
  Waterston, 113
Sinus node, in transposition, 293
Sinus tachycardia, postoperative, 72
Situs solitus, 91
Smeloff-Cutter valve, 421
Sones technique, 6
Splenic syndromes, 91, 159
St Jude medical valve, 422
Starr-Edwards valve, 420
Sternotomy,
  median, 18, 22, 89
Sternum,
  division of, for reoperation, 607
Stress tests, 32
Subclavian angioplasty,
  in coarctation, 372
  for ipsilateral Blalock-Taussig shunt, 112
Subclavian artery,
  H type shunt to pulmonary artery, 111
  aberrant, 390, 391
  shunt to pulmonary artery, 108, 111

Subpulmonary obstruction, transposition with, 298
Subpulmonary stenosis, with Fallot's tetralogy, 235
Supraventricular tachyarrhythmias, 564
    postoperative, 74
Swiss cheese defect, 218, 297
Systemic-pulmonary anastomoses, creation of, 23

Tachycardias, 564 (see also specific arrhythmia)
    ectopic foci of, 580
    postoperative, 72
Temperature, monitoring, 37
Tetralogy of Fallot, 221, 254
    anatomy, 233–238, 340
    associated malformations, 236
    atrioventricular septal defect with, 159, 172, 236
    conduction tissue axis in, 234
    coronary artery anomalies in, 250
    double-outlet right ventricle with, 235
    morphology of, 233, 240
    overriding of aorta, 235
    prognosis, 117
    right aortic arch with, 388
    right ventricular outflow tract obstruction, correction of, 249
    straddling tricuspid valve with, 236
    subpulmonary stenosis in, 235
    surgical treatment, 239–251
        Blalock-Taussig PTFE prosthetic shunt, 243
        closure of previously constructed shunts, 241
        closure of VSD, 245, 247
        coronary artery anomalies, 250
        intracardiac repair, 244
        left Blalock-Taussig anastomosis, 242
        operations, 241
        Pott's anastomosis, 243
        preoperative considerations, 239
        previous operations and, 239
        resection of infundibular muscle, 247
        right Blalock-Taussig anastomosis, 241
        right outflow tract obstruction, 249
        transatrial-pulmonary artery correction, 247
        transventricular repair, 244
        Waterston anastomosis, 243
    ventricular septal defect in, 234
        closure of, 245, 247
Thoracic aortic aneurysms, 509–525
    ascending, 512
    descending, 519
    incisions for, 23
Thoracotomy,
    anterolateral, 28
        closure, 31
        incision, 28
        intercostal layer, 30
    lateral, 89
    posterolateral, 23
        closure, 27
        intercostal layer, 25
        muscle layers, 23
        position of patient, 23
Thromboembolism, from prosthetic valves, 415, 417, 420
Total anomalous pulmonary venous connection, 15
    anatomy, 122–128
    cardiac type, 124
        surgical repair, 134
    diagnosis, 130
    infracardiac and infradiaphragmatic, 125
        surgical repair, 136
    mixed type, 137
    obstructive lesions, 127
    supracardiac type, 124
        surgical repair, 131

Total anomalous pulmonary venous connection (cont.)
    surgical repair, 129–137
        complications, 137
        indications, 130
        postoperative care, 137
        preoperative, 130
        results of, 137
        technique, 131
    to right atrium, 125
Tracheostomy, postoperative, 72
Transposition of great vessels,
    anatomical correction of, 328, 340
        coronary arteries, 334, 335, 336
        great arteries, 333
        indications for, 328
        postoperative care, 340
        preoperative considerations, 328
        preparation of left ventricle, 329
        pulmonary banding in, 331
    anatomy, 92, 291
    associated malformations, 299, 310
    atria in, 292
    atrial appendages juxtaposition in, 313
    atrioventricular junction in, 294
    cardiac catheterization in, 15
    coarctation of aorta with, 299, 310
    complete,
        anatomy of, 291–300
        with subpulmonary obstruction, 298
        with ventricular septal defect, 297
    conduction pathways in, 292
    coronary arteries in, 296
    D, 295
    diagnosis, 301
    double outlet right ventricle with, 291
    incision for, 28
    L, 295
    left ventricular outflow tract, obstruction with, 311
    Mustard's operation for, 301–311
        additional lesions, 310
        complications, 308, 312
        indications, 301
        pericardial baffle, 306, 307
        pericardial patch, 302, 303
        preoperative, 301
        reoperation, 309
        results, 308
        technique, 302
    nodes in, 292
    persistent ductus arteriosus with, 299, 310
    pulmonary artery banding in, 117, 121
    reoperation for, 309
    Senning operation for, 312–318
        indications, 313
        principles of, 313
        technique, 314
    simple, 292
    ventricles and arteries in, 294
    ventricular septal defects with, 310, 313
    with intact ventricular septum, 328
    with left ventricular outflow tract obstruction, 319–327
        complications, 325
        indications for surgery, 319
        preoperative considerations, 319
        with intact septum, 326
        Rastelli operation, 320
Trauma, 497–504
Tricuspid atresia,
    anatomy of, 184–190
    cardiac catheterization in, 15
    classical type, 185
    double inlet ventricle and, 173

Tricuspid atresia (*cont.*)
  Fontan operation for, 192, 193
  right aortic arch with, 388
  variants of, 188
Tricuspid valves,
  anatomy, 94, 95
  damage from myxoma, 556
  Ebstein's anomaly affecting, 204
  annuloplasty, 212
  imcompetence, following Mustard's operation, 308
  in pulmonary atresia, 253
  replacement, in Ebstein's anomaly, 213
  straddling, 221
    in transposition, 297
    with tetralogy of Fallot, 236
Trisomy, 21, 162
Two-dimensional cross-sectional echocardiography, 11

Uhl's anomaly, 254
Ultrasound, 11
Univentricular hearts, *see* Double inlet ventricle
Upstairs-downstairs hearts, 103
Urinary output, 37

Valves,
  anatomy, 94
  prostheses, 415–424
    allograft (or homograft), 416
    biological, 415, 416–419
    bioprosthetic, 417
    Bjork-Shiley, 421, 430, 449
    Carpenter-Edwards, 418
    choice of, 423
    Duromedics, 422
    endocarditis from, 610
    Hall-Kaster, 422
    Hancock, 417
    Ionescu-Shiley, 419
    Lillehei-Kaster, 422
    mechanical, 415, 420–422
    omniscience, 421
    replacement of, 609
    Smeloff-Cutter, 421
    St Jude medical, 422
    Starr-Edwards, 420
    types of, 415
  traumatic rupture, 503
Valvular heart disease,
  anaesthesia in, 46–49
  cardiac catheterization in, 13
  pressure volume loops, 47
Valvular regurgitation, quantification of, 14
Valvular stenosis, grading, 13
Vena cava, tumour of, 562
Ventilation, during bypass, 59
Ventricles,
  architecture of, 102, 103
    influence on conduction tissues, 103
  assessment of function, 5
  dissection of, 609
  double inlet, *see* Double inlet ventricle
  function, during bypass, 41
  hypertrophy, 48
  singles, 173
  in transposition, 294
Ventricle, left, *see* Left ventricle
Ventricle, *see* Right ventricle
Ventricular arrhythmias, postoperative, 74
Ventricular fibrillation, 65
Ventricular hamartoma, 559
Ventricular myxomas, 557
Ventricular outflow tracts,
  anatomy, 104, 105

Ventricular outflow tract obstruction, left, *see* Left ventricular outflow tract obstruction
Ventricular outflow tract obstruction, right, *see* Right ventricular outflow tract obstruction
Ventricular septal defects, 5, 101, 117
  anatomy of, 215–221, 223
  atrioventricular canal defects, 220
  atrioventricular conduction axis, 215
  categorization of, 216
  closure of, in pulmonary atresia, 262
  in coarctation, 368
  defects of membranous septum, 224
  defects of muscular septum, 218, 230
  doubly committed subarterial, 220
  Ebstein's anomaly with, 207
  in Fallot's tetralogy, 234
    closure of, 245, 247
  functional classification, 223
  hypertrophic subaortic stenosis and, 445
  malalignment defects, 221
  perimembranous, 216
  physiology of, 223
  postinfarction, 489, 492
  pulmonary atresia with, 236, 254, 258–266
    closure of VSD, 262
    corrective procedures, 262
    diagnosis, 258
    heart failure in, 261
    indications for surgery, 251
    management of collateral arteries, 259
    multifocal blood supply, 261
    operations for, 260
    palliative procedures, 260, 266
    preoperative considerations, 258
    relief of peripheral stenosis, 260
    results of treatment, 246
    right ventricular outflow tract enlargement, 260
    systemic-to-pulmonary artery shunt in, 260
  repair of, 222–232
    closure of defect, 231
    conduction axis and, 215
    exposure of defect, 230
    indications for, 223
    location of defect, 224
    operations for, 224
    placement of sutures, 225
    results of, 232
    right atrial approach, 228
    right ventricular approach, 224
  spontaneous closure, 223, 237
  supracristal, 220, 232
  transposition with, 297, 310, 313, 320
  traumatic, 503
Ventricular septal fibroma, 561
Ventricular septum,
  necrosis of, 611
  rupture, 503
Ventricular tachycardia, 564
  in left ventricular aneurysm, 483
  treatment of, 8, 581, 582
Ventriculoarterial concordance, 177
  in coarctation, 368
  in Fallot's tetralogy, 235
  in pulmonary atresia, 253
  in transposition, 291
Ventriculoarterial junction, anatomy, 104
Ventriculography, 6
Vessels, surgical access to, 17–31
Vosschulte aortoplasty, 377

Waterston shunt, 113, 243
Wolff-Parkinson-White syndrome, 8, 207, 209, 570